Breast MRI

Elizabeth A. Morris, MD

Director of Breast MRI, Associate Attending Radiologist, Breast Imaging Section, Department of Radiology, Memorial Sloan-Kettering Cancer Center; Associate Professor, Department of Radiology, Weill Medical College of Cornell University, New York

Laura Liberman, MD, FACR

Director of Breast Imaging Research Programs, Attending Radiologist, Breast Imaging Section, Department of Radiology, Memorial Sloan-Kettering Cancer Center; Professor, Department of Radiology, Weill Medical College of Cornell University, New York

Editors

Breast MRI
Diagnosis and Intervention

With Forewords by Larry Norton, MD, and
Beryl McCormick, MD, Clifford Hudis, MD, and
Patrick I. Borgen, MD

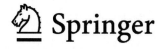 Springer

Elizabeth A. Morris, MD
Director of Breast MRI
Associate Attending Radiologist
Breast Imaging Section
Department of Radiology
Memorial Sloan-Kettering Cancer Center
and
Associate Professor
Department of Radiology
Weill Medical College of Cornell
  University
New York, NY 10021
USA

Laura Liberman, MD, FACR
Director of Breast Imaging Research
  Programs
Attending Radiologist
Breast Imaging Section
Department of Radiology
Memorial Sloan-Kettering Cancer Center
and
Professor
Department of Radiology
Weill Medical College of Cornell
  University
New York, NY 10021
USA

Library of Congress Cataloging-in-Publication Data
Breast MRI: diagnosis and intervention / [edited by] Elizabeth Morris, Laura Liberman.
       p.   ;   cm.
Includes bibliographical references and index.
ISBN 0-387-21997-8 (hardcover : alk. paper)
1. Breast-Magnetic resonance imaging.   I. Morris, Elizabeth, MD.   II. Liberman, Laura.
[DNLM: 1. Breast Diseases–diagnosis.   2. Magnetic Resonance Imaging–methods.
3. Breast–pathology. WP 815 B82844 2004]
RG493.5.M33B744 2004
618.1'907548—dc22   2004050441

ISBN 0-387-21997-8   Printed on acid-free paper.

*To my parents, Jocelyn and James, who inspire
me and made dreams come alive, and
To my husband, Giles Hunt, who makes life
rich with laughter and love and supports me
endlessly, and
To my daughter, Abigail, who makes it all
worthwhile*

EAM

*I dedicate this book to my husband, David
Charles Perlman MD, my children, Daniel Joseph
Perlman and Nina Beth Perlman, and my parents,
Robert and Judith Liberman, for their love and
support in this and all things.*

LL

Foreword I

The book you are about to read is certainly important in itself, as it is an authoritative, practical, and scholarly guide to one of the most rapidly changing and increasingly valuable areas in breast medicine. But its true significance is best appreciated from the long-term historical perspective.

The advances in diagnostics and therapeutics that have transformed our modern world are the results of a revolution in biomedical philosophy that, while starting in the first centuries of the Common Era, is still in progress. This slow but inexorable ascendancy of the organ-based medical tradition of the Arabian-Persian-Hebrew schools and consequent decline of the ancient Greek reliance on manipulation of humors ("feed a cold; starve a fever") has brought functional anatomy into the very center of our thinking. Yet what began with vague concepts of gross organs and organ systems has now progressed into highly sophisticated cell biology, biochemistry, and genetics, even while structure-function linkage has been preserved as the rational core. We have learned to describe phenomena in increasing levels of detail, from the whole tissue down to the level of the single molecule. The process has spun off dramatic improvements in detection, prognostication, and intervention, and promises much, much more.

Seen in this context, the rise of magnetic resonance imaging of the breast is a vital contemporary example of an enduring historical development. The twentieth century saw both the emergence of breast surgery as the first treatment capable of curing some cases of breast cancer and its enhancement by radiation therapy and systemic drug administration. Breast imaging coevolved both to guide the therapeutic hand and to improve the diagnostic hand, thereby vastly augmenting the value of all three treatment modalities. But what we read in these pages is not just a chronicle of advances in the art of visualizing a mass. We are thrust into the middle of a sea change in our ability to assess—simultaneously and non-invasively or minimally invasively—the structure and function of the cells from which cancers arise and are sustained.

Hence, contemporary technology is beginning to provide what twenty centuries of medical progress has sought, a melding of anatomy, physiology, and therapeutics in real time and to strikingly beneficial effect. Fundamental concepts of the normal and cancerous breast are being challenged. Venerable terms like *preneoplastic stroma*, *preinvasive carcinoma*, *multifocality*, and *margin assessment* are being redefined. Our access to the earliest events in breast disease, the molecular events, is opened wider. Where all of this will lead is, of course, unknowable, but the direction is clear: clearer and deeper and more integrated understanding, all in the service of better management. That is the big picture, and that is what these pages really signify.

Larry Norton, MD
Memorial Sloan-Kettering Cancer Center
New York, NY

Foreword

Foreword II

Breast cancer is a major health problem for American women and it accounted for almost 40,000 deaths in 2003. Unlike many other forms of cancer, awareness among women of the risks associated with breast cancer is high and derives from many sources including health education programs promoting screening, extensive media coverage, and first-hand knowledge from friends or relatives with the diagnosis.

Despite this public awareness, our best screening tool, mammography, has a false-negative rate of 10% to 25%, depending on the series. Hundreds of women who participate in screening are falsely reassured that they are breast cancer free each year. Furthermore, mammography has limitations in its ability to accurately establish the extent of disease in the breast for some subsets of women undergoing treatment. For example, it may underestimate the extent of lobular carcinoma in up to 25% of cases. It is in this climate that interest has focused on MRI as an adjunct to mammography.

MRI has been a valuable imaging tool for many parts of the human anatomy since the early 1980s, but it was not widely used for imaging the breast until recently. Fewer than 5 years ago, the US Public Health Service Office on Women's Health organized a meeting to design and develop a research plan for optimization and clinical evaluation of breast MRI. At the time of the meeting, individual clinicians had research experience within a few specific areas of MRI, but the main conclusions of the meeting were that dissemination of breast MRI into the clinic had been slow, there was an urgent need for a lexicon similar to the BI-RADS™ system developed for reading mammograms, and breast MRI required dedicated breast equipment systems.

As detailed in this textbook, significant progress has been made in the development of MRI for the breast. MRI is now recognized as the most sensitive imaging modality for breast cancer, and it has been shown to provide clarity in many clinical situations in which dense breast tissue is not imaged well with routine mammography or with ultrasound. It has been particularly useful in demonstrating the extent of biopsy-proven cancers, especially invasive lobular cancers and ductal carcinoma in situ, which historically were not well imaged with conventional breast techniques. In such situations, the MRI may be useful in guiding both the surgeon and the patient regarding the appropriate choice of breast conservation versus mastectomy.

The sensitivity of MRI can be a challenge as well as a boon. In women with biopsy-proven cancer, MRIs obtained after wide local excision with pathologically close or involved margins may reveal enhancement that could represent a small volume of tumor that is not clinically relevant and has been sterilized in the past with breast radiation, or it could represent surgical artifact. Research in this area is ongoing and will be critical in broadening the utility of this modality.

The specificity of MRI-enhanced lesions in the breast is moderate. Until recently lesions imaged only on MRI and not on breast ultrasound or mammography were technically difficult to biopsy because ferromagnetic needles (MRI unsafe) could not be used in the localizing process if a magnet was required. Now, with several clinical systems commercially available using nonferromagnetic needles (MRI safe) instead of ferromagnetic devices to localize these lesions and sample tissue, better data will be generated. Also, breast imagers have learned a great deal regarding the timing and sequencing of the images.

At present, the clinical impact of breast MRI is uncertain. In a center with dedicated equipment and equally dedicated radiologists, it is probably useful for women with biopsy-proven breast cancers to exclude additional unsuspected disease. As noted previously, MRI can demonstrate the extent of disease in the breast, thereby assisting in decisions regarding appropriate primary surgery. For women who present with biopsy-proven breast cancer in an axillary node but for whom no primary lesion can be identified through physical examination or mammography, MRI can often direct the surgical team to an index lesion in the breast.

For patients with larger but technically resectable breast cancers who elect neoadjuvant chemotherapy in an effort to convert from mastectomy to breast conservation, MRI is an excellent tool to track the response of the index lesion to chemotherapy and determine if and when a limited surgical procedure is feasible.

In special situations, MRI may be useful for screening. For young women with strong family histories of breast cancer, or who carry a known genetic marker for this disease, mammography may be less useful because of their dense breast tissue. In this situation MRI may provide information that complements conventional screening.

As MRI technology improves and more is learned from clinical trials and retrospective studies, the application and utility of this modality should become clearer. It appears likely that MRI of the breast will play an increasingly important role in the diagnosis and management of selected patients with breast cancer.

Beryl McCormick, MD
Clinical Director and Attending Radiation Oncologist
Department of Radiation Oncology
Memorial Sloan-Kettering Cancer Center
New York, NY

Clifford Hudis, MD
Associate Attending and Chief Breast Cancer Medicine Service
Memorial Sloan-Kettering Cancer Center
New York, NY

Patrick I. Borgen, MD
Chief, Breast Service
Department of Surgery
Co-Director, Breast Cancer Disease Management Team
Member, Memorial Hospital for Cancer and Allied Diseases
Memorial Sloan-Kettering Cancer Center, New York
and
Associate Professor of Surgery
Cornell University Medical College
New York, NY

Preface

Breast magnetic resonance imaging (MRI) is creating a revolution in breast diagnosis and intervention. In the last decade, breast MRI has evolved from being an investigational technique to a clinically valuable tool for breast cancer detection and diagnosis. Individuals who perform or refer patients for breast imaging studies need to understand the indications for breast MRI, how to obtain and interpret the images, outcomes of breast MRI in specific scenarios, and how to perform biopsy of lesions detected by MRI only. This book was created to fill that need.

This book is organized into two Parts. Part I, the text, starts with the basics, including a historical overview, technique, how to set up a breast MRI program, the normal breast, the axilla, the breast MRI lexicon, and kinetic analysis. MRI features of benign lesions, ductal carcinoma in situ (DCIS), and invasive breast cancer are discussed in detail. Uses of breast MRI are presented, including high-risk screening, breast cancer staging, assessment of residual disease, MRI after breast cancer treatment, evaluation of silicone breast implants, and other clinical scenarios. The emerging technology of breast MRI spectroscopy is discussed. Specific chapters address MRI-guided interventional procedures, including step-by-step instructions on how to perform MRI-guided needle localization and MRI-guided vacuum-assisted biopsy, and suggestions for challenging cases. The final chapter discusses the potential for breast MRI in percutaneous ablation of breast cancer in the future.

Part II is an atlas of breast MRI. Case examples illustrate the normal breast as well as malignant lesions (distribution of tumor, staging, metastasis, invasive cancer and also have a strong family history of breast cancer and in women who have specific histologies (e.g., invasive lobular) in the index cancer. When breast MRI is used, it should supplement, but not replace, mammography.

For radiologists embarking on a breast MRI program, it may be helpful to start with women who have proven breast cancer, to look for additional ipsilateral and contralateral disease. An essential component of any breast MRI program is the ability to perform localization and biopsy of lesions identified only by MRI. It is invaluable to include mammography technologists experienced at stereotactic biopsy in MRI-guided interventional procedures. Physicians who perform breast MRI should track the results at their own institutions and share this information with their referring clinicians, so that patients can be appropriately counseled. A negative breast MRI does not spare the need for biopsy of a lesion that is suspicious based on mammography or physical examination. It should be remembered that breast MRI is expensive, that some women (e.g., those with claustrophobia, pacemakers, or aneurysm clips) may not be candidates for breast MRI, that there is variability in technique, interpretation, and insurance reimbursement, and that no studies have shown breast MRI to save lives.

This book would not have come to life without the help of many people. Thanks to Robert J. Albano and Margaret Burns at Springer and Barbara Chernow of Chernow Editorial Services for their vision and insight. We thank Hedvig Hricak, MD, our Chairman, for her support. We are grateful to Richard I. DeWitt of Medical Graphics for his meticulous work with the illustrations. We thank Jacqueline Hughes, our office manager, and Jennifer Guido, our research study assistant, for their hard work and dedication. Thanks to Cynthia M. Thornton, mammography supervisor, and Youngduk Paik, Indira Gonzalez, Karen Larson, and Anita M. Sanchez, mammography technologists, for their invaluable contributions to our breast MRI-guided interventional procedures. We thank Richard C. Fischer, MRI supervisor, and C. Gregory Nyman, MRI technologist, who helped us create and maintain our breast MRI program. Thanks to our colleagues in the Departments of Radiology, Surgery, Medical Oncology, Radiation Oncology, Clinical Genetics, and Pathology, with whom we are lucky to work every day. And we gratefully thank D. David Dershaw, MD, Chief of the Breast Imaging Section at Memorial Sloan-Kettering Cancer Center, our colleague, mentor, and friend, who has created an environment that encourages the asking of questions and the seeking of answers.

Laura Liberman, MD, FACR
Elizabeth A. Morris, MD

Contents

Contributors

Andrea F. Abramson, MD
Attending Radiologist, Breast Imaging Section, Department of Radiology, Memorial Sloan-Kettering Cancer Center; Associate Professor, Department of Radiology, Weill Medical College of Cornell University, New York, NY 10021, USA

Lia Bartella, MBChB, FRCR
Clinical Assistant Radiologist, Breast Imaging Section, Department of Radiology, Memorial Sloan-Kettering Cancer Center; Assistant Professor, Department of Radiology, Weill Medical College of Cornell University, New York, NY 10021, USA

Wendie A. Berg, MD, PhD
Breast Imaging Consultant, Lutherville, MD 21093, USA

Nanette Bracero, MD
Clinical Research Investigator, Memorial Sloan-Kettering Cancer Center, New York, NY 10021, USA

D. David Dershaw, MD, FACR
Director, Breast Imaging Section, Attending Radiologist, Department of Radiology, Memorial Sloan-Kettering Cancer Center; Professor, Department of Radiology, Weill Medical College of Cornell University, New York, NY 10021, USA

Alexandra Heerdt, MD, MPH
Associate Attending, Breast Service, Department of Surgery, Memorial Sloan-Kettering Cancer Center; Assistant Professor, Department of Surgery, Weill Medical College of Cornell University, New York, NY 10021, USA

Nola M. Hylton, PhD
Professor, Department of Radiology, University of California, San Francisco, CA 94143, USA

Jennifer B. Kaplan, MD
Clinical Assistant Radiologist, Breast Imaging Section, Department of Radiology, Memorial Sloan-Kettering Cancer Center; Assistant Professor, Weill Medical College at Cornell University, New York, NY 10021, USA

Rachel Katz-Brull, PhD
Research Fellow, Department of Radiology, Center for Advanced Imaging, Harvard Medical School/Beth Israel Deaconess Medical Center, Boston, MA 02466, USA

Christiane K. Kuhl, MD, PhD
Director, MRI Section, Professor, Department of Radiology, University of Bonn, D-53105 Bonn, Germany

Joo Young Melissa Lee, MD
Staff Radiologist, Department of Radiology, Montclair Breast Center, Montclair, NJ 07042, USA

Robert E. Lenkinski, PhD
Director, Experimental Radiology and 3T Magnetic Resonance Imaging/ Spectroscopy Program, Department of Radiology, Beth Israel Deaconess Medical Center; Professor, Department of Radiology, Harvard Medical School, Boston, MA 02466, USA

Laura Liberman, MD, FACR
Director of Breast Imaging Research Programs, Attending Radiologist, Breast Imaging Section, Department of Radiology, Memorial Sloan-Kettering Cancer Center; Professor, Department of Radiology, Weill Medical College of Cornell University, New York, NY 10021, USA

Jennifer H. Menell, MD
Assistant Attending Radiologist, Breast Imaging Section, Department of Radiology, Memorial Sloan-Kettering Cancer Center; Assistant Professor, Department of Radiology, Weill Medical College of Cornell University, New York, NY 10021, USA

Elizabeth A. Morris, MD
Director of Breast MRI, Associate Attending Radiologist, Breast Imaging Section, Department of Radiology, Memorial Sloan-Kettering Cancer Center; Associate Professor, Department of Radiology, Weill Medical College of Cornell University, New York, NY 10021, USA

I
Principles and Practice

1
Breast Magnetic Resonance Imaging: Historical Overview

Joo Young Melissa Lee and Elizabeth A. Morris

Contrast-enhanced magnetic resonance imaging (MRI) of the breast was first performed in the late 1980s in women with biopsy of proven carcinomas. Heywang and colleagues[1] demonstrated that breast carcinomas showed significant enhancement following the administration of contrast material. Most tumors demonstrated contrast enhancement within the first 5 min. However, further investigations showed that not only do malignant lesions enhance, but benign lesions can also show a similar degree of enhancement. Thresholds for significant enhancement were used with normalized units of enhancement to attempt to differentiate more reliably between the different tissues; however, overlap existed.[2] Therefore, multiple differing attempts were made at developing more defining characteristics to distinguish benign from malignant processes.

1. Dynamic Approach

The earliest MRI studies of the breast were performed with a T1-weighted spin echo sequence before and after intravenous gadopentate dimeglumine (Gd-DTPA) with an imaging time of at least 5 min and a slice thickness of 5 mm. With the development of fast T1-weighted gradient echo pulse sequences, imaging of the breast in thinner contiguous sections along with dynamic MRI of the whole breast became feasible. With this new technique, it became possible to repeat the same image at short time intervals and therefore characterize a lesion's enhancement over a shorter interval of time. Using these data, a signal intensity curve can be generated and, thereby, the curve's rate and velocity can be analyzed.

Studies with faster imaging techniques demonstrated that the initial phase of rapid contrast uptake during the first 2 to 3 min contained valuable information to distinguish between benign and malignant tissue. Subsequently, a flurry of studies was performed using these new techniques. Using a two-dimensional (2D) gradient echo sequence, Kaiser and colleagues[3] found that malignancies showed a sudden increase in signal intensity of 100% within the first 2 min. Gradual, mild contrast uptake was seen in benign tissue. Fibroadenomas showed intense enhancement but at a much slower rate than carcinomas. A series performed by Stack and coworkers[4] had similar findings, with malignant lesions showing a steep increase during the first 60 s, followed by a smaller, more gradual increase over 4 to 8 min. Benign tissue only showed a gradual increase in signal intensity at a slower rate, while fibroadenomas demonstrated a marked increase in signal intensity over an 8-min period. Several different attempts were made by other investigators by varying the imaging parameters and changing the enhancement criteria to improve specificity. Boetes and colleagues[5] used a turboFLASH subtraction technique and classified lesions as suspicious if they enhanced within 11.5 s after the aorta opacified. Gilles and coworkers[6] used a T1-weighted spin echo sequence with subtraction imaging and obtained an acquisition time of 47 s. They classified any enhancement concomitant with early normal vascular enhancement as a positive finding for malignancy, obtaining a sensitivity of 95% and specificity of 53%. However, the validity of all these criteria was questioned by later investigators, who found even higher signal intensities in benign lesions such as fibroadenomas.[7,8] These investigators found that while cancers tend to enhance faster than benign lesions, there is still a clear overlap in enhancement rates of benign and malignant lesions.

2. Time Intensity Curves

In a more recent study, Kuhl and colleagues[9] analyzed not only the enhancement pattern of a lesion in its early phase, but also in the intermediate and late phases. By using a 2D dynamic technique, they qualitatively analyzed the shape of the time-signal intensity curve of suspicious lesions over time and described three different curves: type I (steady) curve corresponds to a straight or slightly curved enhancement pattern with the enhancement progressively increasing over time; type II (plateau) curve levels off after the initial sharp level of enhancement; and a type III (washout) curve has a drop in signal intensity after the initial upstroke, indicating washout of contrast. These curves were generated on only focal mass-like lesions that appeared morphologically suspicious and showed a signal intensity increase of more than 60% on the first postcontrast images. A region of interest was placed in the area of the most rapid and strongest enhancement and was quantified by the change in signal intensity before and after the injection of Gd-DTPA. A type I curve was rated indicative of a benign lesion, type II was suggestive of malignancy, and type III was indicative of a malignant lesion. Using these curves, they achieved a sensitivity of 91% and specificity of 83%.

Although this technique appears promising, limitations exist that must be taken into consideration. First, only those lesions that showed suspicious enhancement or suspicious morphology characterized as ill-defined or irregular contoured borders were included in the study, thus limiting lesions such as ductal carcinoma in situ, which may not demonstrate rapid enhancement or present as a mass-like lesion. In addition, studies have also shown that carcinomas can present as small focal masses with visually well-defined margins[10] or present as rim-enhancing masses,[7] lesions that would not have been included in Kuhl's study.

False-positive results are associated with the exclusive use of the dynamic technique, particularly with fibroadenomas and lymph nodes. Although some studies have shown less intense enhancement with fibroadenomas,[3,4] other studies have shown early intense enhancement.[7,11] This possible disparity between studies may be explained by the histologic variability of fibroadenomas. In Orel's series, she notes she had "young" fibroadenomas that exhibited marked, rapid enhancement. This variability of enhancement of fibroadenomas may be related to degree of fibrosis of the tumor as depicted in a study by Brinck and coworkers[12] He showed that the amount of fibrosis within a fibroadenoma correlates with the degree of enhancement following intravenous Gd-DTPA. Fibroadenomas with increased fibrosis on histopathology have less intense enhancement following intravenous contrast, which may account for the variability between studies.

Another potential false-positive result is intramammary lymph nodes. Intramammary lymph nodes with lymphoid hyperplasia have also proven to demonstrate rapid enhancement following contrast administration, thus mimicking carcinoma. Gallardo and colleagues[13] presented three cases of enlarging breast masses seen on MRI that showed strong and rapid uptake, raising the suspicion for malignancy and, therefore, biopsy was performed. Pathology ultimately yielded a diagnosis of lymphoid hyperplasia.

3. Morphologic Approach

The dynamic approach to differentiating benign and malignant lesions has not been fully corroborated by other studies. Some investigators have found no significant difference in the enhancement characteristics between benign and malignant lesions.[7,8,10] In a study of 74 lesions, Harms and colleagues[11] showed significant overlap between malignant and benign lesions such as fibroadenomas, sclerosing adenosis, and proliferative fibrocystic change, obtaining a sensitivity of 94% and specificity of 37%. In this study, Harms and colleagues suggest that analyzing a lesion's morphologic characteristic may help to improve the specificity of MRI. Similar to its use in mammography and ultrasound, border characteristics such as well defined or spiculated may be a useful adjunct to enhancement features.

Subsequently, Orel and coworkers[7] evaluated both the morphologic and enhancement characteristics of suspicious breast lesions. They used a fat-saturated spoiled gradient echo sequence to acquire high-resolution images along with temporal information. Their data confirmed some of the previous studies that signal intensities and enhancement characteristics overlapped between benign and malignant lesions, particularly fibroadenomas. Although carcinomas had a tendency toward more rapid enhancement and washout, there was still a significant overlap with enhancement patterns of fibroadenomas. In her morphologic analysis of lesions, Orel discovered architectural features were helpful in differentiating between benign and malignant lesions. Carcinomas exhibited irregular borders and rim enhancement, while fibroadenomas often had lobulated borders, with nonenhancing internal septations. In a study of 192 patients, Nunes and colleagues[14] exclusively analyzed architectural features to develop a tree-shaped interpretation model to distinguish benign from malignant lesions. Masses with irregular borders and rim enhancement were associated with carcinoma, while masses with lobulated borders and internal septations were associated with fibroadenomas. Nonmass enhancement was also described, which included ductal and regional enhancement. Ductal enhancement correlated with ductal carcinoma in situ, while regional enhancement was not particularly predictive of either benign or malignant disease.

4. Combination of Dynamic and Morphologic Approaches

Currently, it is realized that both dynamic and morphologic data can be helpful in the assessment of breast MRI lesions. In an attempt to optimally use both morphologic and temporal features, Kinkel and colleagues[15] used a three-dimenional (3D) sagittal fat-suppressed T1-weighted fast gradient-recalled echo sequence to obtain high spatial resolution MRIs. Semidynamic information was acquired by obtaining three sets of images at three time-points following the administration of intravenous contrast. The signal intensity on the first postcontrast image acquired at 2 min and 30 s was then compared with the second set of images acquired at 7 min and 30 s. Enhancement kinetics were analyzed visually without the use of a region of interest. *Washout* was defined as any visual decline in signal intensity from the first set of images to the second. *Plateau* enhancement was defined as stabilization in signal intensity, and *progressive* enhancement was defined as an increase in signal intensity between the two sets of images. The morphologic parameters included lesion type (mass vs. nonmass), mass margin, internal enhancement, and T1- and T2-weighted unenhanced visibility. The combination of evaluating the margin (smooth vs. irregular or spiculated) and washout pattern of a lesion resulted in a sensitivity and positive predictive value of 97% and specificity and negative predictive value of 96%. The limitation of this study was that the lesions evaluated were known palpable masses or suspicious findings seen on mammography; therefore, nonmass enhancement, which can often be seen with ductal carcinoma in situ, was not fully evaluated.

In a more recent study by Liberman and coworkers,[16] only lesions exclusively detected on MRI were analyzed by using the three time-point technique with T1-weighted 3D fat-suppressed fast spoiled gradient echo sequence. Morphology of the lesions and visual assessment of the enhancement kinetics were analyzed. For mass lesions, features that correlated with carcinoma were spiculated margin, rim enhancement, and irregular shape. For nonmass lesions, segmental, clumped, linear, and ductal enhancement was predictive of malignancy. The visually assessed kinetic patterns were not significant predictors of carcinoma, but it was noted that washout was more likely in the presence of invasive carcinomas versus ductal carcinoma in situ.

5. Conclusion

Two different concepts have evolved to try to improve the specificity of MRI. One focuses on high spatial resolution to analyze a lesion's morphologic characteristic, and the other focuses on temporal resolution to analyze a lesion's enhancement pattern. With the technology previously available, both of these features cannot be simultaneously optimally analyzed.[17] When a dynamic technique is used, spatial resolution will be sacrificed, thus compromising its sensitivity for small and multifocal breast carcinomas. Efforts to develop a technique that combines both rapid acquisition with preservation of high spatial resolution and complete integration of both kinetic and morphologic features have succeeded. Newer techniques (parallel imaging) use multiple MRI received coil elements to encode spatial information in addition to traditional gradient encoding. By reducing gradient encodings, shorter scan times can be achieved. Parallel imaging is beginning to be used in the breast with excellent results and has allowed optimization of both spatial and temporal resolution so that all features of breast lesions can be optimally assessed.

References

1. Heywang SH, Hahn D, Schmidt H, et al. MR imaging of the breast using Gd-DTPA. *J Comput Assist Tomogr.* 1986;10: 199–204.
2. Heywang SH, Wolf A, Pruss E, et al. MR imaging of the breast with Gd-DTPA: use and limitations. *Radiology* 1989; 71:95–103.
3. Kaiser WA, Zeitler E. MR imaging of the breast: fast imaging sequences with and without Gd-DTPA-preliminary observations. *Radiology* 1989;170:681–686.
4. Stack JP, Redmond OM, Codd MB, et al. Breast disease: tissue characterization with Gd-DTPA enhancement profiles. *Radiology* 1990;174:491–494.
5. Boetes C, Barentsz JO, Mus RD, et al. MR characterization of suspicious breast lesions with a gadoliniun-enhanced turboFLASH subtraction technique. *Radiology* 1994;193: 777–781.
6. Gilles R, Guinebretiere JM, Lucidarme O, et al. Nonpalpable breast tumors: diagnosis with contrast-enhanced subtraction dynamic MR imaging. *Radiology* 1994;191: 625–631.
7. Orel SG, Schnall MD, LiVolsi VA, et al. Suspicious breast lesions: MR imaging with radiologic-pathologic correlation. *Radiology* 1994;190:485–493.
8. Stomper PC, Herman S, Klippenstein DL, et al. Suspect breast lesions: findings at dynamic gadolinium-enhanced MR imaging correlated with mammographic and pathologic features. *Radiology* 1995;197:387–395.
9. Kuhl CK, Mielcareck P, Klaschik S. Dynamic breast MR imaging: are signal intensity time course data useful for differential diagnosis of enhancing lesions? *Radiology* 1999; 211:101–110.
10. Siegmann KC, Muller-Schimpfle M, Schick F, et al. MR imaging-detected breast lesions: histopathologic correlation of lesion characteristics and signal intensity data. *AJR Am J Roentgenol.* 2002;178:1403–1409.
11. Harms S, Flamig DP, Hesley KL, et al. MR imaging of the breast with rotating delivery of excitation off resonance: clin-

ical experience with pathologic correlation. *Radiology* 1993;187:493–501.

12. Brinck U, Fischer U, Korabiowska M, et al. The variability of fibroadenoma in contrast-enhanced dynamic MR mammography. *AJR Am J Roentgenol.* 1997;168:1331–1334.

13. Gallardo X, Sentis M, Castaner E, et al. Enhancement of intramammary lymph nodes with lymphoid hyperplasia: a potential pitfall in breast MRI. *Eur Radiol.* 1998;8: 1662–1665.

14. Nunes LW, Schnall MD, Orel SG, et al. Breast MR imaging: interpretation model. *Radiology* 1997;202:833–841.

15. Kinkel K, Helbich TH, Esserman LJ, et al. Dynamic high-spatial-resolution MR imaging of suspicious breast lesions: diagnostic criteria and interobserver variability. *AJR Am J Roentgenol.* 2000;175:35–43.

16. Liberman L, Morris EA, Lee MJ, et al. Breast lesions detected on MR imaging: features and positive predictive value. *AJR Am J Roentgenol.* 2002;179:171–178.

17. Orel SG. Differentiating benign from malignant enhancing lesions identified at MR imaging of the breast: are time-signal intensity curves an accurate predictor? *Radiology* 1999;211: 5–7.

2
Breast Magnetic Resonance Imaging Techniques

Nola M. Hylton

Magnetic resonance imaging (MRI) of the breast is finding wider clinical application as an adjunct diagnostic procedure to mammography and ultrasound. Because of its high sensitivity and effectiveness in dense breast tissue, MRI can be a valuable addition to the diagnostic work up of a patient with a breast abnormality or biopsy-proven cancer. The major limitation of breast MRI is the low-to-moderate specificity, which in combination with high sensitivity can lead to unnecessary biopsy, patient anxiety, and cost. Nonetheless, there are consistent findings emerging that show contrast-enhanced MRI to be effective for early detection of cancer in high-risk women, and superior to mammography for identifying and demonstrating the extent of diffuse and multifocal breast cancer.[1–4]

There are a number of clinical indications for which breast MRI is believed to add value to the conventional clinical and diagnostic work up, including (1) evaluation of patients with axillary carcinoma and negative mammographic and clinical findings, (2) evaluation of women with questionable mammographic findings and previous breast surgery to distinguish postsurgical scar from recurrent carcinoma, and (3) staging of the extent of a cancer diagnosed by percutaneous needle biopsy. Other indications are less well accepted and are being evaluated largely in the research setting. The sensitivity of MRI to breast carcinoma, particularly in dense breast tissue, has led to the emerging role of MRI in breast cancer screening for women identified to be at high risk. Early results from a number of trials in the United States, Canada, the Netherlands, and Europe show between 2% and 4% cancer yield on screening MRI in the high-risk population.[5–7] Many of the cancers discovered by MRI were occult on mammography and clinical examination. A number of important questions remain to be answered before MRI can be recommended for screening of high-risk women, including the appropriate risk level at which screening should be recommended, and the appropriate screening interval.

The high staging accuracy of breast MRI has led to its use for assessing tumor response to neoadjuvant chemotherapy. Magnetic resonance imaging can contribute in several ways to the management of patients receiving preoperative chemotherapy, including the determination of initial extent of disease for proper staging, early identification of poor responders, and identification of the presence and extent of residual disease for surgical planning. Magnetic resonance imaging measurements of tumor response may have predictive value for disease recurrence and responsiveness to novel therapeutics.[8–10] This potential is being explored in a number of clinical trial venues.

The various clinical indications for breast MRI can place different requirements on how the examination is performed. Clearly, a bilateral examination must be used if screening is the purpose, while unilateral imaging may be appropriate for some diagnostic indications to maximize spatial resolution for better morphologic assessment. In addition to these types of considerations, the emphasis of temporal and spatial resolution, fat suppression, and other factors may be influenced by radiologist preference.

The major challenge for breast MRI is the need to improve the specificity of the technique to avoid the unnecessary procedures and patient anxiety that follow a false-positive finding. This may come about through better integrated biopsy methods, new contrast agents with greater specificity, and/or computer-aided methods to aid radiologic interpretation.

1. MRI Versus Mammography

Mammography has an established role in breast cancer screening and diagnosis. Mammography is an X-ray method that has been optimized for evaluation of breast tissue and the detection of breast cancers, while minimizing radiation dosage. The MRI signal is based on different physical principles than mammography and reflects the density of water protons in tissue and their magnetic inter-actions with molecules in their local environment. The MRI signal is strongly influenced by these magnetic inter-actions, which affect how quickly the water protons can return to equilibrium (a process characterized by the T1 and T2 relaxation times) after receiving radiofrequency (RF) energy from an external source (the RF coil). Para-meters of the MRI technique can be adjusted to change the weighting of the T1 and T2 relaxation times, thus allow-ing image contrast to be manipulated. The MRI signal can also be sensitized to physiologic conditions, such as local water diffusion, blood flow, blood oxygenation, and pH levels. In the application to breast imaging, MRI is per-formed using a T1-weighted technique that is sensitive to the accumulation of gadolinium-based contrast agents, which act to shorten T1 and increase signal intensity. Thus, an early (within 2 min) and significant signal increase in an area of breast tissue indicates a greater density and/or higher leakiness of microvessels, which can be a reflection of tumor angiogenesis. While most breast malignancies show such a signal enhancement, not all signal enhance-ments represent cancer, leading to the high sensitivity, but low-to-moderate specificity of breast MRI.

The different physical properties of mammography and magnetic resonance imaging support their complementary role in breast imaging (Table 2.1). With mammography, X-rays are projected through the thickness of the breast in two orthogonal directions (cranial-caudal and lateral-medial oblique) to minimize the problem of overlapping structures. Mammography is relatively quick to perform and inexpensive. Decades of experience with large-scale breast cancer screening programs and the more recent federal implementation of mammographic quality stan-dards have led to optimized performance of mammogra-phy equipment and radiologic interpretations in high-volume centers.

Two attractive features of MRI for application to breast imaging are its three-dimensional format and strong soft-tissue contrast. These features allow the anatomical struc-ture of the breast to be viewed in great detail. The anatomic detail alone, however, is not sufficient for making a diag-nostic assessment. Malignant lesions are often indistin-guishable from normal and benign structures on T1-weighted or T2-weighted imaging. Cancer detection is aided by the use of a contrast agent, as described earlier. The increased density and leakiness of microvessels asso-ciated with cancer growth can be detected by an early, sig-nificant increase in the signal intensity after contrast is injected.

Contrast-enhanced MRI is not, however, sensitive to microcalcifications, which can be an early indication of breast disease and is a frequent finding on mammography. While calcium deposits can occasionally be seen on MRI as tiny signal voids, breast MRI is not a reliable method for detecting microcalcifications. Signal intensity changes with contrast injection are an indication of an altered microvasculature, a separate and distinct manifestation of breast disease than microcalcifications. Conventional mammography is not a sensitive indicator of increased microvasculature associated with tumor neo-angiogenesis. This again supports the complementary role of mammog-raphy and breast MRI.

2. Technical Requirements for Performing Breast MRI

Magnetic resonance imaging is by nature a very multi-parametric technique involving trade-offs between image characteristics such as contrast, signal-to-noise ratio, reso-lution, field–of view, and scan time. Other parameters can also be varied, including orientation (transaxial, sagittal, or coronal), format (unilateral or bilateral), and use of fat suppression. Each of these variables has implications for the ability of MRI to detect and characterize small lesions in the breast. Because of the high degree of flexibility in choosing the imaging parameters, there is a great deal of variation in imaging techniques described in the literature, making it difficult to compare results and determine the true performance of breast MRI.

Two important technical requirements for breast MRI are the use of a dedicated breast coil and administration of a contrast agent when looking for breast cancer. A con-trast agent is not required to look for implant rupture or leakage. For implant evaluation, T2-weighted fast spin echo techniques using inversion recovery for fat sup-pression and chemical saturation of the water signal can produce images of silicone only. However, noncon-trast methods are not effective for detecting breast malignancies.

TABLE 2.1. Complementary Features of Mammography and MRI

Feature	Mammography	MRI
Signal basis	X-ray	Water proton NMR
Format	2D projection	3D multislice
Breast compression required	Yes	No[a]
Contrast injection required	No	Yes
Examination time	Short (5–10 min)	Long (30–45 min)
Demonstrates calcifications	Yes	No
Effective in dense breast tissue	No	Yes

[a] Mild compression can be used to stabilize breast.

Abbreviations: 2D, two-dimensional; 3D, three-dimensional; NMR, nuclear magnetic resonance.

3. Imaging Coils

State-of-the-art breast coils typically consist of multicoil arrays with a geometric design that provides a high signal-to-noise ratio over an area covering both breasts, with extension beyond the chest wall and into the axilla in the majority of patients. Other considerations in the design of breast coils include patient comfort and open access to the breast for performing MRI-guided wire localizations and needle biopsies. While general surface coils can produce high-quality breast images, they are likely to suffer more from poor homogeneity and inconsistent image quality than a dedicated breast coil. Patient comfort is a significant issue in the design of breast coils because of the need to image in the prone position with the upper torso elevated. The space constraint often results in discomfort to the patient's neck and shoulders.

4. Patient Preparation and positioning

As clinical usage of breast MRI increases, consistency of performance becomes more important. In addition to using a dedicated breast coil, attention to patient positioning can contribute to better examination performance. Because of the relatively long duration that patients are required to remain still, generally without sedation, it is advisable to make patients as comfortable as possible before the start of the examination. Breast MRI examinations are performed with patients lying in the prone position, with both breasts hanging freely in the bilateral openings of the breast coil support. Prone positioning helps to minimize the effects of respiratory motion, although the pendant shape of the breast in this position differs from the compressed shape when the patient is upright during mammography or the flattened shape when the patient is supine during surgical procedures. Depending on the individual, patients may find it more comfortable to keep both arms above their head, by their sides, or one in each position. Placement of an intravenous catheter for contrast agent or access to an injection site in the arm or on the hand for manual injection may require that at least one arm be positioned above the head. Following adjustments of position for patient comfort, the position of the breast should be checked again to ensure that each breast is hanging as completely and deeply as possible within the respective coil opening with the nipple pointing straight down. Distortions of the breast or only partial placement of the breast in the coil well can result in signal hotspots, poor image quality in the regions of the chest wall and axilla, and anatomical distortions that make image interpretation difficult. Inconsistent positioning on sequential examinations of the same patient can make it difficult to compare findings.

Breast MRI that is performed to evaluate a patient for breast cancer requires the use of a contrast agent. Non-contrast MRI is not sensitive to the presence of breast carcinoma and is not considered to be diagnostic. Breast MRI is most commonly performed using one of the gadolinium-based low-molecular-weight MRI contrast agents that are currently approved for human use. Gadolinium is a T1-shortening agent and the accumulation of gadolinium in tissue following intravenous injection reflects alterations in vascular density or permeability that can indicate cancer. The majority of studies reported in the literature use either a single dose (0.1 mmol/kg body weight) or double dose (0.2 mmol/kg body weight) of contrast agent. Both dose levels have demonstrated efficacy with little strong data to support one dose over the other. Because the cost of contrast agent is not insignificant, a single dose is most often recommended. Contrast is usually administered via an indwelling catheter as either a bolus injection or infusion. The mode of injection has implications for pharmacokinetic modeling of the signal intensity changes, but either method can be used. Consistency of the contrast injection method is most important and use of a power injector is recommended, when possible.

5. Image Acquisition Methods

As with all MRI applications, image quality will be affected by the choice of acquisition parameters, including the field-of-view and image matrix (which determine resolution), the timing parameters, and the number of signal averages. For dynamic contrast-enhanced techniques, relatively short scan times are needed to sample the time course of signal enhancement after contrast is injected. For breast cancers the peak enhancement occurs within approximately the first 2 min after bolus injection. Thus, to adequately sample the washin and washout of contrast, image acquisition needs to be repeated at 1 min or shorter intervals for the first several minutes when signal intensity change is most rapid. The time course of the signal intensity can be analyzed using a two-compartmental model of the exchange of contrast agent between the intravascular and extravascular/extracellular space. With knowledge of the arterial input function (AIF; signal change measured in a nearby large artery) and the initial tissue T1 value, the two pharmacokinetic constants, the exchange constant k_{trans} and the fractional blood volume fBV, can be solved. These constants have physiologic relevance to the angiogenic phenotype of cancer and have been shown to be predictive of tumor grade, metastatic potential, and response to treatment.[11–16] Less rigorous methods that do not require the measurement of AIF or T1 can be made with certain assumptions and approximations. Other methods for analyzing the signal intensity time curves are based on empirical measurements of quantities such as area under the curve (AUC), initial slope of enhancement, or signal enhancement ratio (SER).[11,17,18]

While some studies suggest that very short scan times are required (on the order of 2–10s) in order for accurate modeling of the pharmacokinetics of contrast uptake,[19] this recommendation does not take into account the averaging of heterogeneous tissue that can result from the accompanying reduction in spatial resolution, volume of coverage, and/or signal-to-noise ratio.

Many advocate that rather than compromise image quality for dynamic scanning, longer scan times be used to improve the resolution and signal-to-noise ratio and to use fat suppression. Scan time requirements can then be relaxed to acquire only 1 to 2 postcontrast images, with the first postcontrast image timed to coincide with the expected peak of enhancement at about 2min. (This is accomplished using a k-space trajectory for which the lower order phase encoding lines are acquired near the 2-min time point.) Three-dimensional, fat-suppressed, fast gradient echo imaging is usually used in this case to acquire high spatial resolution breast magnetic resonance images. Assessment of the degree of enhancement and lesion morphology is used to make the diagnostic interpretation.

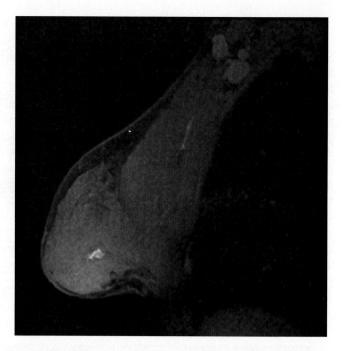

FIGURE 2.2. Unilateral sagittal image through the lesion shown in the left breast of the bilateral image in Figure 2.1. The higher spatial resolution demonstrates the well-circumscribed nature of the lesion and the internal dark septations that are characteristic of fibroadenomas. (Reproduced with permission from American College of Radiology (ACR). ACR BI-RADS®–Magnetic Resonance Imaging. In: *ACR Breast Imaging Reporting and Data System, Breast Imaging Atlas.* Reston, VA. American College of Radiology; 2003.)

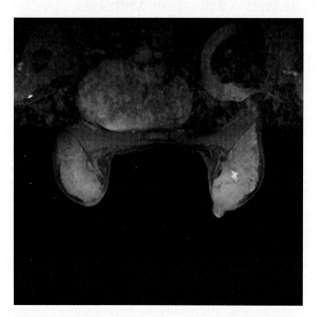

FIGURE 2.1. Bilateral MRI acquired in axial orientation shows a brightly enhancing mass corresponding to a fibroadenoma in the left breast of a patient with very dense breast tissue. Note aliasing of signal from the arms and image blurring due to motion artifact seen posterior to chest wall. Assignment of the phase encoding direction to the left-right direction minimizes artifact-related image degradation in the breast tissue. (Reproduced with permission from American College of Radiology (ACR). ACR BI-RADS®–Magnetic Resonance Imaging. In: *ACR Breast Imaging Reporting and Data System, Breast Imaging Atlas.* Reston, VA. American College of Radiology; 2003.)

Numerous studies have been published regarding the diagnostic usefulness of morphologic features, showing the presence of rim-enhancement, spiculated margins, and linear or ductal shapes, to be indicative of malignancy. Other features, including smooth margins and the presence of dark internal septations, are associated with benign disease. The ACR BI-RADS™ reporting system for breast MRI has recently been published and illustrates many of the morphologic findings encountered on contrast-enhanced breast MRI.

Figures 2.1 through 2.3 illustrate some of the tradeoffs that accompany the choice of imaging parameters. The bilateral axial magnetic resonance image in Figure 2.1 was acquired as part of a screening examination and demonstrates an enhancing mass in the left breast of a woman with very dense breast tissue. There were no significant findings in the right breast. In cases of diffuse or regional enhancement, symmetry or asymmetry with the contralateral breast can be helpful in deciding the significance of the finding. Figure 2.2 shows a sagittal section through the same lesion as in Figure 2.1, taken from a unilateral breast examination of the same patient performed 1wk after the screening examination. The well-circumscribed margin of the lesion

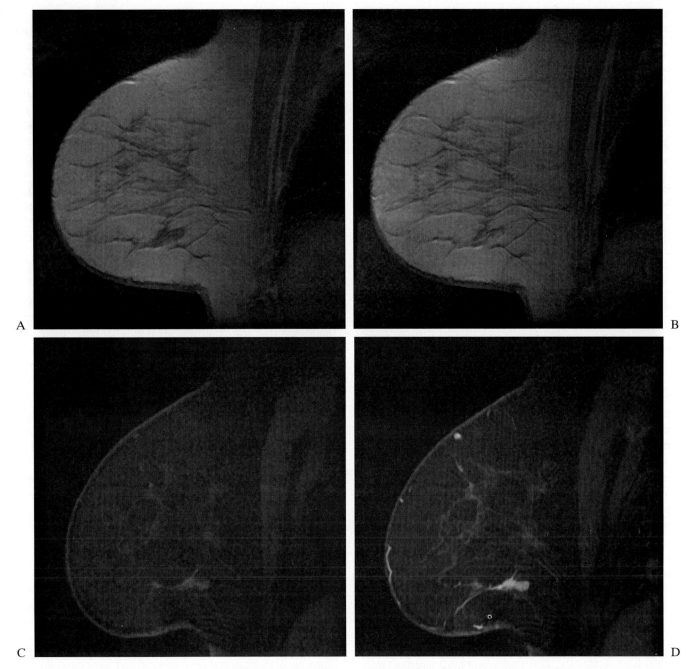

FIGURE 2.3. Pre-(left) and post-(right) contrast images from dynamic two-dimensional (A) and high-resolution three-dimensional (C) examinations of the same patient using pulse sequence parameters similar to those listed in Table 2.2. The post-contrast dynamic image (B) corresponds to the 30-s postcontrast time point. The enhancing mass in the lower central breast showed rapid contrast enhancement and washout on the dynamic series, and was found to be an invasive ductal carcinoma. The irregular lesion shape, presence of spicules, and heterogenous internal enhancement pattern are better appreciated on the high-resolution section (D). (Reproduced with permission from American College of Radiology (ACR). ACR BI-RADS®– Magnetic Resonance Imaging. In: *ACR Breast Imaging Reporting and Data System, Breast Imaging Atlas*. Reston, VA. American College of Radiology; 2003.)

and presence of dark internal septations are better demonstrated on the high resolution image and are characteristic of the confirmed diagnosis of fibroadenoma. In Figure 2.3, pre- and postcontrast images from dynamic and high-resolution studies in the same patient are compared. Rapid enhancement and washout was measured in the lesion on the dynamic series, while the spiculated margins of the lesion are better appreciated on the high spatial

TABLE 2.2. Example Pulse Sequences for Dynamic and High-Resolution Breast MRI

	Dynamic	High Resolution
Acquisition type	2D	3D
Pulse sequence type	Spin echo	Gradient echo
TR	≤100 ms	≤20 ms
TE	4.5 ms	4.5 ms
Flip angle	90°	≤45°
Field of view		
Unilateral	16–22 cm	16–22 cm
Bilateral	32–40 cm	32–40 cm
Matrix size	128 × 128	256 × 192
Slice thickness	3–5 mm	1–2 mm
Number of slices	5–10	32–128
Fat suppression	Subtraction	Chemical saturation or selective water excitation
Scan time	≤1 min	2–4 min

General guidelines for all examinations: use breast RF coil, avoid anterior/posterior phase direction, avoid strong compression.
Abbreviations: 2D, two-dimensional; 3D, three-dimensional; TE, echo time; TR, repetition time.

resolution image. Both findings are highly suggestive of malignancy.

The relative diagnostic usefulness of the pharmacokinetic parameters acquired at moderate spatial resolution versus morphologic feature assessment using volumetric imaging and maximized spatial resolution is difficult to establish and is still being debated. As breast MRI technology advances, these two strategies are converging. Improved techniques that combine both kinetic and morphologic information will also be aided by the availability of longer circulating contrast agents that are under development. Examples of pulse sequence specifications for dynamic and high-resolution techniques are listed in Table 2.2. More recent advances in MRI technology should also contribute to improved breast imaging. Parallel imaging has become available on a number of commercial scanners and allows the simultaneous acquisition of two separate volumes centered on the left and right breasts. This effectively enables bilateral, high-resolution imaging. Novel k-space sampling strategies using spiral or radial trajectories can also lead to gains in efficiency and better immunity to motion. Hybrid techniques are also being introduced that acquire interleaved k-space trajectories that can be separately reconstructed to produce high temporal resolution/low spatial resolution images for dynamic analysis, or can be combined and reconstructed to produce low temporal resolution/high spatial resolution images.[20] Thus, the same data set can be used optimally for both kinetic and morphologic analysis.

6. Fat Suppression

Active fat suppression can improve the detectability of small enhancing lesions, but generally adds to the total scan time. Fat suppression is generally performed by taking advantage of the spectral separation between the fat and water resonances. With chemical saturation techniques, a spectrally selective RF pulse is used to suppress the fat peak prior to issuing the normal excitation RF pulse. Fat therefore does not contribute to the subsequent signal measurement. The fat suppression pulse effectively lengthens the TR, and thus the total scan time. Conversely, water-only excitation pulses can be used, such as is used in the RODEO technique.[21] Other methods, such as periodic inversion pulses, are used to achieve fat suppression with reduced time penalty. Because the spectral separation between fat and water increases with field strength, spectral saturation fat-suppression techniques work more effectively at higher field strengths. In general, these techniques require field strengths of 1 Tesla or higher.

Image subtraction can be used to achieve the effect of fat suppression, but caution should be used in interpreting subtracted images. Subtracted images should be interpreted in conjunction with original unsubtracted images. Image subtraction removes all nonenhancing tissue and, thus, normal and nonenhancing tissue structures are no longer apparent in the subtracted image. For example, enhancement surrounding a biopsy cavity might appear as a rim-like enhancement with a centrally nonenhancing center. Image subtraction cannot be used if significant patient movement occurs between pre- and postcontrast images. Slight patient motion may not be easily detected, but can result in bright and dark edges that correspond to the misregistration between pre- and postcontrast images. Care should be taken to assure that small bright structures are not the result of slight misregistration.

7. Image Postprocessing

One breast MRI examination can generate hundreds of images. A complete diagnostic review has to consider both the spatial relationship of features on multiple slices as well as how those features change over time with the passage of contrast. Postprocessing is used to reduce the number of images for review. Subtraction is one level of postprocessing that can be used to highlight the enhancing features in the image. As mentioned earlier, subtraction is commonly used as a passive method of fat suppression. Another useful postprocessing tool is the maximum intensity projection (MIP), a ray tracing method that projects the brightest pixel value along each parallel ray projected through the volume of data, onto a two-dimensional surface. Maximum intensity projection images can be created from multiple angles and displayed sequentially in a cine loop to give a three-dimensional representation of the image volume. The MIP is most often used with magnetic resonance angiography to create projection images of vascular structures such as the carotid arteries. However, the MIP is also effective for contrast-enhanced, fat-suppressed images of the breast because the brightest structures are likely to be vessels and enhancing tissue. The contrast on MIP images can be enhanced if image subtraction is performed prior to creating the MIP image. Maximum intensity projection images are very effective for demonstrating the distribution of disease in the breast in relation to the skin, nipple, chest wall, and large vessels. The MIP is not reliable for evaluating the internal pattern of lesions or possible extension of disease to the chest wall

or skin. These assessments should be made from the individual slice images. There are numerous commercial software packages available for visualization and display of medical images and most offer capabilities to perform volume rendering, cut-away views, and color-coded displays, in addition to MIP rendering.

Quantitative information can be extracted from MRIs by making measurements in user-defined regions of interest (ROIs), or by creating parametric maps in which an

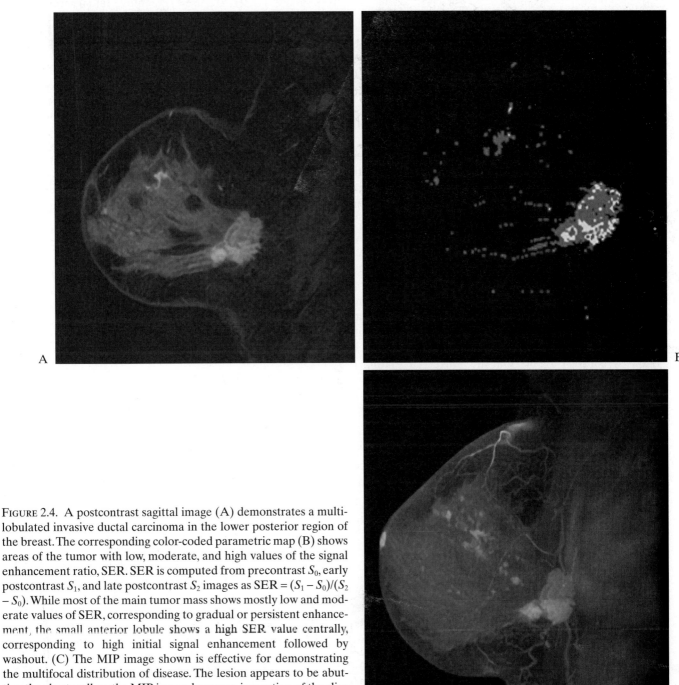

FIGURE 2.4. A postcontrast sagittal image (A) demonstrates a multilobulated invasive ductal carcinoma in the lower posterior region of the breast. The corresponding color-coded parametric map (B) shows areas of the tumor with low, moderate, and high values of the signal enhancement ratio, SER. SER is computed from precontrast S_0, early postcontrast S_1, and late postcontrast S_2 images as SER = $(S_1 - S_0)/(S_2 - S_0)$. While most of the main tumor mass shows mostly low and moderate values of SER, corresponding to gradual or persistent enhancement, the small anterior lobule shows a high SER value centrally, corresponding to high initial signal enhancement followed by washout. (C) The MIP image shown is effective for demonstrating the multifocal distribution of disease. The lesion appears to be abutting the chest wall on the MIP image; however, inspection of the slice image reveals that the lesion and chest wall are separated by a layer of fatty tissue.

image is created from the calculated value of the parameter of interest at every pixel. For example, values of k_{trans}, derived from the signal intensities over a time series of images collected before and after contrast injection can be mapped to a color scale with blue denoting low values of k_{trans} and higher values moving increasingly toward red.

Figure 2.4(A) shows one section through a lobulated mass in the lower, posterior region of the breast, corresponding to an invasive ductal carcinoma. The corresponding parametric map in Figure 2.4(B) shows low (dark gray), moderate (medium gray), and high (white) values of the signal enhancement ratio (SER) parameter. Signal enhancement ratio is computed from precontrast S_0, early postcontrast S_1, and late postcontrast S_2 images as SER = $(S_1 - S_0)/(S_2 - S_0)$. The heterogeneous pattern of enhancement can be appreciated from the SER map. Figure 2.4(C) is the MIP image created in the lateral-medial direction from the full set of 60 sagittal slices acquired immediately following contrast injection. The MIP is effective for demonstrating the size, shape, and location of the mass, as well as the multifocal disease distributed in other regions of the breast. What is not appreciated on the MIP is the heterogenous interior of the lesion and the separation between the mass and chest wall. Both are better illustrated on the individual slice image of Figure 2.4(A).

Ultimately, the standard breast MRI examination will likely include both an optimized data acquisition and integrated postprocessing. Computer-aided tools for diagnosis may also contribute to improved performance of breast MRI. Such systems are currently under development and incorporate image registration, parametric analysis, and diagnostic thresholds for detecting and characterizing malignancies. Improvements in performance may also be gained by contrast agents that are longer circulating or specifically targeted to cancer cells.

References

1. Bedrosian I, Mick R, Orel SG, et al. Changes in the surgical management of patients with breast carcinoma based on preoperative magnetic resonance imaging. *Cancer* 2003;98: 468–473.
2. Esserman L, Hylton N, Yassa L, et al. Utility of magnetic resonance imaging in the management of breast cancer: evidence for improved preoperative staging. *J Clin Oncol.* 1999;17:110–119.
3. Fischer U, Kopka L, Grabbe E. Breast carcinoma: effect of preoperative contrast-enhanced MR imaging on the therapeutic approach. *Radiology* 1999;213:881–888.
4. Kneeshaw PJ, Turnbull LW, Smith A, et al. Dynamic contrast enhanced magnetic resonance imaging aids the surgical management of invasive lobular breast cancer. *Eur J Surg Oncol.* 2003;29:32–37.
5. Kuhl CK. High-risk screening: multi-modality surveillance of women at high risk for breast cancer (proven or suspected carriers of a breast cancer susceptibility gene). *J Exp Clin Cancer Res.* 2002;21(Suppl 3):103–106.
6. Leach MO, Eeles RA, Turnbull LW, et al. The UK national study of magnetic resonance imaging as a method of screening for breast cancer (MARIBS). *J Exp Clin Cancer Res.* 2002;21(Suppl 3):107–114.
7. Morris EA, Liberman E, Balloon DJ, et al. MRI of occult breast carcinoma in a high-risk population. *AJR Am J Roentgenol.* 2003;181:619–626.
8. Esserman L, Kaplan E, Partridge S, et al. MRI phenotype is associated with response to doxorubicin and cyclophosphamide neoadjuvant chemotherapy in stage III breast cancer. *Ann Surg Oncol.* 2001;8:549–559.
9. Wasser K, Klein SK, Fink C, et al. Evaluation of neoadjuvant chemotherapeutic response of breast cancer using dynamic MRI with high temporal resolution. *Eur Radiol.* 2003;13: 80–87.
10. Delille JP, Slanetz PJ, Yeh ED, et al. Invasive ductal breast carcinoma response to neoadjuvant chemotherapy: non-invasive monitoring with functional MR imaging pilot study. *Radiology* 2003;228:63–69.
11. Daniel BL, Yen YF, Glover GH, et al. Breast disease: dynamic spiral MR imaging. *Radiology* 1998;209:499–509.
12. Hayes C, Padhani AR, Leach MO. Assessing changes in tumour vascular function using dynamic contrast-enhanced magnetic resonance imaging. *NMR Biomed.* 2002;15:154–163.
13. Nagashima T, Suzuki M, Yagata H, et al. Dynamic-enhanced MRI predicts metastatic potential of invasive ductal breast cancer. *Breast Cancer* 2002;9:226–230.
14. Knopp MV, Weiss E, Sinn HP, et al. Pathophysiologic basis of contrast enhancement in breast tumors. *J Magn Reson Imaging.* 1999;10:260–266.
15. Stomper PC, Winston JS, Herman S, et al. Angiogenesis and dynamic MR imaging gadolinium enhancement of malignant and benign breast lesions. *Breast Cancer Res Treat.* 1997;45: 39–46.
16. Esserman L, Hylton N, George T, et al. Contrast-enhanced magnetic resonance imaging to assess tumor histopathology and angiogenesis in breast carcinoma. *Breast J.* 1999;5: 13–21.
17. Mussurakis S, Buckley DL, Bowsley SJ, et al. Dynamic contrast-enhanced magnetic resonance imaging of the breast combined with pharmacokinetic analysis of gadolinium-DTPA uptake in the diagnosis of local recurrence of early stage breast carcinoma. *Invest Radiol.* 1995;30:650–662.
18. Hylton NM. Vascularity assessment of breast lesions with gadolinium-enhanced MR imaging. *Magn Reson Imaging Clin N Am.* 1999;7:411–420, x.
19. Henderson E, Rutt BK, Lee TY. Temporal sampling requirements for the tracer kinetics modeling of breast disease. *Magn Reson Imaging.* 1998;16:1057–1073.
20. Song HK, Dougherty L, Schnall MD. Simultaneous acquisition of multiple resolution images for dynamic contrast enhanced imaging of the breast. *Magn Reson Med.* 2001; 46:503–509.
21. Harms SE, Flamig DP. MR imaging of the breast with rotating delivery of excitation off resonance: clinical experience with pathologic correlation. *Radiology.* 1993;187:493–501.

3
Setting Up a Breast Magnetic Resonance Imaging Program

Elizabeth A. Morris

Breast magnetic resonance imaging (MRI) programs can be set up and structured in a variety of ways. Much depends on the local environment, which not only includes the patient population and referral patterns, but also the equipment available and demands made on the MRI unit. Nonetheless, there are some commonalities that are found in most programs. The role of the interpreting radiologist is crucial in creating a successful program as this person acts as the pivot. Incorporation of breast MRI into daily workflow can prove challenging as many logistical problems may arise. It can be helpful to be aware of potential problems and issues in advance. These are discussed in this chapter.

1. Patient Issues

Breast MRI patients have issues that are fairly unique and not found in other patients undergoing MRI. When a women finds herself in the MRI suite for an examination of her breasts it is usually because she has a known cancer, has a very high risk for cancer, or has a problem on her mammogram for which she needs further testing. As a result, these patients are anxious and tense. There are several aspects to scheduling and performing the MRI examination that can alleviate this anxiety.

Flexibility in scheduling MRI examinations can go a long way in decreasing anxiety on the part of the patient. The longer the patient has to wait to schedule an MRI examination, the more anxious she will get, especially if she has a known cancer or a problem on the mammogram. If your program has a dedicated breast MRI machine this likely will not be a problem. As we share our equipment with other types of cases, we have found it helpful to designate daily preoperative breast MRI slots to accommodate breast MRI patients. This approach has allowed us to image patients quickly so that weeks do not elapse before the patient has the examination. A perception that breast disease is important and that breast problems pose unique

issues can be an important factor in providing quick access to imaging.

Information about the MRI procedure can also help decrease anxiety. Some centers provide patients with fact cards about what to expect before, during, and after the procedure (Table 3.1). Designating a person, such as a nurse or assistant, to inform and counsel patients can be invaluable, if there are resources for such a person. If there are no resources for such a person, this job may fall to the radiologist or referring physician. Counseling can be particularly helpful when women are undergoing MRI examination for the first time. Ensuring that there are no absolute contraindications for MRI, such as pacemaker, tissue expander, cochlear implant, and so forth, before the patient arrives in the MRI suite is helpful. Also, explaining in advance the necessity of injecting contrast avoids explanations at the time of the examination, as well as unearths any prior history of reaction to contrast.

Before the patient undergoes the MRI examination, the patient and the referring physician should possess a clear understanding of potential outcomes. Recognition of the possibility of follow-up MRI and possible biopsy due to findings on the MRI is essential and, it is hoped, avoids drastic clinical decisions such as surgery based on MRI findings alone. Often the patient is sent for MRI examination without the understanding that it is a complementary test that may generate additional testing with ultrasonography or mammography. It is hoped that educating referring physicians and patients alike will correct these misperceptions.

As MRI is an adjunctive test that should complement mammography and is only used in specific clinical situations, patient self-referral for breast MRI should be discouraged. Physician referral can also sometimes be problematic, particularly at the start. It may be helpful initially to designate a single radiologist to screen and protocol all referred breast MRI cases to ensure that the appropriate patients are being scanned. This would include requests from clinicians who may not initially

TABLE 3.1. Patient Fact Card
_____

Breast MRI

INTRODUCTION

MRI, magnetic resonance imaging, is a diagnostic procedure to view areas of the body without using X-rays. Magnetic fields and radiowaves are used to detect the size and location of tumors using a large, donut-shaped magnet. Breast MRI is used after a mammogram if more detail is necessary because the doctor suspects there may be disease that the mammogram cannot detect. You cannot have a breast MRI if you have a breast tissue expander or cardiac pacemaker.

PREPARATION

• If you have a condition that makes it difficult for you to lie still in an enclosed area (claustrophobia), or if lying on your stomach with your arms stretched out above your head for 30 to 60 minutes without moving is difficult, tell your doctor before the breast MRI so that medication can be prescribed to help ease any discomfort you may have.
• No other preparation is required. You may take your medication(s) as usual.

TIME

The examination takes up to 40 minutes for both breasts.

PROCEDURE

• You will need to take off your jewelry, bra, and any other clothing items that contain metal, such as zippers or metal buttons.
• You will be able to store your belongings in a locker provided for you.
• Do not take any watches or any card with a magnetic strip (such as a credit card) into the MRI machine, as they may not work once exposed to the magnetic field.
• Before your breast MRI, the procedure will be explained to you, and any questions you have will be answered.
• An intravenous line (IV) will be placed in a vein to give you an injection of a contrast medium called gadolinium-DTPA. The contrast makes it possible to see any abnormality in the breast. The IV will be removed at the end of your procedure.
• You will be asked to lie on your stomach on the MRI table. Once you are positioned, it is extremely important that you do not move during the examination. Your breast will be placed into two holes in the table and will be immobilized by compression paddles.
• You may request earphones so that you can listen to music or earplugs to make you more comfortable and to reduce the clicking sound you will hear from the MRI machine.
• You will be able to talk with the MRI technologist at any time during the examination. If you become very uncomfortable in the MRI machine, tell the technologist.

AFTER THE PROCEDURE

• The site where the contrast medium was injected will be covered with an adhesive bandage (Band Aid®).
• A report of the scan will be sent to your doctor within a few days after your test.
_____

Copyright 1999 Memorial Sloan-Kettering Cancer Center, 1275 York Avenue, New York, NY 10021. Revised 2001.

understand the importance of careful patient selection. We found it helpful not only to approve all initial cases but also followed up with periodic reminders in the form of a memo to referring physicians about appropriate indications.

2. Personnel Issues

Targeting an MRI technologist who can ensure standardization and quality of the breast MRI examination can be extremely useful. This person should also have interpersonal skills that can decrease the anxiety of the breast MRI patient. The quality of the examination is dependent on patient cooperation so a technologist who can reassure the patient is crucial. Patient movement can render the examination uninterpretable. Additionally, if fat suppression is used, a technologist who knows how to troubleshoot problems can decrease the number of call-backs and repeats that may need to be performed.

It is absolutely essential that the technologist position the breast in the breast coil. It cannot be emphasized enough that the patient is unable to position herself cor-

rectly. The technologist must ensure that the breast has been centered in the coil so that artifact is reduced and that the breast is pulled away from the chest wall as much as possible so that the maximum amount of breast tissue is contained within the coil. If the technologist is a man, it may be helpful to have a woman in the department perform this task.

Expert technical support is especially helpful for interventional procedures. For example, during interventional procedures we have found it useful to not only have the MRI technologist for scanning but also have a mammography technologist for positioning, set up, and disposal of materials. If breasts are able to be positioned adequately in the coils, and support personnel are on hand to help with the procedure, simultaneous interventional procedures such as localization or biopsy may be more easily performed.

3. Breast MRI Protocols

Breast MRI is best used for patients with known cancer or those at high risk for developing cancer, therefore not all patients are candidates. Having a clear list of indications goes a long way in the education of referring clinicians. It may be helpful to have a *point* radiologist who approves all initial examinations until referring clinicians develop a sense of appropriate cases to refer to breast MRI. At the beginning it may be useful to scan patients with known cancers to develop a sense of confidence and build a knowledge base. Also, these patients are likely going to the operating room regardless and any additional information that the MRI examination provides will likely only help them.

To maximize the breast MRI examination using the chosen sequence on your scanner, there will be some necessary training of the technologists and experimenting with the sequence. This is to be expected when starting a new service and may need to be factored into the schedule. Until the process becomes streamlined and second nature to the technologists, monitoring the examinations will most likely be needed. A certain critical caseload may need to be in place until confidence in the reproducibility of the examination is ensured.

Depending on how you choose to perform breast MRI examinations, availability of the radiologist may be an issue. If you choose to perform problem-solving detailed studies in which the protocol may vary depending on the clinical problem, then this will require the radiologist's time. Much of what you choose to do will depend on patient volume and availability of a radiologist.

In our practice, a busy clinical service, streamlining the examination for rapidity and reproducibility without constant monitoring was paramount.

We have found protocols that are fixed and streamlined increase throughput. All of our nonresearch examinations, regardless of the clinical indication, are performed with the same protocol. It is now rare that a radiologist needs to monitor an examination as we try to ensure all necessary information is obtained on every patient via close communication beforehand with the referring clinicians and the MRI technologists.

We have found it helpful to review and protocol each case in advance. This way, we can be sure that the patient has had the appropriate work up to date and that all necessary information is available for the time of interpretation. It can also clarify protocols for implant patients, who might be undergoing both a rupture evaluation and an assessment of the breast parenchyma with intravenous contrast. In these cases, the patient and referring physician need to know that these are two separate examinations with differing imaging protocols.

4. Scheduling Considerations

When performing MRI for breast cancer evaluation, a shift in the traditional MRI schedule may be needed. This can help develop continuous referral from surgical and oncological colleagues. In addition to building in flexibility for preoperative cases, flexibility in scheduling other patients can be important. Evaluation of breast lesions has traditionally moved faster than in other areas of medicine. Breast centers are set up for *same-day* service. Asking a patient to wait 2 weeks for an MRI appointment may be perceived as a long delay even though it may be reasonable in other circumstances.

When deciding how to allot your time on the scanner, it may be helpful to *batch* the breast MRI cases, particularly if you examine women at high risk and have a dedicated screening program. We have found this extremely helpful to have the nonemergent cases come for scanning on the weekend. They are comforted seeing other women undergoing the same examination and are usually not sharing the waiting room with acutely ill hospital patients. Additionally, the MRI technologist can develop a rhythm and increase throughput of patients, making the examination more efficient. The breast coil can be maintained on the table and the infusion pump can be easily refilled.

5. Patient Preparation

Similarly, obtaining detailed clinical information from referring colleagues can make a difference in the interpretation of the breast MRI examination. When the radiologist protocols the examination in advance, additional information can be obtained. Also, when the patient arrives in the MRI suite, the patient and nurse fill out a questionnaire together (Table 3.2). This ensures capture of important information, such as prior surgical history of the breasts, any pertinent family history, and menstrual history.

It is helpful to record the patient's last menstrual period and if the patient takes hormone replacement therapy. We generally do not schedule patients based on their menstrual history if there is an acute problem or if the patient is presurgical. However, if the patient does not have a pressing need, such as our high-risk screening patients, we will make all efforts to schedule in the second week of the menstrual cycle. We have found that educating referring physicians about the menstrual changes that can be seen on MRI has been helpful in eliminating the problem of having to repeat an examination due to menstrual changes. In order to educate the referring physician, our schedulers initially ask the referring physician's office if the patient was premenopausal or postmenopausal and if premenopausal, if she would be in the second week of her cycle. If the schedulers are unable to perform the task, the point radiologist who approves all initial breast MRI examinations can easily inquire about menstrual history.

Scars from prior benign breast biopsies and prior breast conservation, as well as palpable abnormalities, are

TABLE 3.2. Patient Questionnaire

Patient name
Medical record number
Age
Referring physician
Date of examination
1. Do you have any breast symptoms? Discharge, lump, pain?   Y   N
2. Does any relative have a history of breast cancer? Age?_____   Y   N
   ___mother ___sister ___grandmother ___other
3. Are you still menstruating?   Y   N
   If yes, date of last menstrual period_____
   If no, year of last menstrual period_____
4. Do you use estrogen replacement therapy?   Y   N
   If yes, for how long?_____
5. Could you be pregnant?   Y   N
6. Have you had prior breast surgery?   Y   N
   If yes, what type?
   ___benign biopsy   __Right __Left
   ___lumpectomy   __Right __Left
   ___mastectomy   __Right __Left
7. Have you had radiation therapy to the breast?   Y   N
   If yes, what side?   __Right __Left
   What year?   _____
8. When was your last mammogram? Date_____
9. Diagram scars or physical findings:

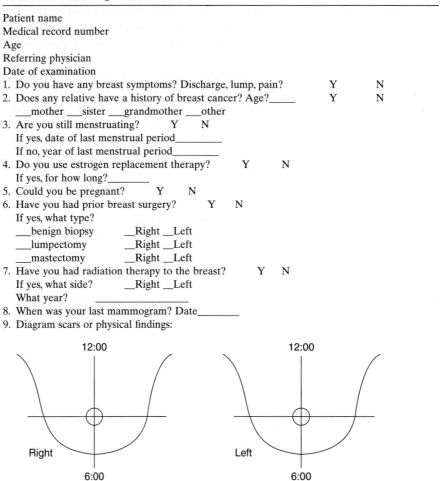

marked with a cutaneous marker such as a fish oil capsule or specialized MRI skin marker. Again, we do not impose any strict criteria about performing the breast MRI examination in relation to surgery. If the patient is undergoing MRI to assess for residual cancer following recent lumpectomy, we try to have the patient images as soon as she is able to lay prone. If the patient is undergoing assessment for recurrent disease, which is usually not an issue in the first 2 years following surgery, we image regardless of the length of time from the surgery, as long as there is strong clinical suspicion.

The nurse generally performs the intake questionnaire, the marking of any abnormalities, and the insertion of the intravenous cannulation in a private room in the MRI suite. If this is unavailable, then privacy with curtains may be sufficient. The dignity of the patient in the MRI suite should be considered whenever possible. For example, when positioning the patient in the breast coil, closing the door to the magnet may be important if there is a lot of traffic in the MRI suite. Also, our male technologists have found it helpful to hold a sheet so that their view is

obscured; this also creates a boundary between the patient and the shaded console window, allowing a sense of privacy. Screens and shades over windows to the console room are another consideration. After the patient is prone, then the technologist can perform the final positioning of the breasts within the coil.

Positioning the breast can be fairly easily performed with an open coil. Closed coils make adequate positioning difficult as one relies mostly on the patient to position her breasts. With an open coil the radiologist or technologist can pull the breast down into the coil, making sure the breast is centrally located to decrease coil artifacts and ensure uniform coverage. Redundant tissue can be eliminated.

Unfortunately, at the time of this writing, breast coils do not come in different sizes. Breasts are not uniform and therefore there are occasions in which the coil may be too small. With an open coil, usually a large breast can be accommodated. With a closed coil and no space for the breast to expand into, significant portions of a breast that exceeds the cup of the coil may be excluded and not imaged, particularly posteriorly and laterally. When communicating with the referring physician in these cases, the limitations of the examination should be emphasized and alternative modalities may be suggested. Overall size limits for patients vary with each manufacturer. It is fairly safe to say that most systems are able to image patients who weigh up to 350 pounds. Usually the limiting factor for most large patients is the size of the bore of the magnet and not the breast coil.

Breast immobilization is an option on some coils. The goal is to not compress the breasts but to gently keep them in place so that patient movement is minimized. When placing the plates a few minutes may be needed to ensure that breast tissue is not displaced posteriorly and therefore excluded from the coil when the plates are affixed. These same plates and grids on some systems can be used for interventional procedures. Positioning is crucial so that the lesion is included in the area that can be accessed by a needle. Mammography technologists are expert at positioning and may be helpful in some cases.

Comfort of the patient is paramount. Having wedges and pillows at the disposal of the person positioning the patient will relax the patient more and ensure a better quality examination. It is better to spend a few extra minutes at the beginning of the examination to be sure that the patient is comfortable than have to repeat the entire examination. In our experience, positioning the arms (by the body or above the head) depends on the comfort of the patient. Clear communication with the patient about the length of the examination and the noises that they will experience will also help. Ear plugs or ear phones for music can decrease the amount of noise while in the magnet. We have found it useful to reassure patients that they are in constant communication with the technologist at all times, alleviating anxiety.

More information provided to the patient only eases the fears about the examination, especially if it is the first time for the patient in the MRI setting. A fact card may prove beneficial and availability of a nurse to answer questions may ally fears. Patient claustrophobia and anxiety can be helped in some cases by medication such as diazepam (Valium®) or alprazolam (Xanax®). We routinely do not give this medication for routine examinations. Medication may be given to patients undergoing magnetic resonance vacuum biopsy and only if the patient is accompanied home.

6. Examination Interpretation

When the breast MRI examination is interpreted, every effort should be made to have the patient's mammograms and ultrasound examinations available. If these are performed elsewhere, it may be helpful to develop a mechanism for submission of these examinations before interpretation. Prior mammograms can be invaluable to document the presence of a lymph node or a stable benign breast mass. If the breast MRI is done for a suspected mammographic problem, the mammogram needs to be correlated with the MRI examination so that an overall recommendation can be issued. Being able to correlate an MRI finding to a mammographic finding may be extremely useful as well as obviate the need for an MRI interventional procedure.

Choices regarding hard copy versus soft copy interpretation depend on available technology. The major benefit of reading soft copy is the sheer lack of numerous sheets of films that can be time consuming to collate, especially if rapid dynamic sequences are obtained. In cases where there are multiple passes, some radiologists will not film every series but will examine the images on a workstation. Picture archival communication systems (PACS) have made the interpretation process much quicker and streamlined. Similarly, improvements in software packages have allowed manipulation of data to be much easier, especially for three-dimensional (3D)volume data sets.

Appropriate window levels can be more easily manipulated with PACS or workstations so that the internal characteristics and borders of a lesion may be better displayed. Additionally, manipulation of the brightness and contrast can be important to general interpretation so that lesions are not overlooked or overcalled. Parametric image analysis with color-coding can be helpful in this regard and can act as an overlay to aid in interpretation. Depending on manufacturer, this may or may not be available. If your system does not have this feature, there are companies who offer systems that perform this type of analysis.

7. Kinetic Analysis

The ease of performing kinetic analysis on images varies with manufacturer, and choices about how to capture this information vary based on time constraints and available hardware. Some radiologists interpret breast MRI at the workstation and manually perform the kinetic analysis on all cases. Others may designate a technologist to place the region of interest over suspicious areas of abnormality and to generate graphs. Others may not perform quantitative kinetics, but rather perform visual kinetics, ensuring uniformity in the window setting.

Kinetic analysis is done on a case-by-case basis in our practice. We will visually assess kinetics initially and then analyze any suspicious areas with a computer aided detection system that produces a color coded map for angiogenesis and curve analysis.

A mechanism to perform time intensity curves (TIC) should be in place in advance. Once again, the choices will depend on the technology available. There are now several software packages available that can perform this function.

8. Communication of Results

Communication with the referring physician about the final recommendation is necessary in breast MRI studies just as it is in mammographic interpretation. At this time there are no requirements by any governmental agency that a patient be informed of her results before she leaves the facility, as there is with mammography. Due to the postprocessing constraints with MRI, it is likely that this will not be an issue in the future. Sometimes patients request their results immediately when they finish the MRI examination. In our practice telling the patient her results is not done for multiple reasons. We do not have the luxury of having a breast radiologist in the MRI suite at the time that the patient is being scanned. Moreover, it is to the patient's benefit that the scan is read with all postprocessing finished as well as with all pertinent prior examinations (such as the mammogram) available, when the radiologist is not rushed to render an interpretation. Because the examinations are usually complicated, radiologists who may be in the MRI suite but not familiar with the case usually do not get involved in the interpretation. Much of how you decide to handle interpretations will depend on the existing practices with referring physicians as well as radiologist availability.

We read all the breast MRI examinations in a batch on the next day, usually in the morning. We have one radiologist every day assigned to interpret the examinations. That radiologist communicates the results directly to the referring physician by telephone or e-mail and the referring physician then communicates the results to the patient. At first, every result was called into the referring physician, however, as we have become busier, only BI-RADS (Breast Imaging Reporting and Data System)[1] 3, 4, or 5 results are communicated to the referring physician.

9. Interventional Issues

Breast intervention under MRI is an essential part of any breast MRI program. Choices in coils will depend on the system that is used. Regardless, the coil should allow both localization and biopsy capabilities. Ideally, the breast should be able to be approached from at least two directions, usually laterally and medially. Magnetic-resonance–compatible needles for both localization and biopsy are now universally available. Choices in biopsy include true cut versus vacuum, as outlined in Chapter 20.

Before embarking on an interventional program it may be useful to determine the number of technologists that will be needed and if these personnel are available. The MRI technologist and mammography technologist each have separate areas of expertise and training and complement each other well. We tend to perform interventional procedures with both technologists. The mammography technologist helps position and is in charge of tray preparation and specimen handling. The mammography technologist ensures continuity for the patient as she will be with the patient during the entire procedure and will perform the postintervention mammogram afterward. The MRI technologist ensures quick image acquisition and set up. MRI technologists may have no experience with intervention, and additional training may be necessary. Advance tray preparation can facilitate and speed up procedures. We have an MRI-compatible cart that is magnet compatible and has a sterile field prepared on the top and all necessary supplies underneath so that replacement of needles or any supplies is not a problem. The mammography technologist is responsible for cleaning the equipment while the MRI technologist sets up for the next patient.

10. Data Gathering

Although there are no absolute requirements at this time for data analysis and limited experience knowing appropriate values for MRI recommendations, it can be extremely helpful for individual practices and individual radiologists to monitor their recommendations for biopsy and 6-month follow up. Although positive biopsy rates vary throughout the world, ranging from 25% to 80%, and depend on a variety of factors, it may be helpful to know where a practice falls in this spectrum. It goes without saying that the radiologist who performs any interventional procedure must correlate the pathologic findings with the MRI findings to ensure that the appropriate area has been removed and that the pathology findings make sense.

11. Practice Growth Issues

Incorporating breast MRI into a radiology practice can be challenging, especially when cases are sporadic. Adequate time for interpretation and correlation with all imaging studies should be factored into the daily schedule. Many practices have appointed a single radiologist to assume the responsibility of the breast MRI program. This works well when the cases are few, however, when the volume increases, more interpreting radiologists will need to be recruited. Most practices find it useful to give the job to a breast imager who is comfortable or interested in MRI. Breast imagers have several advantages; for example their preexisting relationship to surgeons and oncologists which can be helpful as breast MRI usually requires coordinated care as breast MRI is not a stand alone test. Correlation with mammography and follow-up ultrasound is often needed and a radiologist who is familiar with these modalities will provide the best comprehensive care. Additionally, the disease process is the same, which helps with concordance and discordance issues when breast biopsies are performed. Finally, MRI interventional procedures such as localizations and biopsies are similar to mammography procedures.

Additionally, time in the schedule for interventional procedures will be necessary. When starting out, we would perform needle localizations early in the morning before the schedule started for the day. However, once these procedures became daily events and once breast MRI biopsies were routinely performed, we designated two daily interventional slots in the middle of the work day. How the schedule works for intervention depends on the operating room schedule as well as the radiologist's additional responsibilities. An increase in breast MRI volume may lead to a need to increase in staff, both technical and professional, or a shift in responsibilities to accommodate the additional time needed to interpret the examinations.

12. Coil Issues

When selecting a breast coil several options are available. An open coil is preferable for facilitation of positioning of the breast. Additionally, a coil that allows feet first is preferable for patients who may be claustrophobic as the head is partially out of the magnet. A coil with immobilization and biopsy capability is essential as intervention is a part of any breast MRI program. The coil should produce homogeneous images and penetrate to the chest wall to ensure adequate visualization of all breast tissue. We currently use an 8-channel MRI Devices (Waukesha, Wis.) immobilization/biopsy coil/system.

13. Selecting the Sequence

When performing imaging for breast cancer the same principles that apply to mammography apply to MRI. The aim is to detect small lesions to facilitate early breast cancer detection. Depending on how MRI is performed the resolution will vary. In general, MRI does not approach the level of resolution that is obtained with mammography. With increase in field strength, resolution may increase; however, at the time of this writing high field magnets (3 Tesla and more) are not universally available. When performing breast MRI there are two ways to analyze the images: assessment of morphology and assessment of kinetics. As both contain valuable information it is hoped that the sequence selected can evaluate both.

Historically, it was necessary to choose between performing high spatial resolution imaging to assess morphology or high temporal resolution imaging to assess function. Luckily, with advances in equipment and software, there is no need for significant compromise. High spatial resolution sequences, such as 3D spoiled gradient

echo recalled imaging, increase sensitivity, particularly with regard to small invasive cancers and ductal carcinoma in situ (DCIS). The 3D sequence is able to image the entire breast, perform fat suppression, and can be performed rapidly to give dynamic information. However, if there is a need for extremely high temporal resolutionimaging, two-dimensional (2D) spin echo sequences are faster though coverage may be limited, spatial resolution is reduced, and fat suppression is not an option.

Newer imaging options are becoming available for the breast that incorporate parallel imaging, making it possible to image the breasts simultaneously so that temporal and spatial resolution is maximized. With parallel imaging the number of phase encoding steps can be reduced by exploiting spatial information from an array of surface coils. The gain can be traded for improved spatial and/or temporal resolution in any pulse sequence.

14. Memorial Sloan-Kettering Cancer Center Sequence

The patient population of a particular institution most likely will drive the protocol that is employed. If there is a large cancer population, high-resolution techniques tend to be favored as the goal is detection of small lesions. For this reason, at our institution, which is a cancer center, we chose to focus more on high-resolution techniques. We are interested not only in detecting invasive carcinomas but also small foci of DCIS. If there is a low incidence of cancer in a population, lesion characterization becomes more important and low spatial resolution and high temporal resolution tended to be favored. Low-resolution techniques also tend toward bilateral imaging, although currently it is possible to image bilaterally with high-resolution techniques due to the improvement in software and hardware.

Early on in our imaging experience, we experienced significant misregistration from patient movement when solely relying on the subtraction images. Therefore, we elected to perform fat suppression and to use

TABLE 3.3. Memorial Sloan-Kettering Cancer Center Protocol Toggle Method

T2-weighted sagittal fat suppressed
T1-weighted sagittal non–fat-suppressed 3D FSPGR
T1-weighted fat suppressed sagittal 3D FSPGR before and following contrast alternating imaging of each breast (total 3 post contrast acquisitions per breast)
TR 17.1, TE 2.4 (in-phase), a = 35°, BW 31.25
256 × 192, 1 NEX, time = 2 min, freq AP
2-mm slice thickness, no gap
Subtraction
Maximum intensity projection

immobilization plates. We still incorporate subtraction imaging into the protocol to evaluate high signal lesions on T1 that may or may not enhance. T2-weighted imaging was chosen to evaluate cysts, lymph nodes, and myxomatous fibroadenomata, all which can be high in signal on T2. Non–fat-suppressed T1-weighted imaging is performed to confirm fat within the presence of the lymph node hilum or within an area of fat necrosis. Three-dimensional fast spoiled gradient echo sequence (FSPGR) sagittal fat suppressed T1-weighted imaging is then performed on the entire breast before and following the administration of gadolinium-DTPA (0.1 mmol/kg). The contrast agent is bloused through an 18- or 22-gauge needle by hand followed by a saline flush. The nurse administers the contrast, explaining to the patient what she can expect to feel. Three postcontrast images are obtained.

Also, it was and still is important to us to perform bilateral imaging as many disease processes of the breast, including cancer, are bilateral. As with mammography, evaluation of symmetry is beneficial as well. Therefore we performed a bilateral examination using a toggle method (Table 3.3) in which we would examine the breast of interest first, then the contralateral breast for a total of six postcontrast acquisitions (three for for each breast). On several of our magnets this is still the method we use. However, on our newest magnet that supports parallel imaging we perform bilateral simultaneous acquisition with high temporal and spatial resolution. In the future as magnets are upgraded or replaced we plan to use parallel imaging for all our breast MRI cases.

Imaging plane is a matter of preference and often has to do more with the scanner and the preloaded options for imaging. Elimination of cardiac motion also often drives the choice. Sagittal and axial planes have the advantage of corresponding to the mammogram so that direct correlation is possible. Additionally, scanning either in the sagittal or axial planes allows demonstration of ductal pathology, which can be truncated if a coronal plane is used. Linear and segmental abnormalities are much more difficult to appreciate in the coronal plane. Coronal plane imaging may also sacrifice the extreme posterior breast tissue, especially the axillary tail.

The 3D volume set of data allows reconstruction in any scan plane so that if an axial scan plane is initially employed, a coronal rendition is also possible. This can be particularly helpful if a questionable lesion is seen in one dimension and further characterization is required. Questionable vessels become immediately apparent on reconstruction, as are mass lesions. As additional projections can be very helpful in characterizing questionable areas, maximum intensity projections (MIPs) are helpful in providing a big picture evaluation. These 3D composite renderings of the entire breast are helpful in assessing the extent of disease and the relationship of structures. They can be extremely helpful in surgical planning.

15. Conclusion

Setting up a breast MRI program involves multiple personnel and deserves adequate time allotment for imaging and interpretation. Referring physician education is crucial in the initial phases so that appropriate cases are referred and realistic expectations are set. Breast MRI may be a problem-solving test, and the patient may not need further evaluation following the procedure. However, it should be recognized that a significant portion of patients undergoing breast MRI evaluation may require follow up or biopsy and that appropriate mechanisms (such as a method to handle suspicious findings) should be in place before embarking on a program. Breast MRI patients either have a known or suspected breast cancer and therefore are higher in anxiety than the average MRI patient. The radiologist who coordinates the breast MRI program should have a strong knowledge of breast disease, be familiar with biopsy and recommendations for follow up, and be able to communicate effectively to referring physicians and patients. In most practices, a breast imager trained in these skills will best serve the breast MRI program.

Reference

1. American College of Radiology. *Breast Imaging Reporting and Data System (BI-RADS)*. 2nd ed. Reston, VA: American College of Radiology; 1995.

4
The Normal Breast

Elizabeth A. Morris

The anatomy of the breast can be exquisitely demonstrated with magnetic resonance imaging (MRI). Areas of the breast that have been previously beyond the limits of conventional imaging, such as the extreme posterior breast and chest wall musculature, can be evaluated. Normal structures, such as vessels and lymph nodes, are clearly seen, particularly with the help of intravenous contrast. An understanding of the normal structures and anatomy of the breast is essential to the proper interpretation of breast MRIs. This chapter describes the normal anatomy of the breast that is evaluated by breast MRI.

1. Breast Anatomy

The breast is a modified skin gland enveloped in fibrous fascia. The superficial pectoral fascia is located just beneath the skin and in the retromammary space. The undersurface of the breast lies on the deep pectoral fascia.[1] Although there are fascial layers between the breast proper and the pectoralis major muscle, the breast is not completely separate from the pectoralis major muscle, as there are penetrating lymphatics and blood vessels [Figure 4.1(A)].

The breast is composed of three major structures: skin, subcutaneous tissue, and breast tissue (parenchyma and stroma). The parenchyma is divided into 15 to 20 lobes or segments that converge at the nipple in a radial arrangement. The ducts from the lobes converge into 6 to 10 major collecting ducts that have openings at the nipple and connect to the outside. Each of these major ducts arborizes back from the nipple and forms a lobe or segment of glandular tissue that is supported by surrounding connective or stromal tissue [Figure 4.1(B)]. The distribution of lobes is not even as there is a preponderance of glandular tissue in the upper outer quadrant of the breast.[1]

Beneath the nipple openings, the lactiferous sinus is visible. The lactiferous sinus is a slight dilation of the ampullary portion of the major duct. The major ducts that converge below the nipple and drain each segment are 2mm in diameter. Each duct drains a lobe made up of 20 to 40 lobules. Each lobule contains 10 to 100 alveoli or acini. Each lobule also consists of branching ducts that divide into subsegmental structures and terminate in the terminal duct lobular unit. The terminal duct lobular unit consists of the terminal duct and the acinus. The glandular tissue and ducts are surrounded by fat and supported by Cooper's ligaments, which are connective tissue elements that arise from stromal tissue and attach to the prepectoral fascia and dermis and support and suspend the breast tissue (Figure 4.2).

High signal intensity can be identified on precontrast II weighted images in ducts that are dilated and contain proteinaceous or hemmorhagic debris, representing areas of ductal ectasia (Figure 4.3). As with mammography, this can be unilateral or bilateral. The areas involved can be focal or diffuse (Figure 4.4). For the most part, these areas of ductal dilation represent benign disease. However, as there is high signal on the precontrast images, it is important to assess whether enhancement occurs. As the ducts are high in signal on both the precontrast and postcontrast images, small areas of enhancement may be overlooked. Subtraction imaging of the precontrast from the postcontrast image on a pixel-by-pixel basis can ensure that small areas of enhancement are not present (Figure 4.5).

The stroma and connective tissue of the breast contain fat, connective tissue, ligaments, blood vessels, lymphatics, lymph nodes, and nerves. The skin of the breast contains hair follicles, sebaceous glands, and apocrine sweat glands.[2]

Visualization of the pectoralis major muscle is as important in MRI as it is in mammography, to ensure that the breast is maximally imaged (Figure 4.6). With adequate penetration to the chest wall, portions of the pectoralis muscles, major and minor, are reliably visualized [Figures 4.1(B) and 4.7]. As with other imaging techniques, complete visualization of the entire breast parenchyma is essential (Figure 4.8). Protocols that exclude portions of the breast are to be avoided. When selecting a protocol and training technologists, it may be important to emphasize

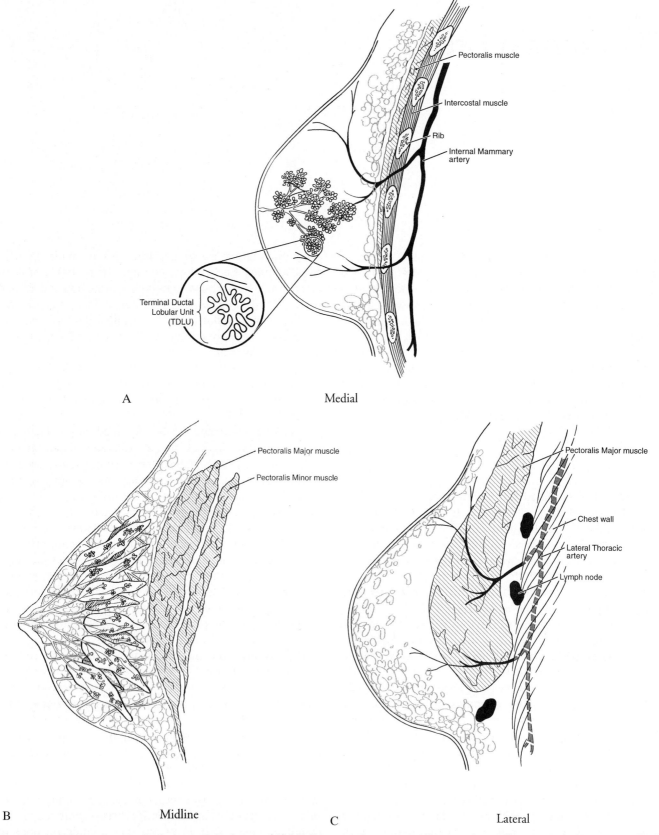

FIGURE 4.1. Schematic of sagittal views of the breast. (A) Medially, the internal mammary artery and branches are seen. The terminal duct lobular unit (TDLU), the site of origin of most of metaplastic, hyperplastic, and neoplastic processes of the breast, is demonstrated. (B) At midline, the pectoralis major and minor muscles are usually seen depending on patient anatomy. Each breast contains approximately 15 to 20 lobes. (C) Laterally, the lateral thoracic artery and branches supply the breast. Level 1 lymph nodes are demonstrated posterior to the pectoralis major muscle.

FIGURE 4.2. Prominent Cooper's ligaments (arrows) in a patient with inflammatory breast cancer. The large central mass is seen as well as focal thickening and enhancement of the skin. This image and all subsequent images were performed on a 1.5 Tesla (T) magnet with a dedicated breast coil using a sagittal fat-suppressed three-dimensional (3D) fast spoiled gradient echo sequence (FSPGR) following intravenous contrast unless otherwise indicated.

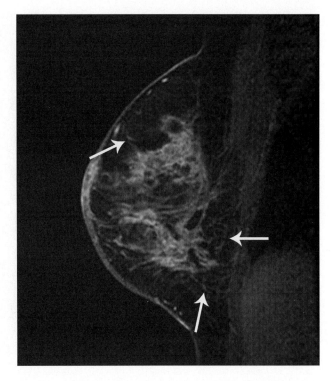

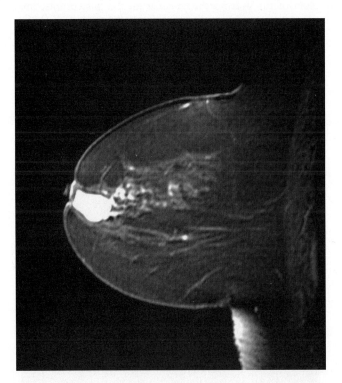

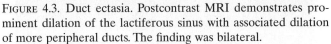

FIGURE 4.3. Duct ectasia. Postcontrast MRI demonstrates prominent dilation of the lactiferous sinus with associated dilation of more peripheral ducts. The finding was bilateral.

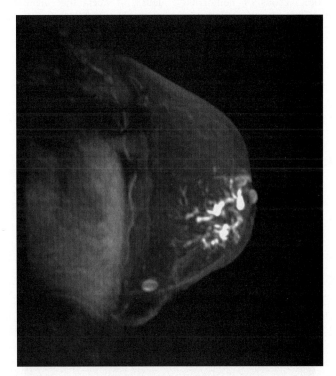

FIGURE 4.4. Maximum intensity projection (MIP) demonstrates segmental duct ectasia. Note markers over the nipple and inferiorly over a palpable abnormality with no corresponding MRI finding.

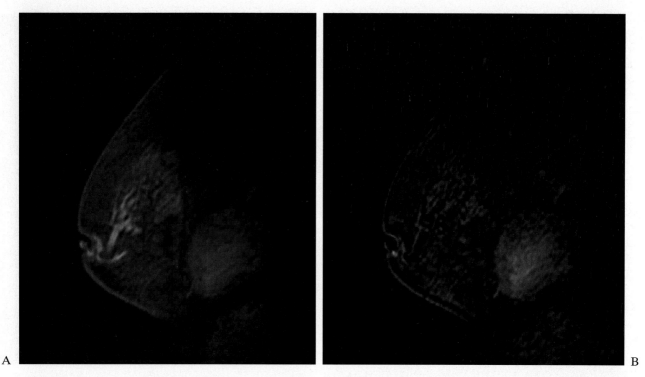

FIGURE 4.5. Benign duct ectasia. (A) Postcontrast sagittal fat-suppressed 3D FSPGR image demonstrates high signal proteinaceous or hemorrhagic debris in ducts that arborize demonstrating one of the lobes of the breast. The precontrast image was identical. Note the convergence in the subareolar region. A marker has been placed on the nipple. (B) Subtraction of the precontrast image from the postcontrast image demonstrates no enhancement of the ductal tree.

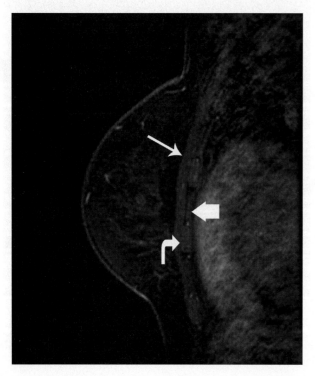

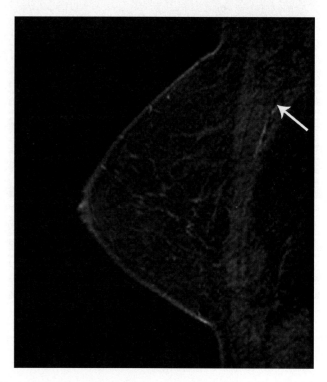

FIGURE 4.6. Medial breast with pectoralis major muscle (arrow) overlying ribs (curved arrow) and intercostal muscles (thick arrow).

FIGURE 4.7. Laterally in the breast the pectoralis minor is visualized (arrow) behind the pectoralis major muscle.

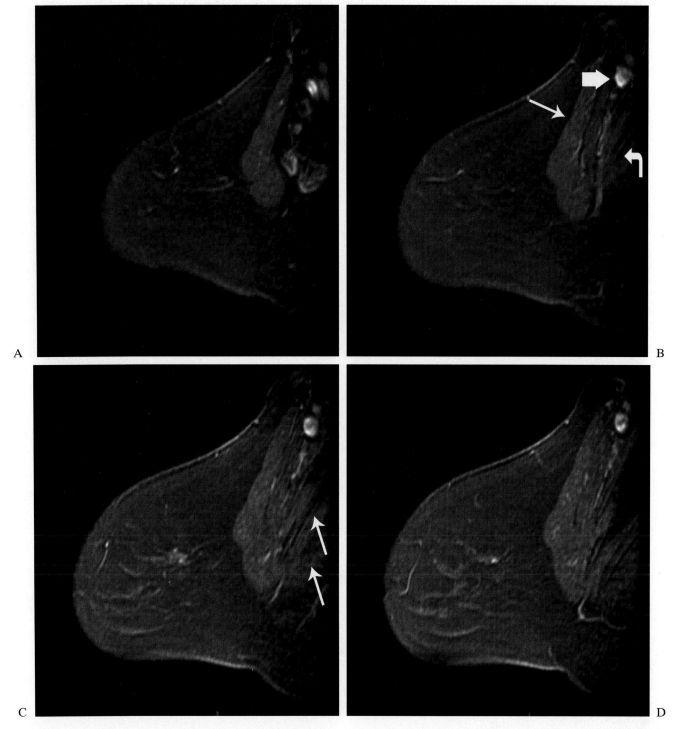

FIGURE 4.8. (A) Multiple normal appearing level I axillary lymph nodes posterior to pectoralis major muscle. (B) Pectoralis major muscle (arrow) and pectoralis minor muscle (curved arrow). Axillary artery identified (thick arrow). (C) Serratus anterior muscle (arrows). (D) Lateral to mid-breast.

(*Continued*)

the inclusion of the axillary tail, inframammary fold, and extreme medial breast tissue as pathology can be hidden in these areas (Figure 4.9). Maximal coverage of the breast includes imaging the axillary tail and high axilla, sites where ectopic breast tissue may be hiding (Figure 4.10). Technologists can also ensure that these areas are imaged by manually pulling breast tissue into the imaging coil.

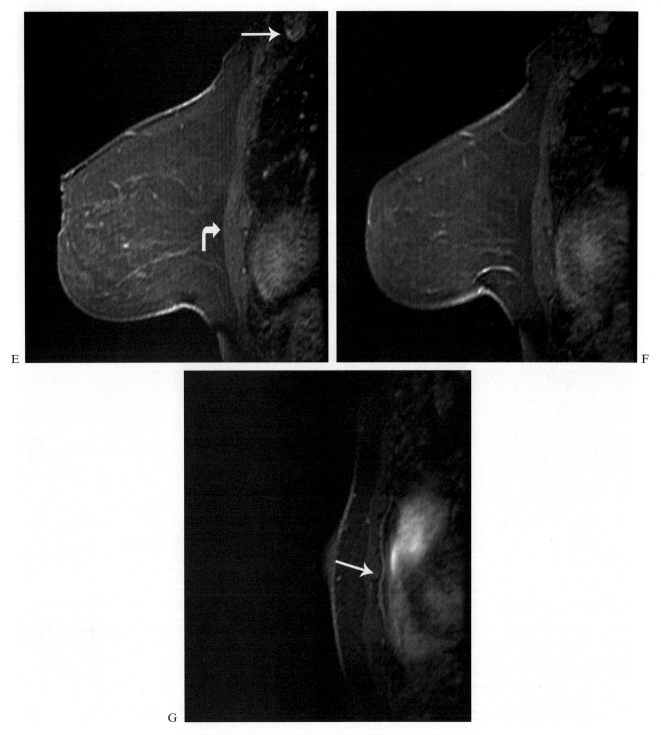

FIGURE 4.8. (*Continued*) (E) Medially, axillary artery can still be seen (arrow). Pectoralis major muscle anterior to chest wall (curved arrow). Note contrast in heart and pulmonary vessels. (F) Medial breast. (G) Internal mammary artery (arrow) anterior to the heart.

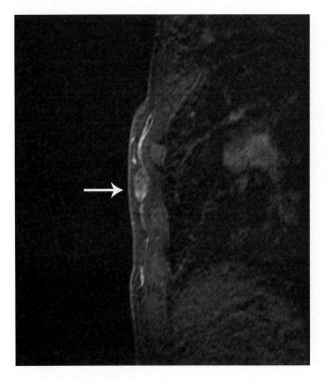

FIGURE 4.9. Medial fibroadenoma (arrow). Field of view should not sacrifice medial breast tissue.

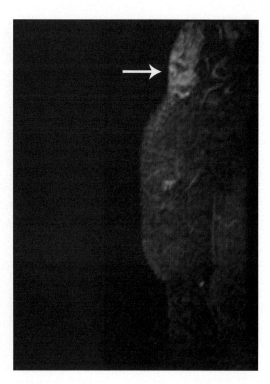

FIGURE 4.10. Ectopic breast tissue in the axillary tail on a lateral image (arrow).

2. Vessels

The breast receives its blood supply from several sources. The lateral thoracic artery [Figures 4.1C and 4.11] arises from the axillary artery and supplies the upper outer quadrant of the breast, constituting approximately 30% of the breast blood supply. Sixty percent of the blood supply arises from the internal mammary artery (Figure 4.12) and its perforating branches, which supply the central and medial aspects of the breast. These are best seen where they penetrate the chest wall close to the sternum (Figure 4.13). The remainder of the blood supply is primarily via the lateral branches of the intercostal arteries. Vessels can be usually distinguished from masses by following the course of the vessel over multiple contiguous sections. Maximum intensity projection (MIP) images can also help to confirm the course of a vessel (Figure 4.14). The supply of vessels to the breast is helpful in understanding the preferential enhancement that can be seen in the upper outer quadrant and along the inferior breast. Generally, the center of the breast is the last to enhance due to the differing blood supply. Bilateral imaging can confirm the impression of benign parenchymal geographic enhancement when the same pattern of enhancement is seen in both breasts.

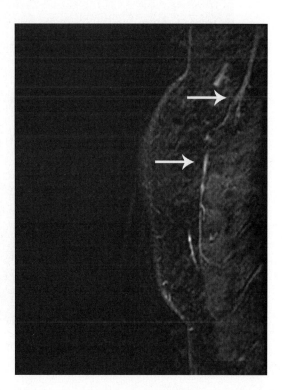

FIGURE 4.11. Lateral thoracic artery (arrow) and branches.

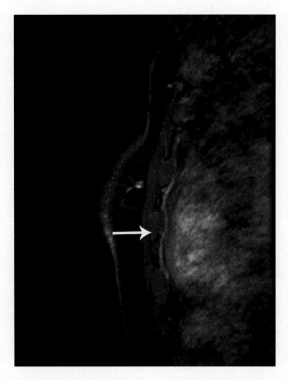

FIGURE 4.12. Internal mammary artery (arrow).

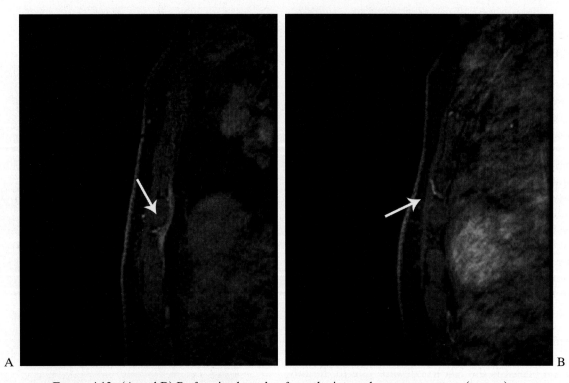

FIGURE 4.13. (A and B) Perforating branches from the internal mammary artery (arrows).

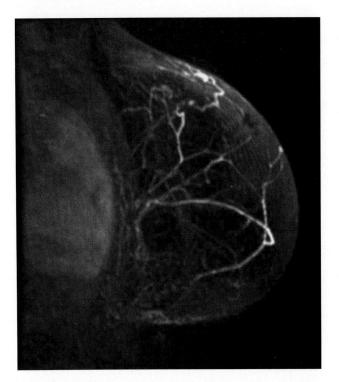

FIGURE 4.14. Maximum intensity projection of breast demonstrates course of vessels.

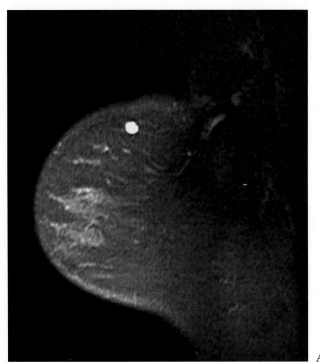

A

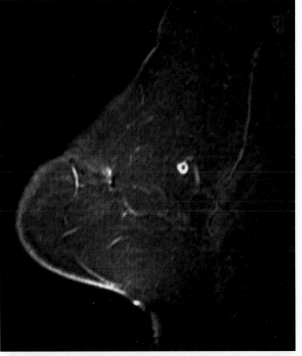

B

3. Lymphatics and Lymph Nodes

Lymphatic drainage of the breast is primarily via the axilla (97%) with the internal mammary chain accounting for the remaining 3%. Level I lymph nodes are found lateral to the lateral border of the pectoralis minor muscle [see Figures 4.1(C) and 4.8(A)]. Level II nodes lie behind the pectoralis muscle, and level III nodes are located medial to the medial border of the pectoralis minor muscle.

Intramammary lymph nodes on mammography are usually seen in the lateral half of the breast along the cone of breast tissue and are found in approximately 5% of women (Figure 4.15). As MRI is able to evaluate more of the posterior breast tissue, and as lymph nodes are highly vascular and enhance intensely, it is not surprising that lymph nodes are seen with more frequency on MRI in locations that are considered atypical for mammography (Figure 4.16). Lymph nodes are easily diagnosed when the characteristic reniform appearance is seen with a fatty hilum. Sometimes vessels radiating into the lymph node hilum can be identified with certainty, also supporting the diagnosis of a lymph node (Figure 4.17). However, lymph nodes can be diagnostic dilemmas[3] when not in the expected location and when morphologic criteria are not typical (Figure 4.18). Dynamic curves can be unreliable as

FIGURE 4.15. (A) Well-circumscribed homogeneous enhancing round mass in the upper outer quadrant does not demonstrate a fatty hilum. Kinetic analysis demonstrated washout kinetics. T2-weighted imaging demonstrated corresponding high signal mass (not shown). Nevertheless, biopsy was performed yielding benign lymph node. (B) Characteristic appearance of lymph node with presence of fatty hilum. Even though a washout kinetic curve was obtained in this lesion, the characteristic morphology allows benign interpretation.

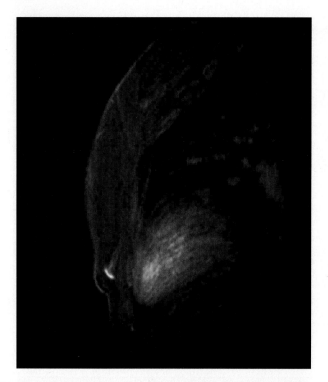

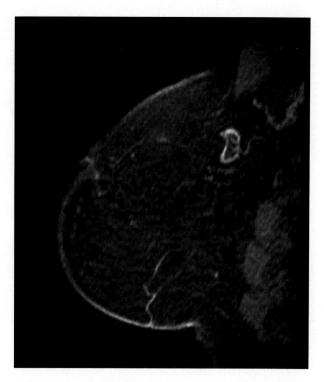

FIGURE 4.16. Lymph node in the posterior medial breast. Presence of vessel extending to hilum and characteristic reniform appearance allows diagnosis.

FIGURE 4.17. Benign lymph node with vessel radiating to hilum.

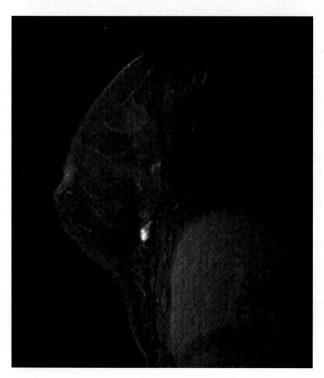

FIGURE 4.18. Lymph node in uncharacteristic location. Lymph node in the posterior central breast with irregular margins and heterogeneous enhancement. If a corresponding high signal mass is confirmed on the T2-weighted sequence these lesions may be followed cautiously.

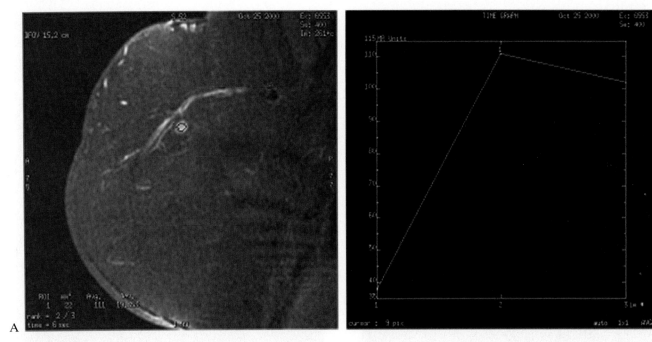

A   B

FIGURE 4.19. (A) Region of interest placed over a round homogeneously enhancing mass in the upper outer quadrant. (B) Kinetic analysis demonstrates washout. As atypical appearing lymph nodes may mimic carcinoma, attention to T2-weighted images can help in confirming the presence of a lymph node. If any doubt persists, biopsy is recommended.

normal lymph nodes can enhance rapidly and can washout, mimicking carcinoma (Figure 4.19). T2-weighted images may be helpful in these cases as lymph nodes may be higher in signal intensity than the normal glandular parenchyma (Figure 4.20). Lymph nodes containing tumor, particularly micrometastases, cannot be reliably diagnosed at this time with the current contrast agents (Figure 4.21).

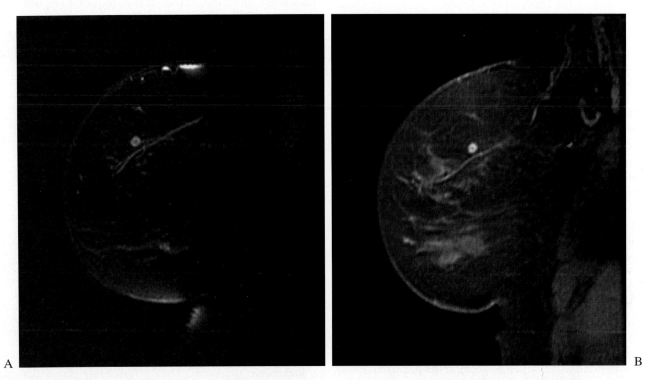

A   B

FIGURE 4.20. (A) T2-weighted image of a lymph node demonstrates high signal. Note lymph node is associated with a vessel and contains a fatty hilum, further confirming benignity. (B) Corresponding postcontrast T1-weighted image.

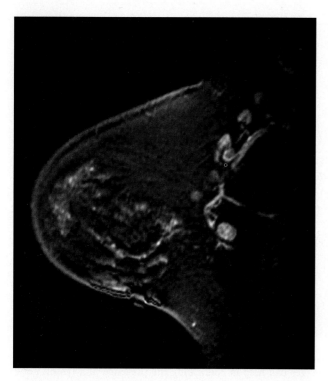

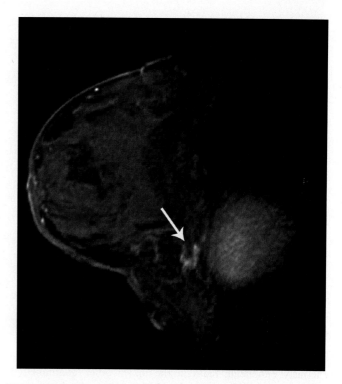

FIGURE 4.21. Benign reactive lymph nodes demonstrate the difficulty of detecting metastases. These lymph nodes are prominent and several do not contain fatty hila nevertheless, they proved to be benign.

FIGURE 4.22. Vessel (arrow) extending through the chest wall was able to be followed over multiple sequential images.

4. Pectoralis Major Muscle

The pectoralis muscles, though attached to the chest wall, are not considered part of the chest wall. This is an important distinction when it comes to staging the patient. If the chest wall is involved, the patient is Stage IIIB and not generally a surgical candidate. On the other hand, if only the pectoralis muscles are involved, then the patient can have surgery with removal of a portion or all of the muscle(s) to achieve negative margins. Tumor involvement of the pectoralis muscles is suspected when abnormal enhancement is noted, indicating tumor involvement. If tumor infiltrates the muscles, staging of the tumor is not changed although surgical planning may be altered. Abutment of tumor to the muscle with loss of the fat plane does not signify muscle involvement.[4]

Sometimes it may be difficult to differentiate tumor involvement between normal enhancing traversing vessels extending through the pectoralis muscle (Figure 4.22). Traversing vessels, however, can be identified on multiple sequential images and their course can be followed (Figure 4.23). Tumor involvement of the pectoralis major muscle generally produces more irregular enhancement. The pectoralis minor muscle, which lies behind the pectoralis major muscle [see Figures 4.1(B) and 4.8(D)], is not generally involved unless there is full-thickness involvement of the pectoralis major muscle. The true chest wall includes the intercostal and serratus anterior muscles as well as the ribs. In order to diagnose chest wall involvement, abnormal enhancement in these structures is required (Figure 4.24).

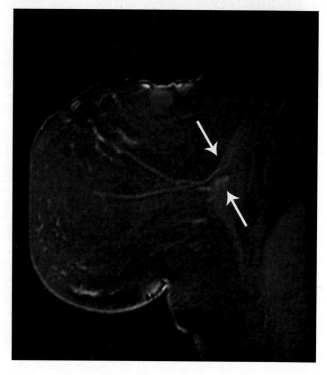

FIGURE 4.23. Vessels (arrows) in the pectoralis major muscle.

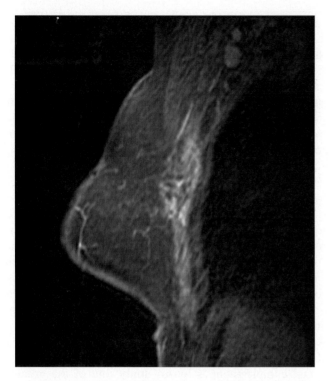

FIGURE 4.24. Chest wall involvement. Note diffuse enhancement of the serratus anterior muscles.

5. Breast Density

Breast density, which is a representation in mammography of the amount of breast parenchyma present in the breast, can be assessed on MRI on both T2- and T1-weighted images. Breasts are characterized using BI-RADS (Breast Imaging Reporting and Data System)[5] criteria: 1, almost entirely fatty; 2, scattered fibroglandular densities; 3, heterogeneously dense; and 4, extremely dense as with mammography (Figure 4.25). Unlike mammography, dense breasts generally do not pose a significant problem on MRI as contrast is used and thin slices are obtained, thus overlapping parenchyma is not a hindrance (Figure 4.25B). There are, however, a small set of patients who exhibit very early rapid enhancement of the parenchyma, which can obscure small enhancing suspicious foci. In these cases, it may be helpful to communicate the lowered sensitivity of MRI to the referring physician.

The breast parenchyma will be altered as the hormonal environment of the breast changes. Age and fluid status will also alter appearance. Both the epithelial ductal tissue and the surrounding connective tissue elements comprising the parenchyma are affected by the hormonal milieu.

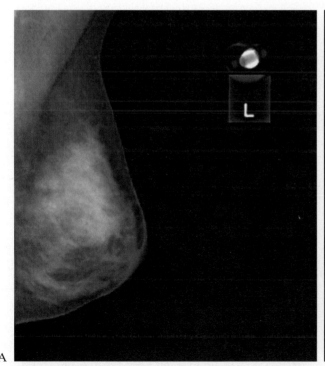
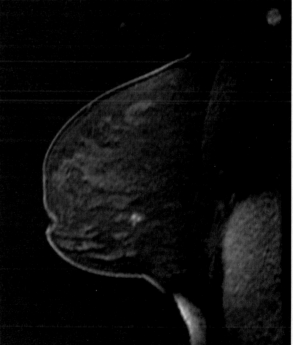

A   B

FIGURE 4.25. (A) MLO view demonstrates dense parenchyma with no abnormalities. (B) Contrast-enhanced MRI in the same patient is positive for a small invasive ductal carcinoma that was likely obscured due to surrounding isodense breast tissue on the mammogram.

Assessment of breast density becomes important when interpreting hormonal changes in the breast, a possible cause of benign parenchymal enhancement. Similarly, fibrocystic change, which can be a cause of false-positive enhancement, occurs more often in dense breasts. By recognizing breast density and the areas in the breast where parenchyma is present, the interpreter can render a more informed opinion.

6. Premenopausal Breast

The premenopausal breast is hormonally responsive.[6] Estrogens cause increased blood flow through breast parenchyma. This phenomenon is mediated by a histamine effect that causes hyperemia, vasodilatation, and capillary leakiness.[7] Contrast enhancement in the breast is dependent on these three factors and, therefore, it is not unexpected that contrast enhancement occurs in a cyclical fashion in the normal premenopausal breast (Figure 4.26)[8] Water displacement studies have shown that breast volume can increase during the second half of the menstrual cycle by 100mL. There is also evidence that in addition to water fluctuations during the menstrual cycle, cyclical changes also affect parenchymal growth.

Enhancement following contrast administration on MRI is related to vascularity, permeability, and capillary leakiness. Therefore, estrogens can cause benign parenchyma to enhance following contrast administration. In premenopausal women, MRI enhancement of breast parenchyma may vary with the phase of the menstrual cycle, greatest in weeks 1 and 4 (Figure 4.27). Enhancement can be stippled in a uniform, diffuse distribution or patchy (Figure 4.28). Enhancement kinetic analysis most often shows gradual increase over time with continuous enhancement. Occasionally these areas of normal hormonally sensitive parenchyma may enhance intensely and in a mass-like distribution (Figure 4.29). For this reason, examination is best performed in midcycle (week 2; between days 7 and 14).

Two studies[9,10] have demonstrated that the majority of young women have enhancement in the breast that may be focal or diffuse. The focal areas of enhancement can mimic malignancy, looking mass-like with well-circumscribed or irregular margins. The majority of these areas, however, have a benign time course: type I or II curves with persistent or plateau kinetics. None had a malignant time curve with rapid washout. When the examination was repeated in mid-cycle, more than half of the areas of enhancement disappeared. Benign background hormonal enhancement is by no doubt one of the greatest challenges facing interpretation of breast MRI, however, if recognized and analyzed (with BI-RADS MRI lexicon) using kinetic information (usually continuous) and morphology (usually non-mass), the correct interpretation can generally be rendered.

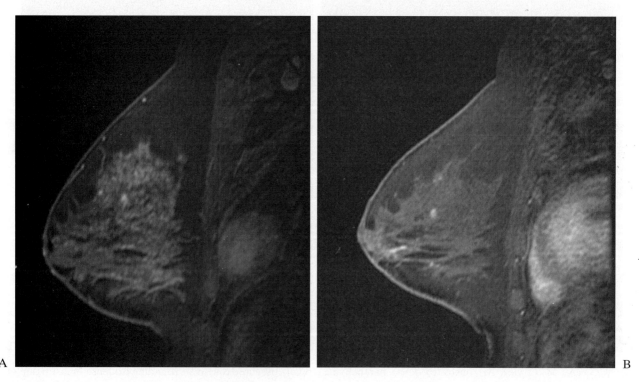

FIGURE 4.26. (A) Initial study in the third week of the menstrual cycle in a premenopausal woman. (B) Follow up several months later in the second week of the cycle demonstrates much less parenchymal enhancement.

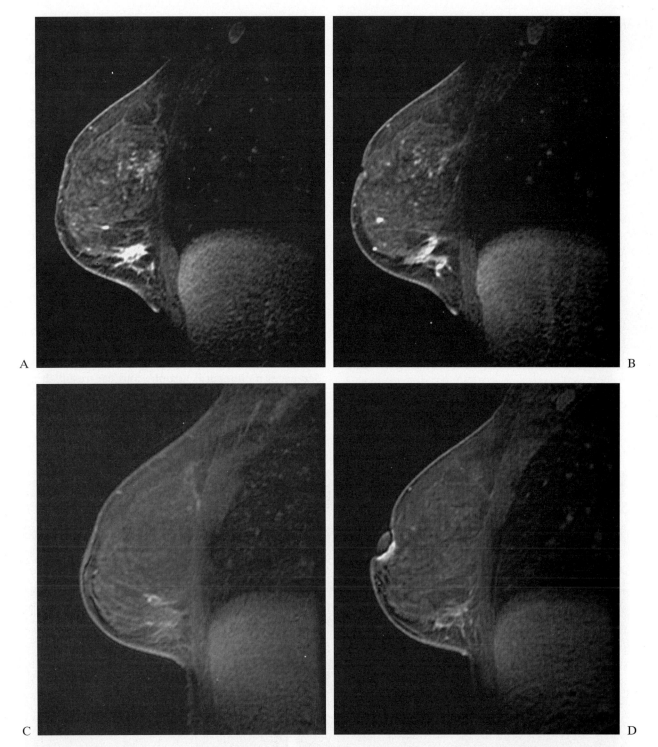

FIGURE 4.27. (A and B) Initial study in the fourth week of the menstrual cycle in a premenopausal woman. (C and D) Follow-up examination in 2 months in the second week of the cycle shows marked decrease in the overall enhancement.

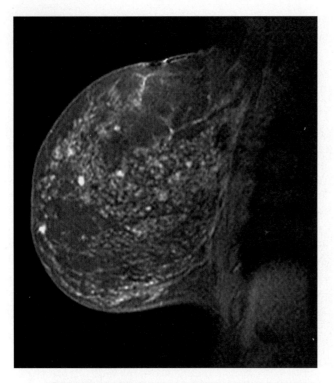

FIGURE 4.28. Diffuse stippled enhancement in a dense breast in a premenopausal patient that was related to hormone effects.

7. Postmenopausal Breast

Menopausal status can affect the breast density.[11] When a patient reaches menopause (usually in her late 40s or early 50s), the body stops producing estrogen and progesterone. The breasts' glandular tissue involutes and shrinks after menopause, replaced by fatty tissue. Therefore, as patients advance in age, in general, breast density decreases as fatty replacement occurs. Structurally, there is a decrease in cellularity and number of lobules as a result of epithelial atrophy. Fibrous connective tissue loses strength and the breasts may sag. This progression can be extremely variable and can affect the breasts in a heterogeneous fashion, leaving some areas of the breast relatively unaffected. Additionally, there is a broad spectrum of breast densities in all ages, with premenopausal patients having fatty breasts and postmenopausal patients having extremely dense breasts. Therefore, although a gross generalization can be made that young women generally have dense breasts that involute with age, this may not apply to a specific individual case.

Administration of exogenous hormonal treatment decreases menopausal atrophy and can result in appearances on MRI of the premenopausal breast (Figure 4.30).[12] This is usually seen with combined hormone replacement

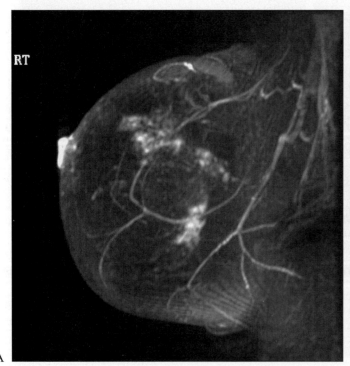

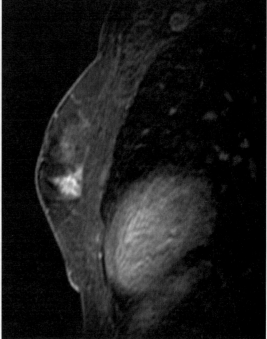

A   B

FIGURE 4.29. (A) Maximum intensity projection image demonstrates patchy areas of mass-like enhancement. The contralateral breast demonstrated similar changes. Kinetic analysis demonstrated continuous enhancement. Therefore it was elected to follow this in several months and re-image in the second phase of the cycle. (B) Mass-like enhancement (result of hormones) disappeared on follow-up examination.

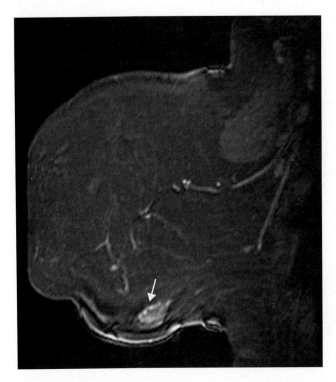

FIGURE 4.30. Postmenopausal patient on hormones for 5 years had areas of mass-like enhancement (arrow) in the inferior breast that regressed but did not disappear after discontinuing exogenous hormone therapy at repeat scanning 6 weeks later. Note adjacent coil artifact inferiority.

therapy with estrogen and progesterone. False-positive results may occur in these circumstances and therefore it is recommended that the patient be off hormones for 6 to 8 weeks before scanning. Usually, if there is an important clinical problem, most centers do not insist that the patient stop hormonal therapy before performing MRI.

8. Chemopreventive Agents

Drugs called antiestrogens and SERMs (selective estrogen receptor modulator) may be able to reduce breast cancer risk. Because estrogen can promote the development of cancer in the breast, drugs that block its action may be helpful in preventing or treating breast cancer. Tamoxifen is a SERM that exerts antiestrogen effects on the breast by binding to the estrogen receptors of breast cells, preventing estrogen molecules from binding to the receptors. By interfering with estrogen receptors in this way, tamoxifen blocks the ability of estrogen to stimulate the proliferation of breast cells. This effect reportedly can decrease enhancement on MRI and decrease breast density in some women (Figure 4.31). As these therapies become more ubiquitous, the effect of imaging studies will need to be rec-

ognized.[13] Parenchymal density as well as parenchymal enhancement in these patients is reduced.

9. Pregnancy

Pregnancy produces extreme changes in the breast parenchyma with associated vascular engorgement. Early in pregnancy, terminal ducts and lobules grow rapidly with lobular enlargement and depletion in fibrofatty stroma. Lobular growth continues throughout pregnancy. Following cessation of lactation, involution of the breast occurs over a period of 3 months.

Evaluation with MRI in the pregnant patient is not advised in the first trimester as the effects of the magnetic field on the fetus at this time are unknown, though depending on the clinical circumstances, the benefits of the information may override the risks. Regardless, in our experience, we have found the utility of MRI in this setting unpredictable at best, as general diffuse intense enhancement is present due to parenchymal enhancement (Figure 4.32). Underlying carcinomas may be obscured to marked intense generalized enhancement. In several cases we have been able to see the primary carcinoma; however, the reliability of detecting additional disease remains unclear (Figure 4.33). No published data address the pregnant patient; all experience is anecdotal at this point.

Similarly, patients who are lactating have diffuse extreme enhancement that poses potential difficulties in interpretation (Figure 4.34).[14] As the issue of pregnancy-related breast cancer (breast cancer diagnosed during pregnancy or within the following year) is significant when a suspicious palpable abnormality is identified in these patients, evaluation with mammography to assess calcifications and with ultrasound to assess masses is favored over the evaluation with MRI. Very few reports of breast MRI in this setting are known at this writing and further study is warranted.

10. Skin and Nipple

Normal skin appears smooth and measures usually 0.5- to 2.0-mm thick, except caudally where it may be slightly thicker due to its usual dependency.[15] Skin should not enhance. Skin scars demonstrate focal skin thickening that does not enhance if mature. Sebaceous cysts can be encountered when performing breast MRI and can enhance when they become inflamed (Figure 4.35). Most often these arise from swollen hair follicles.

The nipple-areolar complex enhances intensely on MRI following contrast administration due to the presence of numerous vessels (Figure 4.36). Normal nipples may show symmetrical enhancement patterns on MRI, even when they are asymmetrical on physical examination.

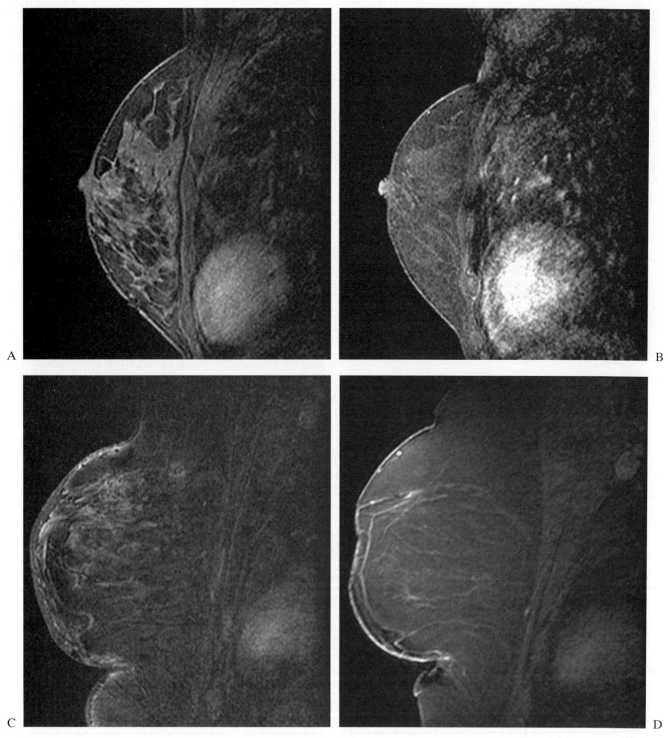

A

B

C

D

FIGURE 4.31. Two examples of loss in breast density following medication with SERMs (selective estrogen receptor modulator). (A) Pretreatment breast density in a 42-year-old woman with contralateral mastectomy. (B) Posttreatment breast density has decreased in the same patient. (C) Pretreatment breast density in a 54-year-old woman with contralateral mastectomy for invasive ductal carcinoma. Skin thickening is due to recent benign breast biopsy. (D) Posttreatment breast density has decreased in the same patient. Note skin thickening resolved.

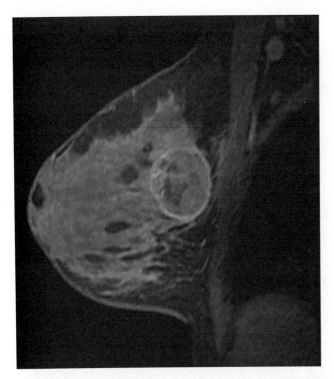

FIGURE 4.32. A 34-year-old patient felt a large mass in the lateral breast several weeks postpartum. Magnetic resonance imaging demonstrates a large partially necrotic rim-enhancing tumor that corresponds to the palpable abnormality. Note intense background enhancement of dense proliferative parenchyma.

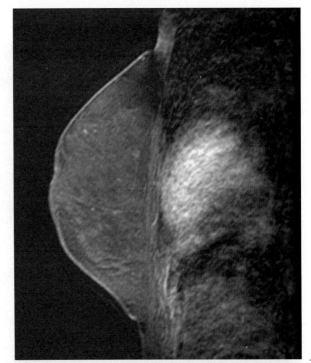

A

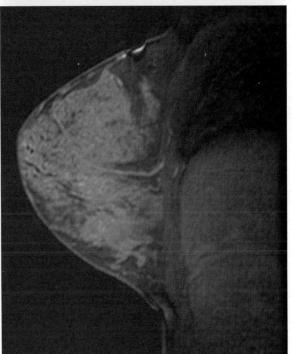

B

FIGURE 4.34. (A) Prior MRI examination in a 33-year-old woman who was on screening protocol. No significant enhancement is identified. (B) The same patient is reimaged while lactating. Note parenchymal proliferation as well as intense enhancement of the lactating breast tissue.

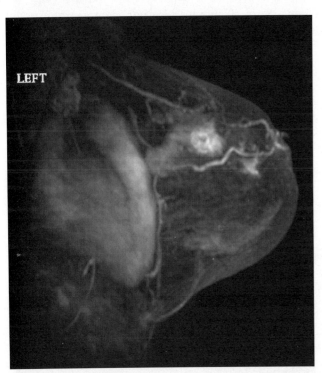

FIGURE 4.33. Maximum intensity projection image of a 39-year-old woman who presented with a lump 1 year following normal delivery. She had been breastfeeding her child from that breast. Maximum intensity projection image shows a highly suspicious mass compatible with carcinoma. Note the background enhancement is not as intense as in the preceding case.

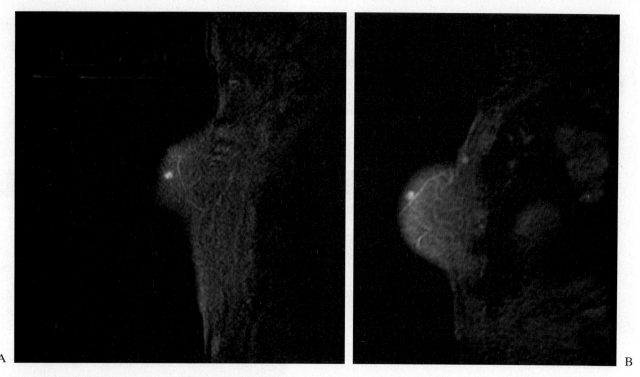

FIGURE 4.35. (A and B) Two examples of sebaceous cysts that demonstrate enhancement. Note that these are directly along the skin surface.

There is usually 1 to 2mm thickness of dermal enhancement with a nonenhancing central area. Rarely, there is linear enhancement passing though the non-enhancing region. Normal nipples do not demonstrate nodular or irregular enhancement along the posterior border (Figure 4.37).[16]

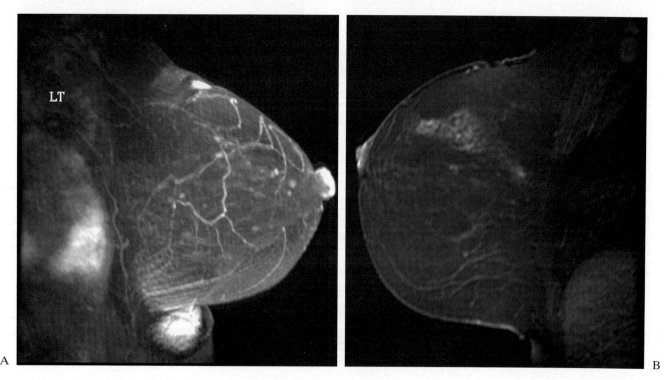

FIGURE 4.36. Nipples on MRI may (A) enhance intensely, (B) mildly, or (C) not at all, depending on blood supply.

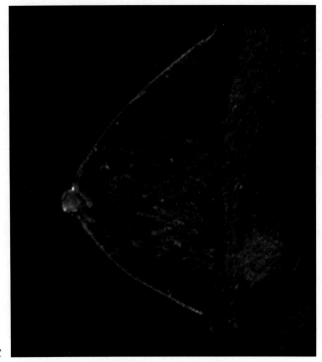

C

FIGURE 4.36. (*Continued*)

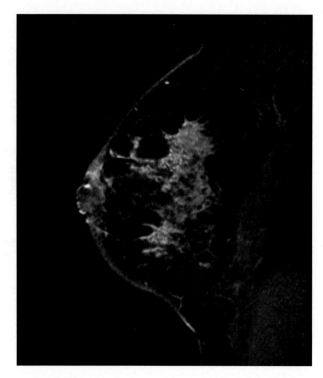

FIGURE 4.37. Abnormal thickened nipple in a patient with inflammatory breast carcinoma.

11. Fat

On non–fat-suppressed T1-weighted precontrast images, fat is high in signal intensity and the breast parenchyma is intermediate signal intensity. Fat can obscure contrast enhancement if not suppressed by some method. Fat suppression can be achieved by subtraction imaging so that the signal from fat is subtracted and only the contrast-enhancing areas of the breast remain. Another method is to perform chemical fat suppression that actively suppresses the signal from fat.

12. Fibrous Tissue and Calcifications

Fibrous tissue is generally low in signal intensity. Foreign objects, such as metallic clips, produce signal void and are very dark. Calcifications, if large enough, can be seen as very low signal. Benign breast calcifications, such as those seen in sclerosing adenosis or fibrocystic changes, are rarely imaged on breast MRI.

13. Conclusion

Normal structures of the breast can be evaluated on breast MRI. Recognition and knowledge of these findings can facilitate interpretation. Some of the challenges in breast MRI include understanding normal structures and normal patterns of enhancement of the breast parenchyma. Hormonal stimulation of the breast, endogenous and exogenous, can be recognized, it is hoped, as benign form morphology and kinetics. Similarly, mistaking benign structures such as lymph nodes for suspicious masses may be lessened if all the pertinent data, including information from all sequences (especially T2 weighted) and any prior imaging comparison such as mammography is considered.

References

1. Harris JR, Lippman ME, Morrow M, Hellman S. *Diseases of the Breast.* Philadelphia, PA: Lippincott-Raven Publishers; 1996.
2. Rosen PP. *Rosen's Breast Pathology.* Philadelphia, PA: Lippincott-Raven Publishers; 1997.
3. Gallardo X, Sentis M, Castaner E, et al. Enhancement of intramammary lymph nodes with lymphoid hyperplasia: a potential pitfall in breast MRI. *Eur Radiol.* 1998;8: 1662–1665.
4. Morris EA, Schwartz LH, Drotman MB, et al. Evaluation of pectoralis major muscle in patients with posterior breast tumors on breast MR images: early experience. *Radiology* 2000;214:67–72.
5. American College of Radiology. *Breast Imaging Reporting and Data System (BI-RADS).* 2nd ed. Reston, VA: American College of Radiology; 1995.

6. Zeppa R. Vascular response of the breast to estrogen. *J Clin Endocrinol Metab.* 1969;29:695–700.

7. Vogel PM, Geariade NG, Fetter BF, et al. The correlation of histologic changes in the human breast with the menstrual cycle. *Am J Pathol.* 1981;104:23–24.

8. Fowler PA, Casey CE, Cameron GG, et al. Cyclical changes in composition and volume of the breast during the menstrual cycle measured by magnetic resonance imaging. *Br J Obstet Gyn.* 1990;97:595–602.

9. Kuhl CK, Bieling HB, Gieseke J, et al. Healthy premenopausal breast parenchyma in dynamic contrast-enhanced MR imaging of the breast: normal contrast medium enhancement and cyclical phase dependency. *Radiology* 1997;203:137–144.

10. Muller-Schimpfle M, Ohmenhauser MD, Stoli P, et al. Menstrual cycle and age: influence on parenchymal contrast medium enhancement in MR imaging of the breast. *Radiology* 1997;203:145–149.

11. Potten CS, Watson RJ, Tickle S, et al. The effect of age and menstrual cycle upon proliferative activity of the normal human breast. *Br J Cancer.* 1988;8:163–170.

12. Reichenbach JR, Przetak C, Klinger G, Kaiser WA. Assessment of breast tissue changes on hormonal replacement therapy using MRI: a pilot study. *J Comput Assist Tomogr.* 1999;23:407–413.

13. Heinig A, Lampe D, Kolbl H, et al. Suppression of unspecific enhancement on breast magnetic resonance imaging (MRI) by antiestrogen medication. *Tumori* 2002;88: 215–223.

14. Talele AC, Slanetz PJ, Edminster WB, et al. The lactating breast: MRI findings and literature review. *Breast J.* 2003; 9:237–240.

15. Wilson SA, Adam EJ, Tucker AK. Patterns of breast skin thickness in normal mammograms. *Radiology* 1982;33: 691–693.

16. Friedman EP, Hall-Craggs MA, Mumtaz H, et al. Beast MR and the appearance of the normal and abnormal Nipple. *Clin Radiol.* 1997;52:854–861.

5
The Axilla

Joo Young Melissa Lee and D. David Dershaw

The most common site of regional involvement of breast cancer is within the axillary lymph nodes. Along with size of the primary carcinoma, the presence of metastatic disease to the axillary lymph nodes is the most important indicator of clinical outcome. Studies of 10-year survival rates have demonstrated that prognosis is directly related to the number of lymph nodes involved.[1-3] As shown in results obtained in the American College of Surgeons' survey, with greater number of nodes involved, there is a progressive decline in survival (Table 5.1). When 1 to 2 nodes are involved, 5-year survival is 62% to 63%, whereas when 5 nodes are involved, survival declines to 47%. With more than 10 nodes involved, survival decreases to 29%. Because knowledge of involvement of lymph nodes is important for staging and treatment planning for patients, techniques to assess the status of these nodes are important.

Additionally, removal of axillary nodes may decrease axillary recurrence of tumor. As axillary recurrence can significantly compromise quality of life with lymphedema and pain, surgical removal or radiation of these involved nodes can be helpful in decreasing the likelihood of this complication.

1. Anatomy

The axillary lymph nodes are divided into three levels that are defined by their relationships to the pectoralis minor muscle: Level I nodes are inferior and lateral to the pectoralis minor muscle; level II nodes are deep to this muscle, and level III nodes are superior and medial to the pectoralis minor (Figure 5.1). The majority of breast cancers spread into these axillary nodes with a small percentage of medially located tumors spreading into the internal mammary lymph nodes. This nodal chain is located parasternally, deep to intercostal muscles, adjacent to the internal mammary vessels.

Metastatic invasion of axillary lymph nodes generally develops in an orderly, progressive pattern, with the nodes of level I first affected, followed by levels II and III. Because of this pattern, as higher levels of the nodal chain are involved, the number of involved lymph nodes increases, and the prognosis worsens. Rarely, there is involvement of higher levels without involvement of lower level lymph nodes. Large series have shown that these *skip metastases* only occur only in approximately 3% to 4% of cases.[4,5] Therefore, if the nodes of level I are free of disease, there is minimal chance of metastatic involvement of lymph nodes in levels II and III.

2. Pathophysiology of Metastatic Disease to Lymph Nodes

Tumor cells usually enter lymph nodes via afferent lymphatics, passing into the marginal sinus, then into the cortex where they first establish themselves. A focus of tumor cells less than 2 mm in diameter on histopathologic analysis is classified as a micrometastasis. Current imaging methods are not able to accurately detect micrometastatic disease. However, as the tumor cells continue to grow within the lymph node, imaging can detect metastatic foci. With this larger tumor burden, the node enlarges, and eventually tumor growth obliterates the fatty hilum. Tumor cells can ultimately break through the cortex leading to extracapsular and extranodal extension and flow into the efferent nodal vessels, at which point they spread into adjacent lymph nodes.[6] With extension of tumor into the pericapsular fat, the contour of the node can become spiculated. This extension suggests a more biologically aggressive tumor, especially in women with three or fewer nodes involved.

TABLE 5.1. Five-Year Results Related to the Number of Pathologically Positive Lymph Nodes

No. of Positive Axillary Nodes	No. of Patients	Survival (%)	Recurrence (%)
0	12,299	72	19
1	2,012	63	33
2	1,338	62	40
3	842	59	43
4	615	52	44
5	478	47	54
6–10	1,261	41	63
11–15	562	29	72
16–20	301	29	75
≥21	225	22	82

Source: Data from Nemoto T, et al. Management and survival of female breast cancer: results of a national survey by the American College of Surgeons. *Cancer* 1980;45:2915–2924.

3. Imaging Methods

3.1. Surgical, Mammographic, and Sonographic Evaluation of Axillary Lymph Nodes

Until recently, imaging of lymph nodes has not played a significant role in staging breast cancer due to the inability to detect micrometastatic involvement. In the past, the gold standard for detecting metastatic involvement of axillary lymph nodes was axillary lymph node dissection, which was often associated with significant morbidity. Despite the ability of axillary dissection to help in locoregional control, it has not been shown to have any impact on the overall survival of the patient.[7]

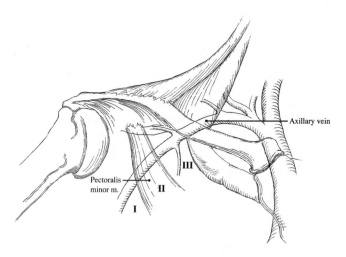

FIGURE 5.1. Anatomy of lymph nodes within the axilla: Level I nodes are located inferior and lateral to the pectoralis minor muscle (PMM), level II nodes are located deep to the PMM, and level III nodes are superior and medial to the PMM.

Increasingly, sentinel lymph node biopsy has become an alternative procedure to evaluate involvement of lymph nodes. Sentinel lymph node imaging uses radionuclide particles and/or a visual tracer to detect the first lymph node draining the tumor site.[8] If histopathologic analysis shows tumor involvement, then a full axillary dissection can be performed. This information is also valuable in determining the need for hormonal therapy or chemotherapy.

Although the assessment is often nonspecific, mammography and sonography can aid in the identification of pathologic lymph nodes. On mammography, abnormal lymph nodes can be identified when they are dense, rounded, or spiculated.[9] On sonography, abnormal lymph nodes lose their hypoechoic cortex and become more rounded, and the fatty echogenic hilum can be obliterated. When abnormal lymph nodes are identified on sonography, fine needle aspiration under sonographic guidance can be performed for definitive cytologic evaluation. This can be very useful as inflammatory, reactive, and metastatic adenopathy can have an identical mammographic and sonographic pattern. The usefulness of mammography has been limited to the evaluation of level I nodes. Level II and III nodes can be imaged sonographically, but the utility of this technique for screening of these nodal levels has very limited experience.

Other cross-sectional imaging modalities can be valuable in assessing the axilla. Computed tomography (CT) can image all levels, but its application is limited by its high radiation doses and thus it would be unusual to use CT for axillary screening. Positron emission tomography (PET) shows a high sensitivity in detecting axillary metastases. However, its specificity is lower. Published sensitivities have ranged from 80% to 95%, while specificities have been reported from 66% to 95%.[10,11]

4. Magnetic Resonance Imaging of Lymph Nodes

Contrast-enhanced magnetic resonance imaging (MRI) of the breast is becoming an integral part of evaluating extent of disease in patients with known breast carcinoma. Contrast-enhanced MRI can identify breast tumors due to their increased tumor vascularity and increased tumor capillary permeability. The same characteristics make it possible to image lymph nodes, which are also intensely vascular and thus can be well seen on contrast-enhanced MRIs. On standard MRI of the breasts, intramammary lymph nodes can be detected as some level I lymph nodes are included in the examination. However, the entire axilla is not fully included in these images as standard breast coils often do not adequately cover this area.

5. Identifying Metastatic Disease

On MRI, normal lymph nodes demonstrate characteristics identical to those seen on other imaging studies: well-circumscribed, reniform masses with a fatty hilum (Figure 5.2). Precontrast T1-weighted sequences without fat saturation can often demonstrate the fatty hilum. On T2-weighted sequences, lymph nodes have intermediate-to-high signal intensity. On postcontrast T1-weighted sequences, they show vivid homogenous enhancement or rim enhancement (Figure 5.3). Size is a nondiscriminating characteristic, as normal lymph nodes with large fatty hila can measure up to 5cm and lymph nodes containing metastatic disease are not necessarily enlarged (Figure 5.4).

Malignant lymph nodes have a more rounded contour as tumor cells grow and expand the lymph node. Eccentric enlargement of the lymph node with focal thickening of the cortex and obliteration of the fatty hilus can occur. They typically demonstrate heterogeneous enhancement (Figure 5.5). However, if tumor has totally replaced the node, diffuse enhancement can also be seen. Lymph nodes

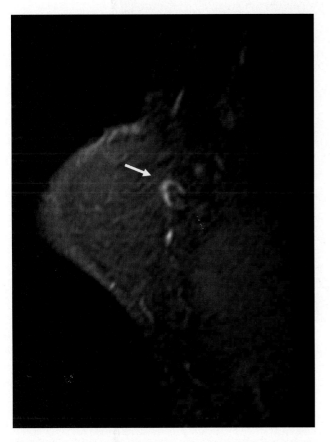

FIGURE 5.2. Sagittal fat-suppressed T1-weighted sequence that demonstrates a normal crescentic-shaped axillary lymph node with a fatty hilum (arrow).

containing metastatic disease are still usually smoothly marginated; however, there also can be gross spiculation and irregularity due to extranodal extension (Figure 5.6).

Malignancies other than breast cancer can spread to the axillary lymph nodes. Lymphomas and leukemias can often cause massive enlargement of lymph nodes. Other common malignancies include lung, melanoma, thyroid, ovarian, and gastrointestinal tumors. These have a similar appearance on MRI to metastatic breast cancer.

Studies have attempted to further distinguish benign from malignant lymph nodes on MRI. Mumtaz et al.[12] classified nodes as abnormal when they enhanced with gadolinium, their size was greater than 5mm, and their signal intensity was higher than soft tissue on short inversion time recovery images. With these criteria, they produced a sensitivity of 90% and specificity of 82%. Kvistad et al.[13] used dynamic enhancement features to distinguish between normal and abnormal lymph nodes. They characterized lymph nodes as being pathologic when their signal intensity increases >100% during the first postcontrast image. With this threshold, they obtained a sensitivity of 83% and specificity of 90%, with an accuracy of 88%. In another study Murray et al.[14] examined lymph node enhancement using a region of interest method and calculated the nodal area. With an enhancement index of >21% and a nodal area of >0.4cm^2, they achieved a sensitivity of 100%, a specificity of 56%, a positive predictive value of 38%, and a negative predictive value of 100%.

Unfortunately, other causes of nodal enlargement can present with patterns identical to that seen with malignant adenopathy. Inflammatory conditions such as rheumatoid arthritis, systemic lupus erythematosus, psoriatic arthritis, and sarcoidosis can cause axillary adenopathy and be indistinguishable from that found with metastatic disease. Gallardo et al.[15] demonstrated that nonmalignant lymph nodes can also rapidly enhance. Biopsy was needed to differentiate hyperplasia from malignant disease in this study.

5.1. Internal Mammary Lymph Nodes

Only a small percentage of cancers drain into the internal mammary lymph nodes. Due to their infrequent involvement, they are not routinely staged. In addition, studies have shown that dissection or irradiation of internal mammary nodes does not improve overall survival.[16] It is, however, an independent additional indicator for a worse prognosis, and therefore when suspected, sampling may be performed on select patients. On MRI, internal mammary lymph node metastasis can be identified along the internal mammary artery and vein in the intercostal space. A relatively recent study has shown that when they measure 5mm in diameter or more, metastatic involvement should be suspected.[17]

J.Y.M. Lee and D.D. Dershaw

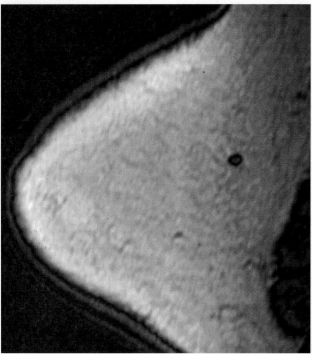

FIGURE 5.3. The appearance of normal lymph nodes on various sequences. (A) Sagittal non–fat-suppressed T1-weighted sequence: intermediate-to-high signal intensity consistent with a fatty hilum. (B) Sagittal fat-suppressed T2-weighted sequence: lymph node has intermediate-to-high signal intensity. (C) Sagittal fat-suppressed postcontrast T1-weighted sequence: homogeneous enhancement of the lymph node.

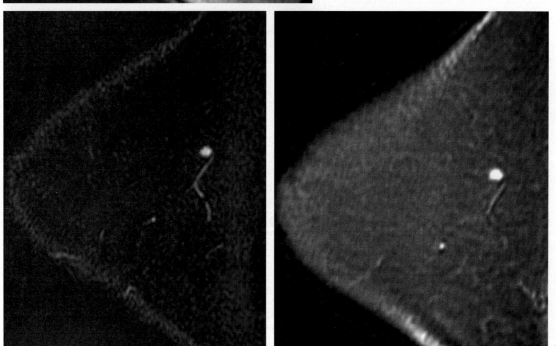

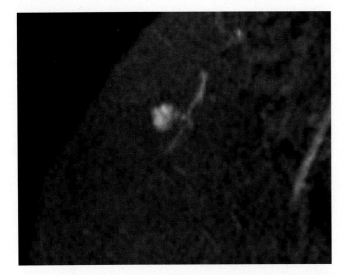

FIGURE 5.4. Metastatic breast carcinoma to an intramammary lymph node. Sagittal fat-suppressed postcontrast T1-weighted sequence shows a small intramammary lymph node with loss of the fatty hilum and irregular margins in this patient with known ipsilateral breast carcinoma.

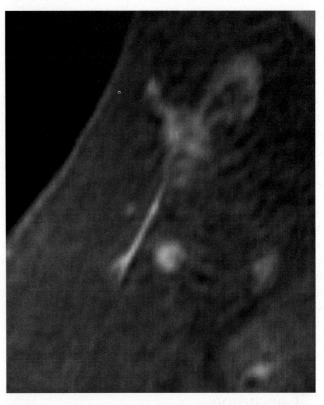

FIGURE 5.6. Metastatic breast carcinoma with spiculated axillary adenopathy. Sagittal fat-suppressed postcontrast T1-weighted sequences show spiculated heterogenously enhancing nodes within the axilla from a patient with known ipsilateral infiltrating ductal carcinoma.

FIGURE 5.5. Example of metastatic breast carcinoma to axillary lymph nodes. (A) Sagittal fat-suppressed postcontrast T1-weighted sequences shows a large irregular enhancing mass (arrow) with a heterogeneously enhancing enlarged axillary lymph nodes (double arrows). (B) Sagittal fat-suppressed postcontrast T1-weighted sequence shows multiple irregular heterogeneously enhancing masses.

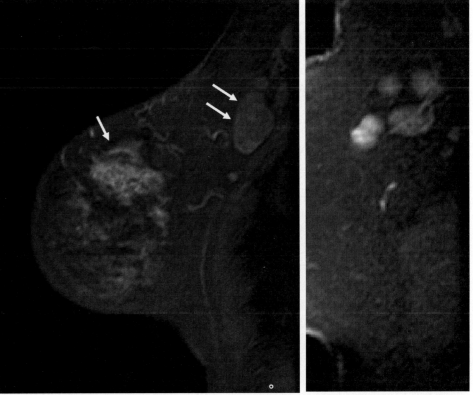

A

B

6. New Contrast Agents

Our current ability to detect small foci of metastasis to lymph nodes is somewhat limited. Recently, dextran-coated ultrasmall superparamagnetic iron oxide (USPIO) particles have been investigated as an alternative contrast agent to evaluate the lymphatic system. These are small iron oxide particles that are intravenously injected and are taken up by normal functioning lymph nodes and inflamed nodes. The macrophages of normal lymph nodes can phagocytose these particles while the lymph nodes with tumor cells are not able to incorporate them. Due to the ferromagnetic properties of iron oxide, normal lymph nodes show a signal intensity decrease on T2*- and T2-weighted sequences because of the effect of magnetic susceptibility. This makes it possible to differentiate benign from malignant lymph nodes. Michel et al.[18] used this agent to attempt to predict the status of axillary lymph nodes with promising results, obtaining a sensitivity of 82% and specificity of 100%. Further large-scale studies with this new contrast agent will ultimately determine its role in preoperative axillary imaging.

7. Conclusion

At present, the preferred method for detecting metastatic disease to the axilla is surgical, using identification and biopsy of the sentinel node. Contrast-enhanced MRI currently does not detect metastatic disease with enough sensitivity and specificity to obviate sentinel node biopsy. Whether MRI will have a role in the detection of metastatic disease to the axilla in the future is uncertain. The need to be able to detect micrometastatic disease by an imaging modality will challenge those who are currently involved in investigation of new contrast agents.

References

1. Valagussa P, Bonadonna G, Veronesi V. Patterns of relapse and survival following radial mastectomy. *Cancer* 1978;41: 1170–1178.
2. Fisher B, Slack NH, Katrych D, et al. Ten-year followup results of patients with carcinoma of the breast in a cooperative clinical trial evaluating surgical adjuvant chemotherapy. *Surg Gynecol Obstet.* 1975;140:528–534.
3. Ferguson DJ, Meier P, Karrison T, et al. Staging of breast cancer and survival rates: an assessment based on 50 years of experience with radial mastectomy. *JAMA.* 1982;248: 1337–1341.
4. Veronesi U, Rilke F, Luini A, et al. Distribution of axillary node metastases by level of invasion: an analysis of 539 cases. *Cancer* 1987;59:682–687.
5. Rosen PP, Martin LL, Kinne DW, et al. Discontinuous or "skip" metastases in breast carcinoma: analysis of 1228 axillary dissections. *Ann Surg.* 1983;197:276–283.
6. Hartveit F, Maehle BO, Halvorsen JF, Tangen M. On the progressive nature of tumour growth in axillary nodes in breast cancer. *Oncology* 1983;40:309–314.
7. Fisher B, Redmond C, Fisher ER, et al. Ten-year results of randomized trial comparing radical mastecomy and total mastecomy with or without radiation. *N Engl J Med.* 1985; 312:674–681.
8. Giulano AE, Kirgan DM, Guenther JM, Morton DL. Lymphatic mapping and sentinel lymphadenectomy for breast cancer. *Ann Surg.* 1994;220:391–401.
9. Dershaw DD, Selland DG, Tan LK, et al. Spiculated axillary adenopathy. *Radiology* 1996;201:439–442.
10. Adler LP, Faulhaber PF, Schnur KC, et al. Axillary lymph node metastases: screening with (F-18)2-deoxy-2-fluoro-D-Glucose (FDG) PET. *Radiology* 1997;203:323–327.
11. Rieber A, Schirrmeister H, Gabelmann A, et al. Preoperative staging of invasive breast cancer with MR mammography and/or PET: boon or bunk? *Br J Radiol.* 2002;75:789–798.
12. Mumtaz H, Hall-Craggs MA, Davidson D, et al. Staging of symptomatic primary breast cancer with MR imaging. *AJR Am J Roentgenol.* 1997;169:417–424.
13. Kvistad KA, Rydland J, Smethurst B, et al. Axillary lymph node metastases in breast cancer: preoperative detection with dynamic contrast-enhanced MRI. *Eur Radiol.* 2000;10: 1464–1471.
14. Murray AD, Staff RT, Redpath TW, et al. Dynamic contrasted enhanced MRI of the axilla in women with breast cancer: comparison with pathology of excised nodes. *Br J Radiol.* 2002;75:220–228.
15. Gallardo X, Sensits M, Castaner E, et al. Enhancement of intramammary lymph nodes with lymphoid hyperplasia: a potential pitfall in breast MRI. *Eur Radiol.* 1998;8: 1662–1665.
16. Veronesi U, Marubini E, Mariani L, et al. The dissection of internal mammary nodes does not improve the survival of breast cancer patients. 30-year results of a randomized trial. *Eur J Cancer.* 1999;35:1320–1325.
17. Kinoshita T, Odagiri, K, Kazuo A, et al. Evaluation of small internal mammary lymph node metastases in breast cancer by MRI. *Radiat Med.* 1999;17:189–193.
18. Michel SC, Keller TM, Frohlich JM, et al. Preoperative breast cancer staging: MR imaging of the axilla with ultrasmall superparamagnetic iron oxide enhancement. *Radiology* 2002;225:527–536.

6
Breast Magnetic Resonance Imaging Lexicon

Elizabeth A. Morris

As contrast enhanced breast magnetic resonance imaging (MRI) becomes more ubiquitous, standardization of terminology has become necessary. To this end, the American College of Radiology (ACR) has sponsored the development of a lexicon that is finalized and is now available. This chapter attempts to illustrate some of the terms that are used in this lexicon. It should be emphasized that this chapter does not replace the ACR BI-RADS™ (Breast Imaging Reporting and Data System) MRI Lexicon. The purpose of this chapter is to familiarize the reader with concepts and terminology in breast MRI interpretation that may be useful.[1-4]

The need for a lexicon becomes apparent when interpreting contrast-enhanced breast MRI as there are many different types of enhancement seen. Because enhancement alone is not sufficient for the diagnosis of malignancy, a method to describe findings is essential. Additionally, each lesion contains information about morphological characteristics as well as information about the dynamics of the contrast enhancement. By analyzing both the morphology and kinetic behavior of a lesion, the specificity of breast MRI is improved. A preliminary lexicon describing both architectural features and dynamic parameters is presented. This chapter focuses on the morphology of both benign and malignant breast lesions seen on breast MRI.

1. Standardization of Terminology

During the past decade, as multimodality breast imaging, including MRI, has become incorporated into the clinical evaluation of the breast, it has become apparent that standardization of terminology is important, particularly across modalities. As with mammography, concise, clear, easily understood language is needed when describing a lesion

seen on breast MRI, so that the description can be understood without the benefit of looking at the actual image. The need for a standardized lexicon for analysis of findings identified on breast MRI is twofold: to concisely describe the findings to facilitate communication between radiologists and referring physicians and to allow analysis of outcomes across institutions to validat management recommendations.

Over the past several years, an international working group consisting of breast MRI experts from around the world has been supported by the ACR to arrive at a consensus lexicon that would describe the findings that are seen on breast MRI.[1-3] One of the goals of the group was to arrive at a consensus regarding architectural and kinetic features that are seen on contrast-enhanced breast MRI. Terms that were proposed by the group are listed in Table 6.1.

The group has expressly tried to incorporate familiar language such as that used in BI-RADS for mammography.[5] When a BI-RADS descriptor could be used, it was applied and new descriptors were developed for findings unique to MRI. By virtue that breast MRI uses contrast and mammography does not, terms to describe the kinetic uptake of contrast by the lesion are unique to breast MRI. Similarly, aspects of morphologic analysis, such as pattern of enhancement, are unique to the breast magnetic resonance examination. The shape and margin analysis is similar to BI-RADS™.

Lesion interpretation in breast MRI relies entirely on lesion enhancement. When analyzing a breast MRI examination, the first step is to establish that the patient received an adequate dose of intravenous contrast. While there are several sophisticated methods that can assess the presence of contrast, the simplest form of confirmation that contrast was received is that vessels in the breast are identified as enhancing structures and contrast is seen in the heart.

Solely identifying an enhancing area on breast MRI as suspicious will not optimize the specificity of breast MRI

Adapted from Morris EA. Illustrated breast MR lexicon. *Semin Roentgenol.* 2001;36:238–249, with permission from Elsevier.

TABLE 6.1. Breast MRI Terms Proposed by the International Working Group of the American College of Radiology

Focus/foci	NonMass enhancement	Other findings
Mass margin	Focal	Nipple retraction
Smooth	Linear	Nipple invasion
Irregular	Ductal	Precontrast high duct signal
Spiculated	Segmental	Focal skin thickening
Mass shape	Regional	Diffuse skin thickening
Round	Multiple regions	Skin invasion
Oval	Diffuse	Edema
Lobular	NonMass enhancement descriptors for all	Lymphadenopathy
Irregular	other types	Pectoralis muscle invasion
Mass enhancement	Homogeneous	Chest wall invasion
Homogeneous	Heterogeneous	Hematoma/blood
Heterogeneous	Stippled/punctate	Abnormal signal void
Rim	Clumped	Cysts
Dark internal septation	Reticular/dendritic	
Enhancing internal septations	Symmetric versus asymmetric for bilateral	
Central enhancement	studies	

and will result in too many false-positive biopsy results. For the best analysis, all features of the lesion should be analyzed, including kinetics as well as morphology of enhancement. By combining kinetic and morphologic information with clinical history and conventional imaging (mammography and ultrasound) findings, a recommendation for biopsy can be made with more assurance.

Because malignant lesions can masquerade as benign and vice versa, there can be overlap in the imaging characteristics of benign and malignant lesions. Because there is overlap, the most definitive method of differentiation between benign and malignant is biopsy, which should be performed for any suspicious finding. This chapter addresses the features that will help the reader determine what is suspicious as well as features of a few classic benign entities on MRI.

2. Technique

There is no gold standard technique for performing breast MRI. Many techniques are available and widely used depending on hardware and software capabilities and personal preferences. T1-weighted sequences obtained before and after gadolinium-DTPA administration are favored. High-resolution techniques optimize lesion morphologic analysis and rapid acquisition is used for assessing enhancement profiles. T2-weighted sequences are useful for identifying breast cysts that can be simple or hemorrhagic, in addition to myxoid fibroadenomas and lymph nodes that can be high in signal intensity. In general, invasive breast carcinomas are not very high in signal intensity on T2 except for mucinous carcinoma or necrotic tumors.[6] Intermediate signal carcinomas can sometimes be

TABLE 6.2. Information Pertinent to Interpretation of the Breast MRI Examination

Patient history	Comparison with prior examinations	3D
Risk	Mammogram	Fat saturation or subtraction
Family history	Ultrasound	Number of postcontrast scans
Personal history	Prior MRI	Time interval between postcontrast
History of prior biopsy (benign or	MRI technique	scans
malignant)	Location of markers and significance	Scan length
Clinical	Field strength	Matrix resolution
Palpable lump/thickening	Contrast media used and dose	Postprocessing techniques
Nipple discharge	Scan plane—sagittal/axial/coronal	Multiplanar reconstruction (MPR)
Known cancer	Slice thickness	Maximum intensity projection (MIP)
Hormonal status	Pulse sequence	Time intensity curves
Menstrual cycle (if pertinent)	Gradient echo	Subtraction
Exogenous hormone replacement	Spin-echo	
therapy	2D	
Recent pregnancy		
Tamoxifen		

Abbreviations: 2D, two-dimensional; 3D, three-dimensional.

seen. Table 6.2 describes information regarding technique that is pertinent to the report.

In addition to providing descriptions of the morphologic and kinetic findings, the MRI report should have a final recommendation to convey the level of suspicion to the referring physician. If a recommendation for biopsy is made, it should be clearly reported in the final impression and a final assessment category should be specified, as in mammography.

3. Breast Histopathology and Magnetic Resonance Imaging

Breast disease pathology is superbly seen and delineated by using breast MRI. To allow identification and characterization of small lesions, slice thickness should be approximately 2mm so that volume averaging is not an issue. Because breast cancer can grow along a duct system extending from the terminal duct lobular unit either into the breast as an invasive mass or extending along the duct system in a segmental fashion to the nipple, breast MRI is exquisitely poised to depict the spread of disease, as long as there is increased vascularity associated with the disease. Three-dimensional maximum intensity projection (MIP) reconstructions can nicely demonstrate such uctal enhancement patterns (Figure 6.1).

Compared with mammography breast MRI is superior at delineating disease extent. Mammography may demonstrate a mass that proves to be an invasive carcinoma that may only be a small component of the total tumor load. Breast MRI not only shows us the invasive component but may also demonstrate the surrounding uncalcified segmental ductal carcinoma in situ (DCIS) from which the invasive carcinoma grew. Multifocal disease is often represented as a segmental area of enhancement representing DCIS in association with several heterogeneously enhancing masses representing the sites where the basement membrane has been crossed and the tumor has invaded the breast.

A basic understanding of cancer growth and spread in the breast aids in the analysis of the morphologic features seen with breast MRI. Similarly, knowledge of the histopathology of benign lesions, such as the different types of fibroadenomas, can aid in the interpretation of benign findings. For example, a slowly enhancing mass may represent a sclerotic hyalinized fibroadenoma, whereas a rapidly enhancing mass may represent a myxoid fibroadenoma. Fibroadenomas may also contain fibrous nonenhancing bands: If these are identified with certainty and all other features appear benign, a benign diagnosis can be made comfortably.

4. Morphologic Features

Morphologic analysis is best performed with high spatial resolution techniques that allow evaluation of the mass shape and border so that suspicious spiculated or irregular masses can be differentiated from smooth benign-appearing masses. Also, with high spatial resolution, the borders and internal architecture of the lesion can be assessed and the pattern of enhancement can be readily characterized.

5. Description of Terms

5.1. Focus/Mass

A focus is a single tiny punctate enhancement that is nonspecific and too small to be characterized. A focus is clearly not a space-occupying lesion or mass (Figure 6.2). An enhancing lesion on MRI can be described as a mass if it displaces tissue and has space-occupying properties. If there are multiple foci in a breast, the term *stippled* can be applied (Figure 6.3).

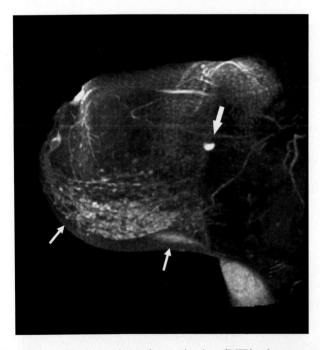

FIGURE 6.1. Maximum intensity projection (MIP) of segmental ductal enhancement in the inferior breast compatible with extensive ductal carcinoma in situ (arrows). All images in the illustrations of the lexicon are performed postcontrast with fat suppression sagittal T1-weighted technique unless otherwise indicated. Note intramammary lymph node (thick arrow).

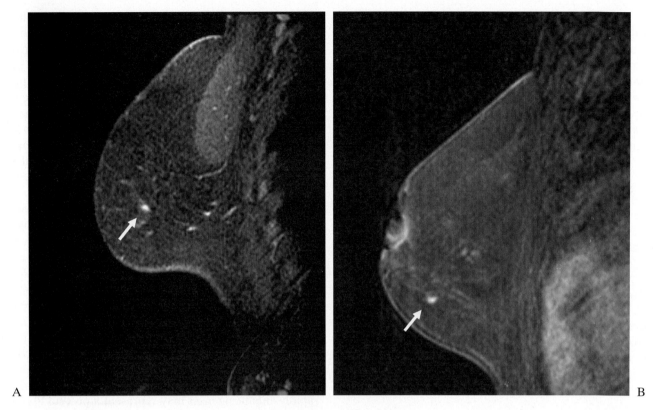

Figure 6.2. (A and B) Foci (arrows).

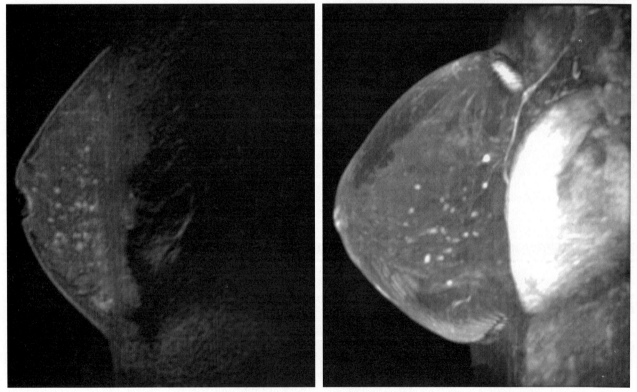

Figure 6.3. (A and B) Stippled enhancement.

5.2. Shape/Margin

The shape and margins of masses can be described. Mass shape can be described as round, oval, lobular, or irregular (Figure 6.4). Margins of masses are smooth, irregular, or spiculated. Spiculated and irregular masses (Figure 6.5) are suspicious for carcinoma, whereas a smooth margin is more suggestive of a benign lesion (Figure 6.6). Margin analysis is dependent on spatial resolution and irregular borders can appear relatively smooth when insufficient resolution is used. Therefore, carcinomas may present with benign imaging features on MRI, particularly when small (Figure 6.7). It should be emphasized that the resolution of MRI is generally not as high as the resolution of mammography and that border definition is not as absolute. Therefore, malignant masses may be more prone to demonstrate benign features on MRI.[7,8]

In general, margin and shape analysis should be performed on the first postcontrast image to avoid

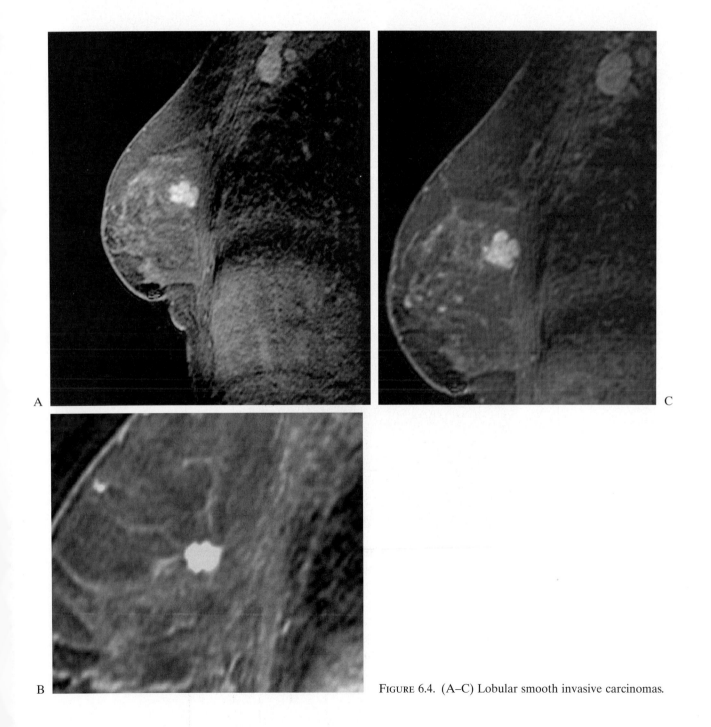

FIGURE 6.4. (A–C) Lobular smooth invasive carcinomas.

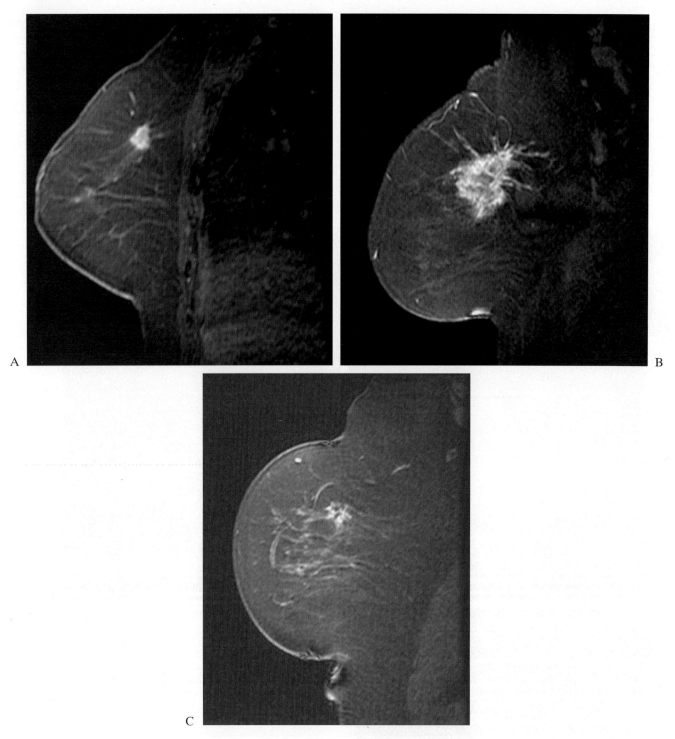

FIGURE 6.5. (A–C) Irregular spiculated invasive carcinomas.

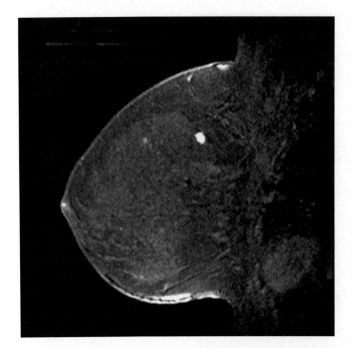

FIGURE 6.6. Oval smooth lymph node.

FIGURE 6.7. Small round smooth carcinoma.

washout and progressive enhancement of the surrounding breast tissue, which can obscure lesion analysis. Additionally, as time elapses after contrast enhancement, the periphery of the lesion may become more indistinct.[9]

5.3. Internal Enhancement

Internal enhancement of masses can be described as homogeneous or heterogeneous. Homogeneous enhancement is confluent and uniform (Figure 6.8). Heterogeneous

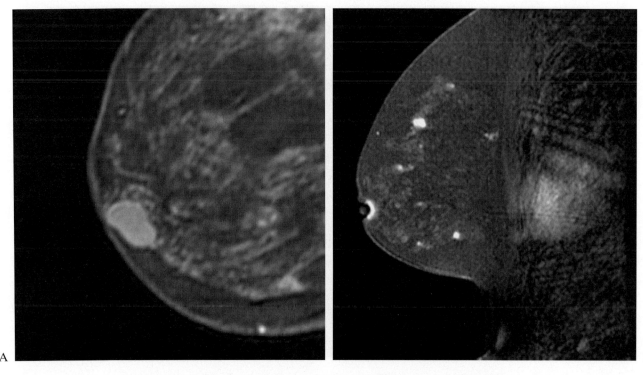

A

B

FIGURE 6.8. Homogeneous enhancement. (A) Fibroadenoma. (B) DCIS.

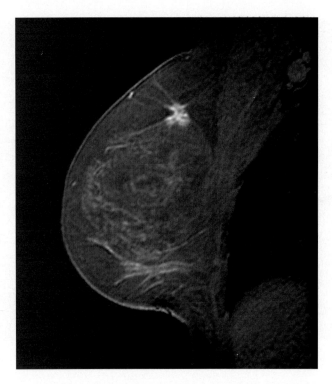

FIGURE 6.9. Heterogeneous enhancement in invasive carcinoma.

enhancement is non-uniform with areas of variable signal intensity (Figure 6.9). Masses may display rim enhancement, a particularly suspicious finding for malignancy (Figure 6.10). Other suspicious findings include enhancing septations (Figure 6.11) or central enhancement (Figure 6.12), though these signs occur less commonly. Homogeneous enhancement is suggestive of a benign process; however, again, in small lesions, one must be careful as

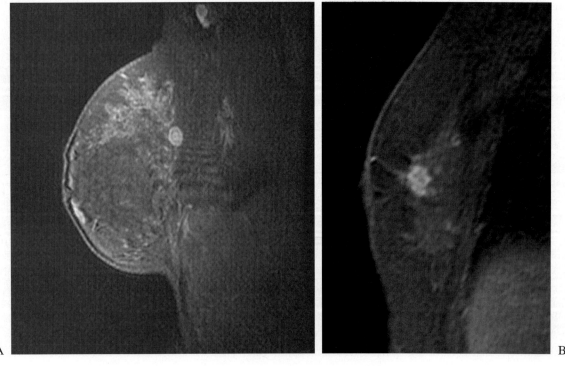

FIGURE 6.10. (A and B) Rim enhancement. Invasive ductal carcinomas.

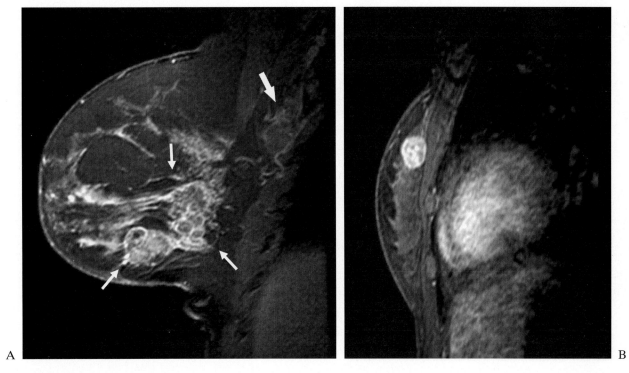

FIGURE 6.11. Enhancing internal septations. (A) Invasive ductal carcinoma (small arrows) and metastatic disease to the axilla (large arrow). (B) Invasive ductal carcinoma.

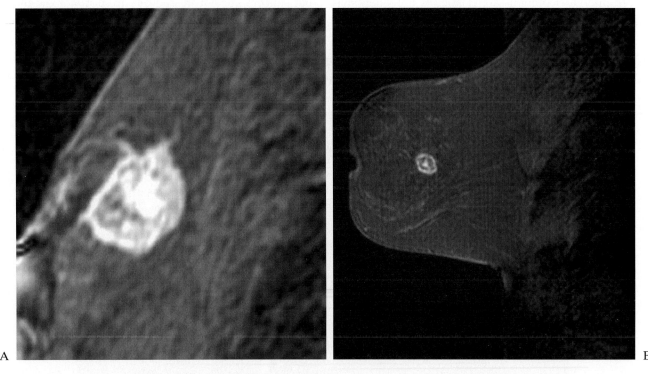

FIGURE 6.12. (A and B) Central enhancement. Invasive ductal carcinomas.

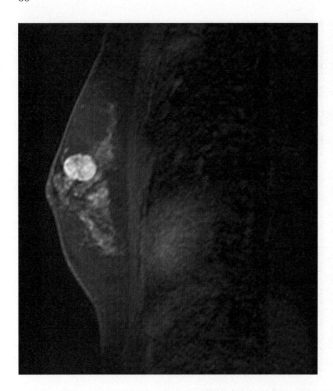

FIGURE 6.13. Dark nonenhancing septations in fibroadenoma.

spatial resolution may limit evaluation. Heterogeneous enhancement is more characteristic of malignant lesions especially if rim enhancement is present.

Dark internal septations are classic for fibroadenomas (Figure 6.13) though are seen in the minority of cases (Figure 6.14). When present, masses can be considered benign with a high degree of certainty (>95% according to Nunes).[10–12] Careful analysis of the lesion is important so that cancers are not missed due to morphologic overlap (Figure 6.15). Similarly, nonenhancing masses are also

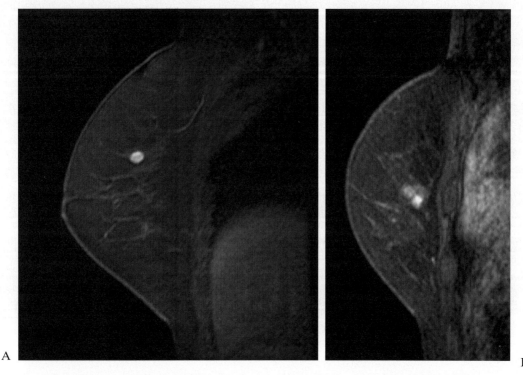

FIGURE 6.14. (A) Smooth mass and fibroadenomas appearing as (B) irregular mass.

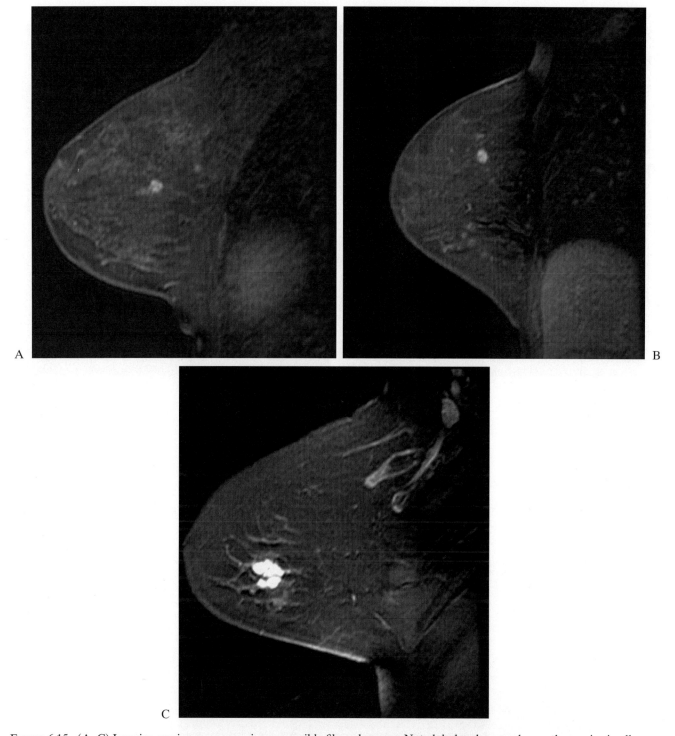

FIGURE 6.15. (A–C) Invasive carcinomas appearing as possible fibroadenomas. Note lobular shape and smooth margins in all cases.

likely benign fibroadenomas that have a high hyaline content (Figure 6.16). Other benign lesions include an inflammatory cyst that enhances peripherally (Figure 6.17) and benign fat necrosis (Figure 6.18) that can exhibit rim enhancement with central low signal indicating fatty content. These latter two lesions should be recognized as potential pitfalls in interpretation of *rim*-enhancing

lesions. The cyst can generally be identified on a T2-weighted image and fat necrosis can often be recognized based on the patient's history and mammographic findings. It may be helpful to include a non–fat-suppressed sequence to assess the central fat content in cases of fat necrosis.

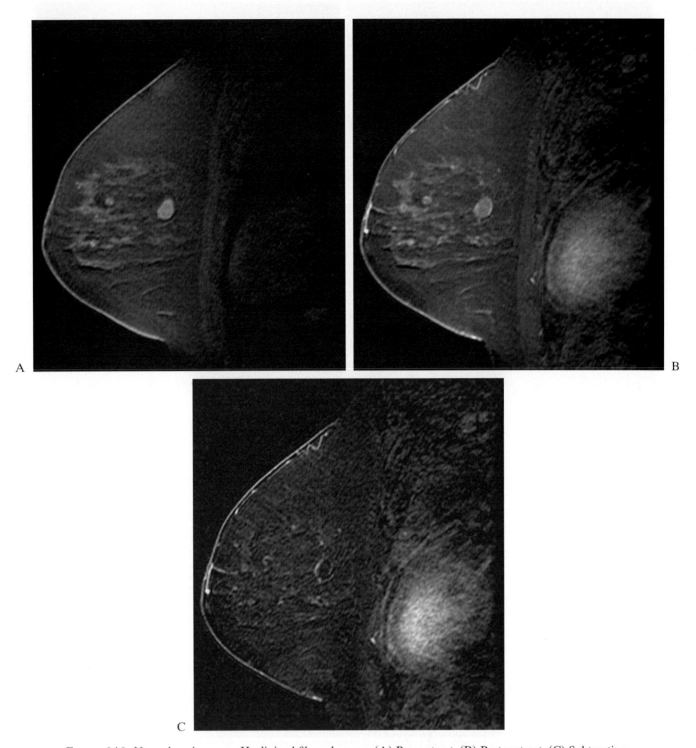

FIGURE 6.16. Nonenhancing mass. Hyalinized fibroadenoma. (A) Precontrast. (B) Postcontrast. (C) Subtraction.

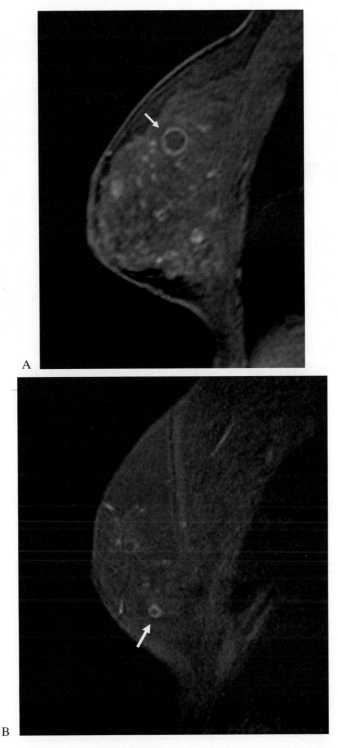

FIGURE 6.17. (A and B) Inflammatory cysts (arrows) in two patients.

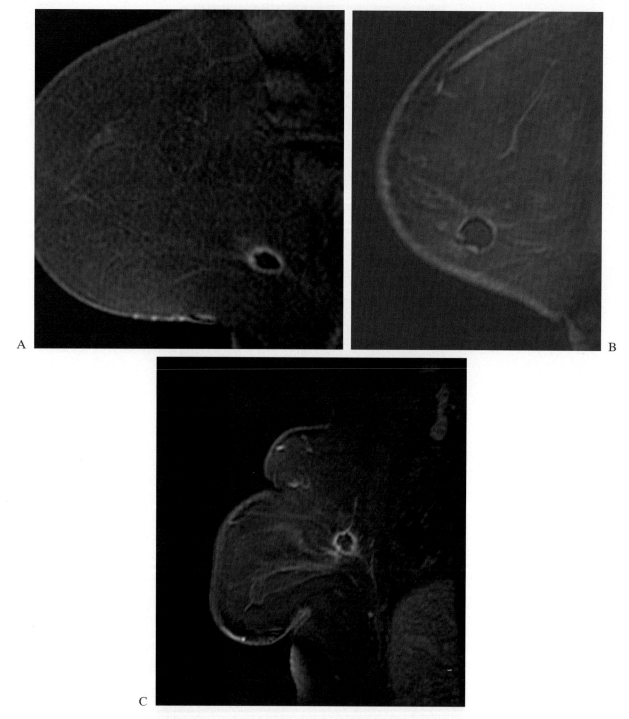

FIGURE 6.18. (A–C) Fat necrosis following surgery.

5.4. Nonmass Enhancement

If the enhancement is neither a focus nor mass, then it is classified as nonmass-like enhancement. Nonmass enhancement is classified according to the distribution of the enhancement and can be described as linear-ductal, linear-nonspecific, regional, segmental, or diffuse. Linear enhancement most often is related to the ductal system (Figure 6.19) although can be seen with nonductal pathology (Figure 6.20). Ductal enhancement corresponds to one or more ducts in orientation and is suspicious for DCIS (Figure 6.21). Ductal-nonspecific would not follow this pattern and is less suspicious for malignancy (Figure 6.22). Segmental refers to enhancement that is triangular in

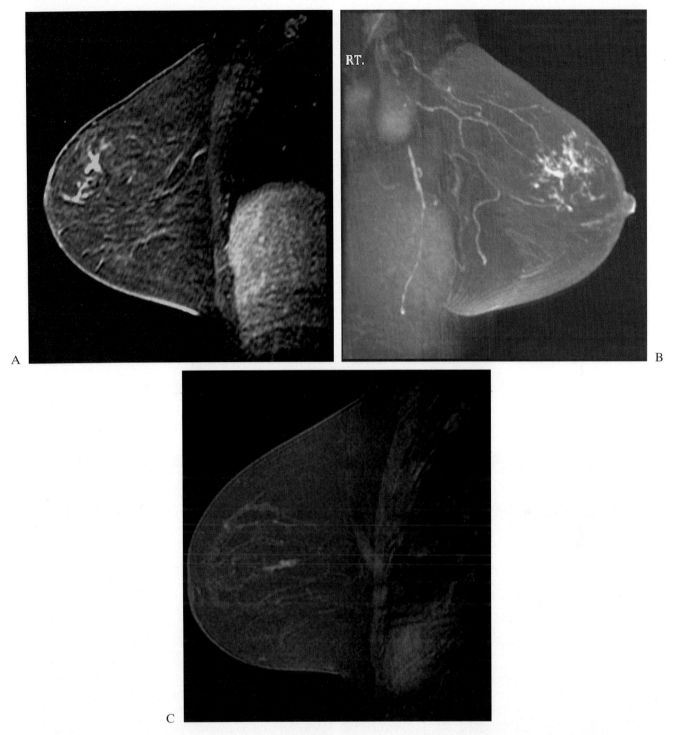

FIGURE 6.19. Ductal enhancement in DCIS. (A) Segmental ductal branching. (B) Maximum intensity projection image of segmental ductal enhancement. (C) Linear irregular enhancement.

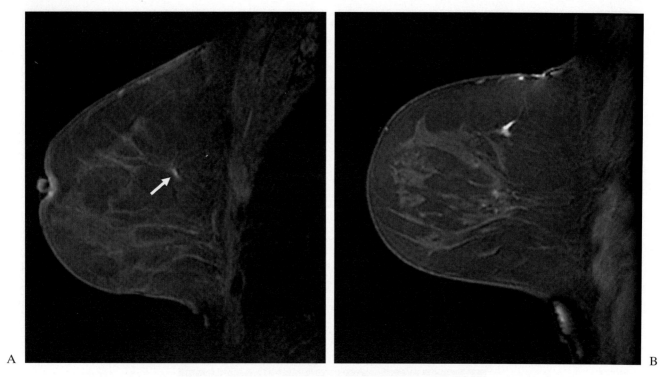

FIGURE 6.20. (A and B) Linear enhancement in scars (arrow) following surgery in two patients.

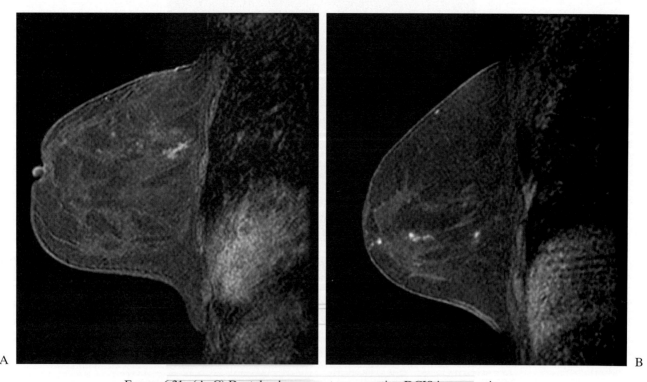

FIGURE 6.21. (A–C) Ductal enhancement representing DCIS in two patients.

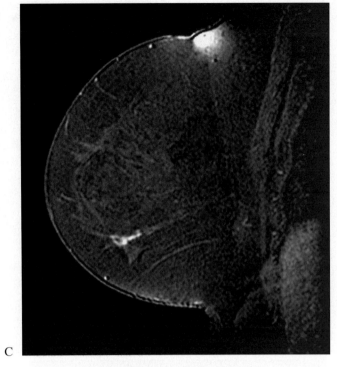

C

FIGURE 6.21. (*Continued*)

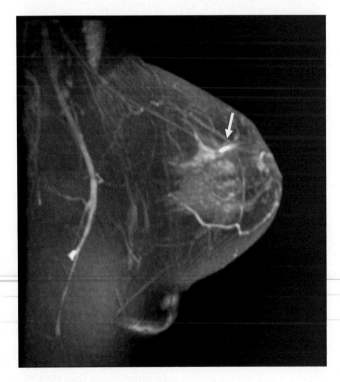

FIGURE 6.22. MIP demonstrating linear enhancement in scar (arrow).

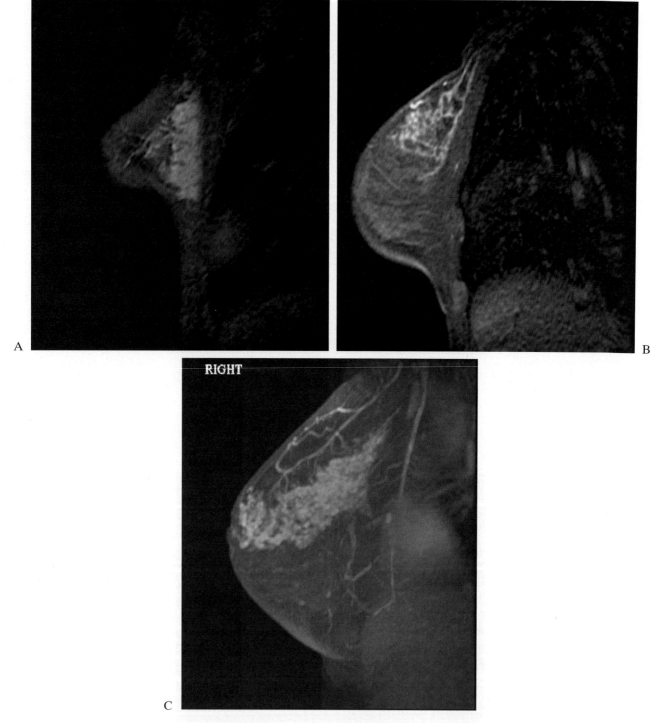

FIGURE 6.23. (A–C) Segmental enhancement representing DCIS in three patients. (C) Maximum intensity projection.

shape with the apex at the nipple and is suspicious for DCIS within a single branching duct system (Figure 6.23). Regional enhancement is enhancement that does not correspond to a single duct system, however, may be within multiple ducts (Figure 6.24).

Linear enhancement can be further described as smooth, irregular, or clumped. As with smooth masses, smooth linear enhancement is suggestive of a benign process. Irregular enhancement refers to any nonsmooth enhancement and may be continuous or discontinuous (Figure 6.25). Clumped enhancement refers to an aggregate of enhancing masses or foci that may be confluent in a cobblestone pattern (Figure 6.26). Linear enhancement is suggestive of DCIS, especially if clumped or irregular (Figure 6.27).

FIGURE 6.24. MIP demonstrating regional enhancement in DCIS.

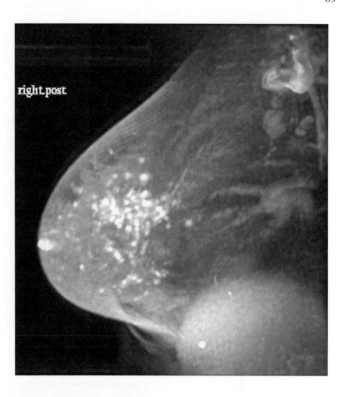

Segmental, regional, or diffuse enhancement can be further described as homogeneous, heterogeneous-stippled/punctate, clumped, septal/dendritic, or non specific. Stippled refers to multiple, often innumerable punctate foci that are approximately 1 to 2mm in size and appear scattered throughout an area of the breast that does not conform usually to a duct system (Figure 6.28). Stippled enhancement is more characteristic of benign normal

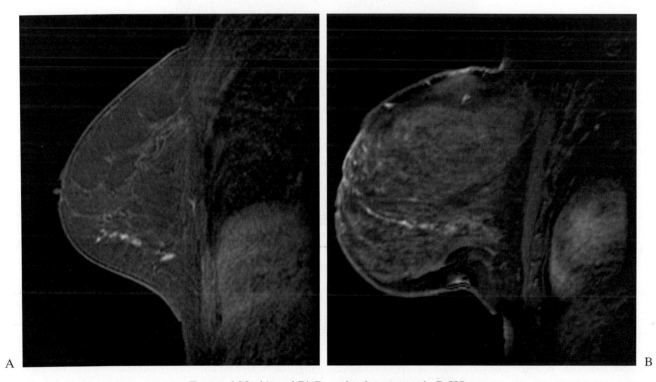

FIGURE 6.25. (A and B) Ductal enhancement in DCIS.

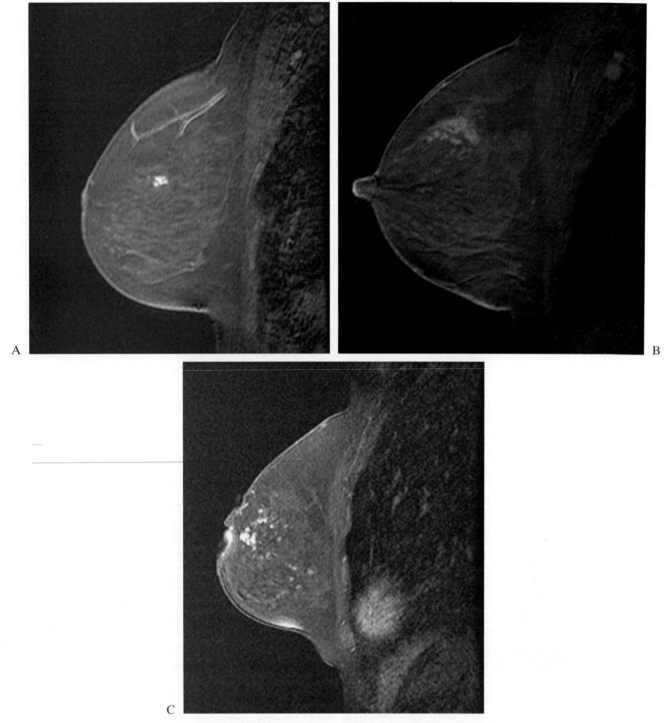

FIGURE 6.26. (A–C) Clumped enhancement in three patients representing DCIS.

variant parenchymal enhancement or fibrocystic changes. Regional enhancement and diffuse enhancement are more characteristic of benign disease such as proliferative changes, although multicentric DCIS may have this appearance (Figure 6.29). Other findings that may be present are listed in Table 6.1 and are demonstrated (Figures 6.30–6.41).

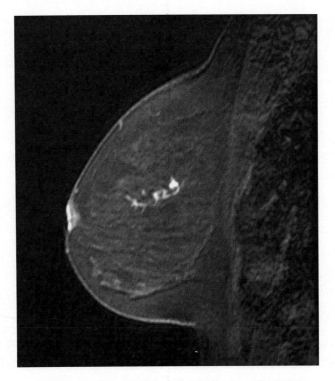

FIGURE 6.27. Linear clumped enhancement in DCIS.

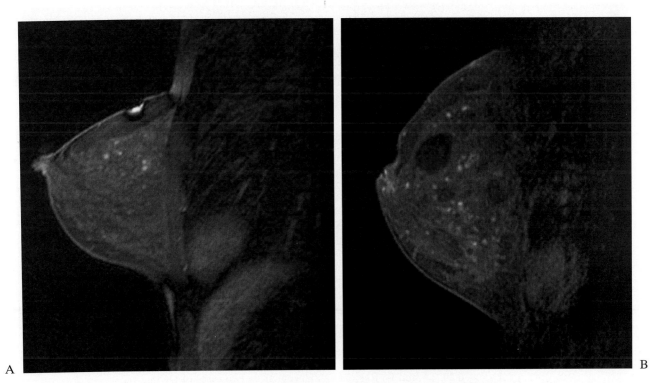

A   B

FIGURE 6.28. (A–D) Examples of stippled enhancement.

(Continued)

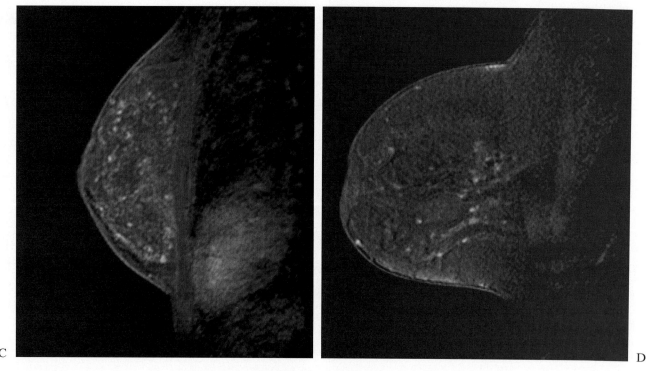

C   D

FIGURE 6.28. (*Continued*)

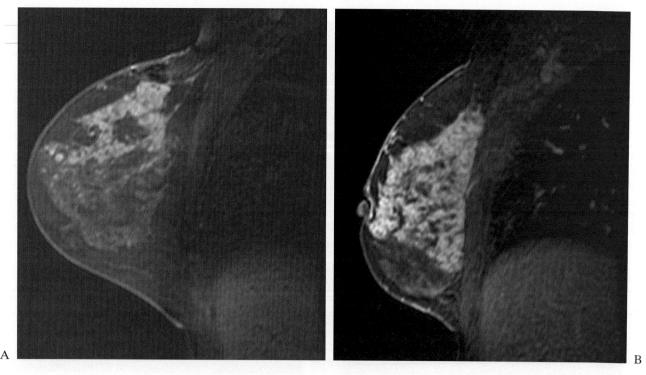

A   B

FIGURE 6.29. (A and B) Regional enhancement in two cases of DCIS.

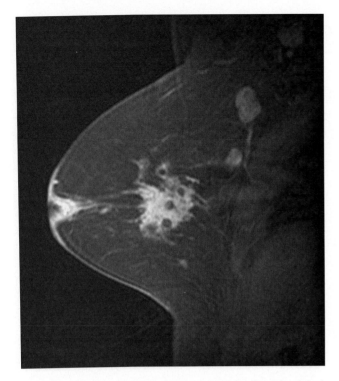

FIGURE 6.30. Nipple retraction due to underlying invasive lobular carcinoma. Note axillary adenopathy.

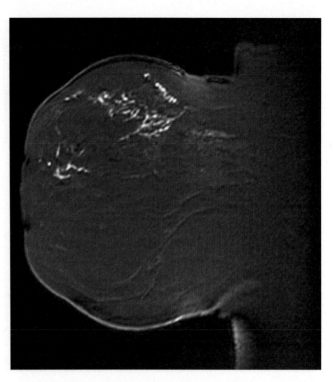

FIGURE 6.32. Duct ectasia. High signal in mildly dilated ducts in a segmental distribution on precontrast images.

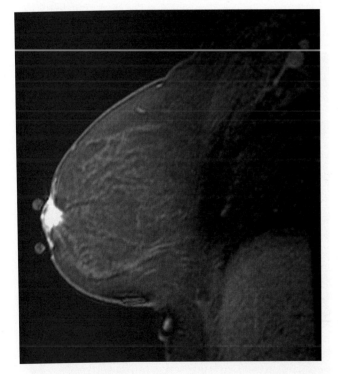

FIGURE 6.31. Nipple invasion. Subareolar invasive ductal carcinoma.

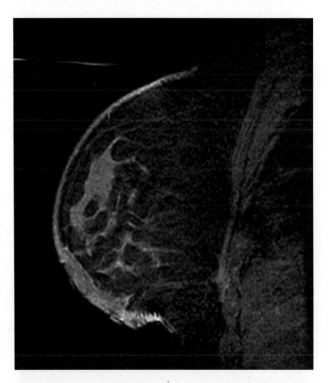

FIGURE 6.33. Focal skin thickening. Status postsurgery and radiation therapy. Note absence of enhancement in skin.

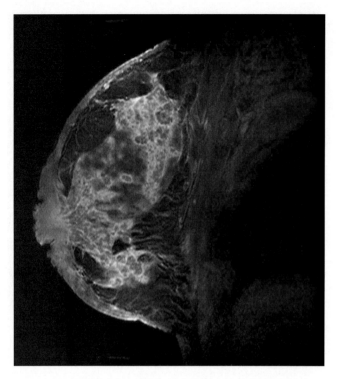

FIGURE 6.34. <u>Diffuse skin thickening with enhancement. Inflam-</u>
<u>matory breast carcinoma.</u> Note reticular dendritic pattern of
enhancement in the breast.

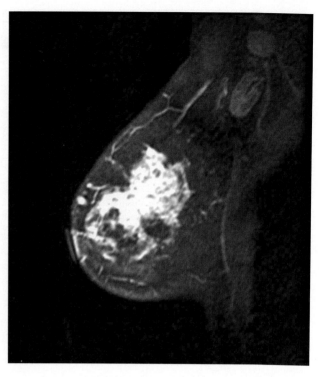

FIGURE 6.36. Locally advanced breast carcinoma with axillary
adenopathy.

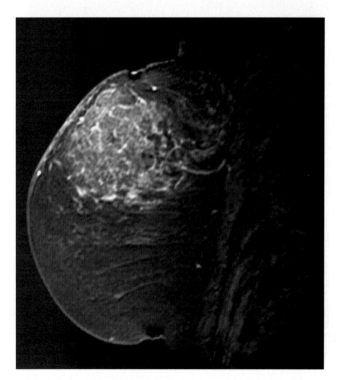

FIGURE 6.35. Focal skin invasion. <u>Underlying inflammatory</u>
<u>carcinoma involving upper breast.</u>

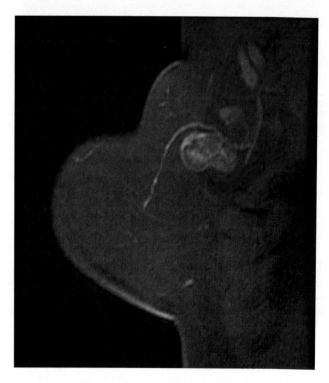

FIGURE 6.37. Axillary adenopathy.

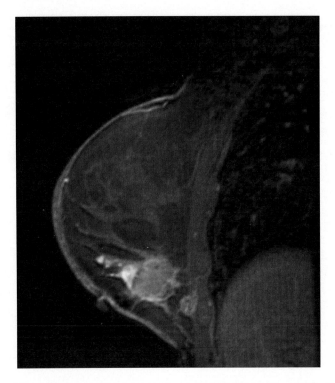

FIGURE 6.38. Chest wall invasion. Note dominant carcinoma in lower breast. Posterior satellite lesion invades intercostal muscle.

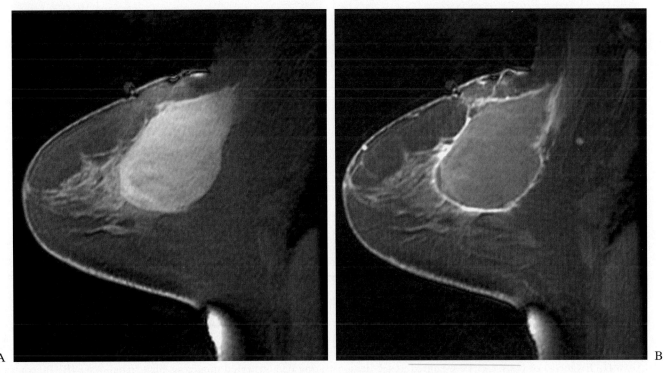

FIGURE 6.39. Hematoma. (A) Precontrast image demonstrates high signal intensity of postoperative hematoma following surgery. (B) Note thin rim of enhancement around hematoma cavity representing immediate postoperative changes.

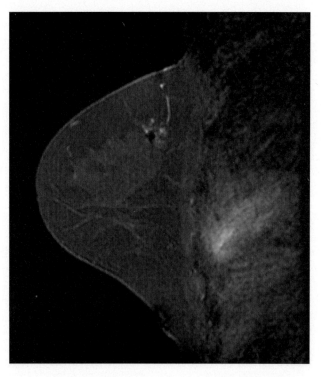

FIGURE 6.40. Abnormal signal void from a metallic clip placed during stereotactic biopsy. Note residual clumped enhancement around the clip indicating residual DCIS.

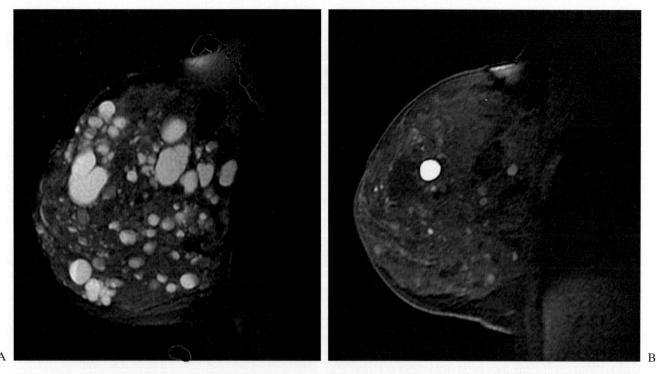

A   B

FIGURE 6.41. Examples of cysts. (A) T2-weighted image demonstrating demonstrated numerous high signal cysts. (B) Precontrast T1-weighted image demonstrates several high signal cysts that have hemorrhagic or proteinaceous content.

6. Value of T2

False-positive biopsy results may be decreased by incorporating information from the T2-weighted images. Cysts, lymph nodes, and certain types of fibroadenomas (myxomatous) are high in signal on T2-weighted images. Although breast adenocarcinomas are generally not high in signal on T2-weighted images, mucinous carcinomas can exhibit high signal and enhance little. Similarly, necrotic tumors may exhibit high signal. However, if the lesion is high in signal on T2-weighted imaging it is more likely to be benign than malignant.

Cysts that are inflammatory and exhibit thin peripheral rim enhancement can be a diagnostic dilemma that is easily solved by referring to the T2-weighted images to confirm the presence of a high signal cyst. Similarly, kinetic uptake of contrast in lymph nodes can mimic breast cancer by exhibiting rapid uptake and early washout. However, if one is able to see a high signal mass on T2 that has morphology suggestive of a lymph node (smooth borders and reniform in shape) a biopsy may be avoided. High cellular fibroadenomas can also be confirmed by assessing the morphological pattern and confirming the high T2 signal.

7. Kinetics

Enhancement kinetics are particularly helpful if the lesion has a benign morphologic appearance. Any suspicious morphologic feature should prompt biopsy and kinetic analysis in these cases, while interesting, is not necessary, as the decision to biopsy has already been made. However, in the case of a well-defined mass that could quite possibly be benign, enhancement kinetic data may help one decide whether biopsy is required or whether it is safe to recommend follow up of the lesion.

To perform kinetic analysis, high temporal resolution is required so that multiple acquisitions can be obtained after the intravenous contrast bolus. In general, the time per sequential acquisition should be under 2 min.

Kinetic techniques analyze the enhancement rate of a lesion by manually placing a region of interest (ROI) over the most intensely enhancing area of the lesion. The signal intensity in the region of interest is then plotted over time. Clearly, the more acquisitions obtained after intravenous contrast administration, the more points on the curve. Additionally, the faster the acquisition, the more potential information obtained about the curve. If multiple ROIs are placed, the most suspicious curve should be reported. The ROI size should be >3 pixels. Signal intensity (SI) increase is measured relative to the baseline signal intensity value.

Three general types of curves are noted that rely less on the absolute value of the enhancement than on the shape of the enhancement curve.[13,14] A type I curve is continuous enhancement increasing with time. A type II curve reaches a plateau phase where maximum signal intensity is reached approximately 2 to 3 min after injection and the signal intensity remains constant at this level. Type III is a washout curve where there has been a decrease in signal intensity after peak enhancement has been reached within 2 to 3 min.

Benign lesions follow a type I curve and malignant lesions follow a type III curve. A type II curve can be seen with both benign and malignant lesions. As with morphologic analysis, malignant lesions can exhibit benign kinetics and vice versa.

8. Suggested Algorithm for Interpretation

An approach to breast MRI interpretation is outlined here (Figure 6.42). Initial evaluation of T2-weighted images is performed to determine if high signal masses, such as cysts, lymph nodes, or myxoid fibroadenomas, are present. Evaluation of the nonenhanced T1-weighted images documents the presence of high signal hemorrhagic or proteinaceous cysts as well as high signal within dilated ducts. The postcontrast T1-weighted images demonstrate the presence of any enhancing masses or nonmass-like areas of enhancement. Morphologic analysis of the architectural features of a mass would then determine if the margins are irregular or spiculated, findings that would be highly suggestive of malignancy. At this point, biopsy would be recommended. A search for the mass by ultrasound may be helpful to allow percutaneous biopsy.

If the mass demonstrates smooth margins and rim enhancement, as rim enhancement is highly predictive of malignancy, biopsy would be recommended as well, once the false-positive causes of rim enhancement, such as inflamed cyst and fat necrosis, have been excluded. Simi-

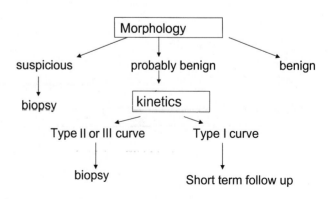

FIGURE 6.42. Algorithm for interpretation.

larly, ductal enhancement that is irregular or clumped will be suspicious for DCIS and biopsy will generally result from this finding.

If, however, the mass is homogeneously enhancing and demonstrates smooth borders, possibly representing a benign finding, kinetic analysis case can be extremely helpful. Kinetics can determine whether this is indeed likely benign (type I curve) or possibly malignant (type II or III curve), prompting biopsy. Because a homogeneously enhancing smooth mass with a type I or II curve has been reported in some malignant lesions, short-term follow up in 6 months may be advisable, if this combination of findings is found to document benignity.

For areas of nonmass-like enhancement, kinetic analysis may be helpful regional enhancement can be found in both benign and malignant breast pathology, such as proliferative changes and DCIS. Kinetic curves may have little use in stippled enhancement, as the tiny foci of enhancement are likely too small for accurate placement of an ROI.

8. Conclusion

The current definitive lexicon for breast MRI incorporates both morphologic and kinetic features of lesions identified on breast MRI. This chapter introduces this material and should not be used as a definitive breast MRI lexicon. It is hoped that terms and concepts presented here will serve as a template to which future lexicon terminology can be added.

References

1. Technical report of the international working group on breast MRI. *J Magn Reson Imaging.* 1999;10:978–1015.
2. Schnall MD, Ikeda DM. Lesion diagnosis working group report. *J Magn Reson Imaging.* 1999;10:982–990.
3. Ikeda DM, Baker DR, Daniel BL. Magnetic resonance imaging of breast cancer: clinical indications and breast MRI reporting system. *J Magn Reson Imaging.* 2000;12: 975–983.
4. Morris EA. Illustrated breast MR lexicon. *Semin Roentgenol.* 2001;36:238–249.
5. American College of Radiology. *Breast Imaging Reporting and Data System (BI-RADS).* 3rd ed. Reston, VA: American College of Radiology;1998.
6. Kawashima M, Tamaki Y, Nonaka T, et al. MR imaging of mucinous carcinoma of the breast. *AJR Am J Roentgenol.* 2002;179:179–183.
7. Kim SJ, Morris EA, Liberman L, et al. Observer variability and applicability of BI-RADS terminology for breast MR imaging: invasive carcinomas as focal masses. *AJR Am J Roentgenol.* 2001;177:551–557.
8. Liberman L, Morris EA, Lee MJ, et al. Breast lesions detected on MR imaging: features and positive predictive value. *AJR Am J Roentgenol.* 2002;179:171–178.
9. Sherif H, Ahmed-Emad M, Oellinger H, et al. Peripheral wash-out sign on contrast-enhanced MR images of the breast. *Radiology* 1997;205:209–213.
10. Nunes LW, Schnall MD, Siegelman ES, et al. Diagnostic performance characteristics of architectural features revealed by high spatial-resolution MR Imaging of the breast. *AJR Am J Roentgenol.* 1997;169:409–415.
11. Nunes LW, Schnall MD, Orel SG, et al. Breast MR Imaging: interpretation model. *Radiology* 1997;202:833–841.
12. Nunes LW, Schnall MD, Orel SG, et al. Correlation of lesion appearance and histologic findings for the nodes of a breast MR imaging interpretation model. *Radiographics* 1999;19: 79–92.
13. Kuhl CK, Schild HH. Dynamic image interpretation of MRI of the breast. *J Magn Reson Imaging.* 2000;12:965–974.
14. Kuhl CK, Mielcareck P, Klaschik S, et al. Dynamic breast MR imaging: are signal intensity time course data useful for differential diagnosis of enhancing lesions? *Radiology* 1999; 211:101–110.

7
Dynamic Breast Magnetic Resonance Imaging

Christiane K. Kuhl

1. Pathophysiological Basis of Dynamic Contrast-Enhanced Breast Magnetic Resonance Imaging

The pathophysiological basis of lesion contrast enhancement in breast magnetic resonance imaging (MRI) has not been fully elucidated yet, but some fundamental facts are known that should help in understanding the technique's specific strengths and weaknesses in terms of lesion detection and differential diagnosis.

It is a well-established fact that malignant lesions release angiogenic factors [e.g., vascular endothelial growth factor (VEGF)] that induce sprouting and growth of preexisting capillaries and induce the de novo formation of new vessels.[1-5] As revealed by histologic and electron microscopic studies, these capillaries exhibit a pathologic vessel wall architecture, with leaky endothelial linings. Therefore, the effect of angiogenic activity is twofold: there is an increased vascularity (vessel density), leading to a focally increased inflow of contrast material, plus an increased vessel permeability, leading to an accelerated extravasation of contrast material at the site of a tumor. Because the regular capillary architecture is lost, arteriovenous shunts are another hallmark of tumor-induced angiogenesis, leading to perfusion shortcuts.

It is currently unclear, however, what exactly determines the degree of contrast material enhancement seen on the MRI. Many studies have been published correlating vessel density with signal intensity changes. The results are contradictory; what can be stated thus far is that vessel density itself cannot be the only contributor.[4,6-17] A possible reason for the inconsistent correlation between MRI-detected enhancement and vessel density or prognostic factors is the fact that the gadolinium-induced signal intensity increase in T1-weighted MRIs is not exactly proportional to the concentration of contrast material that accumulates in a lesion [unlike, e.g., in iodinated contrast agent enhanced computed tomographic (CT) imaging in which

there is a direct correlation between contrast agent concentration and Hounsfield units]. In MRI, lesion enhancement is determined by a variety of contributing factors, including vessel permeability, but also contrast material diffusion rates, composition of the interstitial tumor matrix, and baseline and postcontrast tissue T1 relaxation times. There have been attempts to measure baseline tissue T1 relaxation times to help account for these confounding factors, but this has not gained broad clinical acceptance, and it is unclear as to whether it actually improves differential diagnosis of enhancing lesions. Because signal intensity in susceptibility-based T2*-weighted first-pass perfusion imaging is more directly related to the concentration of gadolinium chelates and, thus, to vessel density and vessel permeability, it has been suggested to use this technique as adjunct to *regular* T1-weighted dynamic imaging to improve differential diagnosis of enhancing lesions.[18-20] Also, macromolecular contrast agents may allow a more close correlation between enhancement rates and microvascular density and capillary permeability.[16,17,21-23]

What is even more problematic from the clinical radiologist's perspective is the fact that a locally increased vascularity and/or capillary permeability is by no means specific for malignant tissues: Almost all benign neoplastic lesions, and many benign nonneoplastic states, go along with a significant hypervascularity or hyperemia.[24-29] Accordingly, contrast enhancement per se or even strong and rapid contrast enhancement is not a feature that is reserved for malignant lesions. Vice versa, a low vascular density can also be found in some malignant changes. Although a nonenhancing invasive breast cancer is so rare that this finding is even worth a case report,[30] tumors with only shallow enhancement do occur in up to 10% of cases, notably in true lobular-invasive cancers[31-33] and in the scirrhotic or desmoplastic type of ductal-invasive breast cancer. Based on histochemical studies it is now assumed that the entire process of angiogenesis differs in these types of breast cancers; there is evidence that in lobular-invasive cancers, angiogenesis is mediated by angiogenic factors other than VEGF.[19] Some well-differentiated invasive cancers (e.g., the tubular type) may go without a significant degree of angiogenesis as well. Moreover, an interaction between tumor cells with the adjacent stroma is not necessarily found in in situ cancers. So while a certain degree of angiogenic activity seems to be a prerequisite for tissue invasion, and, thus, is closely associated with malignant growth, this is not necessarily to be expected for ductal carcinoma in situ (DCIS). Accordingly, contrast enhancement of DCIS can be predicted to vary even more than that of invasive cancers.[34,35]

These pathophysiologic facts explain already that vascularity, and, hence, contrast enhancement, patterns can vary, such that a clear-cut differential diagnosis based on contrast enhancement should prove impossible. It is quite evident that contrast enhancement itself cannot be more specific or more sensitive than the biological (or pathophysiologic) basis it stands for: hypervascularity, or lack thereof, is not pathognomonic for malignant, or benign, lesions. Yet, suprisingly enough, the differential diagnostic power of evaluating lesion contrast enhancement is somewhat better than one might expect given the nonspecific distribution of vessel densities among benign and malignant lesions. The explanation for this phenomenon is probably the fact that it is not the mere number of vessels, but rather the entirety of vessel architecture, permeability, and tissue relaxation times that determines contrast enhancement, and, thus, differential diagnosis in dynamic breast MRI.

2. Technical Issues

2.1. How It All Evolved

After the introduction of gadolinium dimeglumine as MRI contrast agent, many different approaches have been developed for MRI of the breast; they are mentioned here, because, as always, knowledge of past history helps with the understanding of present controversies. Heywang and coworkers were the first to use gadolinium dimeglumine for MRI of the breast.[36] They reported strong contrast enhancement of breast cancers, whereas the normal parenchyma exhibited only weak (if any) enhancement. Heywang suggested a technique that, today, would be called a *semi-dynamic* acquisition: She acquired one precontrast and two postcontrast image stacks; the main reason for obtaining the second postcontrast stack was to ensure detection of lesions with delayed enhancement that may have been missed on the first postcontrast image. Imaging was performed with limited temporal and (with respect to the scanner technology that was available at that

time) relatively high spatial resolution. Because temporal resolution was not the main focus, a three-dimensional (3D) gradient echo technique could be applied.

The approach launched by Kaiser and coworkers was designed to track the rapid signal intensity changes that occur in the early postcontrast period.[37] The technique they proposed could be called the archetype of dynamic breast MRI: They suggested acquiring one precontrast and a series of postcontrast image stacks including both breasts at the highest possible temporal resolution that was achievable at that time (60s). Rapid imaging at that time allowed only a limited spatial resolution, and acquisition of only a small number of sections (5–10), such that only a part (not even half) of the parenchymal volume was covered. Because rapid imaging was necessary, image subtraction was used to suppress the signal from fatty tissues, rather than applying time-consuming active fat-suppression techniques.

Harms and coworkers' concept[38] was based on the well-established fact that malignant lesions exhibit characteristic morphologic features that allow a distinction from benign lesions. To improve analysis of subtle morphologic details, they advocated a technique that may represent the *archetype* of static breast imaging: They suggested imaging of one single breast with high spatial resolution before and after contrast material injection. Because temporal resolution was no issue in this approach, 3D gradient echo imaging was used, and fat suppression ensued by means of (rather time consuming) spectral prepulses.

The two fundamental schools that evolved (and that were also separated geographically) were the *dynamic school* and the *static school*. The dynamic school (most popular in European countries) attempted to distinguish benign and malignant lesions by their enhancement characteristics at high temporal resolution (classically 60s per dynamic scan); usually, both breasts were imaged in the axial or coronal plane, with limited in-plane resolution. On the other end, the static school (most popular in the United States) attempted lesion classification by evaluating morphologic features of enhancing lesions at high spatial resolution; usually, only one breast was imaged at a time in the sagittal plane. Due to the severe technical constraints, particularly during early breast MRI, it was necessary to choose between either temporal or spatial resolution, just depending on the diagnostic criterion that was given priority.

The different approaches are a mere reflection of the fact that breast MRI is technically extremely challenging; the diverging demands of an optimal temporal and spatial resolution for the detection and classification of enhancing lesions can hardly be met with today's equipment. Because researchers had to cope with the technical shortcomings of their respective equipment, they started doing breast MRI at the two ends of the spectrum of imaging techniques that are suitable for breast MRI. It is important to understand that these different approaches must not be misunderstood as being contradictory or as being competitors for the ultimate truth; they have to be understood within the clinical and technical context of the time when they were written and published.

2.2. Where We Are Today

Today, owing to the technical progress that has been made, it is possible to integrate these demands rather than compromising on one or the other. Therefore, modern concepts of breast MRI strive to consider both lesion morphology and contrast enhancement kinetics.[26,39–45] As a consequence, today, there is considerable agreement in terms of what constitutes an appropriate pulse sequence for breast MRI:

- A useful pulse sequence for dynamic breast MRI must offer an appropriate temporal resolution, not only to enable the analysis of enhancement kinetics, but also to improve the delineation and assessment of marginal status of enhancing lesions: Only in the early *arterial* phase, an optimal lesion-versus-parenchyma contrast is obtained. Already by the third postcontrast minute, the rapidly diffusable gadolinium chelates lead to a signal loss (washout) in the cancers and a progressive enhancement of the adjacent normal glandular tissue. This reduces the contrast between the lesion and the surrounding parenchyma, and often enough, the contrast is entirely cancelled out by the fourth postcontrast minute (Figure 7.1). So for the assessment of morphologic details, early postcontrast imaging is necessary. In addition, it has been repeatedly shown that only after the first postcontrast minute the enhancement rates of benign and malignant lesions differ significantly,[46] whereas this difference is already cancelled out in the second or third postcontrast minute.
- A dynamic breast MRI protocol must offer appropriate spatial resolution; however, it is difficult to tell what exactly is appropriate. A simple rule of thumb applies: The more, the better [provided sufficient overall signal-to-noise ratio (SNR)].
- A dynamic breast MRI protocol must cover the entire volume of the fibroglandular tissue of (preferably) both breasts.
- Because bilateral imaging requires a large field of view (FOV), homogeneous fat suppression via active fat saturation techniques is difficult to achieve; usually, it is unreliable. Also, active fat suppression usually needs extra acquisition time, which would mean an additional burden for the temporal-versus-spatial trade off. Accordingly, fat suppression in bilateral dynamic breast MRI is usually achieved by image subtraction.

3. Choice of Pulse Sequences

3.1. What Types of Pulse Sequences Are Suitable?

For dynamic imaging, both two-dimensional (2D) and 3D gradient echo acquisition schemes are suitable (*2D* in this context means *multislice 2D*, i.e., all sections are acquired at the same time as one stack). Fast or Turbo gradient echo imaging has not been advocated for breast MRI. Similarly, EPI pulse sequences are considered not appropriate for dynamic breast imaging, because the accumulation of phase errors may cause significant artifacts; they have been successfully used for ultrafast dynamic imaging, but they are usually not suitable for morphologic analysis. It is questionable whether the strong susceptibility effects associated with echo planar imaging (EPI) acquisition would interfere with the detection and morphologic assessment of small lesions that are embedded in fatty tissue.

A good T1 contrast (T1-weighting) of the pulse sequence is important to fully exploit the effects of contrast agents. As the echo times (TEs) are more or less given by field-dependent in-phase settings of fat and water resonance frequencies, improving the sequences' T1 contrast is only possible by reducing the repetition time (TR). The flip angle has then to be adapted to the TR; in general, it must be set smaller with shorter TRs. When compared with 2D gradient echo, 3D pulse sequences offer an inherently better T1 contrast (mainly due to their substantially shorter TRs) and a higher SNR, which can be traded for improving spatial resolution (in particular thinner section thickness) compared with 2D imaging. And yet, in spite of the obvious technical advantages of 3D imaging, we stick to using 2D gradient echo for our dynamic series. This is because we found that 3D imaging suffers significantly more from image degradation due to all kinds of artifacts (pulsation, susceptibility, ghosting), and it rather *exaggerates* enhancement associated with benign proliferative changes (focal adenosis). Two-dimensional gradient echo is a more stable pulse sequence that offers a calm background and excellent image quality, and with conservative enhancement compared with 3D.

3.2. Some Aspects Regarding Choice of Repitition Time

In general, TR should be as short as possibly achievable; it should be lower than 300 to 350ms in 2D pulse sequences; in 3D, TR is already inherently short (10–20ms). One problematic side effect is that in 2D imaging, the TR increases in direct proportion to the number of sections of a given

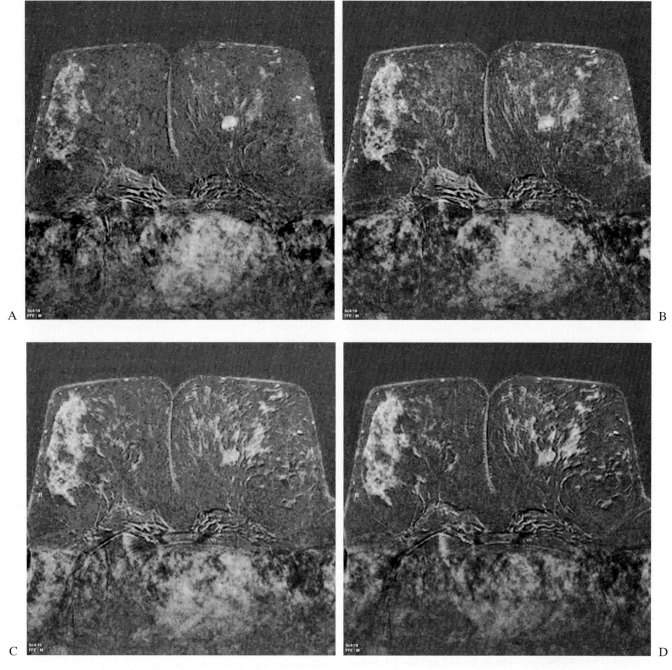

FIGURE 7.1. Impact of temporal resolution of a dynamic series. (A–F) First through sixth postcontrast subtracted image through a dynamic series in a 49-year-old patient with duct-invasive breast cancer in her left breast. Note the strong washout of contrast agent in the cancer, leading to a SI decrease in the postinitial and late postcontrast phase compared with the first postcontrast image (A). Note the progressive enhancement of the normal fibroglandular tissue around the cancer. Note that visibility of the lesion decreases over the dynamic series: Lesion delineation is best during the early postcontrast phase and is almost cancelled out in the third postcontrast minute.

dynamic scan. So the upper TR limit of 350ms also sets the upper limit for the number of sections that can be acquired during one dynamic scan; usually, not more than 35 sections can be accommodated in a TR of 300 to 350ms. With thin sections (e.g., 3mm), this translates into a cranio-caudal coverage of $35 \times 3mm = 105mm$, which is usually just sufficient to cover the entire breast parenchyma in the cranio-caudal direction. To help avoid missing any

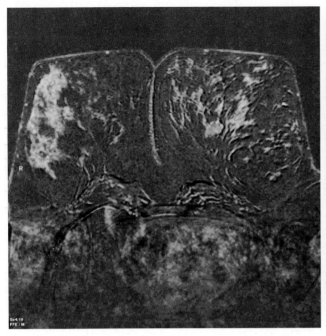
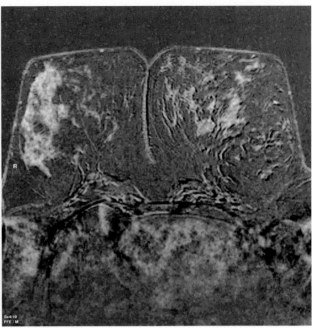

E

F

FIGURE 7.1. (*Continued*)

parenchyma by the dynamic stack, we acquire an extensive set of localizer images that help locate the position and the spatial extent of the parenchymal volume. The radiology technologists are specifically trained to position the dynamic stack exactly matching the (often angulated) position of the parenchyma; if there is doubt, one dynamic scan is run (i.e., 2 min are invested) to check and make sure that all parenchyma is included.

3.3. What to Know About Echo Time

Regarding echo times, TE should be chosen to match the field strength specific in-phase echo time settings: This is less important, but still recommended for pulse sequences with *active* fat suppression (fat saturation) techniques as well. *In phase echo time* is referred to as the time point at which both fat and water spins have the same position in space, that is, they rotate in phase. This is important, because failure to adhere to in-phase echo times will cause signal cancellations at fat/water tissue interfaces. In phase echo time is 4.6 ms at 1.5 Tesla (T), 2.3 ms at 3.0 T, 6.9 ms at 1.0 T, and 13.8 ms for 0.5 T. Because 13.8 ms is a very long TE that is long enough to slow down acquisition speed at 0.5 T, an alternative is to use a TE of 3.0 ms, which goes along with an acceptably small phase difference between fat and water.[47,48]

3.4. Temporal Resolution: How Fast Is Fast Enough?

Regarding temporal resolution, ideally, it should be kept at about 60 s per dynamic acquisition, but up to 120 s per dynamic seem acceptable. Reducing acquisition time further, that is, improving temporal resolution further below *60-s timeline* will probably not offer additional kinetic information if no pharmacokinetic analysis is attempted and is, in our view, unnecessary. We strongly recommend setting the temporal resolution somewhere between 60 and 120 s, and invest all remaining MRI system resources into spatial resolution.

3.5. Spatial Resolution

Spatial resolution should be as high as possibly achievable within 60 to 120 s. Unlike temporal resolution (in which a further increase beyond the 60-s limit would not bring about additional diagnostic information), improving spatial resolution will always be advantageous (provided acceptable SNR levels are maintained). For a bilateral approach, that is, FOV of about 350 mm, an imaging matrix of at least 400×512 should be used. The section thickness should not exceed 3 mm; 1 to 2 mm would be ideal, but with 2D imaging, such a small section thickness is virtually not achievable due to SNR limitations. No gap between sections should be used; this holds true both for 2D and 3D. With a 405 × 512 imaging matrix and a FOV of 320mm, the noninterpolated in-plane spatial resolution is 0.6 × 0.8mm, which is equivalent to many *high resolution* unilateral protocols.[38,39,49–51] Single breast imaging does not necessarily always offer higher spatial resolution than bilateral protocols; you need to compare the actual, noninterpolated pixel sizes to find out.

3.6. What Imaging Plane Is Preferable?

Regarding the imaging plane orientation for bilateral breast MRI, it is not feasible to cover both breasts in the sagittal orientation with current pulse sequence technology. Emerging imaging technologies such as VIBRANT, which is based on parallel imaging techniques, may change this in the next future, but so far, the only option for bilateral imaging is axial or coronal.

There are certain advantages and disadvantages for both planes: The advantage of a coronal orientation is that one can use a rectangular FOV of approximately 60%, which translates into an immediate 60% reduction of the acquisition time. Therefore, this pulse sequence may be useful for 1.0T systems where, due to the relatively long in-phase echo time of almost 7ms, temporal resolution is even more difficult to achieve. However, it usually takes more sections to cover the breast in the anterior-posterior (AP) direction (i.e., coronal imaging) compared with the cranio-caudad (CC) direction (i.e., axial imaging), such that the eventual gain in acquisition speed will not be as high.

The disadvantage of coronal imaging is the fact that most of the blood vessels travel in the AP plane, such that it may become difficult to distinguish a focal lesion from a cross-section of a vessel; often enough, maximum intensity projection (MIP) reconstructions are necessary to distinguish vessels from lesions. With axial imaging, vessels travel in plane, so that they are easily identified as such.

Another aspect is the following: Breathing motions occur mostly in the AP plane, that is, tangentially, *through-plane* for coronal imaging. During in- and expiration, the patient *dives* in and out a given coronal section. This goes along with circular subtraction artifacts that are difficult to interpret and handle. With axial imaging, breathing motion and gross patient motion (which occurs mostly in the left-right direction) will rather stay within the imaging plane of a given section. Therefore, a lesion tends to be displaced *within* a given section, as opposed to being displaced through plane with coronal imaging. This is important, because a lesion that is displaced in-plane is usually still amenable to kinetic analysis (based on analysis of non-subtracted images), whereas this is virtually impossible for a lesion that moves through plane.

One last disadvantage of coronal imaging is the fact that some key anatomic structures for breast imaging are cut through-plane: the nipple and the chest wall. Nipple and chest wall invasion are important clinical contraindications for breast conservation, therefore, an accurate assessment is very important. Axial imaging provides in-plane imaging of these structures, thus facilitating the analysis.

3.7. How We Do It

The dynamic imaging protocol used at our institution may serve as an example for a pulse sequence that strives to offer a good compromise between spatial and temporal resolution (Figure 7.2): It is a 2D multislice gradient echo

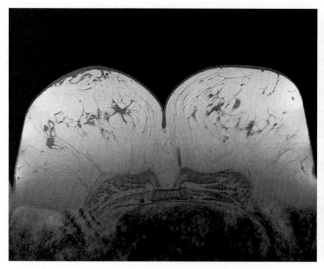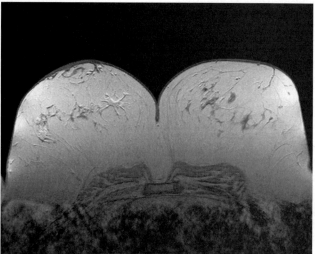

FIGURE 7.2. The University of Bonn Dynamic Breast MRI Protocol in a patient with multicentric duct-invasive cancer of the right breast. (A) Precontrast, (B) first postcontrast.

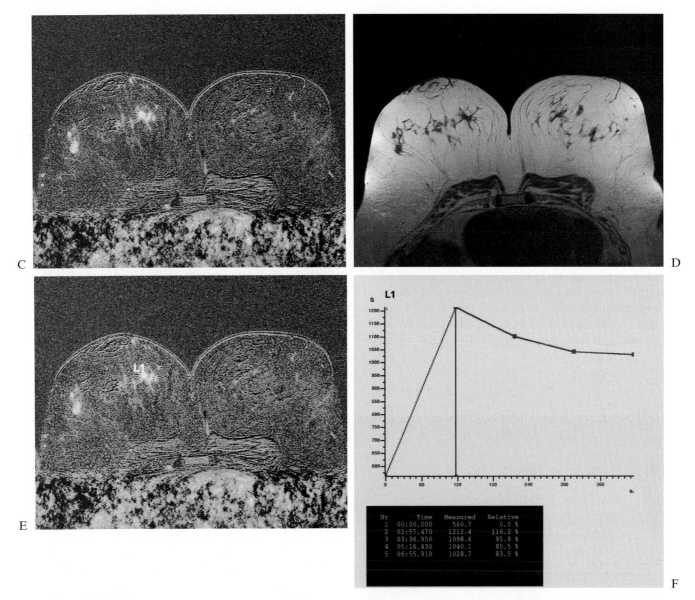

FIGURE 7.2. (*Continued*) (C) First postcontrast subtracted, (D) T2-weighted TSE image, (E) subtracted image with ROI, and (F) signal intensity time course. This is a T1-weighted 2D multislice gradient echo series, TR/TE/FA 290 ms/4.6 ms/90°; 405 × 512 imaging matrix over a 350 FOV, 3-mm section thickness, 110 s acquisition time per dynamic frame, one precontrast and four postcontrast frames (one postcontrast is displayed); fat suppression by subtraction. Note the high anatomic detail, the high "arterial phase" contrast between the enhancing lesions and adjacent normal fibroglandular tissue, and the clear washout time course in the kinetic assessment.

series in the axial orientation, with TR/TE/FA (facet angle) of 300/4.6/90°, a 405 × 512 imaging matrix, a receiver bandwidth of 180 Hz, a field of view of 290 to 310 mm, a section thickness of 3 mm or less (depending on the size of the breast), no gap, with 33 sections; temporal resolution is 1:55 s per dynamic stack. One set of images is acquired before contrast, and another four image stacks after bolus intravenous injection (injection rate of 3 mL/s) of

0.1 mmol/kg gadolinium dimeglumine, followed by a saline flush of at least 20 cc. In addition, we would always acquire non–fat-saturated T2-weighted tissue skin electron beam (TSE) images with identical geometric features as the T1-weighted dynamic series, and in particular with very high spatial resolution. This is because T2 TSE images help classify rapidly enhancing lesions (differential diagnosis myxoid fibroadenoma versus breast cancer).[52]

4. Generating the Source Data for Kinetic Analysis: Region of Interest Placement

In order to evaluate the enhancement pattern of a lesion, a region of interest (ROI) is placed selectively into the enhancing lesion, carefully avoiding inclusion of nonenhancing tissue. The emerging quantitative signal intensity (SI) values are used to plot the *SI time course*. Most MRI systems offer the possibility to manually draw ROI in the images of the dynamic series.

There are some important issues to remember: The goal is to identify the part of the lesion with strongest and fastest enhancement and to place the ROI *selectively* into this area. The goal is *not* to obtain an average of the tumor, but to obtain enhancement kinetics of the most vital tumor parts, because only these ones yield meaningful information, that is, information that is useful for differential diagnosis.[53] There is some disagreement in this aspect, because there are authors who suggest encircling

the entire lesion,[46,54,55] because they have made the experience that with broader or more selective ROI placement, enhancement rates of benign and malignant lesions will decrease or increase to the same degree, with the relative difference between them preserved. However, while the assessment of enhancement rates does not suffer from encircling ROIs, the shape of the signal time course (signal intensity behavior in the postinitial and late postcontrast-phase) *does* change with broader ROIs. Specifically, a washout will only be observable with selective ROIs; with encircling ROIs, the washout will be changed toward less suspicious curve types such as plateau or even a persistent enhancement (Figure 7.3). To achieve a selective ROI placement, the following guidelines should be observed:

- It is necessary to identify the area where enhancement starts first; therefore, one should use the very first postcontrast scan for ROI positioning. One should use very wide window settings on the subtracted or nonsubtracted images, because with narrow windowing, the

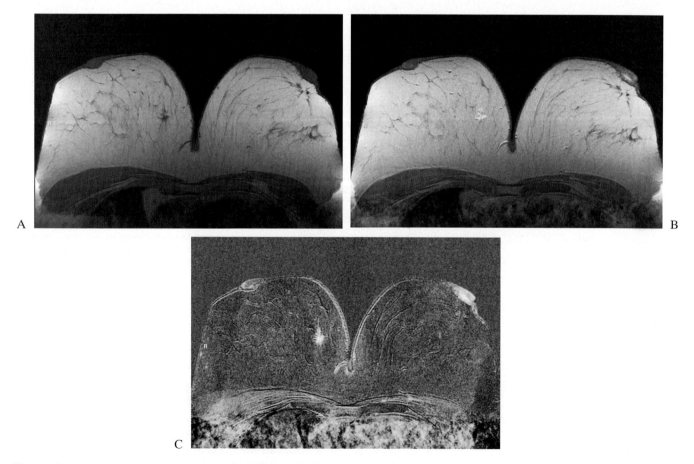

FIGURE 7.3. Impact of ROI placement on the kinetic assessment. (A) Precontrast, (B) first postcontrast, (C) first postcontrast subtracted image in a 53-year-old patient with tubular cancer in her right breast.

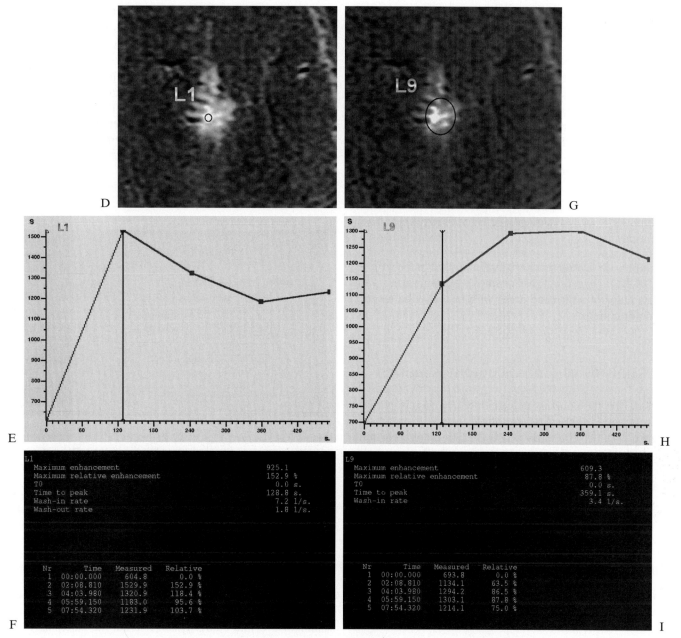

FIGURE 7.3. (*Continued*) (D–F) Kinetic analysis with an appropriately sized and correctly positioned ROI. Note the small size of the ROI, which selectively encloses strongly enhancing parts of the lesion. Note the characteristic "malignant" time course (washout phenomenon in the corresponding signal time course in E). Note the strong and fast contrast enhancement, yielding a washin rate of 153% in F. (G–I) Kinetic analysis with an inappropriate ROI, which encircles the entire lesion. Note that the same lesion exhibits a "benign" time course (persistent type in H). Note the substantially lower washin rate of 63% in I.

entire lesion will have seemingly the same signal intensity, even if there are significant differences regarding enhancement within the lesion.

• It is important to use small ROIs (which include only 2 or 3 pixels in small lesions). This is necessary to sample selectively the part of the lesion that shows strongest enhancement; many enhancing lesions, and in particular breast cancers, are heterogeneous regarding their internal enhancement. If the entire lesion is encircled by an ROI, rapidly enhancing (presumably vital) tumor parts are averaged together with slowly enhancing (nonvital, fibrotic or necrotic) tumor parts. Usually, strongest enhancement and, more importantly, areas with positive washout phenomenon are found only in the peripheral parts of the lesion, corresponding to the vital, invading parts of the tumor.

- It is important to make sure that the ROI is within the lesion in during the entire dynamic series; if the patient moves, it is possible that the lesion moves out of the ROI, which can produce fake "washout" phenomena once the nonenhancing, normal parenchyma is at the site where the lesion was before. The position of the breast with respect to the ROI position on all dynamic images should be checked. If the breast moves out of the ROI, the emerging data cannot be used for diagnosis.
- Whether the ROI actually includes an enhancing lesion, and not a vessel next to a lesion, should be carefully checked. This can best be achieved by generating MPR or MIP images, or by viewing the adjacent sections.

There is dedicated software available that helps with the task of ROI placement, for example, by generating parametric maps in which the areas with fastest enhancement are color coded.

5. Analysis of Enhancement Kinetics

Considering the contrast enhancement pattern during the dynamic series, three different phases can be distinguished (Figure 7.4): (1) The early phase (between contrast injection and the second postcontrast minute), (2) the postinitial phase (3rd to 4th postcontrast minute), and (3) the late phase (later than the 4th postcontrast minute). The kinetic criteria that relate to the different phases are as follows:

5.1. Criteria Relating to the Early Postcontrast Phase

In the early postcontrast phase, *washin rates* (or *enhancement velocities*) are quantified using the following equation:

$$[SI_{postcontrast} - SI_{precontrast} / SI_{precontrast}] - 100$$

where $SI_{postcontrast}$ is the SI of the lesion in the first postcontrastpostcontrast image (usually, 60–120s after injection), and $SI_{precontrast}$ is the SI of the lesion before contrast. This value provides the relative (percentage) SI increase of a lesion that is reached within the early postcontrast phase.

For diagnostic purposes, the enhancement rate is then again classified into slow, intermediate, and fast; unfortunately, there are no universally applicable definitions of the three categories—any variation of pulse sequence parameters, but also field strength of the magnet, timing of contrast enhancement, start of the first postcontrast scan, and vendor-related issues, will impact the actual enhancement

rates that are obtained. This means that for every MRI system and every pulse sequence, the threshold between what one would call rapid or slow enhancement needs to be determined anew. A way to do this is by imaging a series of known breast cancers, measure their enhancement (or washin) rate, and use this as reference for fast enhancement. With increasing experience, it will usually be possible to judge from the visual appearance of a lesion in the first postcontrast image whether or not it qualifies for rapid enhancement or not, thus avoiding time-consuming quan-

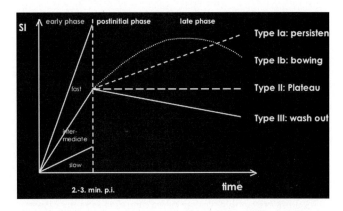

FIGURE 7.4. Different phases of the signal time course of a dynamic series and the respective kinetic criteria. We distinguish three phases: (1) initial postcontrast phase (injection of contrast agent until the second postcontrast minute), (2) postinitial phase (second through third postcontrast minute), (3) late postcontrast phase (4th through 8th postcontrast minute). In the initial postcontrast phase, enhancement rates (washin rates) are calculated. They correspond to relative enhancement within the first or second postcontrast minute. For differential diagnostic purposes, the quantitative data are classified as slow, intermediate, or fast. In the postinitial and late postcontrast phase, the time course of signal intensity is rated visually according to the following scheme: Type Ia ("persistent enhancement"), enhancement continues over the entire dynamic series; the emerging curve is a (more or less) straight line. Peak enhancement is achieved in the last postcontrast scan (and would probably be even later if we acquired more dynamic scans). Type Ib ("persistent with bowing"), enhancement continues over almost the entire dynamic period, but the rate is slowed down during the late postcontrast phase, resulting in a flattening (bowing) of the curve. Peak enhancement is achieved during the late postcontrast phase, and may plateau thereafter or show a very slow decline that starts in the late postcontrast phase. Type II ("plateau curve"), enhancement reaches a steady state after the initial phase. Accordingly, peak enhancement is already reached directly after the early phase, and there is not much SI variation during the intermediate and late postcontrast phases. Type III ("washout curve"), enhancement decreases again directly after the strong signal increase in the early phase. This means that peak enhancement occurs in the first or second postcontrast scan, and already in the third postcontrast image, SI is reduced again.

tification. This, however, requires that subtracted and non-subtracted images are *always* hardcopied or viewed with standardized and fixed window settings.

Many more kinetic features have been described that relate to the early postcontrast phase. Examples are steepness of slope and onset of enhancement. The latter is measured in seconds, with reference to the opacification of, for example, the aorta. What is common to these criteria is that they can only be evaluated in time resolved breast MRI studies, where there are many dynamic scans (i.e., data sampling points) during the early postcontrast phase, as opposed to one (or a maximum of two) dynamic scans with *regular* dynamic imaging. Because time-resolved studies usually do not cover the entire parenchyma, or they do so with a very limited in-plane spatial resolution,[55–59] they did not gain broad clinical acceptance, neither did the respective kinetic features.

5.2. Criteria Relating to the Postinitial and Late Postcontrast Phase

While the SI changes in the early postcontrast phase are usually quantified (*percent signal change*), those that occur in the postinitial and late postcontrast phase are virtually always evaluated qualitatively. This means that the time course is evaluated by simply looking at the curves (SI vs. time plots) and deciding whether, after the early phase, the SI continues to increase, or stays the same (plateaus), or decreases (washout).

Software is available that also quantifies the SI loss (if it is present) relative to peak enhancement, or the time point of peak enhancement, or the slope of the curve (with a negative slope in washout and a positive in progressively enhancing lesions), or the washout rates, but these criteria have not gained broad clinical acceptance, mainly because they are again only obtainable with time-resolved imaging, and, possibly, also because they do not add diagnostic information from what is available by simply classifying the curves according to the previously mentioned simple pattern.

Regarding the visual analysis of lesion time course, one way to classify the enhancement pattern in the postinitial and late postcontrast phase is as follows[53] (Figure 7.4):

- Type 1a (*persistent enhancement*) is a time course in which enhancement continues over the entire dynamic series; the emerging curve is a (more or less) straight line. Peak enhancement is therefore achieved in the last postcontrast scan (and would probably be even later if we acquired more dynamic scans).
- Type 1b (*persistent with bowing*) is a time course in which enhancement continues over almost the entire dynamic period, but the rate is slowed down during the late postcontrast phase, resulting in a flattening (bowing) of the curve. Peak enhancement is achieved during the

late postcontrast phase, and may plateau thereafter or show a very slow decline that starts in the late postcontrast phase.

- Type 2 (*plateau curve*) is a time course in which enhancement reaches a steady state after the early phase. Accordingly, peak enhancement is already reached directly after the early phase, and there is not much SI variation during the intermediate and late postcontrast phases.
- Type 3 (*washout curve*) is a time course in which enhancement decreases again directly after the early phase. This means that peak enhancement occurs in the first or second postcontrast scan, and already in the third postcontrast image, SI is reduced again.

6. Pharmakokinetic Modeling

There are several scientific papers on using pharmakokinetic modeling of the signal time course data acquired during the dynamic series.[57–63] There is, however, no evidence to suggest that pharmakokinetic modeling would add diagnostic information beyond what is obtained with the analysis of plain enhancement rates and visual assessment of curve types. Also, most pharmakokinetic models require very rapid sampling of SI data, thus again interfering with the acquisition of image matrices that would allow a state-of-the-art analysis of lesion morphologic features. There are hardly any pharmakokinetic software packages that are commercially available and ready for clinical use. All in all, pharmakokinetic modeling is not used on a broader clinical scale.

7. Understanding Published Literature: Survivors and One-Hit Wonders of Kinetic Approaches

Many more dynamic approaches to image (and kinetics) interpretation have been developed and published in the literature. To help the reader understand the different ways to interpret the dynamic information, here is a summary:

The oldest approach for quantification of lesion enhancement was published by Heywang and coworkers.[36,64] They suggested quantification of a "normalized enhancement ratio" by assessing the lesions' signal intensity relative to that of fatty tissue. The underlying concept is that the SI of fatty tissue should not change after injection of contrast material, such that it can be used as internal reference. After analyzing normalized lesion signal intensities (NU) in a cohort of 144 patients with benign and malignant breast diseases, they proposed a classification scheme that was based on lesion peak signal intensity increase. Accordingly, their approach to differential diagnosis would be based on the question: "How strongly does the lesion enhance?" Using this criterion, they reported a sensitivity of 100% (71/71), and specificity of 27% (20/73). Once relatively popular, the concept of the *normalized units* has meanwhile been largely replaced by calculating early-phase enhancement (washin) rates (see following discussion). The semidynamic pulse sequence has been abandoned by the authors after more rapid 3D sequences had become available. In a way, however, if one disregards the kinetic modelling aspects, the 3TP method (*3 time point method*) suggested by Degani and Fuman-Haran and coworkers[39,49] is based on a similar concept.

Kaiser and coworkers suggested a quantification of lesion enhancement as well.[37] However, they proposed to normalize enhancement not with respect to the signal from fatty tissue, but with respect to baseline lesion signal intensity, according to the enhancement equation mentioned previously. In a preliminary study of 25 patients, they found that breast cancers exhibit higher enhancement rates, causing a strong signal increase in the early postcontrast period. For differential diagnosis, enhancement velocity (relative SI increase per minute in the early postcontrast period) was suggested. Kaiser found that malignant lesions revealed an enhancement velocity beyond a threshold of 100% (i.e., doubling signal intensity within the first postcontrast minute). Accordingly, the authors suggested establishing the differential diagnosis based on the question: "How fast does the lesion enhance in first postcontrast minute?" Using this approach in a preliminary series of 25 patients, Kaiser reported a sensitivity of 100% (6/6). Unfortunately, however, the authors failed to validate their data in a larger series of patients. In several further review articles that were published in the first half of the last decade, Kaiser and coworkers stated that sensitivity and specificity of their approach was 99% and 98%, respectively. Notwithstanding the rather poor validation, this imaging technique and its associated criteria have gained considerable popularity. Stomper and coworkers, using the same technique on a small series of patients, reported a sensitivity of 92% (23/25), but achieved only a moderate specificity (61%, 16/26). Currently, most of the clinical papers on dynamic contrast-enhanced breast MRI use a similar technique as the one proposed by Kaiser, albeit with higher spatial resolution and with coverage of the entire breast.

Boetes and coworkers suggested a dynamic technique focusing on temporal resolution as well. They found that differential diagnosis could be achieved by determining the onset of lesion enhancement relative to the aortic enhancement. Accordingly, their approach to differential diagnosis would be based on the question: "When (relative to the aorta) does the lesion start to enhance?" They used an ultrafast imaging technique that sacrificed coverage of the entire breast in favor of a single-section, ultrafast bilateral image acquisition based on turbo gradient echo sequences with a temporal resolution of 2.3s.[56] In their cohort, malignant lesions started to enhance 11.5s after bolus arrival in the descending aorta, whereas benign lesions showed a later onset. Using this criterion in 87 lesions, Boetes and colleagues achieved a sensitivity and specificity of 95% (62/65) and 86% (19/22), respectively. However, since then, this technique has not been used in any further paper published by this or another group, suggesting that the ultrafast single section technique is probably difficult to integrate into a clinical breast MRI protocol. Also, Schorn and coworkers tried the same technique and the same diagnostic criteria on a series of 35 lesions (15 malignant, 20 benign). In their series,[65] they could not reproduce a statistically significant difference concerning the progression of enhancement (centripetal, centrifugal) or the onset of lesion enhancement for benign and malignant lesions.

Fischer and coworkers and our group suggested that not only the early postcontrast period, but also the intermediate and late postcontrast phase yields diagnostically useful information[24,53]: Lesions with persistent signal intensity increase (type 1a, 1b) were more likely to be benign, whereas lesions with signal intensity plateau (type 2) or with a washout (type 3) tended to be malignant. Accordingly, this approach to differential diagnosis would be based on the question: "What happens after the early postcontrast phase?" Using this criterion, in a cohort of 266 contrast-enhancing lesions, qualitative evaluation of signal intensity time courses alone (irrespective of other findings related for example to enhancement rates or morphology) yielded a sensitivity of 91% (92/101) and a specificity of 83% (137/164), suggesting that there is diagnostic information inherent to time course analysis. It should go without saying, however, that time course analysis should not be used as a stand-alone criterion, but rather be embedded into the process of differential diagnosis. The assessment of curve types, in particular the use of a washout as criterion for malignancy, has gained wide acceptance and has been used in most of the recently published clinical papers on dynamic contrast-enhanced breast MRI.

All the different approaches mentioned previously were triggered by the experience that breast cancers do exhibit contrast enhancement, but that many benign lesions do so as well. Consequently, to improve lesion classification, it is necessary to assess additional lesion features. The many different ways to assess contrast enhancement kinetics, and the various terms describing kinetic parameters that have been listed should not be misunderstood as discrepancy or scientific inconsistency. Rather, they stand for different ways to look at the same phenomenon: The early, rapid, and strong signal intensity increase (and subsequent washout) that occurs in breast cancers. Alike, the many different thresholds that have been published to establish *cut-off values* for *suspicious* enhancement should not be misunderstood as giving proof of an inherent inconsistency of the dynamic approach: The threshold values will vary greatly with the field strength, pulse sequence, and timing of contrast material injection. As such, they are not valid except for the particular technical setting and patient cohort in which and for which they have been established.

8. How To Use Information Obtained from Dynamic Data

Owing to the biologic and histologic heterogeneity of breast lesions mentioned previously, it should be self-explanatory that it is not possible to interpret dynamic breast MRI studies by means of a simple enhancement cut-off value or threshold. To avoid false-negative decisions, a threshold must be set at relatively moderate enhancement values; however, myriad benign lesions will reach suprathreshold enhancement as well. In addition, some invasive and in particular intraductal breast cancers (see following discussion) may go along with only moderate angiogenic activity and, thus, with only moderate or shallow enhancement. So because there are benign lesions with strong enhancement, and malignant lesions with only moderate enhancement, dynamic data (enhancement velocity, degree, or onset of enhancement and so forth) must not be used as stand-alone diagnostic criterion. Instead, they should be integrated in the process of differential diagnosis to expand (rather than narrow) the armamentarium of differential diagnosis in breast MRI.

8.1. How We Do It

For interpretation of dynamic breast MRIs, we first refer to the initial postcontrast image stack and search for lesions with significant (i.e., supraglandular) enhancement, because lesions that appear at this phase are associated with a significant probability of malignancy. Once such a lesion is identified, we relate to its morphologic features. We use the terminology presented in the MRI lexicon as published by the "lesion diagnosis working group."[66,67] Only thereafter, and as an addendum, kinetics are evaluated.

The first step is to decide whether we deal with a focal mass or a nonmass-related enhancement.

A focal mass has usually a clear correlate on precontrast T1- and T2-weighted images and reveals *space occupying* behavior (Figure 7.5). In nonmass-related enhancement,

no lesion is visible on precontrast images, but the existing parenchyma itself seems to enhance (Figure 7.6). The differentiation of *mass* and *nonmass enhancement* is important and has about the same diagnostic implications as the distinction between *mass* (or mass with calcifications) versus *calcifications alone* on a mammogram. In mass-related enhancement, the differential diagnosis is (benign or malignant) tumor. In nonmass-related enhancement, the differential diagnosis is between DCIS or fibrocystic disease/normal tissue.

If a mass is identified, we first define its shape (round, oval, irregular, stellate), then its margins (smooth, non-smooth, spicules); internal architecture is also evaluated (homogeneous, heterogeneous, rim enhancement, low SI internal septations). Malignant lesions (invasive cancers) tend to have irregular or even stellate shape, non-smooth borders or even spicules, and a heterogeneous internal architecture or even rim enhancement (Figure 7.7).

If a nonmass-related enhancement is identified, we first define its distribution (focal, multifocal, diffuse, regional, segmental, linear/branching), then internal architecture (homogeneous, heterogeneous, or clumped/cobblestone pattern; Figure 7.8). Malignant lesions with nonmass-related enhancement (DCIS) tend to appear as solitary focus of enhancement, or as regional, segmental, or linear-branching enhancement; just like in a mammogram, the distribution of calcifications helps distinguish suspicious from less-suspicious calcifications. If the enhancement is regional or segmental, internal architecture can be evaluated and is typically *clumped*.

Only after the morphologic analysis as described previously, we would evaluate enhancement kinetics (although one may argue that there is some *kinetic bias* in our diagnosis, because we use the first postcontrast image to search for lesions with significant enhancement; this implies that our main attention is focused on lesions with enhancement that is at least sufficient to provide a significant signal intensity increase in the first postcontrast image).

We measure washin rates or classify enhancement visually according its appearance on the first postcontrast subtracted image. To do this, we use standardized window settings. Malignant lesions tend to exhibit strong and fast enhancement; in our setting, this means an enhancement of 90% or more in the first postcontrast minute. If lesions shows rapid or intermediate enhancement, we plot the signal intensity time course to visually assess the postinitial and late postcontrast SI changes (persistent, plateau, washout). Often, a wash out is *not* visually appreciable because the degree of SI decrease during washout is much smaller compared with the initial SI increase during the early phase of enhancement (i.e., on the subtracted images, the lesions continue to appear bright

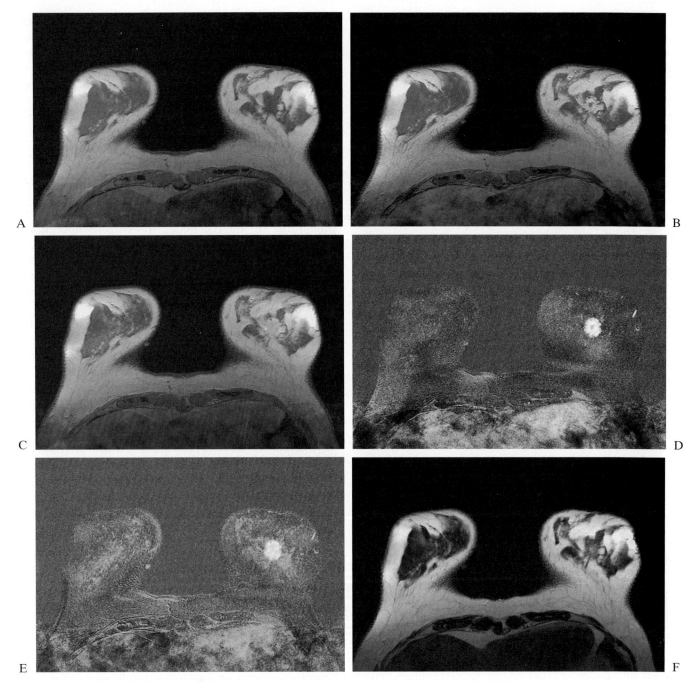

FIGURE 7.5. Mass-related enhancement in a duct-invasive cancer (left breast). (A) Precontrast T1-weighted gradient echo sequence (GE) of the dynamic series. (B) Early postcontrast T1-weighted GE of the dynamic series. (C) Postinitial postcontrast T1-weighted GE of the dynamic series. (D) Early postcontrast subtracted. (E) Postinitial postcontrast subtracted. (F) T2-weighted TSE image. Note that the lesion has a clear correlate on the precontrast T1-weighted GE (A) images. Note the mass effect in pre- and postcontrast images (A–E) and T2-weighted images (F). This is the classic breast MRI appearance of invasive breast cancer. Note the irregular margins and the strong enhancement in the early postcontrast phase (B and D) with washout in the postinitial phase, visible as signal intensity loss (C and E). Note the rim enhancement in the early postcontrast phase (B and D) while this appearance is lost in the postinitial phase (C and E) due to centripetal enhancement. Relatively high signal intensity on T2-weighted image (F)—this would, in this case, not reduce the level of suspicion. As morphology (including internal architecture) and enhancement kinetics are both suspicious, the lesion can be classified as BI-RADS 5.

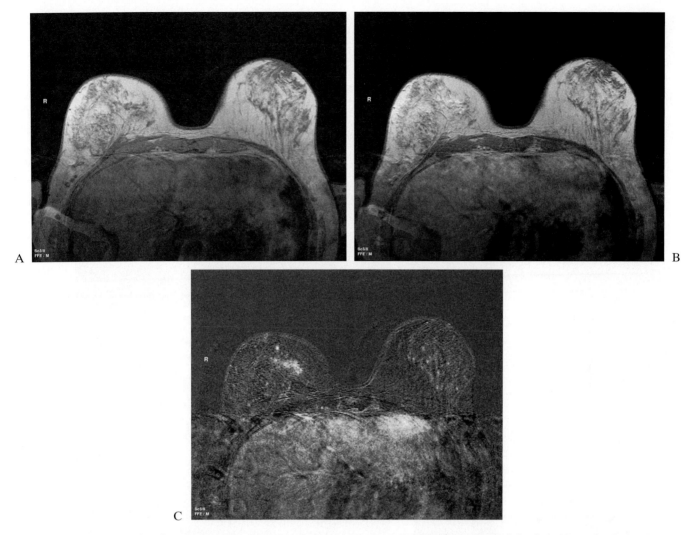

FIGURE 7.6. Nonmass-related enhancement. Nonmass-related enhancement in a DCIS (right breast). (A) precontrast T1-weighted GE of the dynamic series. (B) Ppostcontrast T1-weighted GE of the dynamic series. (C) Ppostcontrast subtracted. Note that the lesion has a no clear correlate on the precontrast T1-weighted GE (A) images. It seems as if the existing parenchymal enhanced after contrast injection. Note the lack of mass effect in precontrast images (A). Note the rather shallow enhancement. Note absence of enhancement in the left breast. Note the segmental configuration of the lesion. With the asymmetric, segmental configuration, the lesion must be classified as at least BI-RADS 4, irrespective of enhancement kinetics.

even if a washout happens, because subtracted images refer to the precontrast signal intensity); in these cases, only the signal time plot reveals that a washout is present. Malignant lesions tend to exhibit a plateau (type 2, about 30%) or even a washout (type 3, about 60%) pattern.

If a lesion shows only slow enhancement, we do *not* necessarily plot the signal time course. The reason is that in lesions with slow enhancement, the time course in the postinitial and late postcontrast period will virtually always be a persistent (type 1a) or (rarely) a plateau (type 2) time course (Figure 7.9). An (admittedly speculative) explanation is that malignant lesions with slow enhancement are usually not particularly hypervascular: for example, they may lack, for one reason or another, angiogenic activity. However, if that is the case, the arteriovenous shunts or the increased capillary permeability that are thought to cause the washout will probably not be present as well. Breast cancers with slow enhancement will usually always show a type 1a time course. So while in lesions with strong enhancement (strong angiogenic activity), there is differential diagnostic information provided by the different curve

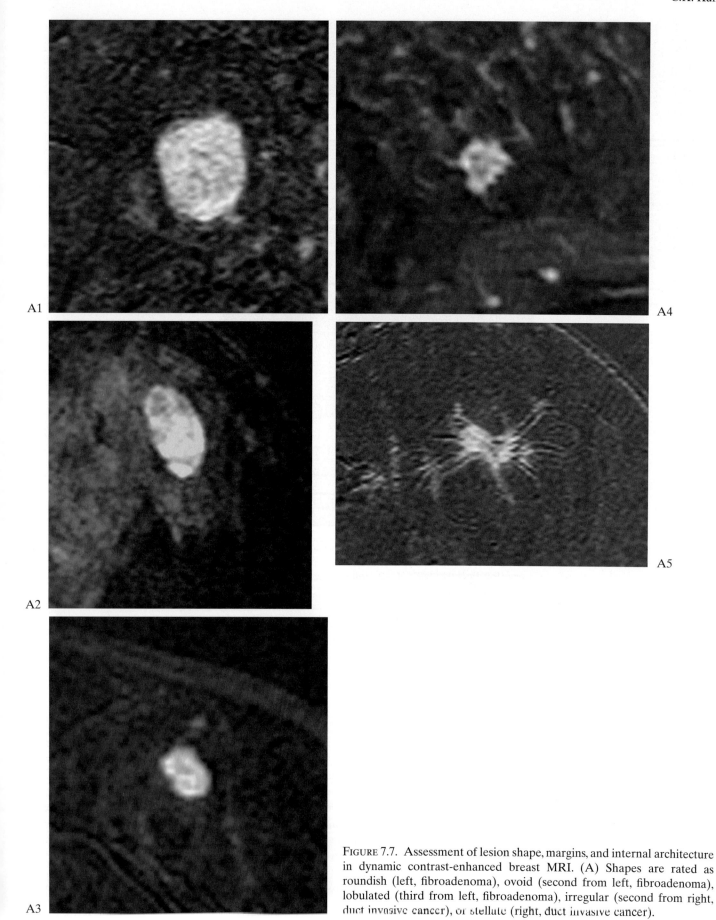

FIGURE 7.7. Assessment of lesion shape, margins, and internal architecture in dynamic contrast-enhanced breast MRI. (A) Shapes are rated as roundish (left, fibroadenoma), ovoid (second from left, fibroadenoma), lobulated (third from left, fibroadenoma), irregular (second from right, duct invasive cancer), or stellate (right, duct invasive cancer).

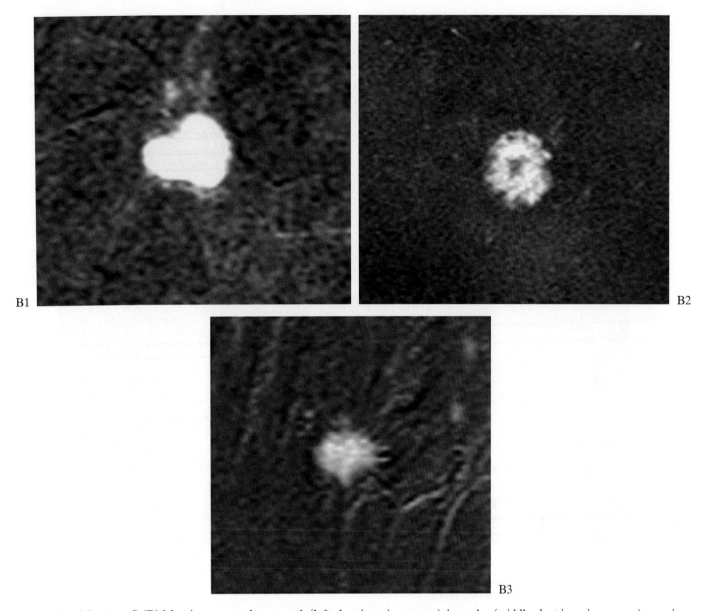

B1

B2

B3

FIGURE 7.7. (*Continued*) (B) Margins are rated as smooth (left, duct invasive cancer), irregular (middle, duct invasive cancer), or spiculated (right, tubular cancer).

(*Continued*)

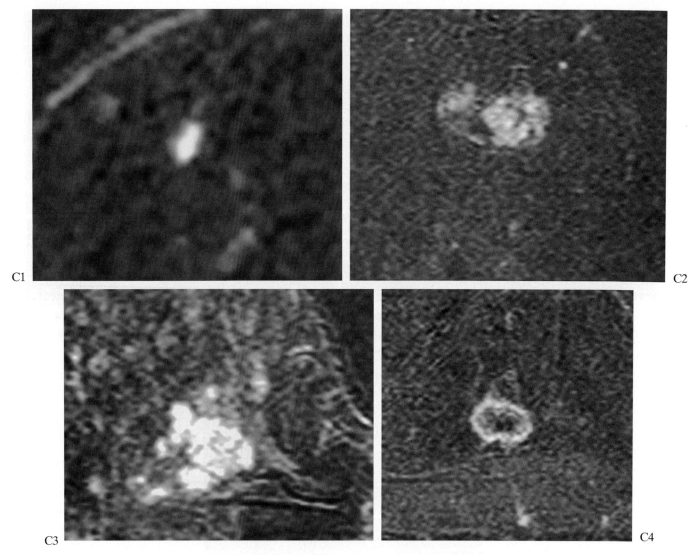

FIGURE 7.7. (*Continued*) (C) Internal architecture is rated as homogeneous (left, fibroadenoma), heterogeneous (second from left, fibroadenoma with regressive changes), internal septations (second from right, fibroadenoma), or rim enhancement (right, medullar invasive cancer).

shapes, this does not apply for lesions with slow enhancement. Accordingly, while in rapidly enhancing lesions, a persistent time course can help diagnose a benign tumor, this does not hold true for lesions with slow enhancement. In short, a time course analysis is only meaningful in lesions with rapid and strong enhancement (washin).

In lesions categorized as *focal mass*, after the kinetic analysis, we would refer to the non–fat-suppressed T2-weighted images[52] and evaluate its signal intensity with respect to the normal fibroglandular tissue (hyperintense, isointense, hypointense). Malignant lesions tend to have isointense or even hypointense signal compared with parenchyma; benign myxoid fibroadenomas and intramammary lymph nodes tend to show hyperintense signal; sclerotic fibroadenomas are as dark on T2-weighted images as invasive cancers, but as opposed to cancers, they do not enhance. Important exceptions to this rule are medullary and mucinous cancer (see following discussion).

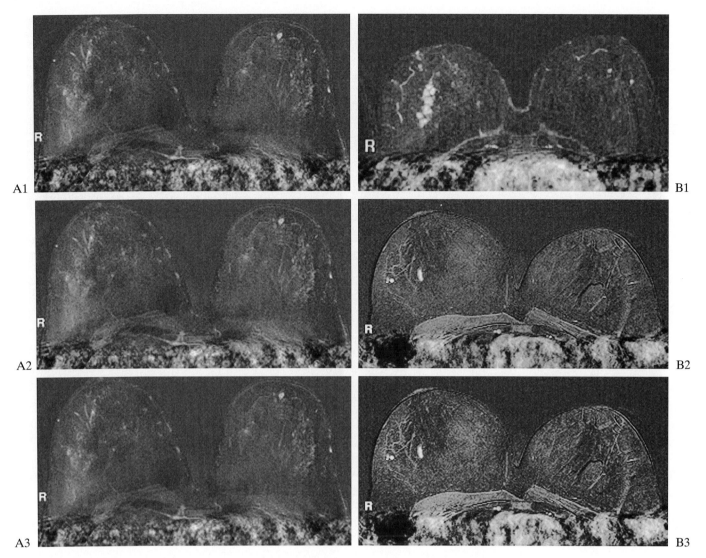

FIGURE 7.8. Assessment of distribution of nonmass-related enhancement in dynamic contrast enhanced breast MRI. (A) Distribution is rated as unifocal (left, papilloma), multifocal (middle, severe bilateral adenosis), diffuse (chronic subclinical mastitis in the left breast), segmental. (B) Segmental (left, DCIS in right breast), linear (middle, DCIS in right breast), or regional (right, DCIS in left breast). The unifocal, multifocal, or diffuse enhancement patterns in A are associated with a low PPV for DCIS and are usually managed by follow up. The segmental and linear and (to a lesser extent) the regional enhancement patterns are associated with a significant PPV for DCIS and are categorized as BI-RADS 4 (if kinetics are nonsuspicious) or BI-RADS 5 (if kinetics are suspicious) and are usually clarified by biopsy.

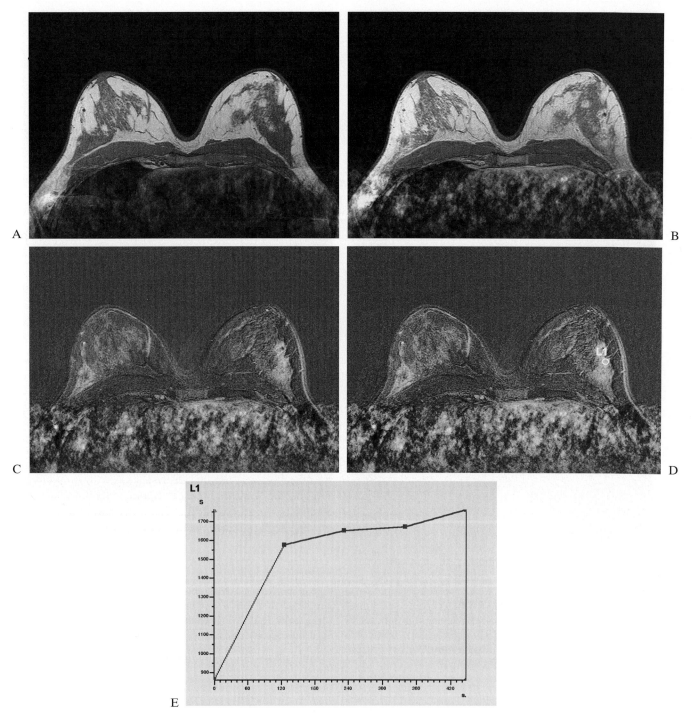

FIGURE 7.9. Invasive breast cancer in the left breast with "benign" enhancement kinetics; physiologic enhancement in the right breast. (A) Precontrast T1-weighted GE of the dynamic series. (B) Postcontrast T1-weighted GE of the dynamic series. (C) Postcontrast subtracted. (D) ROI placement. (E) Signal time course. Poorly differentiated breast cancer (G3) in the left breast in a 42-year-old patient. Note the relatively shallow enhancement and persistent time course. Note, however, the irregular shape of the mass, its irregular margins, and its heterogeneous internal architecture. Compare the slowly enhancing cancer in the left breast with the enhancement in the right breast. In the right breast, there is nonmass-related, regional enhancement in the lateral aspects of the outer quadrant. This is the typical site and aspect of physiologic glandular enhancement.

9. Lesion Categorization: How We Integrate Morphologic and Kinetic Information

- If an enhancing focal mass shows clear malignant features on morphologic assessment (i.e., a stellate shape or borders with spicules or a rim internal architecture), the lesion is usually categorized as BI-RADS 5 irrespective of enhancement kinetics.
- If a lesion is classified as *nonmass related* and shows a segmental enhancement with granular internal architecture or linear-branching enhancement, we recommend biopsy irrespective of kinetics; if these lesions exhibit rapid enhancement and/or washout, they are called BI-RADS 5; with slow or intermediate, persistent or plateau enhancement, the lesions are called BI-RADS 4 (Figure 7.10).
- If a focal mass shows indeterminate or suspicious morphology, but none of the previously mentioned features. For example, if it shows irregular shape and nonsmooth

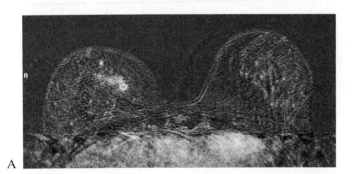

A

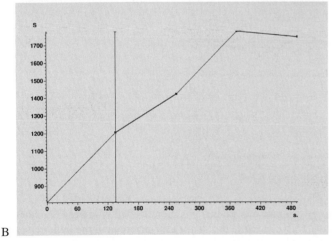

B

FIGURE 7.10. Intraductal cancer in the right breast with "benign" enhancement kinetics. (A) Ppostcontrast subtracted image with ROI in the DCIS seen in Figure 7.6. (B) Corresponding signal time course. There is only shallow and slowly progressive enhancement in this lesion. However, the configuration of the lesion (segmental enhancement) correctly suggests presence of DCIS. Ductal carcinoma in situ can show this type of "benign" enhancement kinetics in up to 40% of cases.

borders and heterogeneous architecture, we refer to kinetics for further categorization. We call it probably malignant if it has a rapid enhancement and washout (BI-RADS 5). We call it suspicious (BI-RADS 4) if it has intermediate enhancement and a persistent or plateau time course. We call it probably benign (BI-RADS 3, hormonal stimulation) and recommend follow up if it shows slow enhancement and a persistent time course, provided there is no suspicious correlate on mammography or breast ultrasound.

- If a focal mass shows benign shape and border characteristics *and* shows a benign internal architecture [low signal intensity internal septations on postcontrast (non)subtracted images and/or T2-weighted images], the lesion is categorized as a BI-RADS 2 irrespective of enhancement kinetics (the NPV of internal septations is higher than the PPV of, e.g., a washout).
- If a focal mass with benign appearing shape and borders lacks internal septations (and only shows homogeneous internal enhancement), categorization depends on kinetics: if it shows persistent or plateau enhancement, it is classified as BI-RADS 2 or 3 (depending on the personal risk status of the patient). If such a lesion shows a washout, we call it suspicious (BI-RADS 4) and recommend biopsy (Figure 7.11).
- We would always refer to the precontrast non–fat-suppressed images in T1- and T2-weighted pulse sequences to identify precontrast high signal intensity within an enhancing lesion, which would be indicative of fat necrosis or lymph node. In lesions with rim enhancement, we carefully check whether the enhancement actually occurs within the lesion (as opposed to around the lesion, the latter being indicative of a complicated cyst, see Figure 7.12).

There are some key features that allow a *definite* diagnosis; all of them are based on lesion morphology (which underscores the importance of having a good spatial resolution). Masses with stellate shape, and/or spicules, and/or rim enhancement, or nonmass-related enhancement with ductal (linear) or segmental configuration (and clumped internal architecture) are called suspicious irrespective of enhancement kinetics.

In turn, a washout usually prompts biopsy irrespective of morphology (usually with a BI-RADS 4 diagnostic category), with the following exceptions: morphologically benign lesions with clearly visible internal low-signal septations (fibroadenomas) or with rim enhancement secondary to internal fatty tissue as revealed by precontrast non–fat-suppressed images (lymph node).

If morphology and kinetics point in the same direction, then the lesion is considered either probably malignant (BI-RADS 5) or benign (BI-RADS 2). If morphology and kinetics point in different directions, then the lesion is considered suspicious (BI-RADS 4) or probably benign

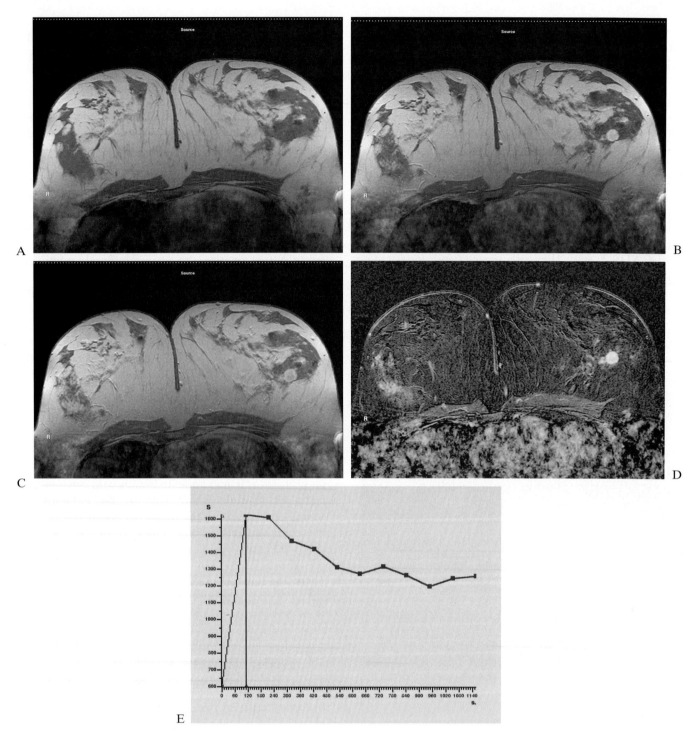

FIGURE 7.11. Invasive breast cancer with "benign" appearing morphologic features. (A) Precontrast T1-weighted GE image of the dynamic series. (B) First postcontrast T1-weighted GE image of the dynamic series. (C) Fourth postcontrast T1-weighted GE image of the dynamic series. (D) Postcontrast subtracted image of the first postcontrast image. (E) Signal time course. Duct invasive cancer with adjacent DCIS in a 56-year-old patient. Note that the tumor exhibits benign morphologic features (roundish or lob- ulated shape, smooth margins, homogeneous internal architec- ture). However, note the strong enhancement in the initial phase, followed by a strong washout of contrast agent which is already appreciable visually (compare C with B) and is also seen on the corresponding signal time course (E). In such a tumor with benign-appearing morphologic features, presence of a washout leads to a BI-RADS 4 category and requires biopsy.

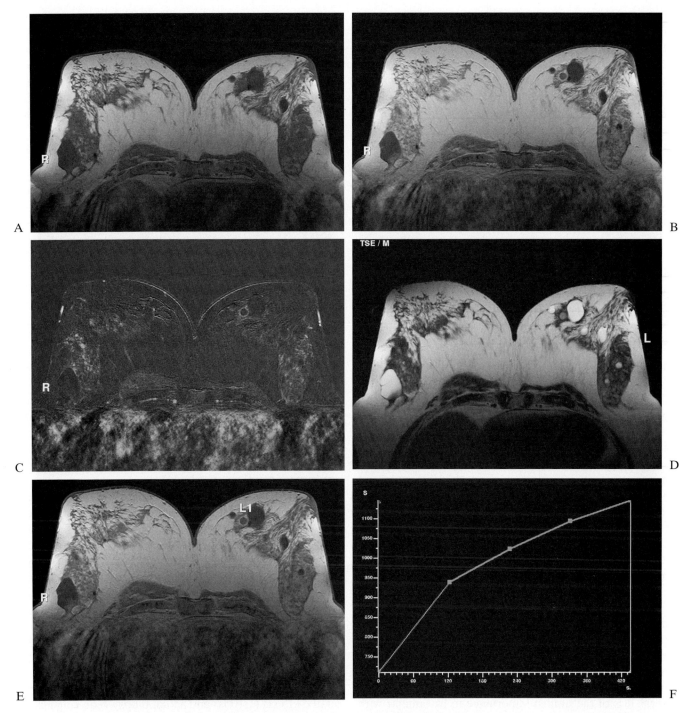

FIGURE 7.12. Significant fibrocystic disease in a 48-year-old patient. (A) Precontrast T1-weighted GE of the dynamic series. (B) Postinitial phase postcontrast T1-weighted GE of the dynamic series. (C) Postinitial phase postcontrast subtracted of the dynamic series. (D) T2-weighted TSE image. (E) T2-weighted TSE image. (F) ROI placement and signal time course. Note the mass with roundish shape in the upper inner quadrant of the left breast. Note that the lesion is hypointense in the T1-weighted precontrast image in A, and moderately hyperintense in T2-weighted image in D (brighter than the fibroglandular tissue, but somewhat darker than the cysts that are present in all quadrants). Note the smooth margins of the lesion in precontrast images (A). Note that the lesion shows a "rim" enhancement in B and C, but note that the enhancement does not occur within the lesion (as delineated in A), but in the tissue *around* the lesion. Note slowly progressive enhancement in the time course (F). This is a cyst with proteinaceous fluid (hence the relatively low SI of this cyst in T2-weighted TSE compared with the signal of the other cysts) and with inflammatory changes around it. With the findings mentioned here, this lesion can be safely categorized as BI-RADS 2.

(BI-RADS 3), depending on the type of criteria as mentioned previously.

These guidelines are not carved in stone, but they have to be adapted to the individual situation by considering clinical findings, the findings in conventional imaging modalities, patient age, her medical history including menstrual status or hormone medication, and, in particular, family history of breast cancer (with particular attention paid to women in families with early onset breast or ovarian cancer or combined breast and ovarian cancer). Still, to help the inexperienced reader to find his or her way through the different diagnostic criteria, a scoring system such as the one proposed by Fischer may be useful.

10. Appearance of the Normal and the Diseased Breast in Dynamic Contrast-enhanced Breast Magnetic Resonance Imaging

10.1. The Normal Breast

As with virtually all glandular tissue of the human body (e.g., salivary glands, pancreas, prostate), the fibroglandular tissue of the breast shows contrast enhancement. Fortunately enough, if one compares the breast fibroglandular tissue with, for example, the pancreas or the parotid gland, enhancement is far less pronounced; this is certainly at least in part due to the fact that the breast parenchyma consists not only of glandular, but also, and to a variable extent, of fibrous and fatty tissue. The comparison with other glands of the human body is, however, still quite instructive because it helps understand what degree of contrast enhancement may be still normal in a breast with predominantly glandular components. In addition, because the breast is a hormone-reactive organ that responds to endogenous (ovarian hormones) or exogenous (replacement therapy) hormonal stimuli, what is looked on as the *normal* breast changes steadily, depending on patient's age, menstrual/menopausal state, and hormonal or antihormonal medication. When starting with breast MRI in general, it is of the utmost importance to be familiar with the variable aspect of the breast parenchyma.

While the fibroglandular tissue usually starts to enhance only in the late postcontrast phase, there are some exceptions to this rule. There are no prevalence data available so far, but based on clinical experience we would propose that about 10% of women (prevalence decreasing with increasing age) exhibit intermediate or strong enhancement already in the postinitial phase, which may interfere with even the mere detection of small breast cancers. Very much like in the mammographically dense breast (i.e., ACR 4 breasts), where breast cancers may be obscured by the parenchyma and where, accordingly, mammographic sensitivity is limited, the strong and multifocal enhancement may obscure enhancing breast cancers. Therefore, we call this an *MRI dense breast*, in order to communicate that the sensitivity (and the negative predictive value) of the respective breast MRI study is limited (Figure 7.13). This is important because it may impact clinical decision making.

Regarding the differentiation of a diffusely growing breast cancer and diffuse parenchymal enhancement: Usually, normal parenchymal enhancement is strongest in the lateral (and upper) aspects of the breast, whereas the inner (and lower) quadrants are relatively spared. Compared with single breast imaging, bilateral imaging is advantageous in this situation because it shows that the enhancement is symmetric and bilateral (Figure 7.13); bilateral diffuse breast cancer is relatively rare.

Particularly in the very young premenopausal patient (at or below the age of 35 years), hormonal influences may also appear as *focal* areas (always nonmass-related enhancement without correlate on precontrast T1- and T2-weighted images) with strong contrast enhancement that may mimic malignant (and benign) lesions. It seems that these *lesions* correspond to the hormone-responsive part of the parenchyma; they should not be mixed up with true, biopsy-requiring lesions. The incidence of these spontaneous contrast-enhancing lesions or *unidentified breast objects* (UBOs) is highest in the first and fourth week of a menstrual cycle, where significantly less enhancement is encountered in the second week.

While in most cases hormone-induced enhancement will be easily classified as such, in particular in very young patients (i.e., younger than 35 years of age), the morphologic (and kinetic) features of hormone-induced enhancement may even mimic malignant lesions. Morphology is usually not pathognomonic. In fact, smooth margins and a benign shape is rare; usually, shape is irregular (but not stellate) and margins are nonsmooth (but no spicules). Enhancement rates are usually intermediate, but can be fast; in the latter case, however, a persistent time course (or a plateau) is seen in the vast majority of cases.[25]

Accordingly, a clear distinction between hormone-related effects (UBOs) and actual biopsy-requiring lesions is often enough difficult, if not impossible (Figure 7.14). Hormonal stimulation should be considered as differential diagnosis *only* in the following settings:

- The patient is premenopausal or on HRT.
- The patient is not on selective estrogen receptor modulator (SERM) therapy (e.g., tamoxifen), with selective estrogen receptor modulators, spontaneous, hormonal-induced enhancement should not occur, such that in these clinical settings, UBO is not an acceptable differential.

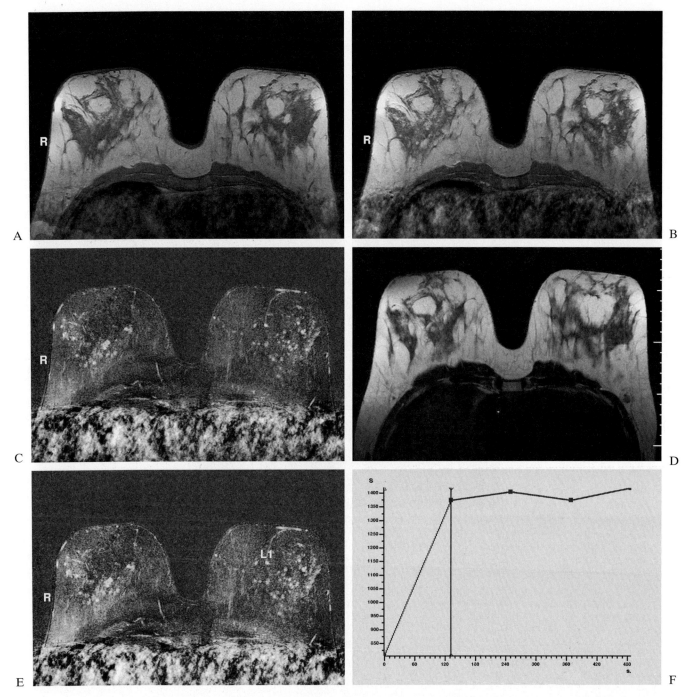

FIGURE 7.13. Diffuse parenchymal enhancement: the MR dense breast. (A) Precontrast T1-weighted GE of the dynamic series. (B) Postcontrast T1-weighted GE of the dynamic series. (C) Post-contrast subtracted. (D) T2-weighted TSE image. (E) ROI placement. (F) Signal time course. Note the multifocal, diffuse enhancement of the entire parenchyma of both breasts. Note the symmetry of lesions. This is what we would call an *MR dense breast*, with the same diagnostic implication as an "ACR 4 parenchymal pattern" has for the mammographic diagnosis. Among the multifocally enhancing lesions, it is virtually impossible to rule out presence of small invasive (or intraductal) cancers. Accordingly, the sensitivity of breast MRI is substantially reduced (as is the sensitivity of mammography in ACR 4 breasts). Also, the diffuse multifocal enhancement has about the same PPV for intraductal or invasive cancers as diffuse calcifications on a mammogram have—in fact, the PPV is low.

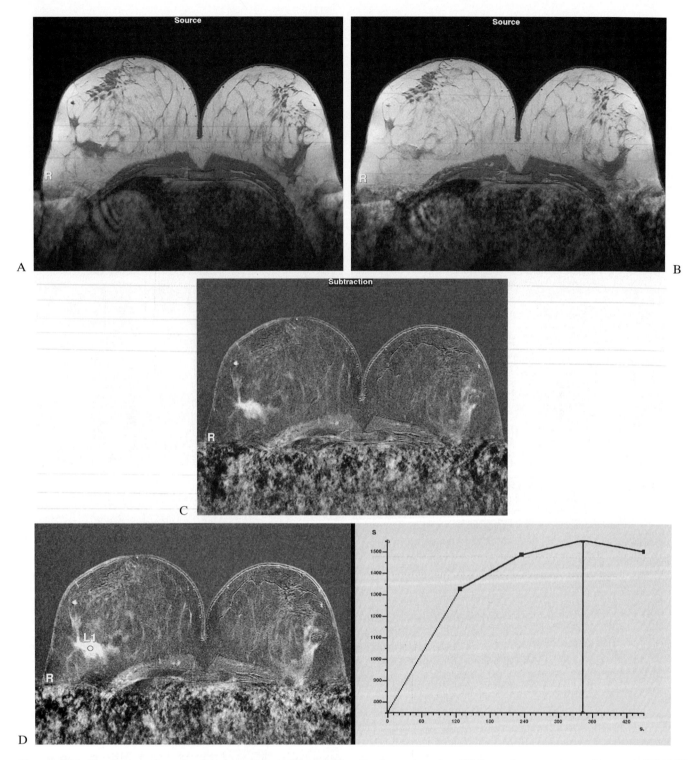

FIGURE 7.14. Focal parenchymal enhancement in a 33-year-old patient: the *UBOs*. (A) Precontrast T1-weighted GE of the dynamic series. (B) Second postcontrast T1-weighted GE of the dynamic series. (C) Second postcontrast subtracted. (D) ROI placement and signal time course.

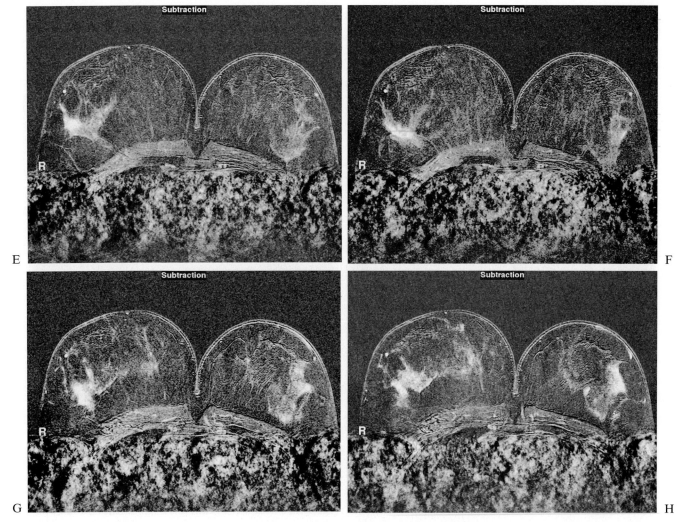

FIGURE. 7.14. (*Continued*) (E–H) Further postcontrast subtracted sections through both breasts. The study was performed in the third week of her menstrual cycle. Note the multiple areas of enhancement, predominantly in the lateral aspect of the outer quadrants, in both breasts. It is "nonmass-related," and it appears irregular, with a fast washin (washin rate: 80%/first minute), but with a persistent curve type. Note that the "lesions" are visible bilaterally, which helps categorize them as "probably hormonal induced." The patient did not have a personal or family history of breast cancer. She had a vague palpable lesion in the upper inner quadrant of the right breast, plus an asymmetric mammographic density in this area; no associated calcifications. The "lesions" visible here had no correlate on mammography, ultrasound, or on clinical examination. They were read as "probably benign" (BI-RADS 3), and the patient was put on 6 months follow up which, in the second week of her menstrual cycle, still revealed enhancement, but in an entirely different geographic pattern. After that, she had a 2-year uneventful followup.

- The lesion has no correlate on mammography or breast ultrasound (directed breast ultrasound with knowledge of MRI findings).
- The lesion corresponds to *nonmass-related enhancement*.
- The lesion does not exhibit a washout time course.

If in a premenopausal patient, an incidental contrast enhancing lesion is seen that fulfills all these criteria, we recommend follow up rather than biopsy.

10.2. Malignant Lesions

10.2.1. Invasive Breast Cancers

The *typical* ductal invasive breast cancer presents as a focal mass with irregular shape (or even stellate shape), irregular borders (or even spicules), and heterogeneous internal architecture (or even rim enhancement) (Figure 7.15). It is important to note that fine anatomic details such as spicules and also rim enhancement in small lesions can

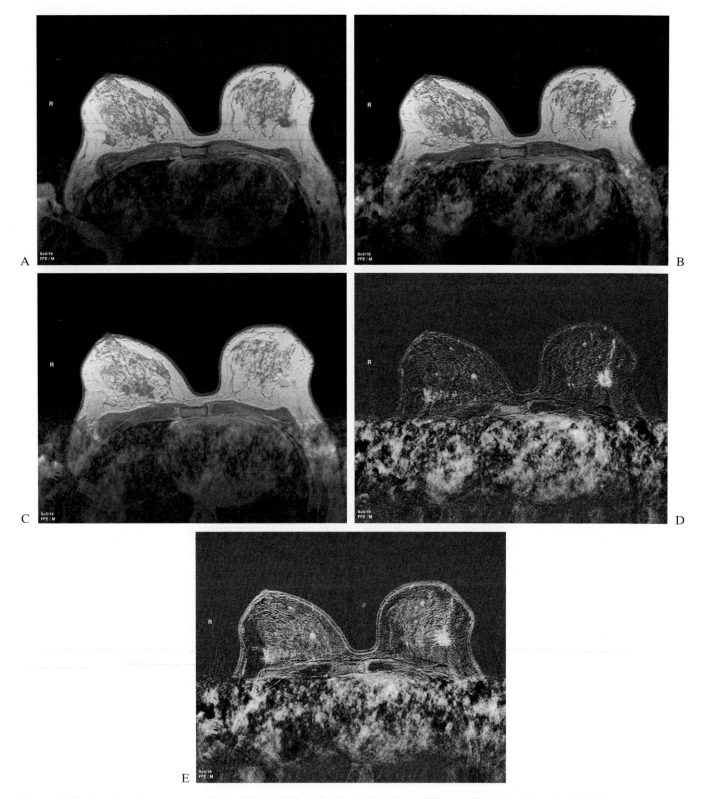

FIGURE 7.15. Invasive breast cancer in a 48-year-old patient. (A) Precontrast T1-weighted GE of the dynamic series. (B) First postcontrast T1-weighted GE of the dynamic series. (C) Fourth postcontrast image of the dynamic series. (D) First postcontrast subtracted image of the dynamic series. (E) Fourth postcontrast subtracted image of the dynamic series.

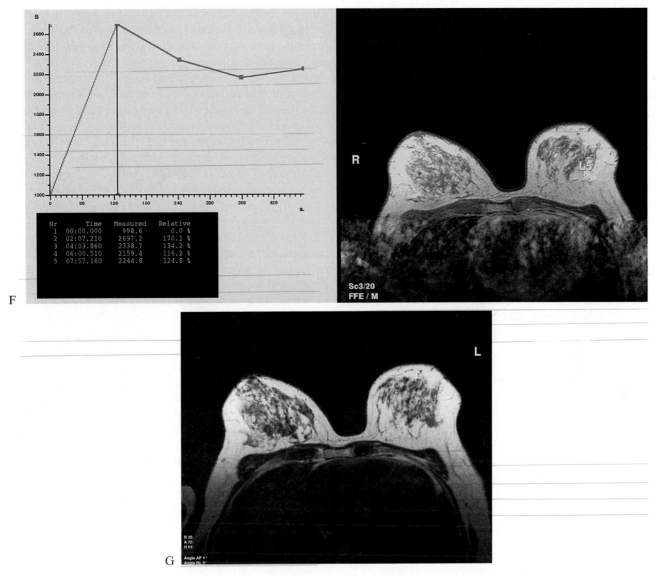

FIGURE 7.15. (*Continued*) (F) ROI placement and signal time course. (G) T2-weighted TSE image. A 48-year-old patient with a mammographically and sonographically visible mass in the upper outer quadrant which was rated as BI-RADS 5. The patient presented for preoperative breast MRI for staging. In the upper outer quadrant of the left breast, there is a suspicious mass. This is the "typical" appearance of an invasive breast cancer in dynamic breast MRI (BI-RADS 5) Note the focal mass is a roundish shape, with spiculated margins, internal architecture reveals rim enhancement (note that the enhancing rim is within the mass, as opposed to the cyst with enhancement in Figure 7.12). Note that rim enhancement is only seen in the early postcontrast phase, whereas there is a progressive filling in over the dynamic series. Note the strong and early enhancement (washin rate is 170% in the first 2min) and the immediate and strong washout. The washout is visible by the time course, but also in the nonsubtracted (compare B and C) and subtracted images (compare D and E). This is due to the very strong washout in this case; often enough, the washout is not perceivable on the images, but is only visualized by the enhancement curves. Note the linear enhancement next to the mass which was due to an intraductal extension. Note the enhancing lesions on the contralateral breast. In fact, the patient had a mammographically and sonographically occult DCIS in her right breast (the DCIS in her right breast is seen in Figures 7.5 and 7.10).

only be appreciated with high spatial resolution imaging (e.g., 512 imaging matrix if a bilateral field of view is used). Washin rates are fast, in our setting well beyond 80% signal increase in the early postcontrast period, followed by a washout (type 3) or plateau (type 2) time course pattern in the postinitial and late postcontrast period. In T2-weighted TSE images, invasive breast cancers tend to exhibit a low SI, isointense or even hypointense, with respect to the adjacent parenchyma.

Most of the invasive lobular breast cancers exhibit the same MRI appearance as ductal invasive cancers: focal mass, irregular morphology, rim enhancement, and so forth. However, in about 10% to 20% of the cases, the tumor grows diffusely, without forming an actual nodule or mass. In these cases, the tumor gradually replaces the existing parenchyma with the typical *single cell* grow pattern. In these cases, lobular breast cancer may present as diffuse, *nonmass-related enhancement*. To make things worse, these types of lobular cancers are not associated with significant angiogenic activity, such that enhancement may be only intermediate, and (rarely) even only low (Figure 7.16). In these cases (and as explained previously), the postinitial and late postcontrast enhancement pattern (curve type) may not be used for further differential diagnosis, because shallow enhancement rates are usually always associated with a persistent time course (type 1a), deceivingly shallow and slow; usually, this is then associated with a persistent, type 1a enhancement pattern. Accordingly, if lobular invasive cancer is in the differential diagnosis, enhancement kinetics can only be used for diagnosis if they are *positive* for cancer (rapid and strong enhancement and washout); if the kinetic pattern is benign or indeterminate, this cannot be used to alleviate the indication to biopsy. Unfortunately, one should be prepared to see lobular breast cancer more often in breast MRI than one would expect it based on its natural prevalence; this tumor is difficult to diagnose mammographically and may cause nonspecific mammographic changes, which may prompt a referral to breast MRI. Accordingly, in our series of breast cancers detected by breast MRI, lobular cancers make up as much as 23% of cases. Still, diffusely growing invasive lobular cancer with slow enhancement is rare; the most important differential diagnosis is chronic (subclinical) mastitis, and sometimes hormone-induced enhancement. Because in most of these cases, the enhancing area is fairly large, it is an easy target for a direct MRI-guided plain or vacuum-assisted biopsy. Also, because hormone-induced enhancement is much more frequent than diffuse lobular cancer, and because it is usually rapidly changing, short-term follow up is a strategy to help avoid unnecessary biopsies.

Medullary invasive cancer is a relatively uncommon entity that occurs in young patients (aged 30–35 years or, rarely, age 39). It has distinct morphologic features that are different from virtually all other invasive breast cancers. On imaging studies as well as on macroscopic and (often enough) even microscopic anatomy, it appears well circumscribed, with smooth, pushing margins. Only on high magnification is the actual invasive growth visualized. Accordingly, it is the most important differential diagnosis versus *myxoid fibroadenoma* if a well-circumscribed focal mass is identified in young patients. What seems particularly helpful in breast MRI as opposed to mammography and breast ultrasound is the fact that internal architecture is usually either heterogeneous (which is rarely seen in fibroadenomas), or there is even rim enhancement. Also, enhancement kinetics can help with the diagnosis: if a washout phenomenon is seen in a well-circumscribed, roundish lesion with strong enhancement, this should prompt biopsy (as long as no internal septations are visible). It is important to consider this diagnosis in patients with a strong family history of breast cancer (in particular patients with family members who were diagnosed with breast cancer at age 35 or younger), or patients in whom a genetic predisposition has been identified (BRCA1 or BRCA2 mutation carriers; Figure 7.17).

Mucinous breast cancer (Figure 7.18) is a highly differentiated breast cancer that usually affects elderly women; it is characterized by abundant accumulation of mucin. Depending on the degree of mucinous components, enhancement rates in dynamic breast MRI vary between fast (for lesions with mainly solid parts and only little mucin) to intermediate (with increasing mucin load) and even almost absent (for lesions that mainly consist of mucin with only a very thin rim of solid tissue around it, see Refs. 30 and 68). In the latter case, the thin rim of solid tissue around the mucin-filled wide interstitial spaces is so fine that it cannot be resolved with MRI. The clue to the diagnosis is the T2-weighted TSE pulse sequence. Here, the mucin-laden cancers appear exceptionally bright, with a signal that is even higher than that of fatty tissue, at least as bright as cysts. So if a lesion with irregular shape and margins, heterogeneous internal architecture (or rim enhancement) and with indeterminate or benign appearing enhancement kinetics exhibits a strikingly bright signal on T2-weighted TSE, mucinous cancer is a differential diagnosis.

Tubular cancer (Figure 7.19) is again a highly differentiated breast cancer (always grade 1) that occurs in middle-aged women. This cancer tends to grow as multifocal or multicentric or even bilateral lesions. Owing to its relatively benign biologic behavior, it is often treated by wide excision; then, however, an accurate staging (e.g., by bilateral MRI) is of utmost importance due to its tendency to multicentric growth. The tumor usually exhibits suspicious morphologic features (spicules, stellate lesions). There is an association between radial scars and tubular cancers; because radial scars exhibit a cancer-like morphology and because they can enhance as breast cancers, it is usually not possible to identify tubular cancer within a radial scar on dynamic breast MRI.

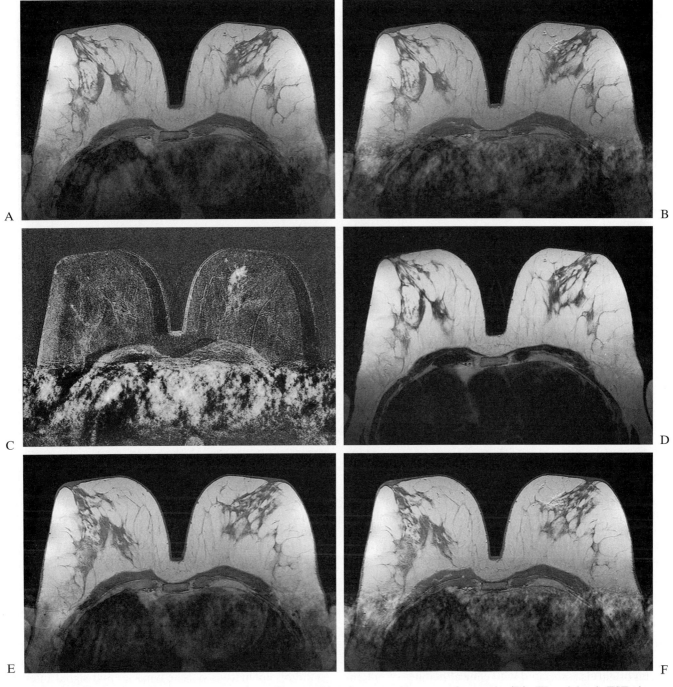

FIGURE 7.16. Lobular invasive breast cancer in a 62-year-old patient. Two consecutive sections of a dynamic breast MRI study: Section 1, (A) precontrast T1-weighted GE of the dynamic series, (B) first postcontrast T1-weighted GE of the dynamic series, (C) first postcontrast subtracted, (D) T2-weighted TSE image. Section 2, (E) precontrast T1-weighted GE of the dynamic series, (F) first postcontrast T1-weighted GE of the dynamic series,

(*Continued*)

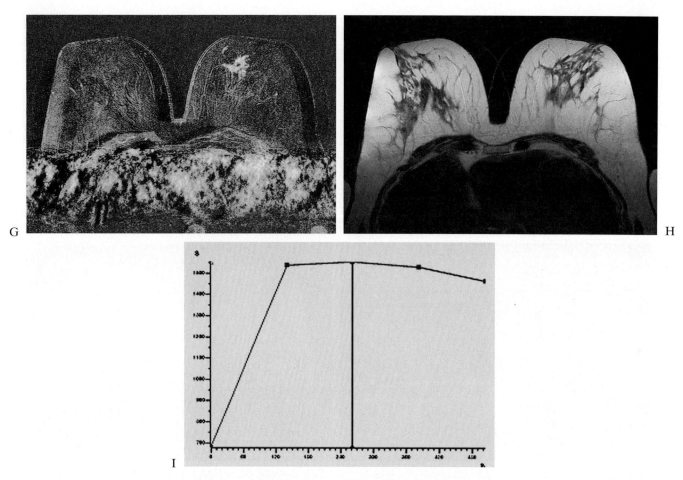

FIGURE 7.16. (*Continued*) (G) first postcontrast subtracted, (H) T2-weighted TSE image, (I) time/signal intensity course. Note the discrete architectural distortion of the parenchyma in the nonsubtracted images. Note the almost "nonmass-related" enhancement that occurs in the upper inner quadrant of the left breast. The existing parenchyma is replaced by tumor tissue—the typical growth pattern of lobular invasive cancer. Note that the tumor grows around fatty tissue, such that there are "inclusions" of fatty tissue in the tumor. This must not be confused with fatty tissue (or bright signal on precontrast T1-weighted images) in focal masses in fat necrosis or in complicated cysts. There is strong early enhancement followed by a plateau time course. The most important differential diagnoses to be mentioned here are lobular invasive cancer, DCIS, and chronic mastitis.

Inflammatory breast cancer (Figure 7.20) is a clinical rather than a distinct pathologic entity. It is diagnosed in cases in which an invasive breast cancer (usually of ductal origin) is associated with clinical findings of inflammation, that is, cutaneous edema and erythema. On histopathology, there is extensive tumor involvement of the lymphatic system. It is important to know that breast cancer that spreads within the lymphatics does not go along with enhancement. This holds true for the primary lymphangitic spread seen in inflammatory breast cancer, but also for lymphatic invasion around a focal breast cancer. Accordingly, depending on the extent of tumor within the lymphatic channels, the breast cancer may exhibit only subtle enhancement (slowly progressive on kinetic assessment), and may even not enhance at all. In the latter cases, there is usually only dermal thickening and edema, interstitial edema (best appreciated on T2-weighted images) and variable cutaneous enhancement. Sometimes the actual tumor stands out against the surrounding edematous parenchyma as low signal intensity mass on T2-weighted TSE images. Because (puerperal or nonpuerperal) mastitis can show the same clinical features and enhancement pattern as inflammatory breast cancer, breast MRI cannot be used to reliably distinguish between these disease entities. The only role of MRI (if any) is to demonstrate the extent of the disease and to monitor response to chemotherapy.

10.2.2. Preinvasive Cancer (DCIS)

Although there are reports in the current literature stating that microcalcifications can be visualized by

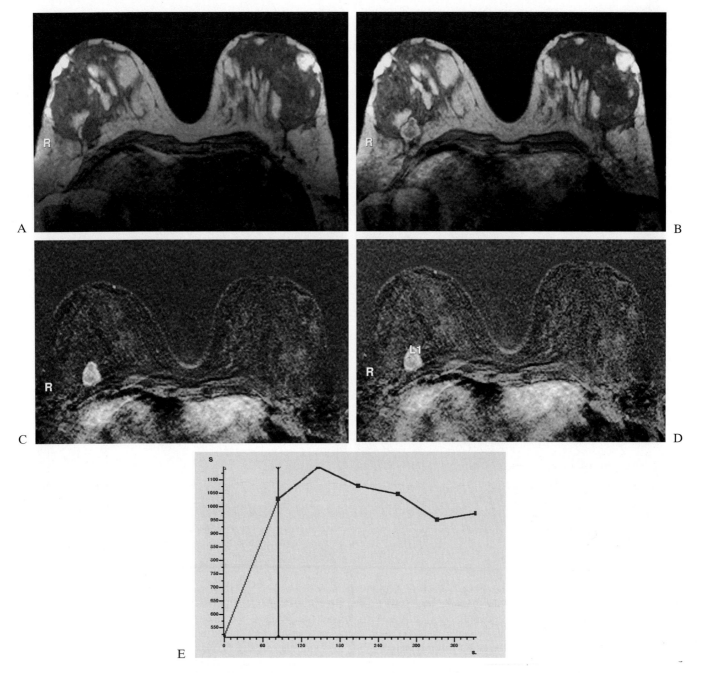

FIGURE 7.17. Medullary invasive breast cancer in a 34-year-old patient at high familial risk for breast cancer. (A) Precontrast T1-weighted GE of the dynamic series. (B) First postcontrast T1-weighted GE of the dynamic series. (C) First postcontrast subtracted. (D) ROI placement. (E) Time/signal intensity course. Note the pear-shaped, ovoid mass with completely smooth borders [borders that abut fatty tissue are best evaluated on pre-contrast, non–fat-suppressed images, i.e. Figure 7.18(A)]. This "benign" morphology with seemingly pushing margins is typical for medullary invasive breast cancer. It is the reason why this medullary cancer (as many others) were interperted as representing probably fibroadenoma on mammography and breast ultrasound. On breast MRI, however, internal (enhancement) architecture and enhancement kinetics help establish the correct diagnosis. Note the pronounced rim enhancement; note the suspicious kinetics with early and strong enhancement, followed by a washout. This helps classify this tumor as BI-RADS 5 [suspicious morphology (internal architecture) plus suspicious kinetics (washout)].

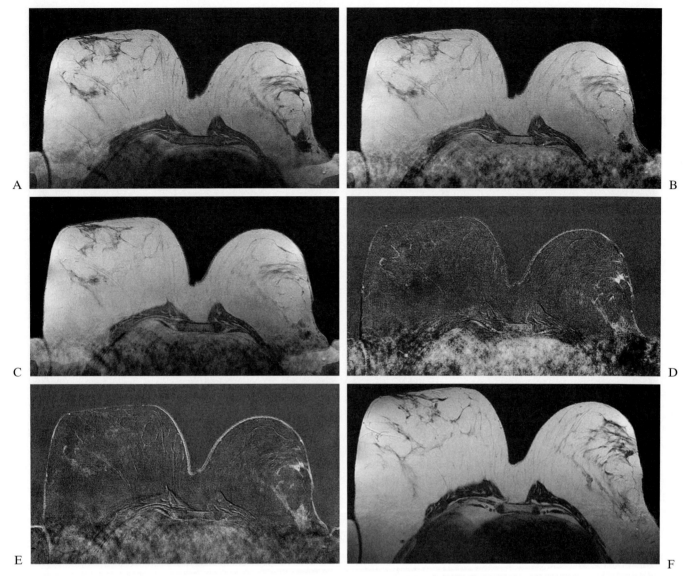

FIGURE 7.18. Mucinous breast cancer in a 71-year-old patient. (A) Precontrast T1-weighted GE of the dynamic series. (B) First postcontrast T1-weighted GE of the dynamic series. (C) Third postcontrast T1-weighted GE of the dynamic series. (D) First postcontrast subtracted. (E) Third postcontrast subtracted. (F) T2-weighted TSE. Note the trifocal breast cancer in (A) two foci in the retro-areolar region, one larger mass in the prepectoral area of the left breast. The two smaller lesions enhance strongly and homogeneously after contrast injection (B and D). However, the larger mass close to the chest wall reveals only very faint enhancement. Accordingly, the mass is hardly visible on postcontrast subtracted images (C) and is only seen in the late post-contrast phase (D). The reason for this is that the large mass is virtually completely filled with mucin, so that there is hardly any solid tumor tissue left. Due to the abundant mucin, the lesion reveals a very high signal on T2-weighted TSE images (F). For the same reason, the mass is hardly visible in T2-weighted TSE images, because in this patient, the mucin is isointense to the adjacent fatty tissue. The two smaller lesions behind the nipple consist of more solid tumor and less mucin; accordingly, they exhibit a lower SI in T2-weighted TSE, and the enhance homogeneously and strongly. Note that the actual extent of disease is best appreciated on precontrast non–fat-suppressed T1-weighted images (A).

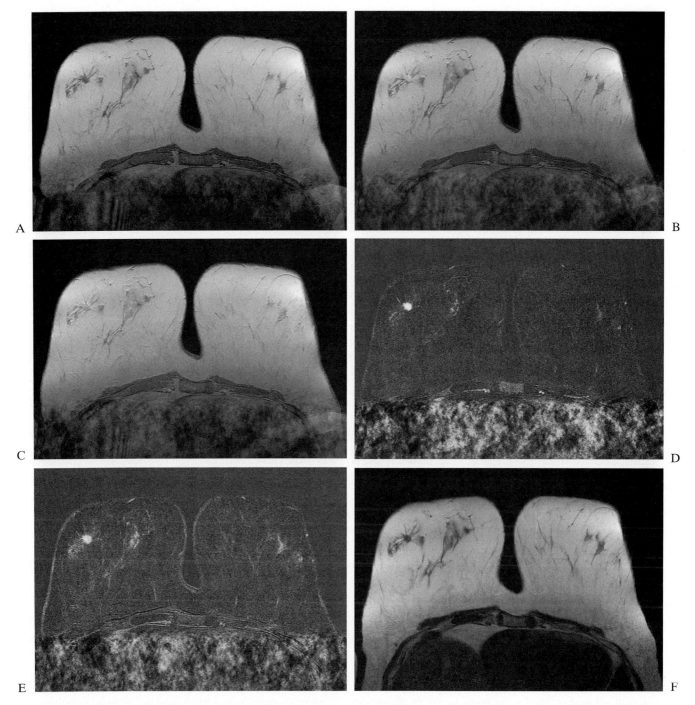

FIGURE 7.19. Multicentric invasive tubular cancer in a 60-year-old patient. Two sections of a dynamic breast MRI study through the lower quadrants (section 1) and the upper quadrants (section 2). Section 1, (A) precontrast T1-weighted GE of the dynamic series; (B) first postcontrast T1-weighted GE of the dynamic series; (C) third postcontrast T1-weighted GE image of the dynamic series; (D) first postcontrast subtracted; (E) third postcontrast subtracted; (F) T2-weighted TSE image. Section 2,

(Continued)

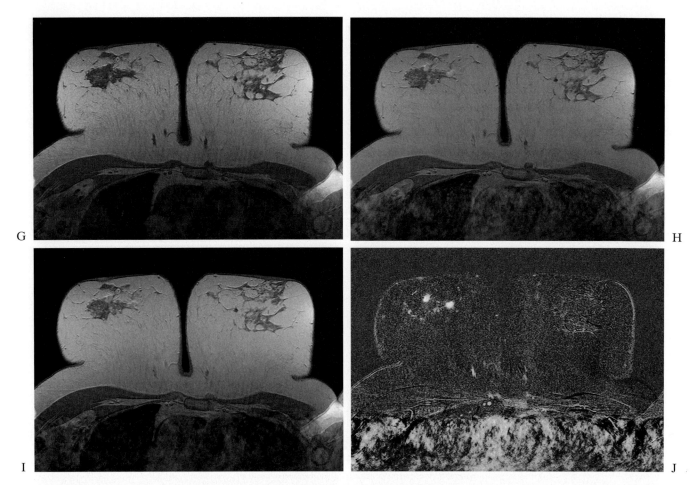

FIGURE 7.19. (*Continued*) (G) precontrast T1-weighted GE of the dynamic series; (H) first postcontrast T1-weighted GE of the dynamic series; (I) third postcontrast T1-weighted GE image of the dynamic series; (J) first postcontrast subtracted. (See Figure 7.20)

high-resolution breast MRI,[69] for current clinical practice, there is ample evidence confirming that microcalcifications (particularly the relevant, tiny ductal calcifications) are not visible on MRI even with high-resolution techniques. Accordingly, while the in situ cancers' propensity to form microcalcification constitutes the basis of DCIS diagnosis in mammography, this feature cannot be exploited for MRI of DCIS.

The criteria pertinent to diagnose invasive breast cancer in dynamic MRI may not be used to diagnose DCIS (or, rather, the absence of a focal mass with strong and early enhancement and washout may not be used to exclude DCIS), probably due to the variable angiogenic activity of in situ cancers, enhancement of DCIS in breast MRI is variable. Only about 30% of DCIS exhibits the typical *carcinoma-type*, strong enhancement and about 50% show

intermediate enhancement, another 15% exhibits slow enhancement, and about 5% do not enhance at all. This means that enhancement rates, but also the degree of enhancement, or the signal behavior in the postinitial and late postcontrast phase may (but not necessarily will) look benign. Diagnostic criteria based on contrast enhancement kinetics are therefore not reliable to exclude DCIS; rather, if they are suspicious, they can be used to confirm the diagnosis.

The actual diagnostic cornerstone of DCIS in dynamic breast MRI is based on lesion morphology or, rather, its configuration (Figures 7.6 and 7.21): the demonstration of nonmass-related enhancement that follows the ductal system, namely linear or asymmetric segmental enhancement (i.e., segmental enhancement that occurs in only one breast, as opposed to bilateral symmetric enhancement

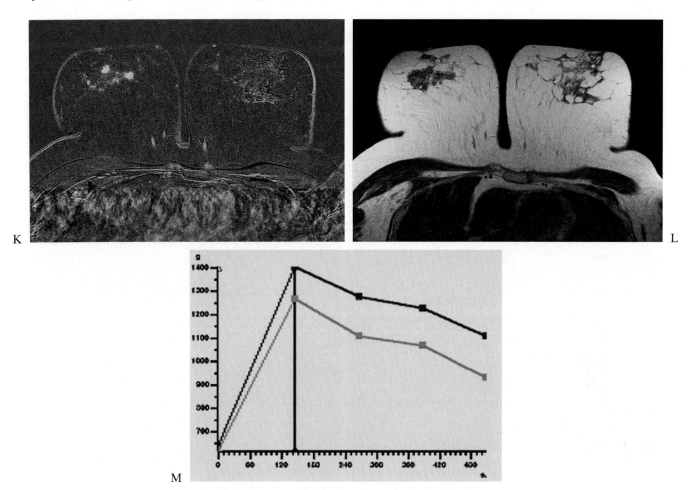

FIGURE 7.19. (*Continued*) (K) third postcontrast subtracted; (L) T2-weighted TSE image; (M) time/signal intensity course. Note the focal mass with roundish shape, spiculated borders [best seen on precontrast, non–fat-suppressed images, i.e., (A), with relatively homogenous internal architecture in the the lower outer quadrant in (A–F). Note the early and strong enhancement, which may sometimes appear segmental and is usually due to hormonal influences). Less often, DCIS is associated with nonmass-related regional or (uni)focal enhancement. An internal *clumped* or *cobblestone pattern* in DCIS with segmental, linear, or regional configuration is typical and should not be mistaken for low signal intensity septations seen in fibroadenomas. followed by a washout, which is visible in nonsubtracted and subtracted images (C and E). This lesion was visible on mammography and breast ultrasound. Note the two further foci in the upper quadrant at the 12 o'clock position, with identical enhancement pattern. Typical multicentric growth of tubular cancer.

which may sometimes appear segmental and is usually due to hormonal influences). Less often, DCIS is associated with nonmass-related regional or (uni)focal enhancement. An internal *clumped* or *cobblestone pattern* in DCIS with segmental, linear, or regional configuration is typical and should not be mistaken for low signal intensity septations seen in fibroadenomas.

It is important to realize that, while a nonenhancing invasive breast cancer is extremely rare (and usually does not need to be considered a relevant differential diagnosis), nonenhancing, that is, MRI occult DCIS does occur in about 5% of cases. This explains why having a recent state-of-the-art mammogram available is considered a prereq-uisite for reading breast MRI studies. On the other hand, it seems that breast MRI can help detect additional, mammographically occult DCIS in a substantial number of patients, both regarding the delineation of intraductal spread in patients diagnosed with invasive cancer, as well as the detection of primary intraductal cancer.[66,69–72]

10.3. Benign Changes

10.3.1. Fibroadenoma

Fibroadenomas represent a frequent finding in breast MRI, much more frequent than is detected on mammog-

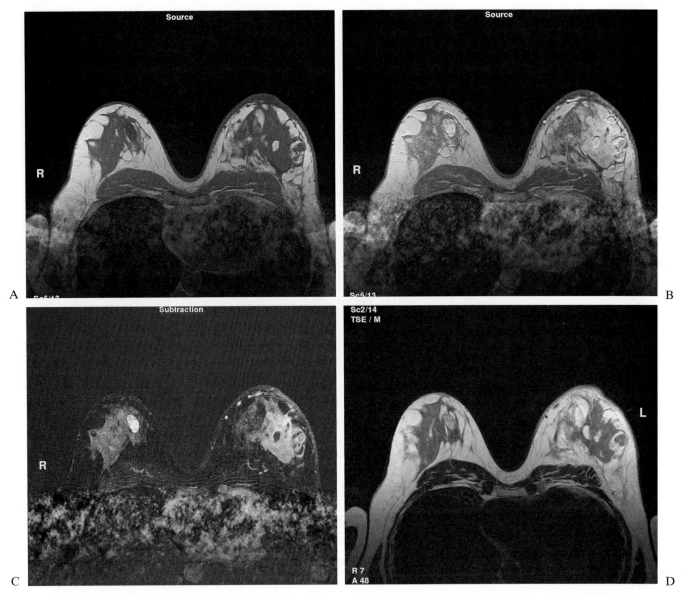

FIGURE 7.20. Inflammatory breast cancer on the left, myxoid fibroadenoma on the right, in a 39-year-old patient at high genetic risk for breast cancer. (A) Precontrast T1-weighted GE of the dynamic series. (B) First postcontrast T1-weighted GE of the dynamic series. (C) First postcontrast subtracted. (D) T2-weighted TSE image.

raphy. Fibroadenomas constitute one of the major differential diagnostic problems for MRI, as they do in mammography or breast ultrasound. There are a variety of diagnostic criteria used in dynamic breast MRI to distinguish fibroadenoma from breast cancer; some of which are quite specific [i.e., they have a high negative predictive value (NPV) for cancer], which is why, in combination, it is often enough possible to confidently classify a fibroadenoma as *definitely benign* (BI-RADS 2; see right breast in Figure 7.20). Still, it will be up to the discretion of the radiologist, up to his or her practice, degree of diagnostic confidence in the individual case, and to his or her personal

preferences in terms of aggressiveness or conservativeness, whether or not, eventually, a biopsy is recommended.

In general, the MRI appearance of fibroadenomas varies strongly with the degree of fibrosis: On one end of the spectrum, there are myxoid fibroadenomas that have large extracellular spaces filled with a gelatinous matrix (Figures 7.20 and 7.22). With increasing age, regressive changes take place; the interstitial matrix undergoes fibrosis, resulting in a sclerotic fibroadenoma on the other end of the spectrum (Figure 7.23).

Ideally, a myxoid fibroadenoma presents as focal mass with ovoid shape, with the long axis parallel to the

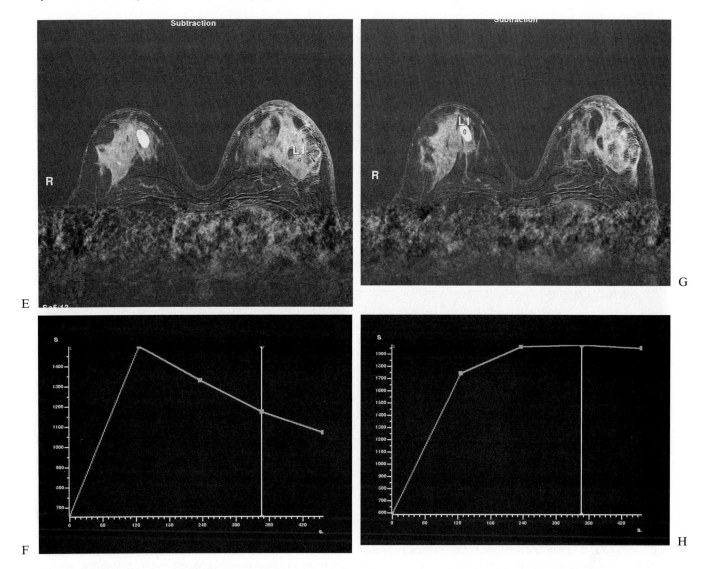

FIGURE 7.20. (*Continued*) (E) ROI in the inflammatory breast cancer with (F) signal time course of the inflammatory breast cancer on the left (G) ROI in the myxoid fibroadenoma on the right with (H) signal time course of the fibroadenoma on the right. Left breast: Inflammatory cancer with diffuse parenchymal and skin edema (note skin thickening in T1-weighted precontrast and T2-weighted TSE images (A and D) and strong contrast enhancement of the skin in B and C. Note the diffuse parenchymal edema with relatively increased signal of the left-sided parenchymal compared to the right side. Note the strong parenchymal enhancement in the early postcontrast phase, followed by a strong washout (F). Note the intramammary lymph node in the upper outer quadrant of the left breast. Right breast: Note the focal mass with oval shape, orientation parallel to Cooper's ligaments. Note the "MR halo" phenomenon, that is, a small streak of fatty tissue around the tumor due to displaced fatty tissue, secondary to the "pushing" tumor margins. Note the smooth borders, internal septations (best visualized on T2-weighted TSE images (D)) and with enhancement kinetics that differ from those of the inflammatory breast cancer on the left: there is strong, but persistent enhancement, corresponding to a type 1a curve, typical for fibroadenoma. In spite of the high genetic risk of the patient and in spite of the fact that there was diffuse cancer on the left, this lesion can be confidently classified as BI-RADS 2. Patient underwent chemotherapy and mastectomy on the left. Follow up of the right breast is over 2 years.

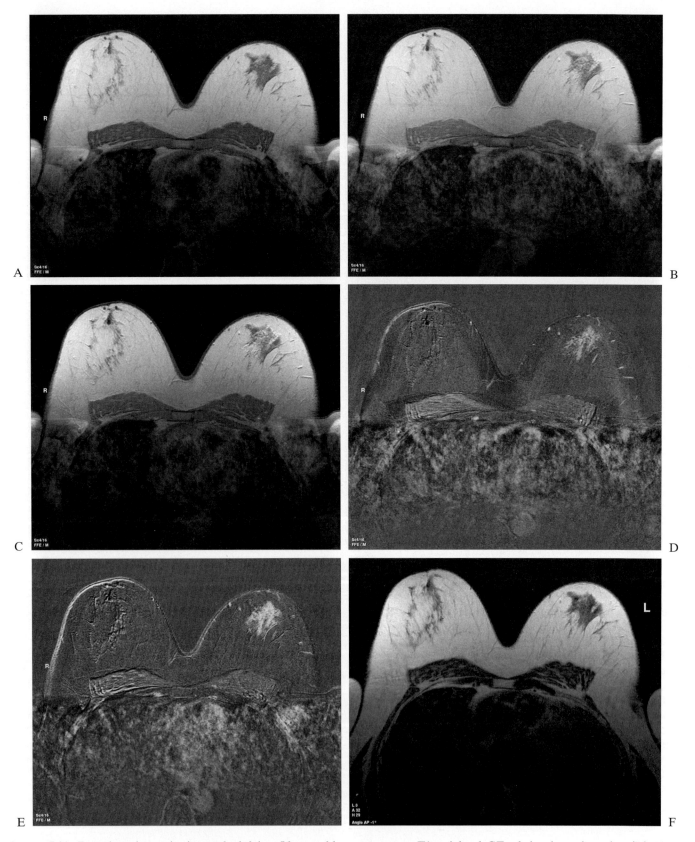

FIGURE 7.21. Ductal carcinoma in situ on the left in a 56-year-old patient who is status post benign breast biopsy on the right. (A) Precontrast T1-weighted GE of the dynamic series. (B) First postcontrast T1-weighted GE of the dynamic series. (C) Second postcontrast T1-weighted GE of the dynamic series. (D) First postcontrast subtracted. (E) Second postcontrast subtracted. (F) T2-weighted TSE image.

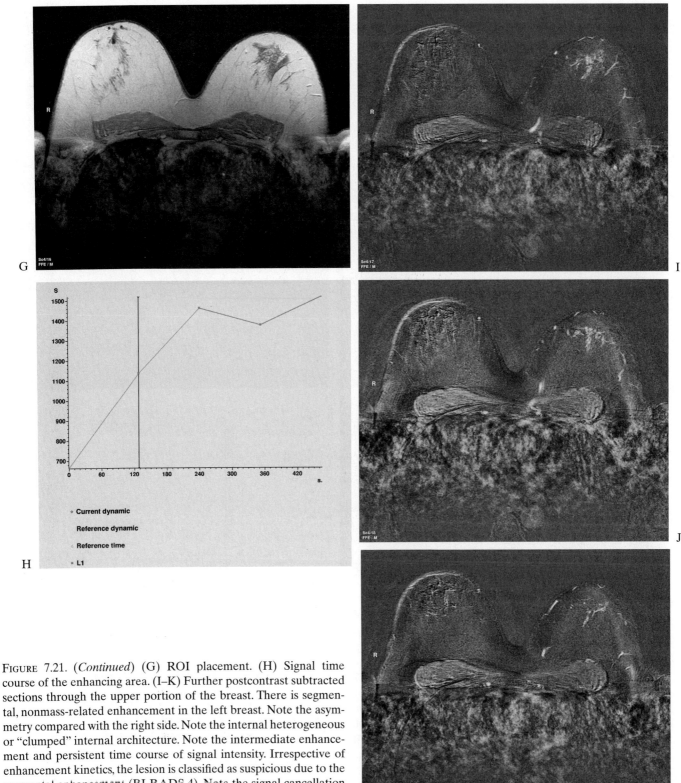

FIGURE 7.21. (*Continued*) (G) ROI placement. (H) Signal time course of the enhancing area. (I–K) Further postcontrast subtracted sections through the upper portion of the breast. There is segmental, nonmass-related enhancement in the left breast. Note the asymmetry compared with the right side. Note the internal heterogeneous or "clumped" internal architecture. Note the intermediate enhancement and persistent time course of signal intensity. Irrespective of enhancement kinetics, the lesion is classified as suspicious due to the segmental enhancement (BI-RADS 4). Note the signal cancellation due to previous benign breast biopsy behind the nipple on the right breast.

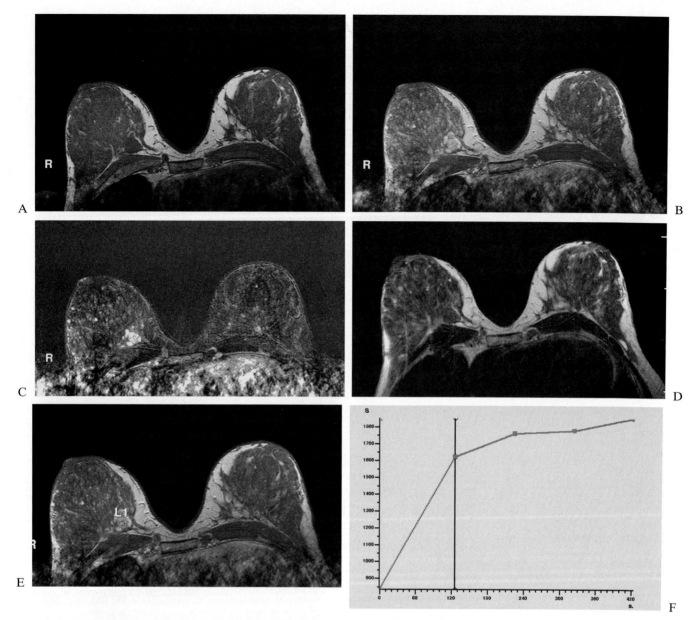

FIGURE 7.22. Fibroadenoma. (A) Precontrast T1-weighted GE of the dynamic series. (B) First postcontrast T1-weighted GE of the dynamic series. (C) First postcontrast subtracted. (D) T2-weighted TSE image. (E) ROI placement. (F) Signal time course. Typical presentation of a fibroadenoma. Note the lobulated shape, smooth borders. Note the "MR halo sign" with displaced fatty tissue around the lesion (visible in non–fat-suppressed precontrast T1-weighted images, i.e., (A)). Note the internal septations visible on non–fat-suppressed and subtracted postcontrast images (B and C). Note the rapid, but persistent enhancement (type 1a time course). Note the heterogeneous signal in the T2-weighted TSE image (D); this fibroadenoma is partially sclerotic. A myxoid fibroadenoma (with homogeneously bright signal on T2-weighted TSE images) is seen in the right breast of the patient in Figure 7.20. With the benign shape, smooth margins, internal septations, persistent enhancement pattern, the lesion can be confidently classified as BI-RADS 2.

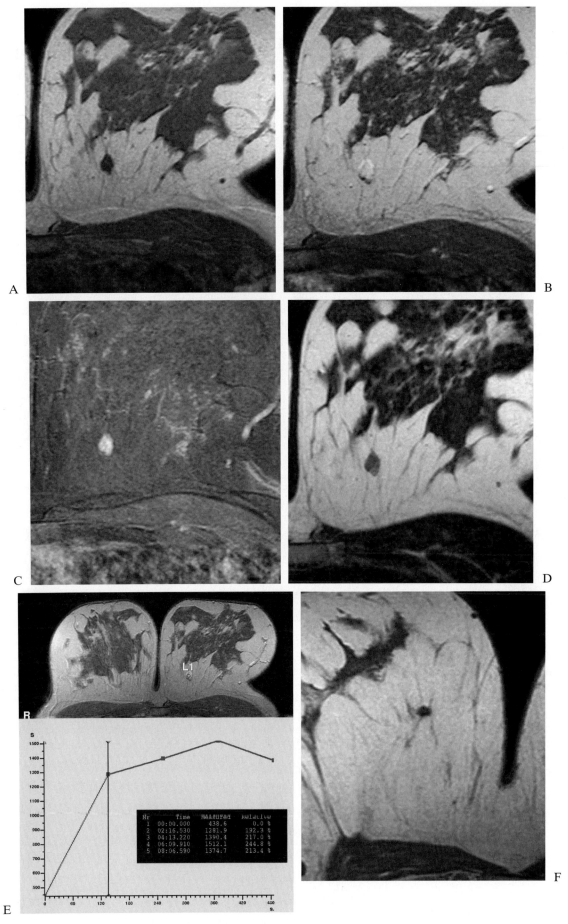

FIGURE 7.23. (*Continued*)

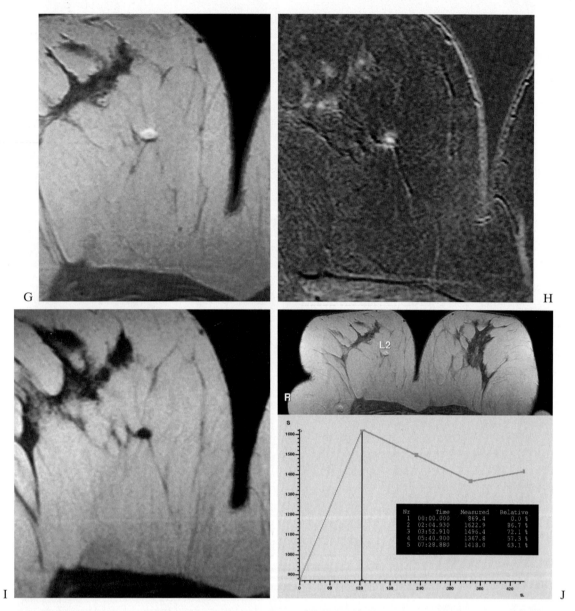

FIGURE 7.23. (*Continued*) Growth pattern with respect to Cooper's ligaments in fibroadenomas and breast cancers. (A–E) Fibroadenoma. (F–J) Duct-invasive breast cancer. (A and F) Precontrast T1-weighted GE of the dynamic series. (B and G) First postcontrast T1-weighted GE of the dynamic series. (C and H) First postcontrast subtracted. (D and I) T2-weighted TSE image. (E and J) ROI placement and kinetic analysis. In A–E, the fibroadenoma presents as focal mass with ovoid configuration. In the non–fat-suppressed precontrast T1-weighted images (A), note that the long axis of the mass is aligned in parallel with the Cooper's ligaments, perpendicular to the chest wall. Note the smooth borders, internal septations, very strong enhancement, but persistent time course, all indicative of fibroadenoma (BI-RADS 2). In F–J, the small (5mm) duct-invasive cancer shows a roundish or ovoid shape. The long axis is horizontal, in parallel to the chest wall, perpendicular to Cooper's ligaments. The small tumor disrupts the natural path of Cooper's ligaments, indicative of invasive cancer. Note the rim enhancement, rapid enhancement followed by washout (BI-RADS 5).

Cooper's ligaments (be aware of the fact that Cooper's ligaments travel in parallel to the outer contours of the breast, i.e., parallel to the chest wall in the dorsal part of the outer quadrants, but perpendicular to the chest wall in the inner and central quadrants; Figure 7.24). The criterion that clinches the diagnosis is internal low-signal septations that are visible on postcontrast images or against the otherwise bright signal on T2-TSE images. These septations are associated with such a high NPV that their presence, together with a benign appearing shape and margin status, justify a BI-RADS 2 categorization of a lesion irrespective of enhancement kinetics. Unfortunately, internal septations are not always seen; with current techniques in dynamic breast MRI, they are visualized in about 30% to 50% of cases, greatly depending on the spatial resolution that is used. More often, a homogeneous enhancement is seen; heterogeneous (patchy) enhancement does occur in case there are regressive changes, which may reduce enhancement in the areas that already underwent fibrosis. With time resolved studies, the enhancement starts in the center of the lesion and progresses from there to the tumor periphery, such that the lesion seems to grow from one dynamic scan to the other (*blooming fibroadenoma*).

In sclerotic fibroadenomas, enhancement is reduced or even absent, and the SI in T2-weighted TSE images is low. As a consequence, internal septations are hardly visible. If enhancement is present, the time course of SI corresponds to a type-1a shape. Enhancement may be somewhat heterogeneous due to regressive clumps of calcifications and the slow progression of enhancement.

According to our experience, the diagnosis can be established with sufficient confidence if all criteria are observable to support the diagnosis of either myxoid or sclerotic fibroadenoma.

10.3.2. Intramammary Lymph Node

Intramammary lymph nodes (Figure 7.25) are a frequent finding in dynamic breast MRI. The typical morphology and location should help establish the diagnosis: Typically, lymph nodes occur in the lateral parts of the upper outer quadrant, in the subcutaneous tissue. With sufficiently high spatial resolution (i.e., 512 imaging matrix), the characteristic internal kidney-shaped architecture is visualized, and the central fatty tissue (the *hilum*) can be identified as bright signal on T1- and T2-weighted (non–fat-suppressed) images. It is important to look at precontrast non–fat-suppressed T1-weighted images to be able to see the central fatty tissue; if one fails to do this, the kidney-shaped lymph node could even be misinterpreted as a focal mass with rim enhancement. This is even more important as enhancement kinetics are usually always *malignant*: Virtually all lymph nodes exhibit a carcinoma-type rapid and fast early phase enhancement, followed by a washout. So it is the typical location within the breast and the typical kidney-shaped morphology with the central fatty tissue that helps one to confidently classify this lesion as a BI-RADS 2.

10.3.3. So-Called Mastopathic or Fibrocystic Changes, Focal Adenosis

In dynamic bilateral breast MRI, so-called mastopathic or fibrocystic changes appear as diffuse, bilateral, patchy, and heterogeneous with multifocal enhancement. The histopathological correlate of the small enhancing dots has been shown to be the focal adenosis, that is, proliferation of the glandular epithelium. It is important to realize that there is no correlation between the kinetic features and the presence or absence of atypias: The enhancement pattern of mastopathic changes does not correlate with the probability of significant histologic lesions. Accordingly, kinetic (or morphologic) features cannot be used to distinguish between regular ductal (or lobular) hyperplasia versus atypical ductal hyperplasia (ADH) or lobular carcinoma in situ (LCIS).

The heterogeneity of enhancement that is seen in patients with fibrocystic disease is due to the presence of areas with predominant epithelial proliferation next to areas with predominant regressive changes (fibrosis) and associated cysts. While the patchy or diffuse enhancement is usually not a diagnostic problem, there are often small dots of nonmass-related focal or multifocal enhancement interspersed within the more or less diffusely enhancing parenchymal tissues. These small foci of enhancement (usually below 4mm in size) are mostly due to small fibroadenomas or nodes of focal adenosis (Figure 7.26). In terms of kinetics, these lesions may look suspicious. They enhance strongly and rapidly in the early postcontrast phase, and in about 10% of cases, they may also exhibit a washout time course in the postinitial phase. Hence, if kinetic pattern is benign, this may help correctly classify these lesions as focal adenosis; if they, too, are suspicious, biopsy is inevitable. In fact, these small enhancing foci are the most important cause for false-positive diagnoses made in breast MRI. In turn, small foci of cancer or DCIS may be masked by enhancement secondary to focal adenosis. The following hints have emerged from clinical practice and may prove helpful.

- If there is *no* correlate for these enhancing foci in mammography and breast ultrasound (which is usually the case), *and* if there is no clinical reason that would advise caution (which would be the case, e.g., if these foci were identified in a patient who presents for preoperative staging of a known breast cancer), we would usually classify these foci as BI-RADS 3 and recommend follow up.
- If bilateral multifocal enhancement is present, it is not useful to attempt quantification or time-course analysis of each and every enhancing spot. Keep in mind that bilateral disseminated multifocal invasive breast cancer is really rare, and that DCIS is usually confined to a

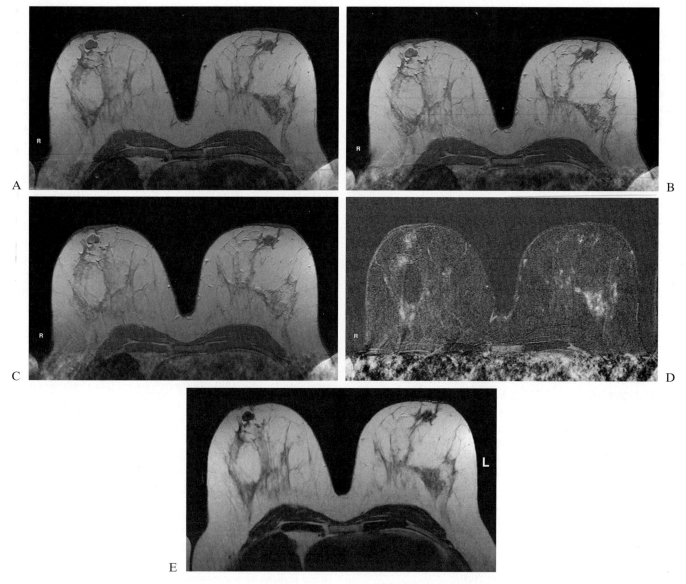

FIGURE 7.24. Sclerotic fibroadenoma. (A) Precontrast T1-weighted GE of the dynamic series. (B) First postcontrast T1-weighted GE of the dynamic series. (C) Late postcontrast T1-weighted GE of the dynamic series. (D) First postcontrast subtracted. (E) T2-weighted TSE image. Note that the focal mass with lobulated shape, smooth borders, which is virtually invisible on early postcontrast subtracted (or fat-suppressed) images in the right breast, because there is only very shallow (if any) enhancement. Therefore, the lesion is best visualized on nonsubtracted (or non–fat-suppressed) images (A, B, or C) or on T2-weighted images (E). Note the very low signal of the lesion in T2-weighted TSE image (E) due to the significant fibrosis.

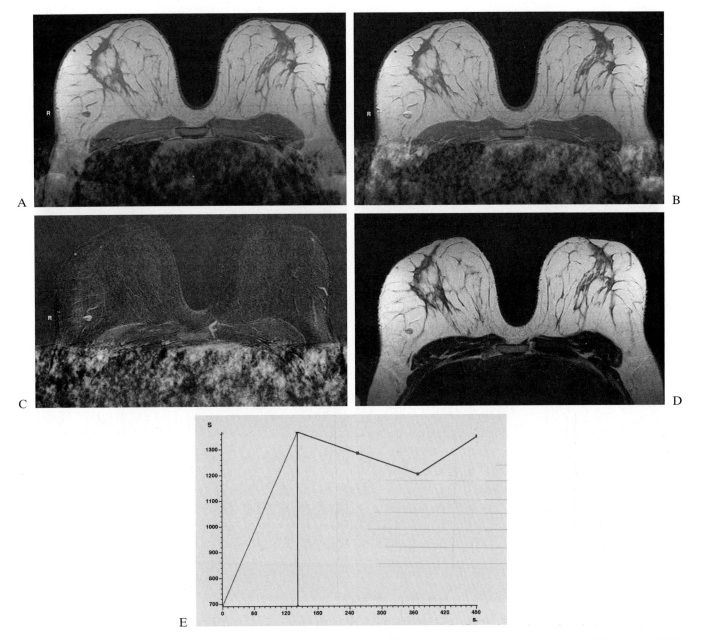

FIGURE 7.25. Intramammary lymph node. (A) Precontrast T1-weighted GE of the dynamic series. (B) First postcontrast T1-weighted GE of the dynamic series. (C) First postcontrast subtracted. (D) T2-weighted TSE image. (E) Signal time course. Note the focal mass with typical oval (or kidney) shape in its typical location (subcutaneous fatty tissue of the upper outer quadrant). Note the "fake" rim enhancement due to the hilum and fatty sinus of the lymph node (to avoid pitfalls, refer to non–fat-suppressed, precontrast T1-weighed images to identify central fatty tissue). Note the lobulated shape, smooth borders. Note the high signal intensity of the lesion in T2-weighted TSE images. Note the very strong and rapid washin, followed by a washout—this is typical for lymph nodes. Virtually all lymph nodes exhibit this enhancement pattern, irrespective of whether they are normal or metastasized. With the typical location, the typical kindey shape, the central fatty hilum, the bright signal on T2-weighted TSE, the lesion is classified as BI-RADS 2 (lymph node). Washout is compatible with the diagnosis of lymph node, which is why a BI-RADS 2 is given, not BI-RADS 3.

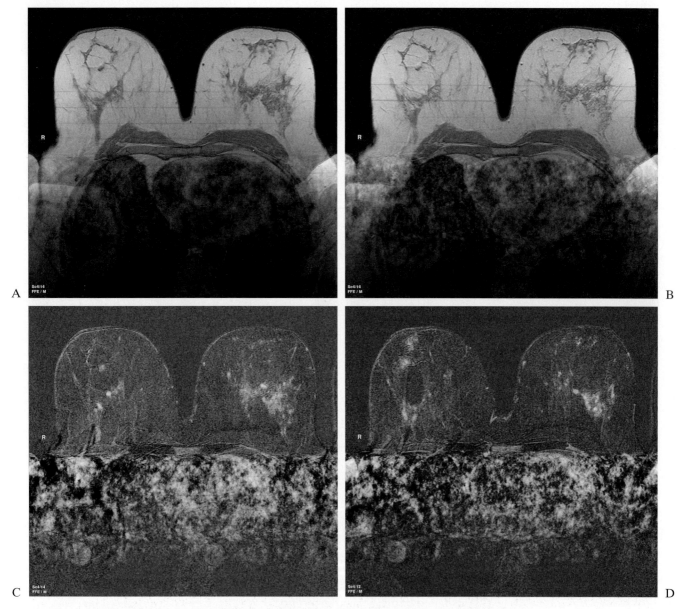

FIGURE 7.26. Diffuse adenosis. (A) Precontrast T1-weighted GE of the dynamic series. (B) First postcontrast T1-weighted GE of the dynamic series. (C) First postcontrast subtracted. (D–G) Four further sections (subtracted images).

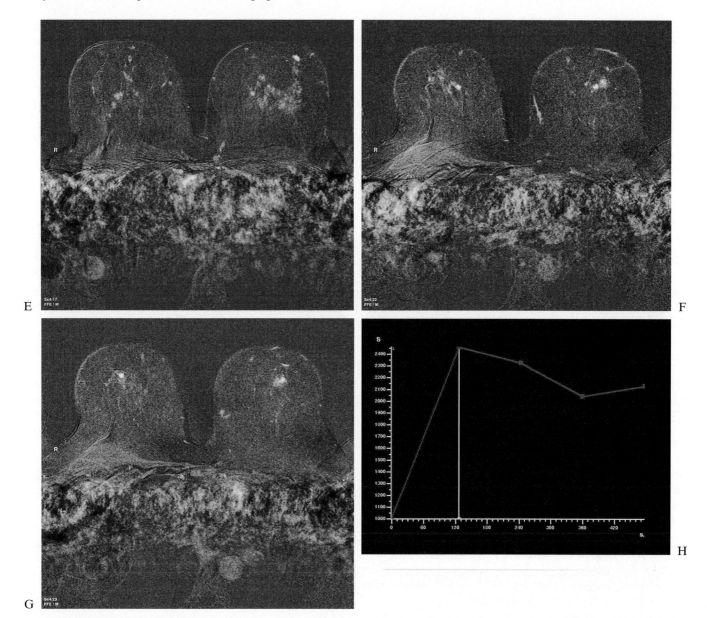

FIGURE 7.26. (*Continued*) (H) Signal time course. Note the multifocal nonmass-related enhancment. Small size of the individual lesions. Early enhancement with biphasic or even washout time course. The nonmass-related lesions are usually too small to be amenable to a meaningful morphologic analysis; enhancement kinetics are not useful as well, because the lesions tend to enhance rapidly, with plateau or even washout enhancement pattern. Accordingly, it is impossible to distinguish small adenosis from small invasive (or intraductal) cancers. This is why the sensitivity of breast MRI regarding the detection of small cancers is significantly reduced in these patients. Follow up for clarification is probably necessary for forensic reasons, but usually will not solve the problem. These enhancing lesions will persist (unlike hormonal-induced enhancement, which can be expected to change its appearance on follow up) even for years.

duct or the territory of a distinct ductal system. So the bilaterality and the symmetry is the clue to the diagnosis and is one important argument for doing bilateral breast MRI.

- On follow ups, enhancing foci due to hormonal effects should change their appearance and location, whereas enhancing foci due to focal adenosis are constant and reproducible over even years of follow up. Therefore, do not expect these foci to resolve or change; they will stay the same.

11. Current Applications of Dynamic Bilateral Breast Magnetic Resonance Imaging

There are several indications for breast MRI; however, it should be noted that at this stage, there are virtually no data available that would allow end-point analyses to be performed on the influence of breast MRI in terms of survival, mortality, morbidity, or quality-of-life issues.

11.1. Clarification of Inconclusive Conventional Imaging Findings

Breast MRI in general offers a wealth of information on the lesion in question, all the physical and biochemical features that determine image contrast on (contrast-enhanced and plain) MRI studies. The many parameters that contribute to lesion appearance translate into a full battery of differential diagnostic criteria. These may be used to distinguish benign and malignant lesions even in cases that are inconclusive on conventional imaging, the most established indication being the differentiation of tumor recurrence versus scar tissue in the follow up of patients who underwent breast conservation therapy.

Specifically *dynamic* breast MRI may be useful to evaluate lesions that appear morphologically benign on conventional imaging studies: The evaluation of time course kinetics introduces a completely independent diagnostic parameter (i.e., tissue perfusion/diffusion/vessel permeability) that can help distinguish benign lesions (e.g., fibroadenoma) from well-circumscribed breast cancer. For example, if a lesion looks benign in terms of morphology, a correct diagnosis may still be possible if signal intensity time courses are evaluated.

It should be noted, however, that if breast MRI is to be used for clarification of mammographically or sonographically suspicious lesions, then it is an important prerequisite that the radiologist is familiar with the specific limitations of all three imaging modalities. It is important to realize that there are specific constellations of mammographic or sonographic findings that may not be clarified by a negative breast MRI, whereas in others, MRI can be

used to obviate the need for biopsy. Clinical scenarios where MRI cannot be used to alleviate the indication to biopsy are, for example, cases with suspicious mammographic microcalcifications: Because sensitivity of breast MRI for in situ cancers is limited, it may not be used to exclude underlying DCIS. Moreover, it should be kept in mind that, in general, percutaneous core biopsy may be more appropriate to definitively clarify conventionally inconclusive lesions.

11.2. Staging

If on conventional imaging studies a solitary focus of breast cancer has been identified and a breast conserving therapy is considered, preoperative breast MRI is indicated to rule out or localize additional breast cancer foci. This is particularly important in patients diagnosed with lobular invasive cancers because these cancers tend to be even more difficult to diagnose mammographically and sonographically and in patients with a strong familiy history of breast cancer because they tend to develop multicentric disease.[71,73,81] In a recent article, Fischer and coworkers report on preoperative dynamic breast MRI for local staging of patients who were candidates for breast conservation.[75] They diagnosed therapeutically relevant additional findings in 16% of cases, and synchronous contralateral breast cancer in as many as 6% of patients.[75] These data were also confirmed by more recent articles by Lee and Liberman[82,84] (Figure 7.27).

Because dynamic breast MRI (as opposed to high-spatial-resolution *static* breast MRI) allows the simultaneous evaluation of both breasts, a screening of the contralateral breast will always be performed at the same time (and in one investigation) as staging for the breast with known cancer.

11.3. Assessing Tumor Response to Neoadjuvant Chemotherapy

Neoadjuvant chemotherapy is increasingly used in patients with locally advanced breast cancer (LABC), both for restoring operability, but also for systemic treatment of possible concomitant lymph node or distant metastases. Conventional imaging techniques, however, offer only a poor diagnostic accuracy for the assessment of chemotherapeutic effects. This is mainly due to the fact that, after effective chemotherapy, tumor tissue may be replaced by diffuse fibrosis. The fibrous tissue may simulate residual tumor on clinical palpation, and it may interfere with an accurate depiction of residual tumor both on mammograms and on breast ultrasound studies. Moreover, not only for reasons of optimizing patient care, but also for economic reasons, it is crucial to reliably identify nonresponders as soon as possible. There is evidence that

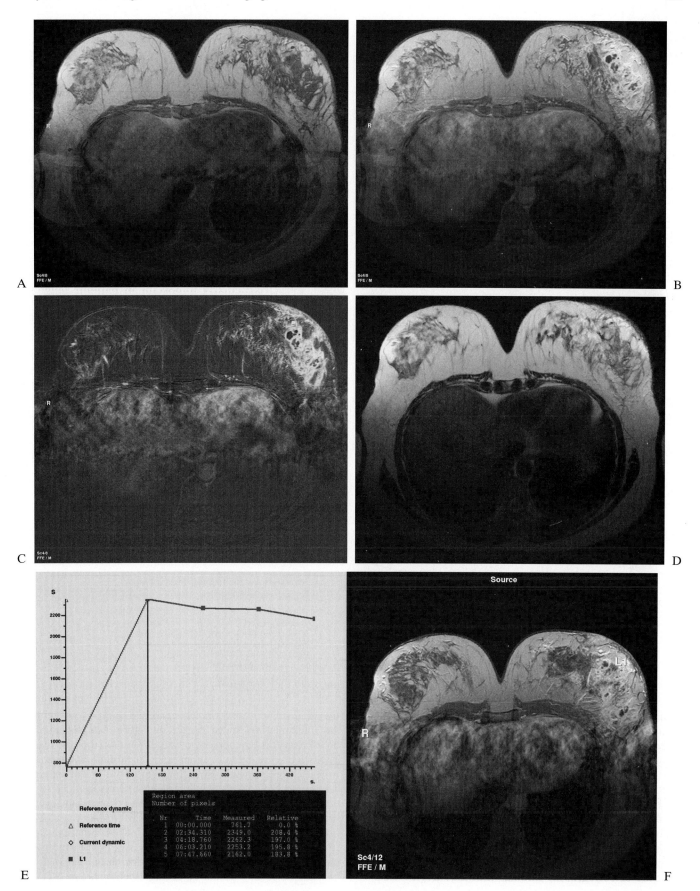

FIGURE 7.27. (*Continued*)

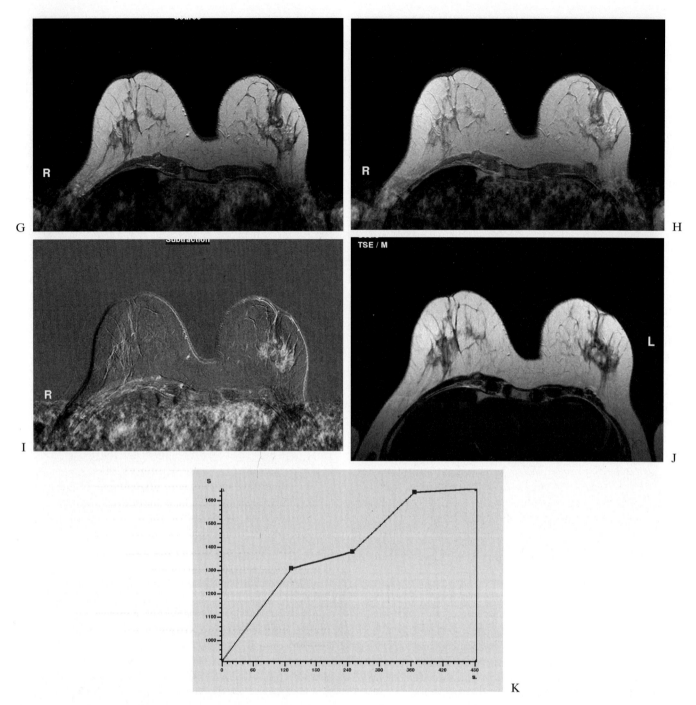

FIGURE 7.27. (*Continued*) Acute and chronic mastitis. (A–E) Acute nonpuerperal mastitis in a 45-year-old patient. (F–J) Chronic mastitis in a 43-year-old patient. (A and F) Precontrast T1-weighted GE of the dynamic series. (B and G) First postcontrast T1-weighted GE of the dynamic series. (C and H) first postcontrast subtracted. (D and I) T2-weighted TSE image. (E and K) ROI placement and kinetic analysis. In A–E, acute mastitis presents as diffuse edema of the entire breast and the skin (best visible on T2-weighted TSE images, D), with diffuse and strong enhancement of the parenchyma and the skin, with formation of abscesses (see areas with rim enhancement in C). Note that enhancement kinetics are indistinguishable from those of inva-sive (e.g., inflammatory) breast cancers. Compare the picture to the inflammatory breast cancer in Figure 7.20. Inflammatory breast cancer is the most important differential to acute mastitis. The two disease entities cannot be distinguished by breast MRI. In F–J, chronic mastitis. Note the architectural distortion due to a huge focal mass with only intermediate enhancement, type 1a time course. Our primary diagnosis (based on mammography, breast ultrasound, and MRI) was diffusely growing (e.g., lobular) invasive cancer. No clinical symptoms of inflammation. Biopsy revealed chronic mastitis. (Lobular) invasive breast cancer is the most important differential diagnosis for chronic mastitis. The two disease entities cannot be distinguished by breast MRI.

dynamic breast MRI is ideally suited to fulfill both of these tasks.

Considering evaluation of chemotherapy response, dynamic breast MRI is able to quantify functional tissue parameters, that is, tumor perfusion, as a surrogate marker for tissue viability in addition to assessing tumor size. Because dynamic breast MRI is able to detect and quantify chemotherapy-induced changes of the perfusion (i.e., viability) of malignant tissues, this can be exploited for assessing tumor response to neoadjuvant chemotherapy. Several groups have investigated if dynamic breast MRI can identify responders or nonresponders. There is some evidence to suggest that after about two chemotherapy cycles, and before a measurable change of tumor size occurred, response to chemotherapy is heralded by a substantial change of contrast enhancement patterns.[85–89] Decreasing enhancement rates, and more importantly a change of the enhancement behavior in the postinitial and late period (washout or plateau converted to type 1a) are the hallmark of early tumor response to chemotherapy. Although the sample size of the respective studies is small, there is sufficient evidence to suggest that assessing breast MRI enhancement kinetics is as least as useful for the early diagnosis of response as is positron emission tomography (PET) imaging, with the additional advantage of providing exact information on tumor size. Given the high clinical and economical relevance of an early identification of nonresponders, this may emerge as a most important application for dynamic breast MRI, provided these findings are validated in a larger group of patients.

Several studies have confirmed that compared with conventional imaging modalities, breast MRI is greatly more sensitive and specific for assessing residual tumor extent after chemotherapy. It should be well understood, however, that although breast MRI may be better than clinical assessment or conventional imaging, it is still far from being perfect. Scattered residual vital cancer cells in the former tumor bed in responders may not enhance after contrast, thus escaping the diagnosis. These tumor remnants do not influence prognosis and, thus, the classification of response. However, if induction chemotherapy is performed with the ultimate goal of breast conservation, breast MRI cannot be used to rule out residual micromanifestations in responders, and it may not be able to identify patients who are amenable to breast conservation after induction chemotherapy.[11,90–94]

11.4. High-Risk Screening

The average lifetime risk for a woman to develop breast cancer is 12%. There are several different conditions that may increase the risk: Women with a personal history of breast cancer, women with a tissue diagnosis of a borderline breast lesion such as ADH or LCIS, women with a history of mediastinal irradiation (e.g., after Hodgkin's disease), and, most notably, women with proved BRCA mutation or with a family history suggestive of hereditary breast cancer. Breast MRI has been advocated to serve as screening tool in all of these clinical situations.[71,95–99] The dynamic approach seems to be particularly useful here for several reasons.

In a screening setting, bilateral imaging is required—dynamic imaging is almost always done with coverage of both breasts, whereas high-spatial-resolution static MRI can only be performed on one single breast at a time (Figure 7.28).

Women with proven or suspected germline BRCA mutation face an 80% to 90% lifetime risk of being diagnosed with breast cancer, and they develop the disease at significantly younger ages (i.e., in their early 30s). Accordingly, these women require an intensified screening that starts at age 25 to 30. In these very young women, however, sensitivity of mammography may be significantly reduced. There is, meanwhile, significant published evidence regarding the role of breast MRI screening for familial breast cancer. Our results (and those of other groups[71,96–99]) document that dynamic breast MRI is clearly superior to mammography and breast ultrasound both for early detection and classification of familial breast cancers.

Specifically, *dynamic* contrast-enhanced breast MRI may be suitable for these women because BRCA1-induced breast cancers tend to exhibit atypical (benign) morphologic features. Even on gross pathology or on low-magnification histology, these tumors may appear completely well circumscribed, with no evidence of infiltration. Accordingly, even with highest spatial resolution imaging, the morphologic features of these tumors may be indistinguishable from that of fibroadenomas. Dynamic breast MRI, however, allows the additional evaluation of enhancement kinetics (surrogate for tissue perfusion or angiogenesis activity; Figure 7.29). In our cohort, 5 of the 9 BRCA-induced cancers revealed a deceivingly benign morphology, but highly suspicious contrast enhancement kinetics with rapid and strong wash in, followed by a washout (type 3). So in spite of the apparently benign morphologic features of hereditary breast cancers, a true-positive diagnosis was possible in all cases based on dynamic MRI. Accordingly, sensitivity of breast MRI versus mammography and breast ultrasound combined was 100% versus 44%.

Another reason why dynamic imaging may be helpful for screening very young women is the issue of hormonal stimulation. As explained, hormone-induced activation of the glandular tissue may produce UBOs, that is, focal contrast-enhancing areas that are not associated with any structural changes of the parenchymal composition, but that are probably caused by the local histamine-like effects of ovarian steroid hormones.[18,28] Because these pseudolesions are able to exhibit scary irregular morphology, they are a notorious cause for false-positive diagnoses in young

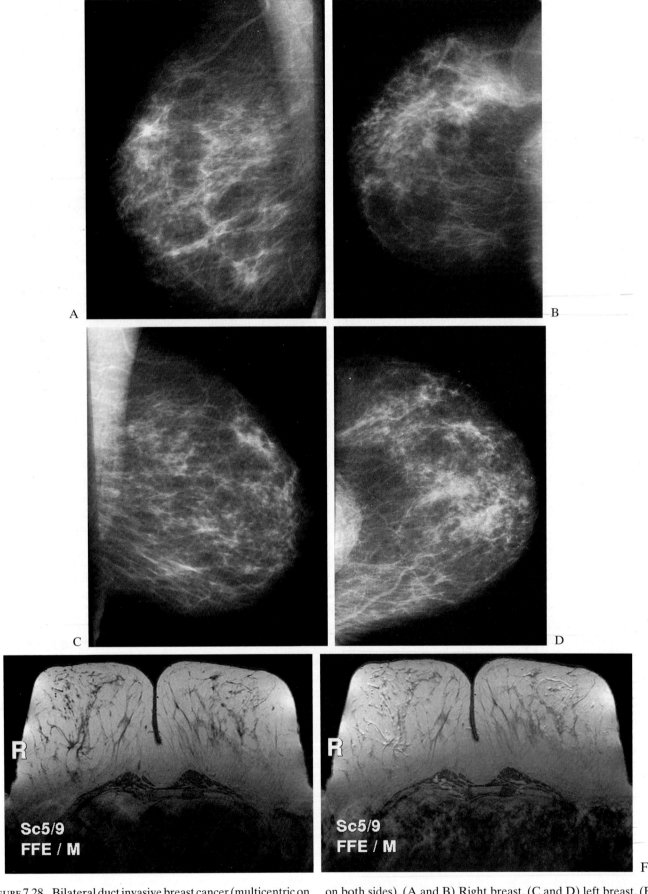

FIGURE 7.28. Bilateral duct invasive breast cancer (multicentric on the right) in a 64-year-old patient presenting for screening without clinical symptoms. (A–D) Screening mammogram (MLO and CC on both sides). (A and B) Right breast, (C and D) left breast. (E and G) Section 1 (through the lower aspects of the lower quadrant) (F) Precontrast T1-weighted image. (F) Postcontrast.

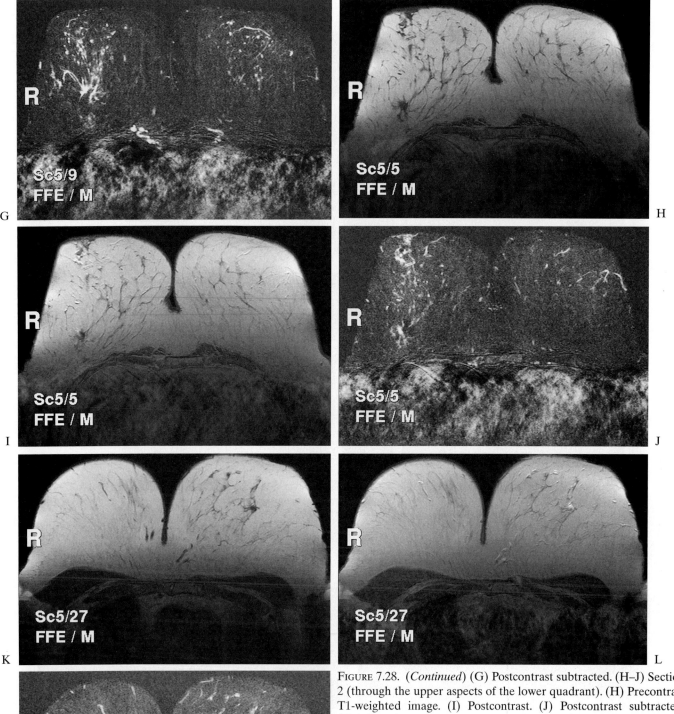

FIGURE 7.28. (*Continued*) (G) Postcontrast subtracted. (H–J) Section 2 (through the upper aspects of the lower quadrant). (H) Precontrast T1-weighted image. (I) Postcontrast. (J) Postcontrast subtracted. (K–M) section 3 (through the upper aspects of the upper quadrants). (K) Precontrast T1-weighted image. (L) Postcontrast. (M) Postcontrast subtracted. Note that the mammogram is not dense (ACR 2 pattern). Note the architectural distortion and stellate mass in the lower outer quadrant on the mammogram of the right breast. Note the possible second tumor visible on the right CC view in the central quadrant of the right breast. The left breast was read normal. Note the stellate mass in the lower outer and central quadrant of the left breast. Note the associated scattered nonmass-related enhancement in a segmental configuration, suspicious for an intraductal extension (EIC) confirmed by biopsy. Note the in contralateral cancer with irregular morphology, strong and early enhancement. The lesion was occult also on directed breast ultrasound of the target area. Magnetic-resonance–guided needle localization and biopsy was performed and revealed a second breast cancer with different histology (duct invasive) compared to the tubular cancer on the right.

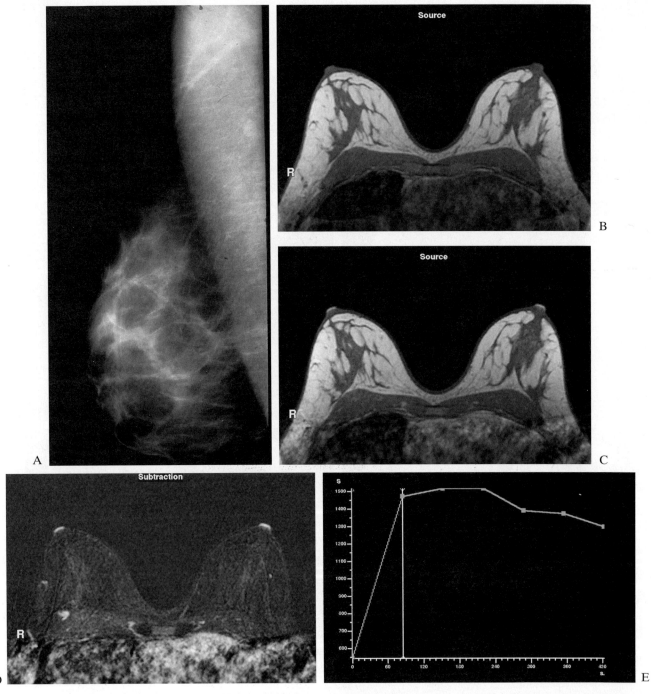

FIGURE 7.29. Screening for breast cancer in a 33-year-old patient with documented BRCA1 mutation. (A) Screening mammogram (MLO of the right breast). (B) Precontrast T1-weighted of the dynamic series. (C) First postcontrast of the dynamic series. (D) First postcontrast subtracted. (E) Signal time course of the enhancing lesion. The mammogram was read normal. Note that the breast is not very dense (ACR 3 glandular pattern). Note the small irregular enhancing lesion in the lower outer quadrant. Note absence of enhancement in the remaining right or left breast, which makes the diagnosis of hormonal stimulation less likely. Note the strong and early enhancement with washout. Because morphology and kinetics are suspicious, the lesion was rated BI-RADS 5. As directed physician-based high resolution (7.5–11 MHz) ultrasound was normal, MR-guided biopsy was performed and revealed a small pT1a duct invasive breast cancer grade 3. N0, M0.

patients. In these cases, *benign* contrast enhancement kinetics can help correctly classify these enhancing areas.

11.5. Assessing Tumor Grade and Prognosis

It has been extensively shown that tumor vascularity, as revealed by histologic vessel density counts, correlates with tumor aggressiveness and malignant (in particular metastatic) potential.[2,3,5,100–103] Because contrast enhancement patterns in dynamic breast MRI seem to be linked with hypervascularity, the intriguing thought came up that dynamic breast MRI might be useful for allowing a *tumor grading* or assessing tumor aggressiveness or prognosis in vivo. Several reports have been published investigating the correlation between contrast enhancement rates or time course features and prognostic factors such as histological grading, lymph node status, S-phase fraction, and modern proliferation indices (oncogenes/tumor suppressor genes) such as c-erbB-1, c-erB-2, p53, or Ki-67. Unfortunately, however, the results of these studies are inconsistent. In two prospective studies, no correlation with any of the criteria used in dynamic breast MRI (enhancement rates, maximum enhancement, washout rates, etc.) has been obtained.[104,105] Yet there are two studies that revealed a highly significant correlation between contrast enhancement in dynamic MRI and prognostic factors:[106,107] Mussurakis reported on a strong correlation of enhancment rates and tumor grading as well as nodal status in 53 patients with invasive breast cancers; Boné and coworkers confirmed these findings in another 50 breast cancer cases.

It is unclear from where the discrepancy between the published studies stems. It is possible that the variability in determining contrast enhancement rates if manually drawn ROIs are used may account for some heterogeneity of results. This is supported by the fact that Mussurakis reports that a statistically significant correlation between enhancement rates and prognostic factors was only obtained if an automatic ROI definition based on parametric images was used.

Studies on contrast-enhanced dynamic breast MRI of explanted adenocarcinoma have been performed using new blood-pool contrast agents, allowing assessment of tumor vessel permeability, and, thus, of tumor angiogenic activity grading. Hopes are high that, once these agents are available for use in human subjects, an actual noninvasive in vivo grading of breast cancers becomes feasible based on preoperative breast MRI.

12. Future Directions

As explained, for optimal clinical results, MRI of the breast should be performed with very high spatial and temporal resolution. Several techniques are emerging that may help

with this task. New image-acquisition strategies (parallel imaging), high-field MRI (3 Tesla and higher), and new contrast media (macromolecular contrast agents) may improve our ability to meet these requirements.

Parallel imaging such as sensitivity encoding (SENSE) is a new approach to MRI acquisition.[108] With multielement surface coils, the spatial sensitivity gradient inherent to surface coils can be exploited for encoding spatial information in parallel with regular phase encoding. Depending on the number of coil pairs, this translates into a proportional increase of acquisition speed (twofold with a SENSE factor of 2, etc.) without change in image contrast. The gain in image acquisition speed can be invested in improving spatial resolution at a given acquisition time or in improving temporal resolution with high-matrix imaging. Although SENSE imaging is fully integrated in routine clinical practice for many body and MRI angiography applications, its use in breast MRI is lagging behind. The reason for this is that, because of the reduced number of phase-encoding steps, using SENSE is associated with a reduction of the SNR by about 30%. With the high-matrix dynamic imaging technique that is required for breast MRI, this results in borderline SNR. An ideal combination is to use SENSE at high field systems (e.g., 3.0T): Magnets operating at 3.0T and higher are becoming increasingly available in the clinical setting. With the inherently increased SNR brought about by high-field systems, SENSE can be used to acquire high-SNR, high spatial-resolution images with a temporal resolution that ensures *arterial-phase* lesion contrast. Another approach to solve the temporal-versus-spatial dilemma is to use contrast media that diffuse less rapidly compared with the small gadolinium (Gd) chelates that are in use today. One of the promising candidates for this purpose is the blood-pool agent Gadomer (Schering, Berlin, Germany). Originally designed as a new contrast medium for MRI angiography (e.g., coronary angiography), it has been shown to provide an arterial-phase type of lesion-to-parenchyma contrast not only for 2min but for a period of about 30 to 45min. This would allow one to take the time for very high spatial-resolution imaging. The resulting Gadomer-enhanced MRIs reveal cross-sectional views through breast cancers with unprecedented anatomical detail: It is to be expected that this will help further improve the positive predictive value (PPV) of breast MRI. In addition, dynamic information could be obtained by doing bolus tracking (first-pass perfusion imaging) with T2*-weighted pulse sequences, as intravascular contrast agents allow a much more accurate evaluation of lesion perfusion compared with the rapidly diffusable Gd chelates.

References

1. Folkman J, Klagsbrun M. Angiogenic factors. *Science* 1987; 235:442–447.

2. Folkman J, Watson K, Ingbr D, Hanahan D. Induction of angiogenesis during the transition from hyperplasia to neoplasia. *Nature* 1989;339:58–61.

3. Hansen S, Grabau DA, Sorensen FB, et al. Vascular grading of angiogenesis: prognostic significance in breast cancer. *Br J Cancer.* 2000;82:339–347.

4. Lewin M, Bredow S, Sergeyev N, et al. In vivo assessment of vascular endothelial growth factor-induced angiogenesis. *Int J Cancer.* 1999;83:798–802.

5. Weidner N, Semple JP, Welch WR, Folkman J. Tumor angiogenesis and metastasis—correlation in invasive breast carcinoma. *N Engl J Med.* 1991;324:1–8.

6. Aref M, Brechbiel M, Wiener EC. Identifying tumor vascular permeability heterogeneity with magnetic resonance imaging contrast agents. *Invest Radiol.* 2002;37:178–921.

7. Boné B, Wiberg MK, Parrado C, et al. Mechanism of contrast enhancement in breast lesions at MR imaging. *Acta Radiol.* 1998;39:494–500.

8. Buadu LD, Murakami J, Murayama S, et al. Breast lesions: correlation of contrast medium enhancement patterns on MR images with histopathologic findings and tumor angiogenesis. *Radiology* 1996;200:639–649.

9. Buckley DL, Drew PJ, Mussurakis S, et al. Microvessel density of invasive breast cancer assessed by dynamic Gd-DTPA enhanced MRI. *J Magn Reson Imaging.* 1997;7:461–464.

10. Frouge C, Guinebretiere JM, Contesso G, et al. Correlation between contrast enhancement in dynamic magnetic resonance imaging of the breast and tumor angiogenesis. *Invest Radiol.* 1994;29:1043–1049.

11. Huber S, Wagner M, Zuna I, et al. Locally advanced breast carcinoma: evaluation of mammography in the prediction of residual disease after induction chemotherapy. *Anticancer Res.* 2000;20:553–558.

12. Knopp MV, Weiss E, Sinn HP, et al. Pathophysiologic basis of contrast enhancement in breast tumors. *J Magn Reson Imaging.* 1999;10:260–266.

13. Muller-Schimpfle M, Noack F, Oettling G, et al. Influence of histopathological factors on dynamic MR mammography. *Fortschr Geb Rontgenstr Neuen Bildgeb Verfahr.* 2000;172:894–900.

14. Stomper PC, Winston JS, Herman S, et al. Angiogenesis and dynamic MR imaging gadolinium enhancement of malignant and benign breast lesions. *Breast Cancer Res Treat.* 1997;45:39–46.

15. Su MY, Cheung YC, Fruehauf JP, et al. Correlation of dynamic contrast enhancement MRI parameters with microvessel density and VEGF for assessment of angiogenesis in breast cancer. *J Magn Reson Imaging.* 2003;18:467–477.

16. Turetschek K, Huber S, Floyd E, et al. MR imaging characterization of microvessels in experimental breast tumors by using a particulate contrast agent with histopathologic correlation. *Radiology* 2001;218:562–569.

17. van Dijke CF, Brasch RC, Roberts TP, et al. Mammary carcinoma model: correlation of macromolecular contrast-enhanced MR imaging characterizations of tumor microvasculature and histologic capillary density. *Radiology* 1996;198:813–818.

18. Kuhl CK, Bieling H, Gieseke J, et al. Breast neoplasms: T2* susceptibility-contrast, first-pass perfusion MR imaging. *Radiology* 1997;202:87–95.

19. Kvistad KA, Rydland J, Vainio J, et al. Breast lesions: evaluation with dynamic contrast-enhanced T1-weighted MR imaging and with T2*-weighted first-pass perfusion MR imaging. *Radiology* 2000;216:545–553.

20. Delille JP, Slanetz PJ, Yeh ED, et al. Breast cancer: regional blood flow and blood volume measured with magnetic susceptibility-based MR imaging—initial results. *Radiology* 2002;223:558–565.

21. Helbich TH, Gossman A, Mareski PA, et al. A new polysaccharide macromolecular contrast agent for MR imaging: biodistribution and imaging characteristics. *J Magn Reson Imaging.* 2000;11:694–701.

22. Pham CD, Roberts TP, van Bruggen N, et al. Magnetic resonance imaging detects suppression of tumor vascular permeability after administration of antibody to vascular endothelial growth factor. *Cancer Invest.* 1998;16:225–230.

23. Schwickert HC, Stiskal M, Roberts TP, et al. Contrast-enhanced MR imaging assessment of tumor capillary permeability: effect of irradiation on delivery of chemotherapy. *Radiology* 1996;198:893–898.

24. Fischer U, V Heyden D, Vosshenrich R, et al. Signalverhalten maligner und benigner Läsionen in der dynamischen 2D-MRT der Mamma. *Fortschr Röntgenstr* 1993;158:287–292.

25. Kuhl CK, Kreft BP, Bieling HB, et al. Dynamic breast MRI in premenopausal healthy volunteers: normal values of contrast enhancement and cycle phase dependency. *Radiology* 1997;203:137–144.

26. Kuhl CK. MR imaging of breast tumors. *Eur Radiol.* 2000;10:46–58.

27. Heywang-Köbrunner SH, Viehweg P, Heinig A, Kuchler C. Contrast enhanced MRI of the breast: accuracy, value, controversies, solutions. *Eur J Radiol.* 1997;24:94–108

28. Müller-Schimpfle M, Ohmenhauser K, Stoll P, et al. Menstrual cycle and age: influence on parenchymal contrast medium enhancement in MR imaging of the breast. *Radiology* 1997;203:145–149.

29. Schnall MD, Ikeda DM. Lesion diagnosis working group report. *J Magn Reson Imaging.* 1999;10:982–990.

30. Fischer U, Kopka L, Grabbe E. Invasive mucinous carcinoma of the breast missed by contrast-enhancing MR imaging of the breast. *Eur Radiol.* 1996;6:929–931.

31. Qayyum A, Birdwell RL, Daniel BL, et al. MR imaging features of infiltrating lobular carcinoma of the breast: histopathologic correlation. *AJR Am J Roentgenol.* 2002;178:1227–1232.

32. Weinstein SP, Orel SG, Heller R, et al. MR imaging of the breast in patients with invasive lobular carcinoma. *AJR Am J Roentgenol.* 2001;176:399–406.

33. Yeh ED, Slanetz PJ, Edmister WB, et al. Invasive lobular carcinoma: spectrum of enhancement and morphology on magnetic resonance imaging. *Breast J.* 2003;9:13–18.

34. Kuhl CK, Mielcarek P, Leutner C, Schild HH. Diagnostic criteria of ductal carcinoma in-situ (DCIS) in dynamic contrast-enhanced breast MRI: comparison with invasive breast cancer (IBC) and benign lesions. *Proc Int Soc Magn Reson Med.* 1998;931.

35. Westerhof JP, Fischer U, Moritz JD, Oestmann JW. MR imaging of mammographically detected clustered microcalcifications: is there any value? *Radiology* 1998;207:675–681.

36. Heywang SH, Hahn D, Schmidt H, et al. MR imaging of the breast using gadolinium-DTPA. *J Comp Assist Tomogr.* 1986;10:199–204.

37. Hulka CA, Edmister WB, Smith BL, et al. Dynamic echo-planar imaging of the breast: experience in diagnosing breast carcinoma and correlation with tumor angiogenesis. *Radiology* 1997;205:837–842.

38. Harms SE, Flamig DP, Hesley KL, et al. MR imaging of the breast with rotating delivery of excitation off resonance: clinical experience with pathologic correlation. *Radiology* 1993;187:493–501.

39. Furman-Haran E, Grobgeld D, Kelcz F, Degani H. Critical role of spatial resolution in dynamic contrast-enhanced breast MRI. *J Magn Reson Imaging.* 2001;13:862–867.

40. Kinkel K, Helbich TH, Esserman LJ, et al. Dynamic high-spatial-resolution MR imaging of suspicious breast lesions: diagnostic criteria and interobserver variability. *AJR Am J Roentgenol.* 2000;175:35–43.

41. Liu PF, Debatin JF, Caduff RF, et al. Improved diagnostic accuracy in dynamic contrast enhanced MRI of the breast by combined quantitative and qualitative analysis. *Br J Radiol.* 1998;71:501–509.

42. Song HK, Dougherty L, Schnall MD. Simultaneous acquisition of multiple resolution images for dynamic contrast enhanced imaging of the breast. *Magn Reson Med.* 2001;46:503–509.

43. Szabo BK, Aspelin P, Wiberg MK, Bone B. Dynamic MR imaging of the breast. Analysis of kinetic and morphologic diagnostic criteria. *Acta Radiol.* 2003 44:379–386.

44. Obenauer S, Schorn C, Stelter B, et al. Contrast-enhanced high in-plane resolution dynamic MRI of the breast. Are there advantages in comparison to standard dynamic MRI? *Clin Imaging.* 2002;26:161–165.

45. Baum F, Fischer U, Vosshenrich R, Grabbe E. Classification of hypervascularized lesions in CE MR imaging of the breast. *Eur Radiol.* 2002;12:1087–1092.

46. Mussurakis S, Gibbs P, Horsman A. Primary breast abnormalities: selective pixel sampling on dynamic gadolinium-enhanced MR images. *Radiology* 1998;206:465–473.

47. Kuhl CK, Kreft BP, Hauswirth A, et al. MR-Mammographie bei 0.5 Tesla: Vergleich von Bildqualität und Sensitivität der MR-Mammographie bei 0.5 T und 1.5 T. *RöFo* 1995;162:381–389.

48. Kuhl CK, Kreft BP, Hauswirth A, et al. MR-Mammographie bei 0.5 Tesla: Die Differenzierbarkeit maligner und benigner Läsionen in der MR-Mammographie bei 0.5 T und 1.5 T. *RöFo* 1995;162:482–491.

49. Degani H, Gusis V, Weinstein D, et al. Mapping pathophysiological features of breast tumors by MRI at high spatial resolution. *Nat Med.* 1997;3:780–782.

50. Leong CS, Daniel BL, Herfkens RJ, et al. Characterization of breast lesion morphology with delayed 3DSSMT: an adjunct to dynamic breast MRI. *J Magn Reson Imaging.* 2000;11:87–96.

51. Nunes LW, Schnall MD, Siegelman ES, et al. Diagnostic performance characteristics of architectural features revealed by high spatial-resolution MR imaging of the breast. *AJR Am J Roentgenol.* 1997;169:409–415.

52. Kuhl CK, Mielcarek P, Klaschik S, et al. Are T2-weighted pulse sequences helpful to assist differential diagnosis of enhancing lesions in dynamic breast MRI? *J Magn Reson Imaging.* 1999;9:187–196.

53. Kuhl CK, Mielcarek P, Klaschik S, et al. Are signal time course data useful for differential diagnosis of enhancing lesions in dynamic breast MR imaging? *Radiology* 1999;211:101–110.

54. Mussurakis S, Buckley DL, Horsman A. Dynamic MRI of invasive breast cancer: assessment of three region-of-interest analysis methods. *J Comput Assist Tomogr.* 1997;21:431–438.

55. Daniel BL, Yen YF, Glover GH, et al. Breast disease: dynamic spiral MR imaging. *Radiology* 1998;209:499–509.

56. Boetes C, Barentsz JO, Mus RD, et al. MR characterization of suspicious breast lesions with a gadolinium-enhanced TurboFLASH subtraction technique. *Radiology* 1994;193:777–781.

57. Choyke PL, Dwyer AJ, Knopp MV. Functional tumor imaging with dynamic contrast-enhanced magnetic resonance imaging. *J Magn Reson Imaging.* 2003;17:509–520.

58. Port RE, Knopp MV, Hoffmann U, et al. Multicompartment analysis of gadolinium chelate kinetics: blood-tissue exchange in mammary tumors as monitored by dynamic MR imaging. *J Magn Reson Imaging.* 1999;10:233–241.

59. Tofts PS, Berkowitz B, Schnall MD. Quantitative analysis of dynamic Gd-DTPA enhancement in breast tumors using a permeability model. *Magn Reson Med.* 1995;33:564–568.

60. Agoston AT, Daniel BL, Herfkens RJ, et al. Intensity-modulated parametric mapping for simultaneous display of rapid dynamic and high-spatial-resolution breast MR imaging data. *Radiographics* 2001;21:217–226.

61. Hoffmann U, Brix G, Knopp MV, et al. Pharmacokinetic mapping of the breast: a new method for dynamic MR mammography. *Magn Reson Med.* 1995;33:506–514.

62. Taylor JS, Tofts PS, Port R, et al. MR imaging of tumor microcirculation: promise for the new millennium. *J Magn Reson Imaging.* 1999;10:903–907.

63. Tofts PS, Brix G, Buckley DL, et al. Estimating kinetic parameters from dynamic contrast-enhanced T(1)-weighted MRI of a diffusable tracer: standardized quantities and symbols. *J Magn Reson Imaging.* 1999;10:223–232.

64. Heywang SH, Wolf A, Pruss E, et al. MR imaging of the breast with Gd-DTPA: use and limitations. *Radiology* 1989;171:95–103.

65. Schorn C, Fischer U, Luftner-Nagel S, Grabbe E. Diagnostic potential of ultrafast contrast-enhanced MRI of the breast in hypervascularized lesions: are there advantages in comparison with standard dynamic MRI? *J Comput Assist Tomogr.* 1999;23:118–122.

66. Hwang ES, Kinkel K, Esserman LJ, et al. Magnetic resonance imaging in patients diagnosed with ductal carcinoma-in-situ: value in the diagnosis of residual disease, occult invasion, and multicentricity. *Ann Surg Oncol.* 2003;10:381–388.

67. Ikeda DM. Progress report from the American College of Radiology Breast MR Imaging Lexicon Committee. *Magn Reson Imaging Clin N Am.* 2001;9:295–302.

68. Miller RW, Harms S, Alvarez A. Mucinous carcinoma of the breast: potential false-negative MR imaging interpretation. *AJR Am J Roentgenol.* 1996;167:539–540.

69. Soderstrom CE, Harms SE, Copit DS, et al. Three-dimensional RODEO breast MR imaging of lesions containing ductal carcinoma in situ. *Radiology* 1996;201:427–432.

70. Ikeda DM, Birdwell RL, Daniel BL. Potential role of magnetic resonance imaging and other modalities in ductal carcinoma in situ detection. *Magn Reson Imaging Clin N Am.* 2001;9:345–356.

71. Kuhl CK, Schmutzler RK, Leutner CC, et al. Breast MR imaging screening in 192 women proved or suspected to be carriers of a breast cancer susceptibility gene: preliminary results. *Radiology* 2000;215:267–279.

72. Liberman L, Morris EA, Dershaw DD, et al. Ductal enhancement on MR imaging of the breast. *AJR Am J Roentgenol.* 2003;181:519–525.

73. Amano G, Ohuchi N, Ishibashi T, et al. Correlation of three-dimensional magnetic resonance imaging with precise histopathological map concerning carcinoma extension in the breast. *Breast Cancer Res Treat.* 2000;60:43–55.

74. Bedrosian I, Mick R, Orel SG, et al. Changes in the surgical management of patients with breast carcinoma based on preoperative magnetic resonance imaging. *Cancer* 2003;98:468–473.

75. Fischer U, Kopka L, Grabbe E. Breast carcinoma: effect of pre-operative contrast-enhanced MR imaging on the therapeutic approach. *Radiology* 1999;213:881–888.

76. Harms SE. Breast Cancer Staging Working Group report. *J Magn Reson Imaging.* 1999;10:991–994.

77. Hiramatsu H, Enomoto K, Ikeda T, et al. The role of contrast-enhanced high resolution MRI in the surgical planning of breast cancer. *Breast Cancer* 1997;4:285–290.

78. Kneeshaw PJ, Turnbull LW, Drew PJ. Role of magnetic resonance imaging in the diagnosis and single-stage surgical resection of invasive lobular carcinoma of the breast. *Br J Surg.* 2002;89:1296–1301.

79. Liberman L, Morris EA, Dershaw DD, et al. MR imaging of the ipsilateral breast in women with percutaneously proven breast cancer. *AJR Am J Roentgenol.* 2003;180:901–910.

80. Munot K, Dall B, Achuthan R, et al. Role of magnetic resonance imaging in the diagnosis and single-stage surgical resection of invasive lobular carcinoma of the breast. *Br J Surg.* 2002;89:1296–1301.

81. Quan ML, Sclafani L, Heerdt AS, et al. Magnetic resonance imaging detects unsuspected disease in patients with invasive lobular cancer. *Ann Surg Oncol.* 2003;10:1048–1053.

82. Lee SG, Orel SG, Woo IJ, et al. MR imaging screening of the contralateral breast in patients with newly diagnosed breast cancer: preliminary results. *Radiology* 2003;226:773–778.

83. Liberman L, Morris EA, Dershaw DD, et al. MR imaging of the ipsilateral breast in women with percutaneously proven breast cancer. *AJR Am J Roentgenol.* 2003;180:901–910.

84. Liberman L, Morris EA, Kim CM, et al. MR imaging findings in the contralateral breast of women with recently diagnosed breast cancer. *AJR Am J Roentgenol.* 2003;180:333–341.

85. Abraham DC, Jones RC, Jones SE, et al. Evaluation of neoadjuvant chemotherapeutic response of locally advanced breast cancer by magnetic resonance imaging. *Cancer* 1996;78:91–100.

86. Balu-Maestro C, Chapellier C, Bleuse A, et al. Imaging in evaluation of response to neoadjuvant breast cancer treatment benefits of MRI. *Breast Cancer Res Treat.* 2002;72:145–152.

87. Delille JP, Slanetz PJ, Yeh ED, et al. Invasive ductal breast carcinoma response to neoadjuvant chemotherapy: noninvasive monitoring with functional MR imaging pilot study. *Radiology* 2003;228:63–69.

88. Gilles R, Guinebretiere JM, Toussaint C, et al. Locally advanced breast cancer: contrast-enhanced subtraction MR imaging of response to preoperative chemotherapy. *Radiology* 1994;191:633–638.

89. Knopp MV, Brix G, Junkermann HJ, Sinn HP. MR mammography with pharmacokinetic mapping for monitoring of breast cancer treatment during neoadjuvant therapy. *Magn Reson Imaging Clin N Am.* 1994;2:633–658.

90. Mumtaz H, Davidson T, Spittle M, et al. Breast surgery after neoadjuvant treatment. Is it necessary? *Eur J Surg Oncol.* 1996;22:335–341.

91. Rieber A, Zeitler H, Rosenthal H, et al. MRI of breast cancer: influence of chemotherapy on sensitivity. *Br J Radiol.* 1997;70:452–458.

92. Trecate G, Ceglia E, Stabile F, et al. Locally advanced breast cancer treated with primary chemotherapy: comparison between magnetic resonance imaging and pathologic evaluation of residual disease. *Tumori* 1999;85:220–228.

93. Wasser K, Sinn HP, Fink C, et al. Accuracy of tumor size measurement in breast cancer using MRI is influenced by histological regression induced by neoadjuvant chemotherapy. *Eur Radiol.* 2003;13:1213–1223.

94. Weatherall PT, Evans GF, Metzger GJ, et al. MRI vs. histologic measurement of breast cancer following chemotherapy: comparison with x-ray mammography and palpation. *J Magn Reson Imaging.* 2001;13:868–875.

95. Morris EA, Liberman L, Ballon DJ, et al. MRI of occult breast carcinoma in a high-risk population. *AJR Am J Roentgenol.* 2003;181:619–626.

96. Warner E, Plewes DB, Shumak RS, et al. Comparison of breast magnetic resonance imaging, mammography, and ultrasound for surveillance of women at high risk for hereditary breast cancer. *J Clin Oncol.* 2001;19:3524–3531.

97. Stoutjesdijk MJ, Boetes C, Jager GJ, et al. Magnetic resonance imaging and mammography in women with a hereditary risk of breast cancer. *J Natl Cancer Inst.* 2001;93:1095–1102.

98. Podo F, Sardanelli F, Canese R, et al. The Italian multicentre project on evaluation of MRI and other imaging

modalities in early detection of breast cancer in subjects at high genetic risk. *J Exp Clin Cancer Res.* 2002;21(Suppl 3): 115–124.

99. Tilanus-Linthorst MM, Obdeijn IM, Bartels KC, et al. First experiences in screening women at high risk for breast cancer with MR imaging. *Breast Cancer Res Treat.* 2000; 63:53–60.

100. Acenero MJ, Gallego MG, Ballesteros PA, Gonzalez JF. Vascular density as a prognostic indicator for invasive ductal breast carcinoma. *Virchows Arch.* 1998;432:113– 117.

101. Costello P, McCann A, Carney DN, Dervan PA. Prognostic significance of microvessel density in lymph node negative breast carcinoma. *Hum Pathol.* 1995;26:1181–1184.

102. Goede V, Fleckenstein G, Dietrich M, et al. Prognostic value of angiogenesis in mammary tumors. *Anticancer Res.* 1998; 18:2199–2202.

103. Karaiossifidi H, Kouri E, Arvaniti H, et al. Tumor angiogenesis in node-negatvie breast cancer: relationship with relapse-free survival. *Anticancer Res.* 1996;16:4001– 4002.

104. Fischer U, Kopka L, Brinck U, et al. Prognostic value of contrast-enhanced MR mammography in patients with breast cancer. *Eur Radiol.* 1997;7:1002–1005.

105. Stomper PC, Herman S, Klippenstein DL, et al. Invasive breast carcinoma: analysis of dynamic magnetic resonance imaging enhancement features and cell proliferative activity determined by DNA S-phase percentage. *Cancer* 1996 1;77:1844–1849.

106. Boné B, Aspelin P, Bronge L, Veress B. Contrast-enhanced MR imaging as a prognostic indicator of breast cancer. *Acta Radiol.* 1998;39:279–284.

107. Mussurakis S, Buckley DL, Horsman A. Dynamic MR imaging of invasive breast cancer: correlation with tumour grade and other histological factors. *Br J Radiol.* 1997; 70:446–451.

108. van den Brink JS, Watanabe Y, Kuhl CK, et al. Implications of SENSE MR in routine clinical practice. *Eur J Radiol.* 2003;46:3–27.

8
Benign Lesions

Andrea F. Abramson

Even if contrast-enhanced breast magnetic resonance imaging (MRI) is reserved for the clinical situations in which the probability of finding a breast carcinoma is high, there is still a greater probability of finding a benign lesion on breast MRI than a carcinoma. An appreciation of benign findings on breast MRI may be crucial to avoid unnecessary biopsies. This chapter reviews the most common benign lesions of the breast and attempts to characterize their appearance on MRI.

1. Mass Lesions

1.1. Noncontrast-Enhanced Images

Conspicuity of mass lesions on fat-suppressed T2-weighted (T2W) images generally depends on the water content of the lesion.[1,2] For example, simple cysts are very conspicuous as they consist almost entirely of fluid surrounded by a thin layer of epithelium. Similarly, myxomatous, cellular fibroadenomas are high in signal on T2W images, but sclerotic, acellular fibroadenomas are not due to the fact that the cellular water content is less.[3] Lymph nodes are often conspicuous on the T2W image due to their cellular content and they appear high in signal.[4] Assessing the T2W images for high signal in the suspected area of a lymph node can often confirm this diagnosis if the characteristic fatty hilum is not apparent. Carcinomas can be high in signal on T2 especially if they are partially cystic or necrotic. This is particulary true for mucinous carcinoma, which has been reported to be high in signal on T2 and may not demonstrate typical malignant enhancement profiles.[5]

Generally, most mass lesions, benign and malignant, are similar in signal intensity, isointense, to surrounding breast parenchyma on fat-suppressed T2W images.[4] Similarly, mass lesions benign and malignant are isointense to parenchyma on T1-weighted (T1W) noncontrast images unless they contain proteinaceous material, such as breakdown products of blood. Cysts with varying amounts of

protein can be high in signal on T1W images before the administration of intravenous contrast.[1,2]

1.2. Contrast-Enhanced Images

Lesions cannot be adequately assessed using T2 or T1 signal characteristics without the use of intravenous contrast. T1-weighted fat-suppressed contrast-enhanced images increase both the sensitivity and specificity of the breast examination by allowing better characterization of lesion morphology, enhancement intensity, and kinetics.[4,6,7] An MRI lexicon has been developed to standardize terminology to be used in reporting breast MRI findings[8] (see also Chapter 6).

Certain MRI findings are highly predictive of benign disease. Shape and borders define masses morphologically. For example, a round or oval shape of a mass has been shown to carry a 97% to 100% predictive value for benignity[7–10] in some series. Other series[11] however have shown that up to 20% of carcinomas can have a benign appearance on MRI with round, smooth appearing margins. It can be safely stated that the classic benign characteristics seen on mammography cannot be easily translated to MRI. Many of the shape and border characteristics that are used in assessment of breast lesions are not as reliably assessed on MRI due to the inherent current lower resolution obtained with MRI compared with that of mammography.[11] Possibly with improvement in protocols, as well as a shift to higher field magnets, increased resolution will be feasible so that morphologic architecture can be optimized.

Masses with smooth or lobulated borders in one series had a predictive value for benignity of 97% to 100%.[7,9,10,12] Caution should be exercised, however, if a smooth or lobulated mass has suspicious internal enhancement or rim enhancement or if the lesion demonstrates washout kinetics. As with mammography, the worst feature of the lesion should be taken into consideration when trying to decide how to manage such a lesion.[8,13] Future series will demonstrate the predictive value of the MRI descriptors when used in multiple settings.

Lack of enhancement is also helpful in distinguishing benign from malignant disease. For example, complete absence of mass enhancement carries a predictive value of 100% for benignity.[4,14,15] Mass lesions that enhance less than surrounding breast tissues usually are benign 93% to 100% of the time.[12] Predictive values for enhancing lesions vary, however; if an enhancing lesion has benign morphology (such as the reniform shape of an intramammary lymph node), the lesion is most likely benign.

Pattern of enhancement is also a considered feature in MRI evaluation of lesions. For example, homogeneously enhancing masses and lobulated masses with nonenhancing septations can carry a 93% to 97% predictive value for benignity in some hands and are usually fibroadenomas.[7,8,11,12,16] Rim enhancement is most predictive of malignancy, usually seen with an invasive carcinoma; however, rim enhancement can be a cause of false-positive findings, sometimes associated with benign inflamed cysts and fat necrosis. The appearance of an inflammatory cyst is usually not a diagnostic dilemma when the rim is thin and regular and the cyst does not enhance. T2-weighted images usually confirm the presence of a cyst.[11]

Enhancement kinetic analysis is less reliable than morphology for evaluation of mass lesions.[14] Quantitatively evaluated signal parameters do not differ significantly between malignant and benign lesions. Generally, though, progressive (or continuous) time intensity curves suggest benign disease.[2,4] Plateau kinetics may be identified in both benign and malignant disease.[17] In both the progressive and plateau curves, there is slower uptake of contrast and no washout. Malignant entities, such as infiltrating lobular carcinoma, medullary carcinoma, and ductal carcinoma in situ (DCIS),[2] can have benign looking curves without washout.

1.3. Fibroadenoma

Fibroadenomas are the most common benign neoplasm of the breast. They may occur in all age groups, but are most common in young women with peak incidence in the 30s. They may be solitary or multiple.[2,3,18] Histologically, fibroadenomas are most often smooth, occasionally lobulated, circumscribed, round, or oval masses. They are comprised of epithelial and stromal elements surrounded by a pseudocapsule.[19] The epithelial component is composed of gland-like, duct-like spaces containing terminal duct and lobular tissues. The stromal elements consist of surrounding connective tissue containing varying amounts of collagen and acid mucopolysaccharides.[20,21] The predominance of epithelial versus stromal components varies with age.[21] The epithelial elements usually predominate in younger women. In older postmenopausal women, the stromal component dominates and may hyalinize or calcify.[3,4,16]

On noncontrast-enhanced T2W images, signal intensity varies depending on the fluid content of the lesion. Cellular, myxomatous lesions, often seen in younger patients, are high in signal[1] (Figures 8.1 through 8.3). Less cellular and sclerotic lesions, seen in older patients, vary from intermediate to low signal intensity[3,16,20] (Figures 8.4 through 8.6).

Fibroadenomas are of low signal on T1W noncontrast images and most often cannot be distinguished from adjacent glandular tissues.[4] On T1W contrast-enhanced images, fibroadenomas are usually round, oval, or lobulated with smooth, circumscribed margins. Cellular, myxomatous fibroadenomas lesions demonstrate uniform and homogeneous enhancement. Forty percent to 60% of enhancing fibroadenomato contain nonenhancing internal septations, which, if seen, are diagnostic for benign fibroadenoma to >95% certainty[7,22] (Figure 8.7). Less cellular, fibroadenomas enhance less or not at all. Sclerotic fibroadenomas do not enhance at all. When there is no enhancement, there is an almost 100% likelihood of benignity. The enhancement kinetic curves generally are continuous or plateau.[4,16]

Phyllodes tumor is a variant of fibroadenoma. This rare tumor has been previously inaccurately called cystosarcoma phylloides or giant fibroadenoma.[18,19] Histologically phyllodes tumors are similar to cellular intracanalicular fibroadenomas. They are distinguished by the presence of epithelial-lined clefts and their rapid growth.[19,23] T2-weighted images show bright intensity from both the cellular and cystic components of phyllodes tumors. T1-weighted contrast-enhanced images demonstrate intense enhancement with continuous or plateau kinetics. Note should be made that a small percentage of these lesions are considered malignant because they recur and can metastasize.[23]

1.4. Papilloma

Papillomas may be solitary or multiple. When solitary, they are usually small (<1 cm) and located centrally near the nipple in a major lactiferous duct; more than half are associated with duct ectasia.[18,24] Seventy percent to 80% of the time, they present clinically with bloody nipple discharge in women 30 to −55 years of age.[19,25,26] When papillomas are multiple, they are more often peripherally located and bilateral. They appear to arise from the terminal ductal lobular unit (TDLU) rather than from a major duct and much less often present as bloody nipple discharge.[20,21] Rarely, the clinical presentation is a palpable mass. There is a controversial slight increased association with carcinoma.[24,26]

Conventional breast imaging modalities are of limited utility. Occasionally, microcalcifications are seen on mammography in the region of the lesion identified on MRI, but usually papillomas are mammographically occult due

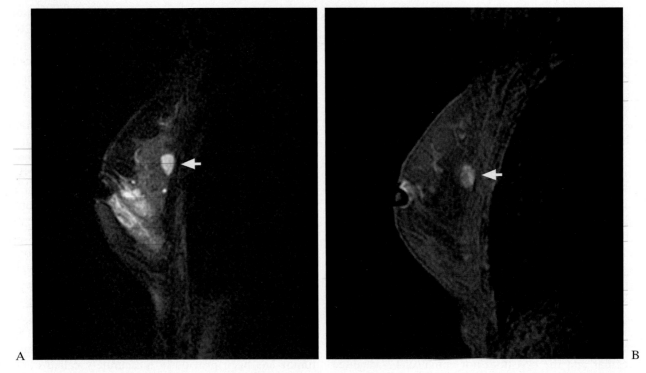

A   B

FIGURE 8.1. Fibroadenoma. A 54-year-old with family history of breast cancer. Ultrasound shows solid, oval, well-circumscribed mass. (A) High signal intensity mass on T2W precontrast image (arrow). This and all following T2W images are fat suppressed.

(B) Heterogeneously enhancing mass on T1W postcontrast-enhanced image (arrow). This and all following T1W images are fat suppressed, unless otherwise noted.

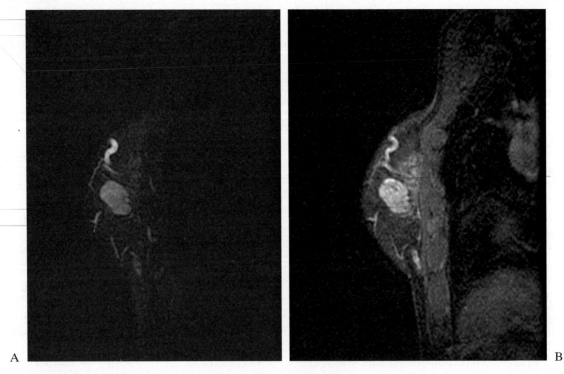

A   B

FIGURE 8.2. Fibroadenoma. A 44-year-old with history of contralateral phyllodes tumor. Mammogram and ultrasound correlate with enlarging mass in upper inner quadrant on MRI. (A)

High signal intensity mass on T2W precontrast image. (B) Enhancing mass on T1W postcontrast-enhanced image. Note absence of nonenhancing septations.

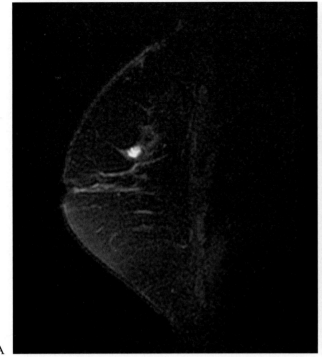

A   B

FIGURE 8.3. Fibroadenoma. A 60-year-old woman. Status post left mastectomy for infiltrating lobular carcinoma. Right breast ultrasound guided core biopsy yielded cellular epithelial lesion. Surgical excision yielded cellular myxofibroepithelial lesion consistent with fibroadenoma. (A) High signal intensity mass on T2W precontrast image. (B) Enhancing mass on T1W postcontrast-enhanced images.

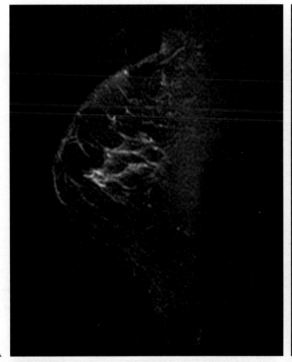
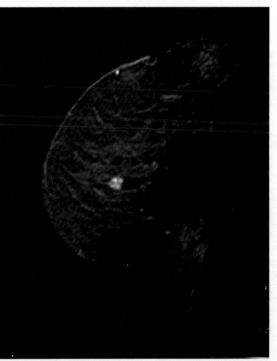

A   B

FIGURE 8.4. Fibroadenoma. A 71-year-old woman. Status post contralateral lumpectomy in distant past for invasive ductal carcinoma. New palpable left axillary adenopathy; lymph node biopsy showed metastatic lobular carcinoma. Magnetic resonance imaging guided needle localization of abnormal enhancement in the lower inner quadrant of the left breast yielded infiltrating lobular carcinoma. Magnetic resonance imaging guided needle localization in the upper inner quadrant yielded fibroadenoma associated with lobular carcinoma in situ and sclerosing adenosis. (A) T2-weighted image does not reveal a mass compatible with a less cellular histolopathology. (B) Enhancing mass with nonenhancing septations on T1W postcontrast image.

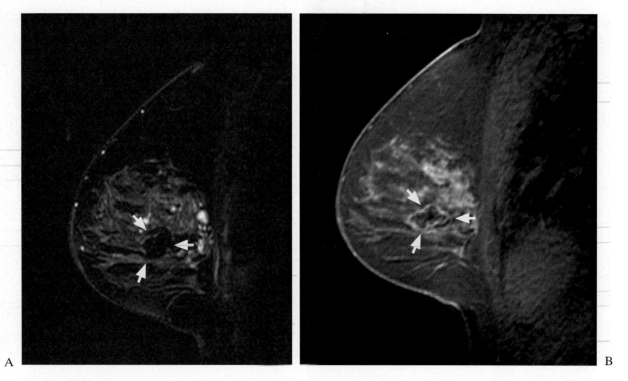

FIGURE 8.5. Fibroadenoma. A 47-year-old woman. Status post right lumpectomy for infiltrating ductal carcinoma, tubular type, and DCIS. Left breast with mammographically stable calcified fibroadenoma. (A) Mass is isointense with signal void of calcifications on T2W image (arrows). Note high signal in cysts. (B) Faint enhancement on delayed T1W postcontrast-enhanced image (arrows).

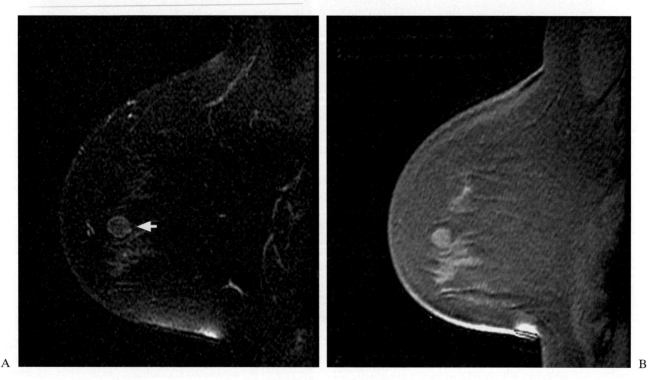

FIGURE 8.6. Fibroadenoma. A 78-year-old, status post contralateral lumpectomy. (A) Circumscribed heterogeneous moderate signal intensity mass on T2W image (arrow). (B) Mass is also identified on T1W precontrast image.

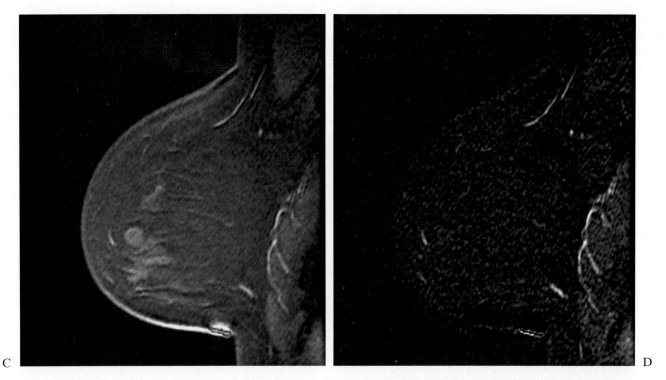

C   D

FIGURE 8.6. (*Continued*) (C) No enhancement on T1W postcontrast enhanced scan. (D) Subtraction image shows no enhancement.

to their small size and central location. A sonogram may show a dilated duct with or without an intraductal mass. Galactography may show a dilated duct containing a solitary frond-like filling defect.[26]

Histologically, papillomas consist of villous, branching, and interanastomosing papillae with a central vascular core, usually connected to the duct wall by a delicate stalk. Papillomas may undergo fibrosis or infarction.[24,25,27] Most

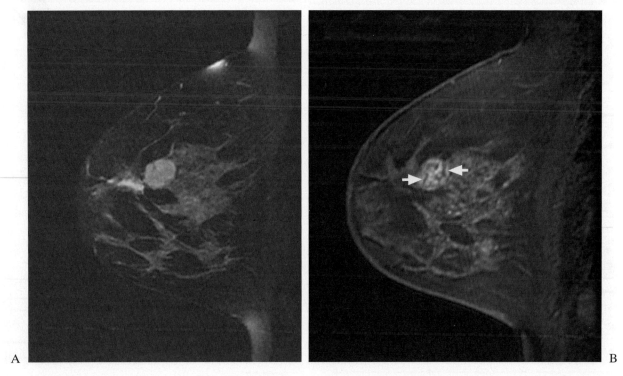

A   B

FIGURE 8.7. Fibroadenoma with nonenhancing areas. A 48-year-old woman. Status post right mastectomy for infiltrating ductal carcinoma. Left breast with palpable mass with mammographic and ultrasound correlates. (A) Mass with high intensity signal on T2W image. (B) Enhancing mass with nonenhancing areas on T1W postcontrast image (arrows).

papillomas are occult on MRI, except when associated with a dilated duct (Figures 8.8 through 8.10). On fat-suppressed T2W images, a high signal intensity dilated central duct may contain a small intermediate signal mass.[25,28]

Papilloma and its associated dilated duct are of low signal intensity on T1W no-contrast images; however, if the duct fluid is hemorrhagic or of high protein content, it will appear bright.[22] On T1W fat-suppressed contrast-enhanced images, papillomas enhance intensely and uniformly as round, circumscribed, often subareolar small masses, except if they are sclerosed and there is no enhancement at all.[3,4,28]

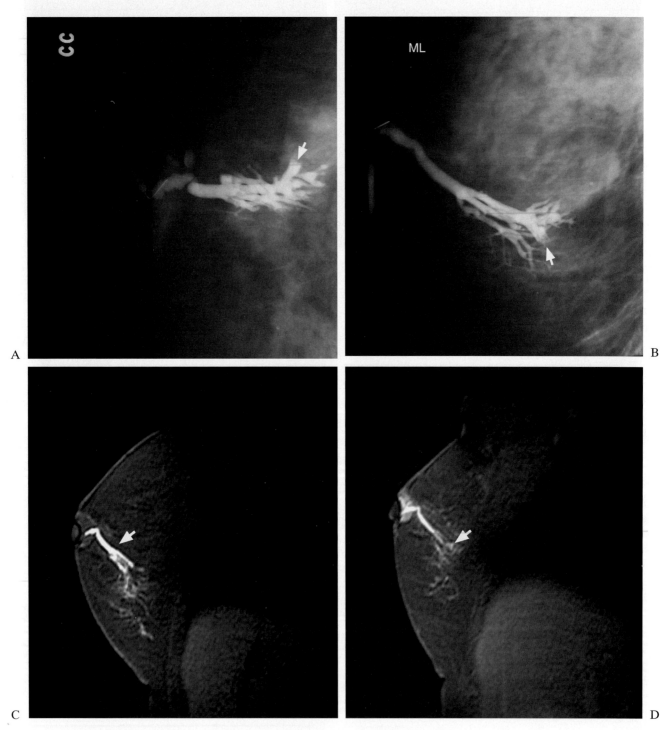

FIGURE 8.8. Papilloma-dilated duct with mass. A 54-year-old with right spontaneous bloody nipple discharge. Ductogram, (A) cranial-caudal and (B) lateral-medial projections, demonstrates filling defect at proximal end of dilated duct (arrows). (C) T1-weighted precontrast image shows high signal proteinaceous or hemorrhagic fluid in a dilated duct (arrow). (D) T1-weighted postcontrast enhanced image demonstrates slight enhancement of the mass filling defect (arrow).

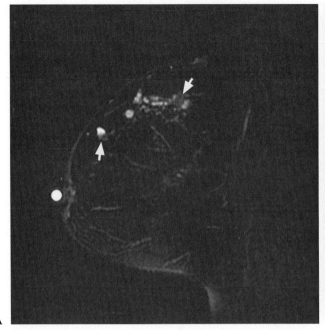

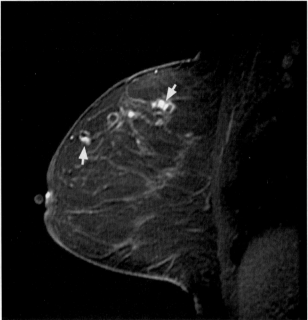

A   B

FIGURE 8.9. Papilloma-papillomatosis. A 55-year-old woman with history of remote contralateral ductal carcinoma in situ. History of multiple papillomas. (A) Multiple high signal intensity areas consisting of dilated ducts seen on T2W image. Arrows demon- strate associated masses that subsequently enhance. (B) T1- weighted postcontrast image demonstrates multiple enhancing masses associated with dilated ducts. Biopsy yielded two scleros- ing papillomas associated with atypical duct hyperplasia (arrows).

1.5. Cysts

Breast cysts are common; they are the most common lesion seen on MRI. Cysts are usually multiple and often wax and wane with the menstrual cycle. True cystic disease occurs most often between the ages of 45 to 55 due to hyperpla- sia of ductal epithelium and dilatation of ducts during the menstrual cycle not balanced by regressive parenchymal changes.[19,20] Histologically, a cyst is a focal dilatation of a duct. It is a fluid collection surrounded by a thin layer of apocrine epithelium. The fluid may be clear and straw- colored, but, if there has been intracystic hemorrhage or

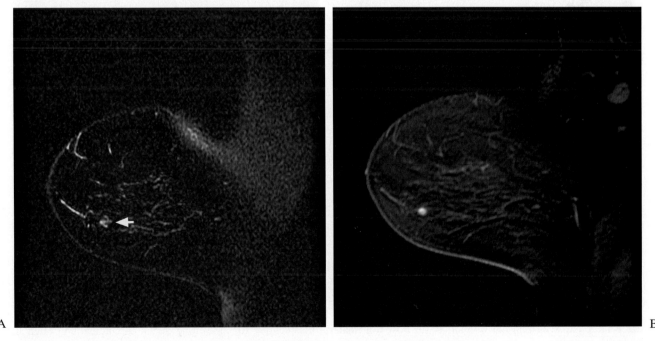

A   B

FIGURE 8.10. Papilloma-solitary lesion. A 48-year-old woman with contralateral infiltrating ductal carcinoma. (A) Moderately signal intensity on T2W-weighted image (arrow). (B) Enhancing mass on T1W postcontrast image.

(Continued)

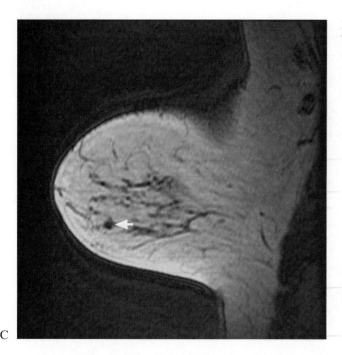

FIGURE 8.10. (*Continued*) (C) Very low signal intensity mass on T1W non–fat-suppressed image (arrow).

C

inflammation, the fluid may be thick or layering,[2] green or black from breakdown products of blood. The wall of the cyst may be thick if there is organized chronic inflammatory cells and fibrosis.

On T2W noncontrast images, simple cysts are characteristically very high fluid-signal, round, sharply circum-

scribed masses (Figure 8.11). On T1W fat-suppressed precontrast images, simple cysts exhibit signal intensity less than or equal to surrounding breast tissue. If the cyst fluid contains protein from blood products, however, intermediate-to-high signal intensity, depending on the protein content, is seen (Figure 8.12). On T1W fat-suppressed

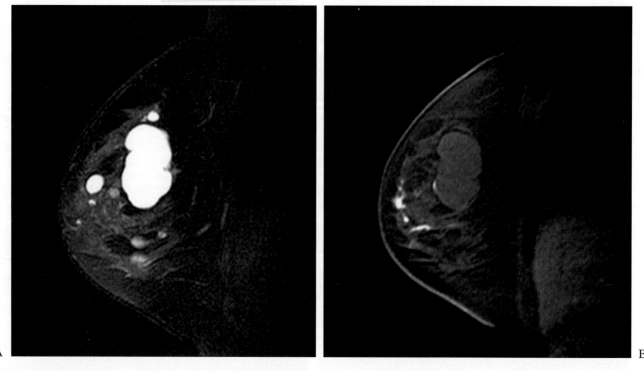

A

B

FIGURE 8.11. Cyst. A 49-year-old woman. Status post contralateral mastectomy for infiltrating ductal carcinoma. (A) High signal intensity circumscribed mass on T2W images. (B) No enhancement on T1W postcontrast image. Note anterior duct ectasia.

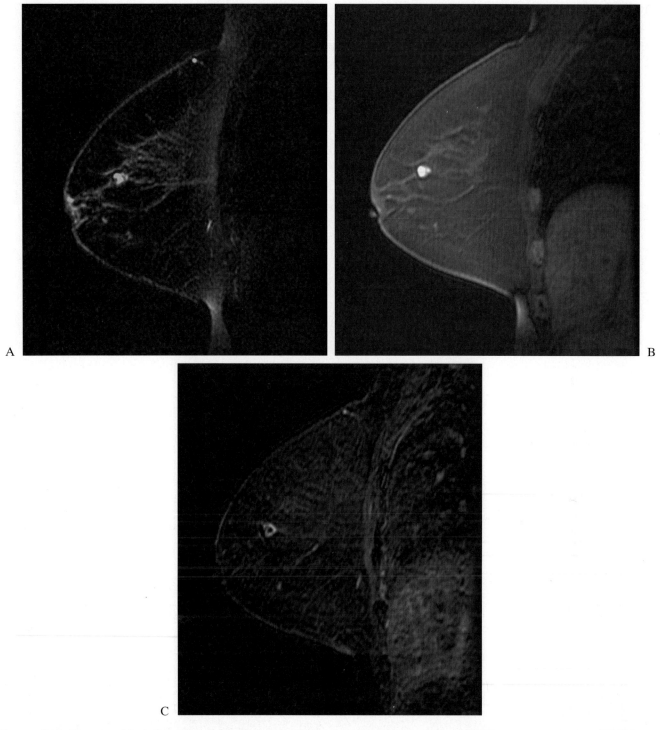

FIGURE 8.12. Hemorraghic inflamed cyst. A 57-year-old with history of contralateral ductal carcinoma in situ. (A) High signal mass on T2W images. (B) Low-to-moderate signal proteinaceous debris within the mass on T1W precontrast images. (C) Subtraction images show only thin rim enhancement.

contrast-enhanced images, simple cysts do not enhance. If there has been inflammation with organization, there may be thin peripheral rim enhancement[9] (Figures 8.13 and 8.14). Caution should be taken to differentiate an inflamed cyst from carcinoma as the latter may exhibit similar MRI features. To be confident of the diagnosis of cyst, the peripheral rim enhancement must be thin and smooth; there must be no central enhancement and the

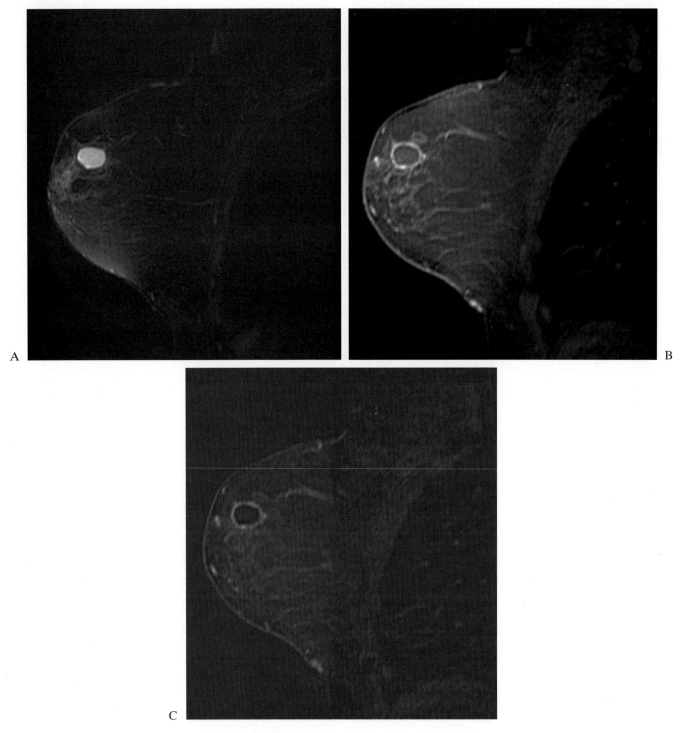

FIGURE 8.13. Inflammatory cyst. A 65-year-old woman with contralateral ductal carcinoma in situ. (A) High signal intensity circumscribed mass on T2W images. (B) Thin rim enhancement on T1W postcontrast images. (C) Thin rim enhancement on subtraction image.

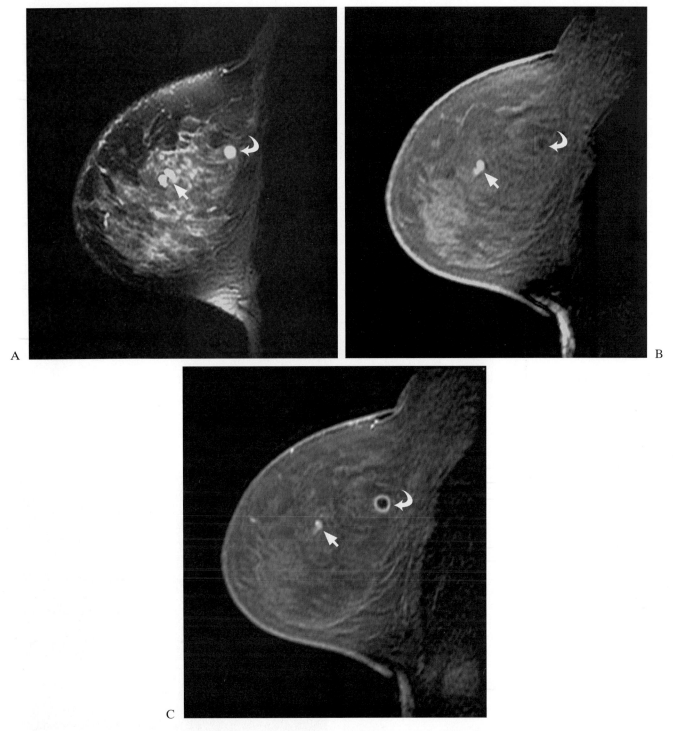

FIGURE 8.14. Inflammatory cyst. (A) High signal circumscribed masses on T2W image (straight and curved arrows). (B) Low-to-moderate signal proteinaceous material in more anteriorly located lesion on T1W precontrast image (straight arrow). (C) More anterior lesion does not enhance (straight arrow) and posterior lesion demonstrates thin rim enhancement on T1W postcontrast image (curved arrow).

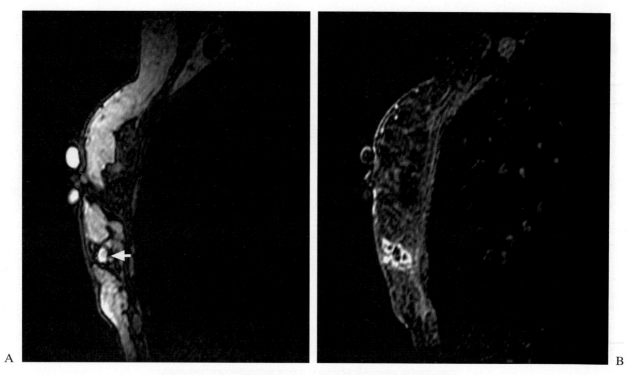

FIGURE 8.15. Fat necrosis. (A) Focal high signal on T1W preconstrast non–fat-suppressed image consistent with fat necrosis (arrow). (B) Subtraction image demonstrates only rim enhancement.

T2W noncontrast images must not demonstrate signal less bright than that of fluid.[9]

1.6. Fat Necrosis

When necrosis of fat cells occurs, from loss of vascular supply from surgery, radiation, or other trauma, enzymes lipolyze the content of adipocytes.[18,21] Histologically, recent fat necrosis consists of a collection of inflammatory cells, lipid-laden macrophages, histiocytes, and hemorrhage.[19] As time goes by the necrotic tissues become surrounded by giant cell granulomatous reaction, much later by fibrosis.[19,21] Saponification of the fat may occur, leading to the presence of calcification. A painless mass may be the clinical presentation.

T1-weighted noncontrast images show very low signal intensity mass of variable shape, surrounded by a rim of variable signal intensity (Figures 8.15 through 8.17). Non–fat-suppressed noncontrast T1W images can be extremely helpful in confirming the impression of fat necrosis by revealing bright fat signal centrally within the enhancing lesion. The appearance of fat necrosis on T1W contrast-enhanced images is variable. The variability in MRI characteristics is due to the various stages in development, maturation, and resolution of fat necrosis. When

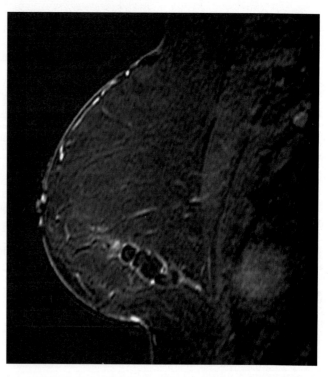

FIGURE 8.16. Fat necrosis. A 58-year-old status post reduction mammoplasty 5 years ago. Slight rim enhancement on T1W subtraction.

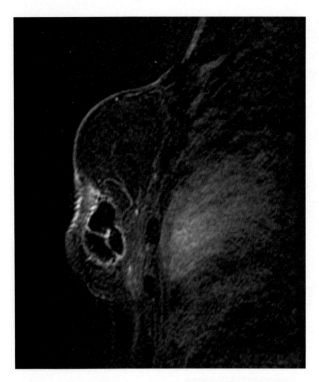

FIGURE 8.17. Fat necrosis. A 49-year-old status post mastectomy with TRAM flap reconstruction in 2001. Now with new palpable mass in TRAM flap. Nonenhancing complex mass with enhancing septations on contrast-enhanced T1W image. Note low signal central, nonenhancing fat.

Contrast-enhanced T1W fat-suppressed images generally show a circumscribed enhancing mass (Figures 8.18 and 8.19). Occasionally, a nonenhancing central hilum can be identified. Kinetic analysis of normal lymph nodes shows rapid enhancement and washout, typical for malignancy. Therefore, lymph nodes can be confused with carcinoma if only the kinetic curves are considered. T2W images demonstrating a high signal mass reassure the presence of a probable lymph node despite the kinetic pattern. Hyperplastic or inflammatory lymph nodes usually cannot be distinguished from metastatic lymph nodes.[30] Extreme irregularity of a lymph node in the axilla can raise the suspicion of metastatic involvement with extranodal extension. A central fatty focus in an oval circumscribed mass confirms the presence of a normal lymph node in a T1W non–fat-suppressed noncontrast imaging series. Preoperative detection of metastases can be performed though is not highly sensitive[31] as small areas of nodal involvement are not assessed.[32] With the widespread use of sentinel lymph node biopsy and the possibility of detection of micrometastatic disease, the sensitivity of MRI in the evaluation of metastatic disease may not be high enough to compete with sentinel node biopsy.

1.8. Hamartoma

These are rare, solitary benign malformations that resemble neoplasms, but result from faulty development of breast tissues. They are circumscribed lesions containing varying amounts and combinations of normal breast tissue, mature fat, adipose tissue, muscle and connective tissue, surrounded by a thin fatty capsule.[19] The nomenclature varies with the dominant component histologically.[18,20] They have a diagnostic mammographic appearance, and MRI is usually not needed for their diagnosis.

On T1W fat-saturated contrast-enhanced images, there may be some slight enhancement if glandular elements are prominent. The fatty capsule may be seen if non–fat suppressed series are used.[4]

the MRI findings are florid, fat necrosis may be indistinguishable from malignancy. There may be a central nonenhancing stellate,[4] irregular mass with surrounding prominent thick, irregular rim enhancement. Enhancing septations may be identified. History of trauma and mammographic features are helpful to distinguish. Additionally, comparison with the mammogram can be invaluable in cases in which fat necrosis is suspected as characteristic oil cysts, calcifications, and distortion can be seen.

1.7. Lymph Node

Lymph nodes are part of the normal anatomy of the breast. They are seen most commonly in the axilla and axillary tail,[27] but they may also be identified in other quadrants, though less commonly in the lower inner quadrant.[29] Magnetic resonance imaging demonstrates lymph nodes in the posterior breast that have heretofore been out of the field of imaging. These can be identified in many normal breasts. Normal lymph nodes are oval and circumscribed and usually measure up to 1.5 cm and may be related to a coursing vessel. Sometimes a vessel extending up to the lymph node hilum is seen. The classic reniform shape and characteristic location can usually confirm the impression of a lymph node.

1.9. Abscess

Abscesses can result from unresolved local infection, caused by obstruction of the duct near the nipple and acute, chronic, or lactational mastitis. They are usually palpable, often subareolar in location and associated with erythema, edema, and induration of overlying skin and pain.[21]

Noncontrast T2W images show focal moderate-to-high signal mass depending on the water content (Figure 8.20). Shape and margins vary from round to irregular. The overlying thickened skin may be intermediate or bright in signal depending on the degree of edema[4] (Figure 8.21).

T1-weighted noncontrast images show the central mass as medium signal with a lower signal capsule surrounding the mass.[4] Contrast-enhanced T1W images demonstrate a

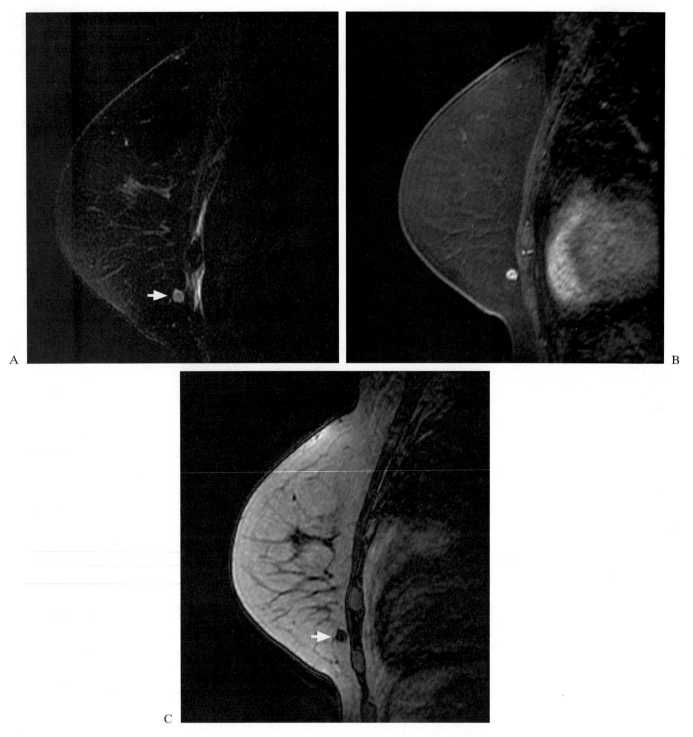

FIGURE 8.18. Lymph node. A 60-year-old woman status post right lumpectomy in 1996. Chest wall recurrence 2001. Computed tomography showed enlarging mass in contralateral breast. (A) Moderately high signal mass identified in lower inner quadrant on T2W image (arrow). (B) Enhancement on T1W postcontrast image. (C) Circumscribed, oval, low signal mass with no central fatty hilum on T1W precontrast non–fat-suppressed image, proved to be posterior intramammary lymph node (arrow).

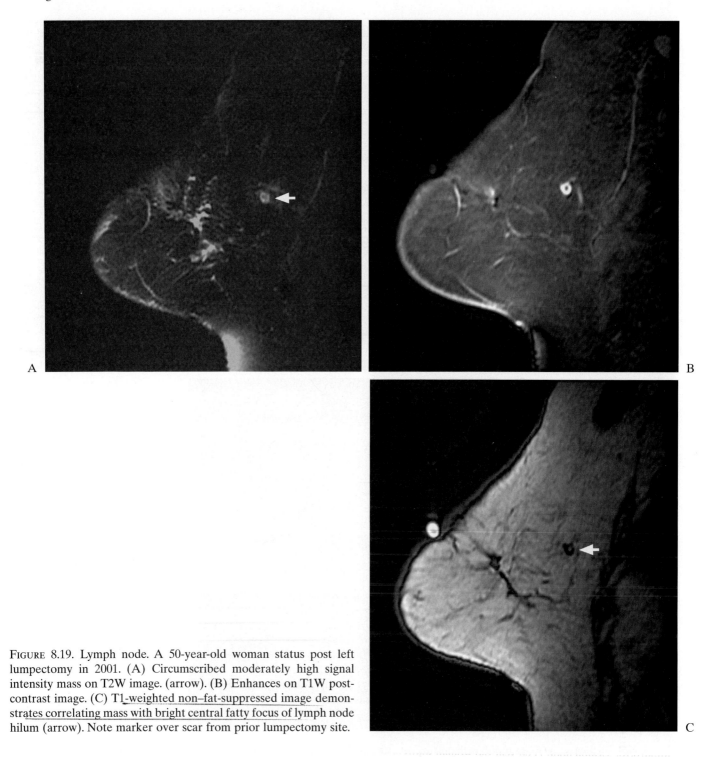

FIGURE 8.19. Lymph node. A 50-year-old woman status post left lumpectomy in 2001. (A) Circumscribed moderately high signal intensity mass on T2W image. (arrow). (B) Enhances on T1W post-contrast image. (C) T1-weighted non–fat-suppressed image demonstrates correlating mass with bright central fatty focus of lymph node hilum (arrow). Note marker over scar from prior lumpectomy site.

nonenhancing central, round, or irregular mass surround by an early intensely enhancing rim. The surrounding inflammatory tissues may enhance moderately and irregularly and may be thickened. Abscess may be confused with malignancy because the enhancement kinetics of the rim and the irregular appearance of the overlying tissues are similar. History and clinical examination will be helpful to distinguish from carcinoma.[33]

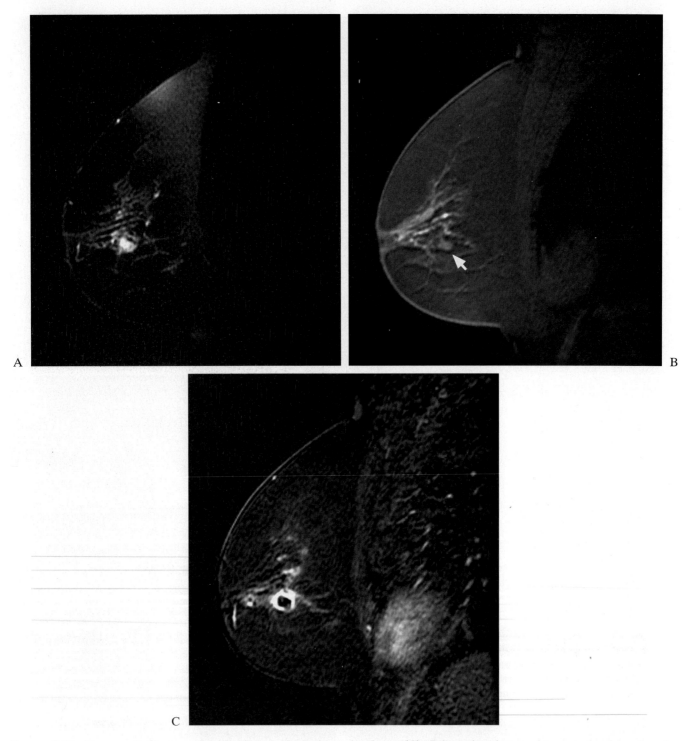

FIGURE 8.20. Abscess. A 51-year-old with history of mastitis. Hypermetabolic lesion identified on PET scan. (A) High signal intensity mass on T2W image. (B) Intermediate signal on T1W precontrast image (arrow). Note high signal proteinaceous debris in ducts. (C) Subtraction image demonstrates irregular rim enhancement. Cannot distinguish abscess from malignancy on magnetic resonance; pathology yielded findings consistent with abscess.

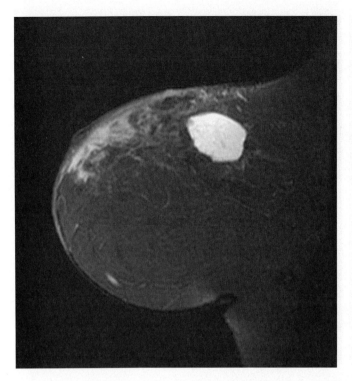

FIGURE 8.21. Abscess cavity with overlying edema on fat-suppressed T2W images.

2. Nonmass Lesions

2.1. Fibrocystic Disease

Fibrocystic disease is the most common, most often bilateral, disorder of the breast. It is the result of distortion and exaggeration of normal menstrual cyclic changes of ductal epithelium and stroma.[18,20,21] Histopathologically, fibrocystic disease, also called *chronic cystic mastitis* or *mammary dysplasia*, is not a single discrete entity. Nonproliferative fibrocystic changes, which are not associated with an increased risk to breast cancer, consist of cysts of varying sizes, stromal fibrosis, and apocrine metaplasia. Proliferative fibrocystic changes include hyperplasia without atypia, papillomas, and sclerosing adenosis. Atypical hyperplasias, such as atypical lobular hyperplasia and atypical ductal hyperplasia, included in the spectrum of fibrocystic disease,[4,19,20,21] may be associated with a slight increased risk for cancer.

Fibrocystic parenchyma is most often difficult to distinguish from normal breast parenchyma on both T2W and T1W noncontrast imaging series (Figures 8.22 and 8.23). This is because fibrocystic parenchyma, like normal parenchyma, has a variable appearance dependent on the water and collagen content of the tissues.[14] The pattern may be similar to that seen on the mammogram. One may identify clusters of small cysts, less than 3mm. On T1W

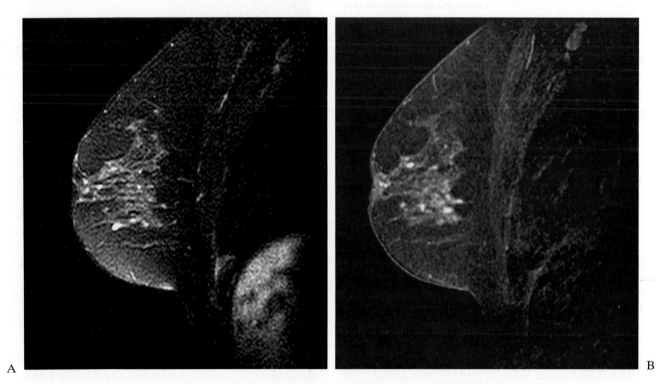

A   B

FIGURE 8.22. Fibrocystic disease. (A) Many small high intensity focus on T2W image. (B) Stippled enhancement on T1W postcontrast enhanced image.

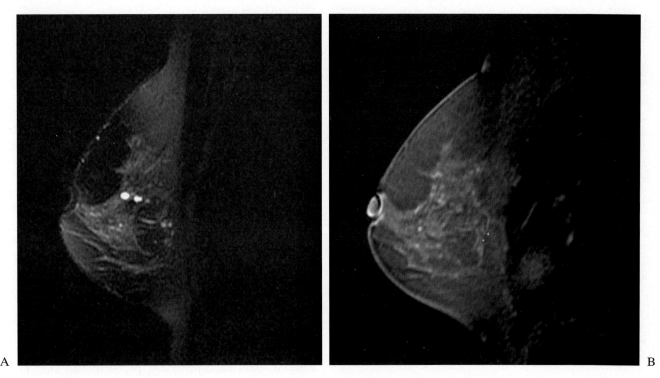

A   B

FIGURE 8.23. Fibrocystic disease. (A) Two circumscribed high signal intensity masses seen on T2W image. (B) T1-weighted postcontrast image demonstrates no enhancement of the cysts and stippled enhancement through the breast.

contrast-enhanced images, however, there may be a prominent presence of stippled regional enhancement.[2,8,12] Occasionally, this pattern may seem to coalesce and appear as a region of clumped enhancement or even as a heterogeneous large mass.[12]

Proliferative changes, such as sclerosing adenosis, may appear as mass-like lesions due to the compression of stroma with distortion or the glandular elements. These patterns are difficult to distinguish from carcinoma or DCIS.[12] Generally, if these patterns vary with the menstrual cycle, least conspicuous in mid-cycle, the diagnosis of fibrocystic disease is more likely. Evaluation of enhancement kinetics can be helpful if continuous or plateau kinetic patterns are observed.[6,14,17]

2.2. Sclerosing Adenosis

Sclerosing adenosis is one of the benign causes of enhancement on MRI. The enhancement may be patchy or more diffuse (Figure 8.24). The MRI enhancement pattern depends on its histologic pattern. Histologically, sclerosing adenosis consists of swirls of desmoplastic proliferation with variable amounts of epithelium and myoepithelium. These may appear in a lobulocentric pattern and may be confused with tubular carcinoma. They also may assume an infiltrative pattern and may be confused with invasive lobular carcinoma. Sclerosing adenosis may also be asso-

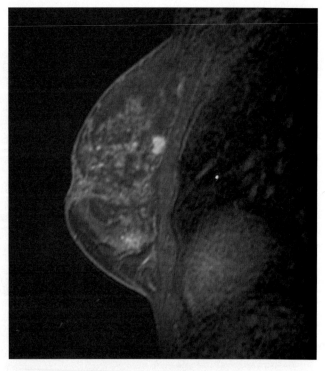

FIGURE 8.24. Sclerosing adenosis. T1-weighted postcontrast image demonstrates irregular enhancement in the posterior breast. There is stippled benign enhancement throughout the remained or the breast. Surgical biopsy yielded nodular sclerosing adenosis.

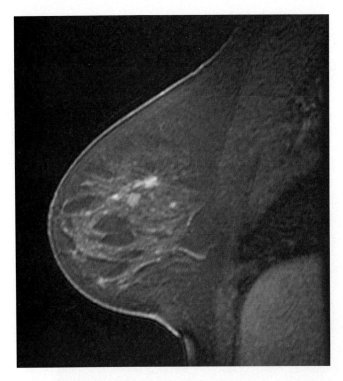

FIGURE 8.25. 46-year old with recent diagnosis of breast carcinoma undergoes contralateral screening breast MRI. A spiculated mass is identified in the 12 o'clock axis of the breast. MR localization and surgical biopsy of the lesion yielded florid fibrocystic changes, including radial scars.

ciated with the stromal components of other benign lesions such as radial scars papillomas, and fibroadenomas.[3,19,21]

2.3. Radial Scar

This lesion has been described in the literature by many names, including radial sclerosing lesion, complex sclerosing lesion, sclerosing papillary proliferation, nonencapsulated sclerosing lesion, and indurative mastopathy. Pathologically, radial scar has a stellate configuration consisting of a central fibroelastic sclerotic core. Radiating from this core are proliferative elements consisting of epithelial hyperplasia, papillomatosis, and sclerosing adenosis. There is a known association with malignancy, usually tubular carcinoma, particularly if the lesion is greater than 2cm in women older than 50 years of age in 25% of cases.[3,19,21]

Imaging features of the radial scar present a diagnostic challenge. The features can appear as a spiculated mass, suggesting the presence of invasive carcinoma on mammogram and ultrasound. On MRI, contrast-enhanced T1-weighted images show an enhancing irregular or spiculated mass that is indistinguishable from carcinoma (Figures 8.26 and 8.27). For this reason, biopsy is required. Enhancement is usually heterogeneous; kinetic patterns are unreliable and can overlap.[34]

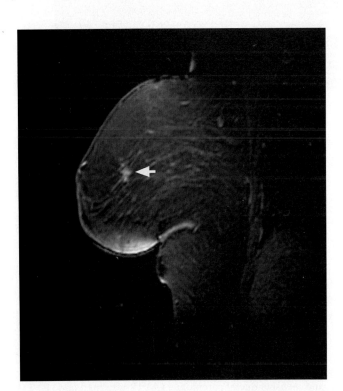

FIGURE 8.26. Radial scar. Small spiculated, enhancing mass on T1W postcontrast images, which yielded radial scar at surgery (arrow). Note suboptimal positioning with inferior skin fold.

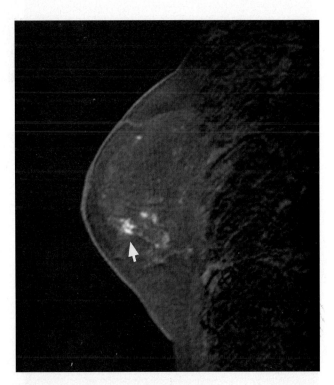

FIGURE 8.27. Radial scar. Small spiculated enhancing mass on T1W postcontrast images, which yielded radial scar at surgery (arrow).

2.4. Parenchymal Scar

Another diagnostic challenge is normal scar versus recurrence of carcinoma in the conserved or reconstructed breast. It is known that if a postsurgical scar is enlarging on mammography, becoming denser or more spiculated over time, recurrence should be suspected. Also, new appearance of clustered pleomorphic calcifications suggests recurrence. Ultrasound may be helpful if, by comparison to a previous study, the hypoechoic parenchymal

scar with or without acoustic shadowing appears larger, more nodular, or speculated.[4]

Contrast-enhanced MRI has been helpful in the evaluation of this problem. The MRI appearance of normal scar evolves over time. Immediately after surgery, there is usually a resolving hematoma that appears bright on T2W noncontrast images. On T1-weighted contrast-enhanced images, there may be vaguely nodular, rim, or linear mild-to-moderate (usually late) enhancement, surrounding the operative bed (Figures 8.28 through 8.30). This is due to the

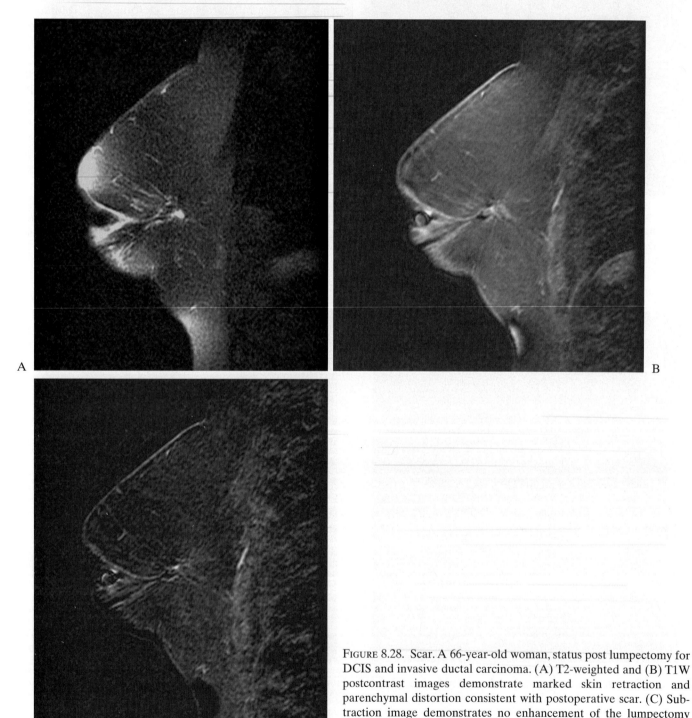

FIGURE 8.28. Scar. A 66-year-old woman, status post lumpectomy for DCIS and invasive ductal carcinoma. (A) T2-weighted and (B) T1W postcontrast images demonstrate marked skin retraction and parenchymal distortion consistent with postoperative scar. (C) Subtraction image demonstrates no enhancement of the lumpectomy bed.

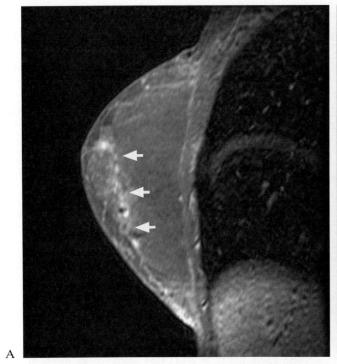

FIGURE 8.29. Scar. Status post reduction mammoplasty. (A) One month postoperative T1W postcontrast enhanced image demonstrates linear, nonductal postoperative change (arrows).

(B) Seven month postoperative T1W postcontrast image shows resolution of immediate postoperative change. Nonenhancing parenchymal scar is identified.

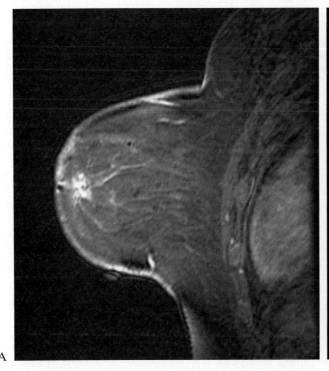
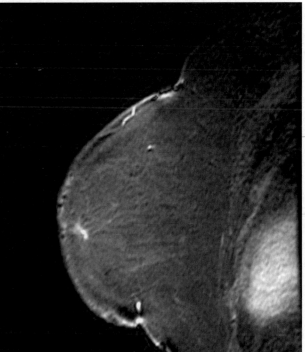

FIGURE 8.30. Scar. Status post surgical benign biopsy. (A) Post surgical T1W postcontrast-enhanced image demonstrates irregular subareolar enhancement. (B) Six-month follow-up T1W contrast-enhanced images shows almost complete resolution of postoperative changes.

presence of granulation tissue with ingrowth of vessels, fibroblasts, and inflammatory response. Enhancement kinetic patterns of early scar and recurrence can overlap as both can demonstrate washout. By 3 to 6 months, however, the normal parenchymal scar has generally matured into nonenhancing dense fibrosis, reliably differentiated from enhancing recurrence on MRI. The appearance of scar in the irradiated breast follows a similar histologic course and 1 year following radiation, there should be no enhancement of the operative bed on T1W contrast-enhanced images or in the remainder of the breast.[4,35–37]

3. High-Risk Lesions

The diagnosis of a high-risk lesion such as lobular carcinoma in situ (LCIS), atypical ductal hyperplasia (ADH), and atypical lobular hyperplasia may be important for a selected patient as these diagnoses confer a specific risk of developing breast cancer. These high-risk markers indicate increased future risk rather than the specific precursor lesion of breast cancer. The future increased risk applies to both breasts equally and not just to the breast where the high-risk lesion was found.

3.1. Lobular Carcinoma In Situ (LCIS)

Since the earliest days of breast MRI, it has been noticed that LCIS can be a cause of false-positive enhancement. On mammography, LCIS is usually found as an incidental finding on pathology when biopsy is performed for calcifications. The familiar characteristic lack of specific imaging findings for LCIS on mammography may not hold true for MRI. Lobular carcinoma in situ has been shown to have features that can be suspicious for malignancy. Although little has been published about the appearance of LCIS on MRI, in our experience LCIS constitutes 10% of suspicious linear ductal enhancement.[38]

3.2. Atypical Ductal Hyperplasia (ADH)

Histopathologically, areas of ADH show some but not all of the characteristics of ductal carcinoma in situ. The risk of developing carcinoma following the diagnosis of ADH is five times the general population. If there is a coexistent family history, the risk increase is increased to 11. In our experience ADH constitutes 9% of suspicious linear ductal enhancement.[38]

References

1. Stark DD, Bradley WG. *Magnetic Resonance Imaging*. St. Louis: CV Mosby Co; 1988.
2. Warren R, Coulthard A. *Breast MRI in Practice*. London: Taylor and Francis; 2002:73–96.
3. Heywang-Kobrunner SH, Dershaw DD, Scheer I. *Diagnostic Breast Imaging*. 2nd ed. Stuttgart: Ehieme; 2001.
4. Heywang-Kobrunner SH, Bech I. *Contrast Enhanced MRI of the Breast*. 2nd ed. Berlin: Springer; 1995.
5. Kawashima M, Tamaki Y, Noriaka T, et al. MR imaging of mucinous carcinoma of the breast. *AJR Am J Roentgenol*. 2002;179:179–183.
6. Liberman L, Morris EA, Benton CL, et al. Probably benign lesions at breast magnetic resonance imaging: preliminary experience in high-risk women. *Cancer* 2003;98:377–388.
7. Nunes LW, Schnall MD, Orel SG, et al. Breast MR imaging: interpretation model. *Radiology* 1997;202:833–841.
8. Morris, EA. Illustrated breast MR lexicon. In: Miller WT, Berg WA, eds. *Seminars in Roentgenology*. Vol. 36: *Breast Imaging*. Philadelphia: Saunders; 2001:238–249.
9. Nunes LW, Schnall MD, Siegelman ES, et al. Diagnostic performance characteristics of architectural features revealed by high spatial-resolution MR imaging of the breast. *AJR Am J Roentgenol*. 1997;169:409–415.
10. Nunes LW, Schnall MD, Orel SG. Update of breast MR imaging architectural interpretation model. *Radiology* 2001;219:484–494.
11. Kim SJ, Morris EA, Liberman L, et al. Observer variability and applicability of BI-RADS terminology for breast MR imaging: invasive carcinomas as focal masses. *AJR Am J Roentgenol*. 2001;177:551–557.
12. Nunes LW, Schnall MD, Orel SG, et al. Correlation of lesion appearance and histologic findings for the nodes of a breast MR imaging interpretation model. *Radiographics* 1999;19:79–92.
13. Liberman L, Morris E, Lee MJY, et al. Breast lesions detected on MR imaging: features and positive predictive value. *AJR Am J Roentgenol*. 2002;179:171–178.
14. Morris EA. Review of breast MRI: indications and limitations. In: Miller WT, Berg WA, eds. *Seminars in Roentgenology*. Vol. 36: *Breast Imaging*. Philapdelphia: Saunders; 2001:226–237.
15. Orel SG. MR imaging of the breast. *Radiol Clin N Am*. 2000;38:899–912.
16. Hochman MG, Orel SG, Powell CM, et al. Fibroadenomas: variety of MR appearances with radiologic-histopatholoic correlation. *Radiology* 1997;204:123–129.
17. Ikeda DM, Hylton NM, Kuhl CK, et al. *ACR-Breast Imaging and Reporting System-Magnetic Resonance Imaging: Illustrated BI-RADS-MR*. Reston, VA: American College of Radiology; 2003:1–43.
18. Bassett L, Jackson VP. *Diagnosis of Disease of the Breast*. Philadelphia: Saunders; 1997:352–354.
19. Rosen PP. *Rosen's Breast Pathology*. 2nd ed. Philadelphia: Lippincott, William, & Wilkens; 2001.
20. Bland K, Copeland EM. *The Breast—Comprehensive Management of Benign and Malignant Diseases*. Philadelphia: Saunders; 1991:91–92.
21. Harris JR, Hellman S, Henderson IC, et al. Benign breast disorders. In: *Breast Diseases*. 2nd ed. New York: JB Lippincott Co; 1991:15–46.
22. Liberman L, Morrris E, Lee MJY, et al. Breast lesions detected on MR imaging: features positive predictive value. *AJR Am J Roentgenol*. 2002;179:171–178.

23. Liberman L, Bonaccio E, Hamele-Bena D, et al. Benign and malignant phyllodes tumors: mammographic and sonographic findings. *Radiology* 1996;198:121–124.

24. Liberman L, Bracero N, Vuolo MA, et al. Percutaneous large-core biopsy of papillary breast lesions. *AJR Am J Roentgenol.* 1999;172:331–337.

25. Rovno HDS, Siegelman ES, Reynolds C, et al. Solitary intraductal papilloma: findings at MR imaging and MR galactography. *AJR Am J Roetgenol.* 1999;172:151–155.

26. Woods ER, Helvie MA, Ikeda DM, et al. Solitary breast papilloma: comparison of mammographic, galactographic and pathologic findings. *AJR Am J Roetengnol.* 1992;159:487–491.

27. Meyer JE, Ferraro FA, Frenna TH, et al. Mammographic appearance of normal intramammary lymph nodes in an atypical location. *AJR Am J Roentgenol.* 1993;161:779–780.

28. Orel SG, Dougherty CS, Reynolds C, et al. MR imaging in patients with nipple discharge: initial experience. *Radiology* 2000;216:248–254.

29. Schmidt WA, Boudousquie AC, Vetto JT, et al. Lymph nodes in the human female breast: a review of their detection and significance. *Hum Pathol.* 2001;32:178–187.

30. Kinoshita T, Tashiro N, Yoshigi J, et al. Inflammatory intramammary lymph node mimicking the malignant lesion in dynamic MRI: a case report. *Clin Imaging.* 2002;26:258–262.

31. Kvistad KA, Rydland J, Smethurst HB, et al. Axillary lymph node mestastases in breast cancer: preoperative detection with dynamic contrast-enhanced MRI. *Eur Radiol.* 2000;10:1464–1471.

32. Yoshimura S, Sakurai T, Oura S, et al. Evaluation of axillary lymph node status in breast cancer with MRI. *Breast Cancer* 1999;6:249–258.

33. Chung SX, Yang I, Sang HB, et al. Differentied diagnosis of MR imaging of pyogenic abscess tuberculous abscess and inflammatory cancer in breast: comparison with mammography and US. *Ultrasound Med Biol.* 1997:23 (Suppl):5150.

34. Lee JM, Liberman L, Morris EA, et al. MR imaging findings of radial scars. *AJR Am J Roentgenol.* 2003;180 (Suppl):51.

35. Lewis-Jones HG, Whitehouse GH, Leinster SJ, et al. The role of magnetic resonance imaging in the assessment of local recurrent breast carcinoma. *Clin Radiol.* 1992;43:197–294.

36. Dao TH, Rahmouni A, Campana F, et al. Tumour recurrence versus fibrosis in the irradiated breast: differentiation with dynamic gadolinium-enhanced MR imaging. *Radiology* 1993;187:751–755.

37. Gilles R, Guinebretiere JM, Shapeero LG, et al. Assessment of breast cancer recurrence with contrast-enhanced subtraction MR imaging: preliminary results in 26 patients. *Radiology* 1993;188:473–478.

38. Liberman L, Morris EA, Dershaw DD, Tan LK. Ductal enhancement on MR imaging of the breast. *AJR AM J Roentgenol.* 2003;181:519–525.

9
Ductal Carcinoma In Situ

Jennifer H. Menell

Ductal carcinoma in situ (DCIS) is malignancy confined to the ducts of the breast and, therefore, is considered a preinvasive form of cancer. Since the advent of widespread mammographic screening, ductal carcinoma is found more frequently and is now responsible for up to approximately one-third of detected breast cancer.[1] The early detection of DCIS is thought to be one of the reasons for the decrease in breast cancer mortality. However, controversy with regard to the importance of DCIS exists because not all DCIS progresses to invasive carcinoma. At this writing, it is not possible to determine which DCIS lesion will ultimately invade; therefore, all DCIS lesions are treated as potentially lethal. However, there is evidence that suggests that approximately 30% to 50% of DCIS will progress to invasive carcinoma.[2] This supports the theory that the treatment of this preinvasive cancer will offer benefit to the patient.

1. Mammography and Ductal Carcinoma In Situ

Traditionally, the mammographic detection of DCIS depends on the presence of suspicious microcalcifications. Ductal carcinoma in situ is calcified in up to 90% of cases.[1,3] However, all breast cancer does not contain calcifications, as only approximately 30% to 40% of invasive breast cancer is calcified.[4] As DCIS is considered to be the predisposing factor for the development of invasive carcinoma, we are, therefore, likely missing DCIS on mammography.

In a study by Dershaw and colleagues,[1] 41% of DCIS were greater than 2.5cm and all were seen as multicentric on mammography. Additionally, contralateral DCIS, in patients with known invasive cancer or DCIS, was seen in 26% of cases.[1] Additionally, Page and coworkers[5] have determined that 28% of women with biopsy yielding

DCIS subsequently develop invasive carcinoma. Therefore, in women with known breast cancer, a higher likelihood of undetected ipsilateral or contralateral cancer exists.

Holland and Hendriks[6,7] suggest that mammography is not always able to detect the actual size of tumor as well as extent of disease in the breast. Previously published series by Holland, Hendriks, and coworkers,[7] examining early stage breast cancer, showed that only 37% of mastectomy specimens demonstrated no surrounding tumor, while 20% had tumor foci within 2cm of the index tumor, and 43% had tumor greater than 2cm from the index tumor. Therefore, a significant number of women have unsuspected and undetected tumor in the same and/or different quadrants of the breast. Because surgical planning relies on the accurate detection of disease, and not all DCIS lesions are calcified and therefore not always detected, additional imaging modalities may prove useful in assessing disease extent, particularly in early stage breast cancer such as DCIS. Magnetic resonance imaging (MRI) has been shown to be more sensitive than mammography in detection of additional sites of invasive cancer as well as in situ cancer.

It has been shown that the most common mammographic appearances of calcifications caused by DCIS are linear/branching, coarse granular, or fine granular calcifications.[3,6,8] The linear calcifications represent casts of calcifications in necrotic tumor along the ducts.[6] However, much overlap exists between the mammographic appearance of DCIS and nuclear grade; therefore, mammographic patterns of calcifications are not able to predict pathology. However, mammographic patterns can indicate the probable aggressiveness of the tumor. For example, Evans and coworkers[9] claim that the findings of casting calcifications typical of necrosis favor a more aggressive subtype of DCIS. Similarly, Slanetz and coworkers[10] have observed that a mass seen mammographically indicates a higher likelihood of well-differentiated cancer, or a lower grade.

2. Magnetic Resonance Imaging and Ductal Carcinoma In Situ

Magnetic resonance imaging has been documented to be capable of depicting up to 100% of invasive breast carcinomas.[11–21] However, the accurate detection of DCIS by MRI has not yet been confirmed. Experience with DCIS and MRI is limited. Previously published series suggest that MRI is less capable of detecting DCIS than invasive cancer with the accuracy in detection of DCIS ranging from 20% to 95% (Table 9.1).[11–13,15,17,20–30] A recently published series by Menell and colleagues[31] at our institution reports a sensitivity of 88% in the MRI detection of DCIS.

Magnetic resonance imaging is capable of detecting not only calcified DCIS, but also noncalcified DCIS, therefore improving the evaluation of disease extent. Magnetic resonance imaging does not identify calcifications. Some reports suggest that the larger calcifications associated with the comedo subtype can be detected as small areas of hypointensity, but these have not been reproduced. In general, DCIS is seen as clumped enhancement in either a focal, ductal, linear, segmental, or regional distribution on MRI.

Magnetic resonance imaging enhancement of DCIS is a complex phenomenon. According to Knopp and coworkers,[32] the pathophysiology behind the enhancement patterns of DCIS is not clear. However, research states that vascular permeability appears to play a more significant role than vascular density in determining specific enhancement patterns.[32] Earlier research by Guidi and coworkers[33] describes two patterns of angiogenesis in DCIS. The first is a diffuse increase in microvessels, while the second is due to increased microvessels to a specific area with possible vascular cuffing.[33] Buadu and colleagues[34] support these results, claim that there is a correlation between the rate of contrast enhancement and microvessel density, and conclude that the analysis of the degree of tumor angiogenesis may help determine various enhancement patterns in benign and malignant lesions. More research should be done to further clarify these issues.

Efforts to document the sensitivity of MRI in the detection of DCIS have been made and the literature reflects wide variations in sensitivities. The range of sensitivities may be due to variations in interpretation and imaging techniques used by different investigators. For example, in a study performed by Fischer and coworkers,[28] DCIS was found in 72% of patients, with only 60% of cases demonstrating a kinetic curve that was suggestive of malignancy. This study, however, based the results using dynamic MRI rather than high-resolution imaging.[28] Similarly, Sittek and coworkers[29] published a study documenting that the sensitivity of MRI in the detection of DCIS was 70%. But, in combination with mammography, the sensitivity increased to 90%.[29] The authors claimed that no reliable pattern of enhancement was identified, as DCIS appeared as multifocal enhancement, as a random finding, or even without enhancement in 30% of cases.[29] However, the study was performed on a 1.0 Tesla (T) magnet, with a lower signal-to-noise ratio. In general, most investigators have found that DCIS does not demonstrate typical enhancement curves.

In a recent study by Hwang and coworkers,[35] MRI was found to be 88% accurate in detecting residual disease, 82% accurate in detecting invasive disease, and 90% in detecting multicentric disease. Furthermore, in patients following surgery, the sensitivity in the detection of residual and multicentric disease was 96% and 86%, respectively.[35] This study also claims that a negative MRI can rule out residual disease, occult invasive cancer, and multicentric disease.[35]

An additional study by Westerhof and colleagues[27] compared mammographically evident calcifications and MRI findings to determine benign from malignant lesions. Again, their low sensitivities were described to be a result of a variable imaging pattern of enhancement by DCIS, and the investigators concluded that calcifications seen by mammography should be investigated using traditional biopsy techniques.[27]

3. Magnetic Resonance Imaging of Mammographically Evident Calcifications

As MRI techniques have been developing over the years, it has been hypothesized that MRI of suspicious microcalcifications could determine the need for biopsy. However, this has not always been the case. For example, Gilles and colleagues[12] described that MRI was not capable of

TABLE 9.1. Sensitivities in the MRI Detection of DCIS

Study	Sensitivity
Orel et al., 1995[11]	4/6 (67%)
Gilles et al., 1995[23]	34/36 (94%)
Boetes et al., 1995[17]	7/8 (88%)
Fobben et al., 1995[20]	2–3/5 (40%–60%)
Soderstrom et al., 1996[24]	5/5 (100%)
Gilles et al., 1996[12]	56/58 (97%) (3 cases of LCIS were included)
Bone et al., 1996[19]	14/17 (82%)
Fischer et al., 1996[28]	25/35 (72%)
Sittek et al., 1997[29]	14/20 (70%)
Orel et al., 1997[22]	10/13 (77%)
Boetes et al., 1997[25]	13/17 (76%)
Westerhof et al., 1998[27]	22/33 (67%)
Viehweg et al., 2000[26]	48/50 (96%)
Zuiani et al., 2002[30]	26/28 (92.85%)
Menell et al., 2003[31]	29/33 (88%)

distinguishing benign and malignant calcifications due to poor specificity. Westerhof and colleagues[27] reported similar results. However, another study by Nakahara and colleagues[36] evaluated mammographically evident calcifications and MRI enhancement patterns and reported a 100% sensitivity for DCIS and DCIS with microinvasion. These results stated that MRI was more reliable than mammography in differentiating benign from malignant calcifications and concluded that microcalcifications without MRI enhancement may not need biopsy.[36] However, as only 40 cases were included in their study, and those cases of DCIS with microinvasion were included, other research must be done to support these findings. Our research at Memorial Sloan-Kettering Cancer Center (MSKCC) also demonstrated that the majority of mammographically evident calcifications associated with DCIS were visualized on MRI.[31] However, we support previous research by Westerhof and coworkers[27] and recommend that mammographically evident suspicious microcalcifications without corresponding MRI enhancement should be biopsied using traditional methods.

Other research demonstrates higher sensitivities in the MRI detection of DCIS, but also identifies limitations in DCIS detection. For example, Viehweg and coworkers[26] concluded that 96% of DCIS lesions were demonstrated by MRI, but only one-half of lesions met the criteria for "typical enhancement" with an early, focal, poorly defined, or ductal pattern. This study concluded that DCIS may frequently demonstrate atypical enhancement patterns.[26] Furthermore, a study by Gilles and coworkers[23] demonstrated contrast enhancement in 94% of DCIS lesions. While this study demonstrates an equally high sensitivity as that of Viehweg and colleagues,[26] one-third of cases of DCIS contained foci of microinvasion, perhaps falsely elevating their sensitivity. Additionally, Orel and colleagues[22] described a 77% sensitivity in the MRI detection of DCIS, and recommended that MRI was able to detect both mammographically evident and occult DCIS. Limitations of MRI, however, included small foci of tumor that may be evident at mammography and pathologic examination, but not visualized with MRI.[22] Our experience at MSKCC demonstrated a sensitivity of 88% in the MRI detection of pure DCIS and excluded cases of microinvasive tumor.[31]

4. False-Negative Results by Magnetic Resonance and Mammography

As previously stated, DCIS is calcified in approximately 90% of cases that are detected mammographically.[1,3] However, only approximately one-third of mammographically evident calcifications is detected in invasive ductal carcinoma.[4] Because DCIS is considered to be, if not always, the predisposing factor for invasive ductal carcinoma,[5,37] we are probably missing a considerable proportion of DCIS on screening mammography.

The false-negative rate for the MRI detection of DCIS has varied in the literature. Reported sensitivities for the MRI detection of DCIS vary from 20% to 95%.[11–13,15,17,20–30] Therefore, the false-negative rate ranges from 5% to 80%. Boetes and colleagues[25] examined false-negative cases of breast carcinoma in MRI, and concluded that MRI missed up to 4% of cases. However, DCIS lesions accounted for the largest percentage of MRI occult lesions, as the false-negative rate for the MRI detection of DCIS was 23.5%.[25] However, our experience has been different. We have found a sensitivity of 88%, with a false-negative rate of 12%, which was better than mammography in both sensitivity and false-negative rate.[31] As our patient population was a high-risk population, more research needs to be done to assess the false-negative rate in a screening population of patients.

5. Nuclear Grade

It has been suggested that the nuclear grade of a DCIS lesion affects enhancement, or even, lack of enhancement. Some previous reports have postulated that high-grade DCIS is detected more easily than low grade.[25,27,28] However, other researchers have concluded that there is no significant difference in the detection of high-versus low-grade DCIS.[11,15,22,23,26] Our experience supports these findings.[31] In fact, our research showed that there was no significant difference in the nuclear grade of DCIS found by mammography or MRI.[31]

6. Significant Ductal Carcinoma In Situ Lesions on Magnetic Resonance Imaging

Just as the description of a significant DCIS lesion on mammography has been documented, so has the appearance of DCIS lesions on MRI. The mammographic determination of DCIS usually depends on the presence and appearance of calcifications, as DCIS lesions infrequently present as masses. The most common pattern of DCIS mammographically is linear/branching calcifications due to tumor necrosis within the ducts.[6]

The most common appearances of DCIS lesions on MRI are documented in Table 9.2. Similar to mammography, linear/ductal enhancement patterns are the most common (Figure 9.1). Segmental, regional, mass, or diffuse enhancement is less common (Figures 9.2 through 9.5). Our experience supports this theory, as 62% of DCIS lesions demonstrated linear/ductal enhancement.[31] Mass enhance-

TABLE 9.2. Enhancement Pattern in the MRI Detection of DCIS

Study	Linear/Ductal	Clumped	Nodular	Focal	Regional	Segmental	Mass	Poorly Defined	Diffuse
Orel et al., 1995[11]	3								1
Gilles et al., 1995[23]	12		4					10	8
Soderstrom et al., 1996[24]	1 (clumped linear)	4							
Gilles et al., 1996[12]				46					10
Orel et al., 1997[22]	6				3		1		
Westerhof et al., 1998[27]	4			18					1
Viehweg et al., 2000[26]	8						12	23	5
Zuiani et al., 2002[30]	3			9		5			
Menell et al. 2003[31]	18				1		10		

ment was only found in 34%, while regional non/mass enhancement was found in 3%.[31]

The imaging sequence employed at our institution includes a localizing sequence followed by a sagittal fat-suppressed T2-weighted sequence [TR/TE 4000/85 (repetition time msec/echo time msec)]. A T1-weighted three-dimensional fat-suppressed fast spoiled gradient echo [17/2.4 (repletion time msec/echo time msec)]; flip angle 35; band width, 31.25 MHz) sequence is then per-

formed before and three times following a rapid bolus injection of gadopentate dimeglumine (Magnevist®). Generally, DCIS lesions are hypointense or isointense to breast parenchyma on fat suppressed T2-weighted images. Ductal carcinoma in situ lesions are not visualized, or are hypointense, on precontrast fat-suppressed T1-weighted images. Ductal carcinoma in situ lesions rapidly enhance following the administration of gadopentate dimeglumine. Assessment of DCIS lesions by visual kinetics is

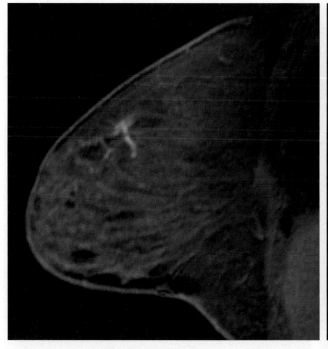 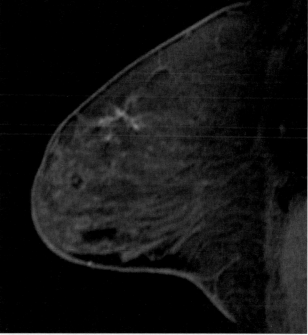

A   B

FIGURE 9.1. A 53-year-old woman status post bilateral breast biopsies yielding DCIS in the right breast, and DCIS with invasion in the left breast. Magnetic resonance imaging performed for extent of disease evaluation. (A and B) MRIs of the right breast [sagittal fat-suppressed fast spoiled gradient echo sequence (FSPGR) T1-weighted postcontrast for this example and all following examples] show linear ductal enhancement separate from the lumpectomy site extending over 1.9 cm in the upper inner quadrant of the right breast on two sequential slices. Ductal carcinoma in situ was found following MRI-guided needle localization and surgical excision.

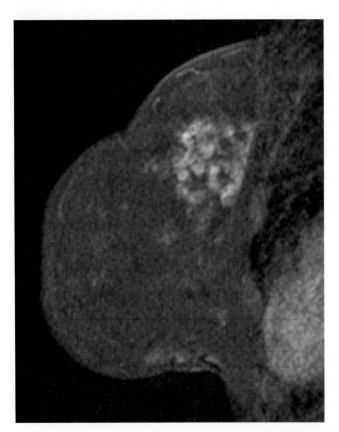

FIGURE 9.2. A 47-year-old woman after stereotactic core biopsy of the left breast calcifications yielding DCIS for extent of disease evaluation. Magnetic resonance imaging of the left breast demonstrates a segmental area of irregular enhancement extending over approximately 4cm in the upper inner quadrant. Mammographic needle localization (not shown) of corresponding calcifications yielded DCIS.

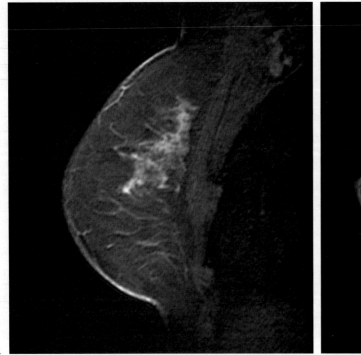

A   B

FIGURE 9.3. A 52-year-old woman with mammographically evident right breast calcifications (not shown) yielding in situ carcinoma, ductal carcinoma, and lobular carcinoma with a tiny focus of invasive lobular carcinoma. Magnetic resonance imaging performed for extent of disease evaluation. (A and B) MRI of the right breast demonstrates regional enhancement in the upper inner quadrant extending over approximately 6cm. Magnetic resonance imaging guided needle localization followed by surgical excision yielded DCIS.

FIGURE 9.4. A 28-year-old woman with a palpable right breast mass yielding invasive ductal carcinoma and DCIS following lumpectomy for MRI for extent of disease evaluation. Magnetic resonance imaging of the right breast demonstrates regional enhancement in the upper inner quadrant of the breast extending toward the nipple over 2.5 cm. Residual DCIS was found at mastectomy.

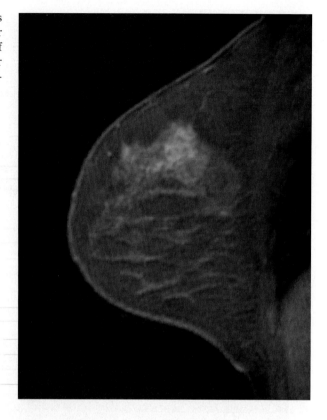

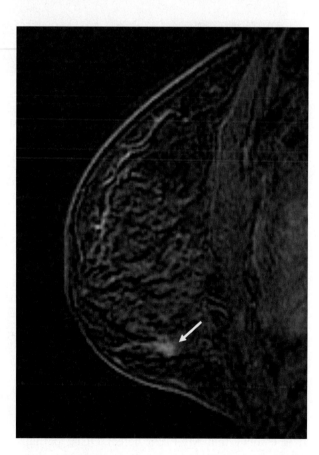

FIGURE 9.5. A 63-year-old woman with palpable right breast carcinoma for MRI evaluation for extent of disease. Subtraction MRI of the left breast demonstrates an 8-mm irregular heterogenously enhancing mass (arrow) in the lower inner quadrant. Magnetic resonance imaging guided needle localization (not shown) followed by surgical excision yielded DCIS.

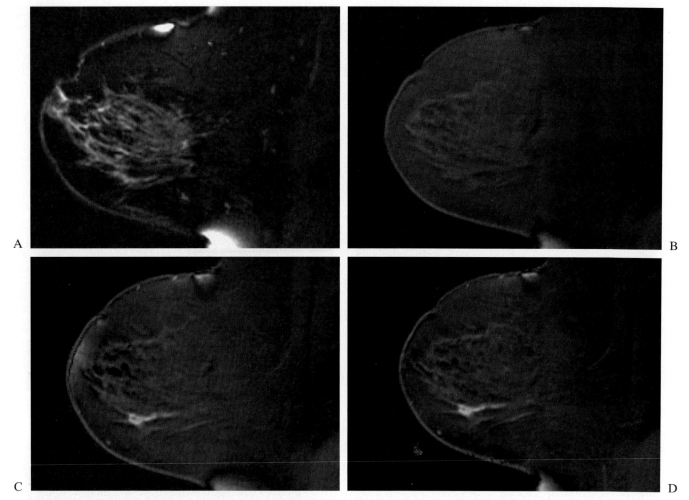

FIGURE 9.6. A 61-year-old woman status post contralateral mastectomy with linear ductal enhancement in the right breast. (A) Sagittal T2-weighted image of the right breast demonstrates a mild amount of glandular tissue. (B) Sagittal T1-weighted image before intravenous contrast administration demonstrates no hyperintense lesions. (C) Sagittal, first postcontrast-enhanced T1-weighted image demonstrates clumped, linear ductal enhancement in the lower inner quadrant. (D and E) Sagittal second (D) and third (E) postcontrast-enhanced T1-weighted images demonstrates persistent clumped linear ductal enhancement in the lower inner quadrant with plateau kinetics. (F) Subtraction image again demonstrates clumped linear ductal enhancement. (G) MRI-guided needle localization was performed yielding ductal carcinoma in situ (arrow denotes artifact from localization wire).

performed at our institution, and plateau kinetics was more frequently encountered than washout kinetics.[31] (Figure 9.6). Zuiani and colleagues[30] support these results as all three patterns of kinetics, washout, plateau, and steady enhancement, were demonstrated in this study.

7. Conclusion

It is evident that MRI can detect DCIS, perhaps even better than mammography. It is also true that mam-mography and MRI are complementary modalities with improved detection of DCIS when both tests are performed. Suspicious calcifications on mammography should undergo biopsy despite a negative MRI, and, conversely, a suspicious linear area of enhancement on MRI should be biopsied despite a negative mammogram. The detection of DCIS has large implications in the setting of screening high-risk patients where detection of early stage breast cancer is essential. Additionally, MRI can be helpful in the evaluation of potential multifocal or multi-centric breast cancer in the patient with recently diagnosed DCIS.

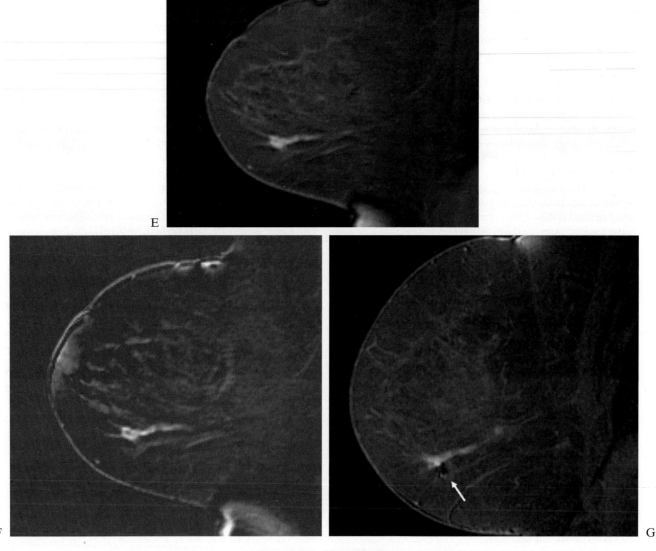

FIGURE 9.6. (*Continued*)

References

1. Dershaw DD, Abramson A, Kinne DW. Ductal carcinoma in situ: mammographic findings and clinical implications. *Radiology* 1989;170:411–415.
2. Recht A, Rutgers EJT, Fentiman IS, et al. The fourth EORTC DCIS consensus meeting-conference report. *Eur J Cancer.* 1998;34:1664–1669.
3. Stomper PC, Connolly JL, Meyer JE, et al. Clinically occult ductal carcinoma in situ detected with mammography: analysis of 100 cases with radiologic-pathologic correlation. *Radiology* 1989;172:235–241.
4. Griff SK, Dershaw DD. Breast cancer. In: Bragg DG, Rubin P, Hricak H, ed. *Oncologic Imaging.* Philadelphia: Saunders; 2002:265–294.
5. Page DL, Dupont WD, Rogers LW, et al. Intraductal carcinoma of the breast: follow-up after biopsy only. *Cancer* 1982;49:751–758.
6. Holland R, Hendriks JHCL. Microcalcifications associated with ductal carcinoma in situ: mammographic-pathologic correlation. Semin Diagn Pathol. 1994;11:181–192.
7. Holland R, Veling SH, Mravunac M, et al. Histologic multifocality of Tis, T1-2 breast carcinomas. Implications for clinical trials of breast-conserving surgery. *Cancer* 1985;56: 979–990.
8. Dinkel HP, Gassel AM, Tschammler A. Is the appearance of microcalcifications on mammography useful in predicting histological grade of malignancy in ductal cancer in situ? *Br J Radiol.* 2000;73:938–944.
9. Evans A, Pinder S, Wilson R, et al. Ductal carcinoma in situ of the breast: correlation between mammographic and pathologic findings. *AJR Am J Roentgenol.* 1994;162:1307–1311.
10. Slanetz PJ, Giardino AA, Oyama T, et al. Mammographic appearance of ductal carcinoma in situ does not reliably predict histologic subtype. *Breast J.* 2001;7:417–421.

11. Orel SG, Schnall MD, Powell CM, et al. Staging of suspected breast cancer: effect of MR imaging and MR-guided biopsy. *Radiology* 1995;196:115–122.

12. Gilles R, Meunier M, Lucidarme O, et al. Clustered breast microcalcifications: evaluation by dynamic contrast-enhanced subtraction MRI. *J Comput Assist Tomogr.* 1996; 20:9–14.

13. Gilles R, Guinebretiere JM, Lucidarme O, et al. Nonpalpable breast tumors: diagnosis with contrast-enhanced subtraction dynamic MR imaging. *Radiology* 1994;191:625–631.

14. Harms SE, Flamig DP, Hesley KL, et al. MR imaging of the breast with rotating delivery of excitation off resonance: clinical experience with pathologic correlation. *Radiology* 1993;187:493–501.

15. Stomper PC, Herman S, Klippenstein DL, et al. Suspect breast lesions: findings at dynamic gadolinium-enhanced MR imaging correlated with mammographic and pathologic features. *Radiology* 1995;197:387–395.

16. Heywang SH, Wolf A, Pruss E, et al. MR imaging of the breast with Gd-DTPA: use and limitations. *Radiology* 1989; 171:95–103.

17. Boetes C, Mus RDM, Holland R, et al. Breast tumors: comparative accuracy of MR imaging relative to mammography and US for demonstrating extent. *Radiology* 1995;197:743–747.

18. Hulka CA, Smith BL, Sgroi DC, et al. Benign and malignant breast lesions: differentiation with echo-planar MR imaging. *Radiology* 1995;197:33–38.

19. Bone B, Aspelin P, Bronge L, et al. Sensitivity and specificity of MR mammography with histopathological correlation in 250 breasts. *Acta Radiol.* 1996;37:208–213.

20. Fobben ES, Rubin CZ, Kalisher L, et al. Breast MR imaging with commercially available techniques: radiologic-pathologic correlation. *Radiology* 1995;196:143–152.

21. Teifke A, Hlawatsch A, Beier T, et al. Undetected malignancies of the breast: dynamic contrast enhanced MR imaging at 1.0T. *Radiology* 2002;224:881–888.

22. Orel SG, Mendonca MH, Reynolds C, et al. MR imaging of ductal carcinoma in situ. *Radiology* 1997;202:413–420.

23. Gilles R, Zafrani B, Guinebretiere JM, et al. Ductal carcinoma in situ: MR imaging-histopathologic correlation. *Radiology* 1995;196:415–419.

24. Soderstrom CE, Harms SE, Copit DS, et al. Three-dimensional RODEO breast MR imaging of lesions containing ductal carcinoma in situ. *Radiology* 1996;201:427–432.

25. Boetes C, Strijk SP, Holland R, et al. False-negative MR imaging of malignant breast tumors. *Eur Radiol.* 1997;7: 1231–1234.

26. Viehweg P, Lampe D, Buchmann J, et al. In situ and minimally invasive breast cancer: morphologic and kinetic features on contrast enhanced MR imaging. *MAGMA* 2000;11: 129–137.

27. Westerhof JP, Fischer U, Moritz JD, et al. MR imaging of mammographically detected clustered calcifications: is there any value? *Radiology* 1998;207:675–681.

28. Fischer U, Westerhof JP, Brinck U, et al. Ductal carcinoma in situ by dynamic MR-mammography at 1.5 T [in German]. *Rofo Fortschr Geb Rontgenstr Neuen Bildgeb Verfahr* 1996; 164:290–294.

29. Sittek H, Kessler M, Heuck AF, et al. Morphology and contrast enhancement of ductal carcinoma in situ in dynamic 1.0 T MR mammography [in German]. *Rofo Fortschr Geb Rontgenstr Neuen Bildgeb Verfahr* 1997;167:247–251.

30. Zuiani C, Francescutti GE, Londero V, et al. Ductal carcinoma in situ: is there a role for MRI? *J Exp Clin Cancer Res.* 2002;21:89–95.

31. Menell JH, Morris EA, Dershaw DD, et al. Determination of presence and extent pure ductal carcinoma in situ by mammography and MR. ARRS 2003 (presented).

32. Knopp MV, Weiss E, Sinn HP, et al. Pathophysiologic basis of contrast enhancement in breast tumors. *J Magn Reson Imaging.* 1999;10:260–266.

33. Guidi AJ, Fischer L, Harris JR, et al. Microvessel density and distribution in ductal carcinoma in situ of the breast. *J Natl Cancer Inst.* 1994;86:614–619.

34. Buadu LD, Murakami J, Murayama S, et al. Breast lesions: correlation of contrast medium enhancement patterns on MR images with histopathologic findings and tumor angiogenesis. *Radiology* 1996;200:639–649.

35. Hwang ES, Kinkel K, Esserman L, et al. Magnetic resonance imaging in patients diagnosed with ductal carcinoma in situ: value in the diagnosis of residual disease, occult invasion, and multicentricity. *Ann Surg Oncol.* 2003;10:381–388.

36. Nakahara H, Namba K, Fukami A, et al. Three-dimensional MR imaging of mammographically detected suspicious microcalcifications. *Breast Cancer* 2001;8:116–124.

37. Rosen PP, Braun DWJr, Kinne DE. The clinical significance of pre-invasive breast carcinoma. *Cancer* 1980;46:919–925.

10
Magnetic Resonance Imaging of Invasive Breast Carcinoma

Lia Bartella and D. David Dershaw

Although magnetic resonance imaging (MRI) has demonstrated variable specificity, multiple investigators have reported sensitivity of this modality for the demonstration of invasive breast cancer approaching 100% in several series.[1-4] The invasive cancers in these studies have predominantly been invasive ductal carcinoma. Both lesion morphology and enhancement kinetics are useful parameters in identifying malignant lesions and several series have suggested that these parameters can individually be strong predictors of malignancy.[5,6] Liberman and coworkers[6] showed that the features with highest positive predictive value for malignancy included spiculated margin, rim enhancement, and irregular shape for masses, and segmental or clumped ductal enhancement for nonmass lesions. Kuhl and coworkers[5] concluded that a washout (type 3) time-signal intensity curve is a strong independent predictor of malignancy.

1. Tumor Neovascularity and Angiogenesis

Angiogenesis, the growth of new blood vessels, is an important natural process occurring in the body, both in health and in disease. In some serious diseases states, the body loses control over angiogenesis. This occurs in some malignancies in which excessive angiogenesis can develop. Tumors cannot enlarge beyond 1 to 2mm unless they are vascularized; beyond these dimensions, oxygen and nutrients cannot diffuse from blood vessels and hypoxia induces apoptosis by activation of *p53*. Neovascularization has a dual effect on tumor growth: Perfusion supplies nutrients and oxygen, and newly formed endothelial cells stimulate the growth of adjacent tumor cells by secreting polypeptides such as insulin-like growth factors, platelet-derived growth factor, granulocyte-macrophage colony-stimulating factor, and interleukin-1.[7] Angiogenesis is requisite not only for continued tumor growth, but also for metastasis. Without access to the vasculature, the tumor cells cannot metastasize. Hence angiogenesis is a necessary biologic correlate of malignancy.[8]

In dynamic contrast-enhanced MRI of the breast, tumor angiogenesis is exploited by the use of intravenous contrast agents producing enhancement of cancerous lesions.[9] Angiogenesis facilitates contrast enhancement in two ways: Increased vascularity leads to an increased contrast inflow and increased vessel permeability leads to accelerated contrast extravasation at the tumor site.[10-12]

Chelates of gadolinium, a lanthanide with three unpaired electrons that has a very strong magnetic field, are the most universally used contrast agents. Chelates such as diaminotetra-ethyl penta-acetic acid (DTPA) strongly bind the gadolinium, which avoids toxicity while allowing access of water molecules to the gadolinium. Gadolinium has several effects due to its strongly paramagnetic nature. It can produce relaxation, a change in the magnetic state of hydrogen atoms in water molecules; as a result, the appearance of tissues dramatically changes. High-contrast-agent uptake in T1-weighted images produce a high signal and cause tissues to appear bright.[13]

Diagnosis of breast cancer uses information evident on contrast-enhanced images that make it possible to discern the morphology of the enhancing lesion and the dynamic behavior of the contrast agent within the lesion. Dynamic information shows the rate at which tissue enhances and the rate at which contrast agent washes out. Several factors affect this process including perfusion, vascular permeability, and the extracellular, extravascular volume. It has been shown that the differences in dynamic MRI enhancement are a direct consequence of microvascular distribution within the neoplasm, so the contrast agent provides a means of investigating tissue vasculature.[14]

Morphological and enhancement patterns of areas of suspicion should be assessed using the criteria described in the MRI lexicon of the American College of Radiology.[15] This facilitates accuracy of assessment, interpretation, and communication of findings.

2. Secondary Signs of Invasive Breast Cancer

The presence of secondary morphologic features increases suspicion of carcinoma. These features include skin and nipple changes and lymphadenopathy. Architectural distortion can be present, extending beyond the limits of the malignancy.

2.1. Skin and Nipple Changes

With progressive enlargement, carcinomas can become adherent to the deep fascia of the chest wall and so become fixed in position. Extension to the skin or fibrosis associated with the tumor can also cause dimpling and retraction. Peau d'orange or skin thickening with an *orange skin* pattern occurs secondary to a local blockage of lymphatic drainage. This appearance of an orange peel is produced by tethering of the skin to the breast by Cooper ligaments. In inflammatory carcinoma, widespread lymphatic involvement is due to diffuse cancer infiltration. This results in swelling, tenderness, and erythema.

On MRI, the skin and nipple routinely enhance. Differentiation of normal from abnormal patterns is facilitated by use of the opposite breast for comparison. The detection of nipple inversion can be impossible if breast positioning does not place the nipple in profile. However, attention should be paid to skin thickness and breast contour to detect focal thickening and distortion. Because the skin and nipple normally rapidly enhance, early enhancement with malignant involvement of these structures is usually not evident.

2.2. Lymphadenopathy

Breast cancer can metastasize both via the lymphatic and the hematogenous routes. Lymphadenopathy can be present at the time of initial diagnosis. The two most frequent locations are the axillary and the internal mammary lymph node chains. Other possible sites include the supraclavicular and cervical nodes, into the chest, and the abdomen. The pattern of lymphatic spread varies according to the site of the initial carcinoma in the breast, although axillary involvement is by far the most common.

Because lymph nodes are vascular, they demonstrate a normal pattern of early enhancement. Differentiation of nodes in the axilla that are normal or contain metastatic disease can be difficult. Asymmetry with the opposite site, absence of central fat, or spiculation of contour suggest possible malignant involvement.

2.3. Architectural Distortion

As well as infiltrating into adjacent glandular and adipose tissue, breast cancers can incite a scirrhous reaction in sur-rounding tissue. This results in architectural distortion that may or may not be due to direct tumor involvement. It is unknown whether lack of enhancement in an area of architectural distortion can reliably exclude malignancy.

On MRI the extent of enhancement of the carcinoma may be more extensive than that appreciated on the mammogram. It is reasonable to assume that peritumoral inflammation can cause enhancement patterns to be more extensive than true tumor involvement.

3. Types of Invasive Breast Cancer

Approximately 80% of breast cancers arise in the ducts, with the most common histology of invasive cancer being invasive ductal carcinoma not otherwise specified (NOS). Specialized subtypes of invasive ductal carcinoma also occur, including mucinous, tubular, medullary, and papillary carcinomas. Tumors composed purely or predominantly of the specialized subtypes are generally better differentiated and have a better prognosis than invasive ductal carcinoma NOS. Less than 10% of breast cancers arise in the lobules of the breast and are invasive lobular carcinomas. Other unusual primary malignant lesions that arise in the breast include lymphoid and hematopoetic malignancies and mesenchymal stromal neoplasms, such as malignant phyllodes tumors and sarcomas. Metastatic lesions can also involve the breast. Features of these lesions and their MRI patterns are discussed below.

4. Invasive Ductal Carcinoma Not Otherwise Specified (NOS)

Invasive ductal carcinoma NOS accounts for 65% to 80% of breast cancers.[16–18] The term *ductal carcinoma* is used because these tumor cells exhibit variable degrees of histologic and cytologic differentiation toward mammary ductal epithelium.[19] Invasive ductal carcinoma is a heterogeneous group of malignant neoplasms with different clinical and biologic characteristics.[18,19] Therefore, it is not surprising that this disease has various morphologies and enhancement patterns. Macroscopically, most tumors are of the scirrhous type and therefore have a spiculated, irregular border. This spiculated lesion is characterized by extensive fibrosis and consists of a central mass that radiates into the surrounding breast tissue. Less frequently, invasive ductal carcinomas are well defined with lobulated shape and circumscribed margins.

Magnetic resonance imaging is highly sensitive in the detection of invasive ductal carcinoma of the breast, although the specificity is somewhat lower. Invasive ductal carcinoma may present on MRI as irregular or spiculated masses with peripheral or rim enhancement (Figures 10.1 and 10.2). Less frequently, these present as smooth masses with lobulated borders. Irregular enhancement within the mass is frequently seen. Small sites of enhancement near a known or suspected cancer should be viewed with caution, and the need for their biopsy should be considered.

Although mass-like enhancement is most characteristic of invasive ductal carcinoma, associated nonmass ductal enhancement should be viewed with suspicion as possibly representing in situ or additional invasive cancer. Regional or diffuse enhancement is less common but can also be seen in invasive ductal carcinoma.[6,20] When cancers are extensive, it can be difficult to differentiate diffuse normal enhancement from diffuse parenchymal enhancement due to carcinoma. Comparison with the contralateral breast facilitates this differentiation.

In our experience at Memorial Sloan-Kettering Cancer Center (MSKCC), carcinoma was present in 25 (25%) of 100 MRI-detected lesions, of which 13 (52%) were DCIS and 12 (48%) were invasive carcinoma.[6] Histology of inva-

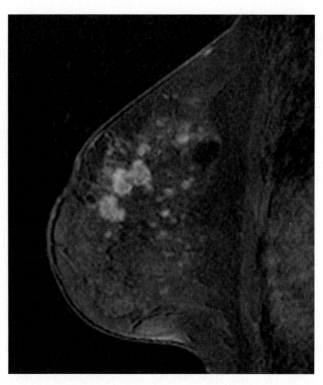

FIGURE 10.2. This 45-year-old woman presented with left nipple retraction. Mammography showed dense breasts with subtle distortion in the left 12:00 axis. No sonographic correlate was found for the distortion. Sagittal, T1-weighted, contrast-enhanced MRI of the left breast shows multiple rim-enhancing masses. Magnetic resonance imaging guided needle localization yielded multifocal infiltrating ductal carcinoma.

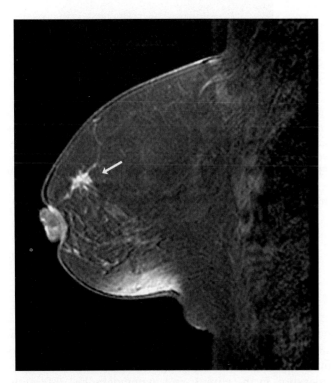

FIGURE 10.1. This 57-year-old woman presented with a left axillary lymph node positive for mammary carcinoma. Sagittal, T1-weighted, contrast-enhanced MRI of the left breast shows a spiculated enhancing mass (arrow), not visible on mammography or ultrasound. Surgery revealed invasive ductal carcinoma (0.8cm) and ductal carcinoma in situ, detected by MRI only.

sive carcinoma was invasive ductal carcinoma in nine (including six with DCIS) and invasive lobular carcinoma in three. Among 12 invasive cancers, 11 were masses and 1 was a nonmass area of regional enhancement. Among the 11 invasive malignant masses, margins were irregular in 5, spiculated in 4, and smooth in 2; shape was irregular in 9 and lobular in 2; enhancement pattern was heterogeneous in 7, homogeneous in 3, and rim in 1.[6]

5. Specialized Subtypes of Invasive Ductal Carcinoma

5.1. Mucinous Carcinoma

Mucinous carcinoma is a specialized subtype of infiltrating ductal carcinoma also known as colloid, mucous, mucoid, or gelatinous carcinoma.[21] Pure mucinous carcinoma accounts for less than 2% of all breast cancers; if one includes tumors with focal mucinous differentiation, the reported frequency of the tumor may be as high as 4%.[21] Mucinous carcinomas are often large and circumscribed but not encapsulated. Histologically, foci of epithelial cells appear to be swimming in lakes of mucin and are connected by bands of connective tissue. This tumor affects an older population and has a better prognosis than infiltrating ductal cancers NOS, especially when smaller than 2cm.[19]

As this cancer is relatively rare, there are no large series addressing its MRI pattern. Some studies have described the MRI features, and these are of a mass lesion with no distinct morphology that allows differentiation from NOS invasive ductal cancers.[22,23] Mucinous carcinoma may also present as a smooth mass mimicking a benign lesion.[20]

5.2. Tubular Carcinoma

Tubular carcinoma, a specialized subtype of invasive ductal carcinoma, accounts for less than 2% of all breast cancers and for approximately 20% of cancers detected by mammography.[24] The median age at diagnosis for women with tubular carcinoma is in the mid-to-late 40s, slightly younger than for breast cancer in general. Tubular carcinomas are highly differentiated infiltrating carcinomas composed of uniform cells arranged in well-developed tubules. They are usually small and rarely metastasize to the axillary nodes, so they carry a good prognosis. On mammography these usually present as small spiculated masses. Reported cases on MRI demonstrated a spiculated mass.[22,23] These tumors cannot be distinguished from spiculated infiltrating ductal carcinomas NOS based on MRI patterns alone (Figure 10.3).

5.3. Medullary Carcinoma

Medullary carcinoma, another specialized subtype of invasive ductal carcinoma, has been defined as "well circumscribed carcinomas composed of poorly differentiated cells with scant stroma and prominent lymphoid infiltration."[19] In most series, medullary carcinomas account for less than 5% of malignant breast tumors, although it does account for higher percentage of cancers in younger women: medullary carcinoma accounted for 10% of cancers diagnosed in women aged 35 years or less.[25] Although some studies have reported medullary carcinoma to be more common among black than white women, this has not been universally confirmed.

In the early literature, medullary carcinomas were described as large, circumscribed tumors that tended to undergo cystic degeneration. Currently, medullary carci-

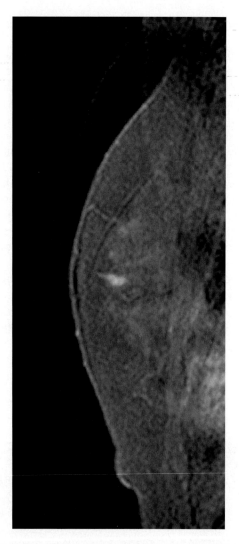

FIGURE 10.3. This 46-year-old patient, who had prior right mastectomy for breast cancer and a normal left mammogram, underwent a high-risk screening MRI of the left breast. Sagittal, T1-weighted, contrast-enhanced MRI of the left breast shows a small spiculated mass. Magnetic resonance imaging guided needle localization yielded a small tubular carcinoma.

nomas are usually smaller than 3cm at diagnosis. The smooth margin and firm consistency of medullary carcinomas may be similar to that of fibroadenomas, often a consideration in the clinical and mammographic differential diagnosis. This tumor often presents as a lobulated or oval dense mass on mammography, with indistinct or circumscribed margins.[26] Reported cases on MRI were of lobulated masses with moderate enhancement.[23]

5.4. Papillary Carcinoma

Papillary carcinoma is a rare specialized subtype of invasive ductal carcinoma in which the invasive component forms papillary structures. Papillary carcinoma accounts for 1% to 2% of breast cancers.[27] The histologic hallmark of all papillary tumors, benign or malignant, is the arborization of fibrovascular stroma supporting the epithelial component. The cytomorphology is distinctive, with the presence of single papillae and three-dimensional papillary clusters similar to those described in papillary carcinoma of the thyroid gland. An absent myoepithelial layer distinguishes papillary carcinomas from benign papillary lesions.[27] If a cystic component is present, the tumor is described as an intracystic papillary carcinoma. The intracystic type can be as large and several centimeters and remain noninvasive. Magnetic resonance imaging characteristics have been described as moderately enhancing mass with irregular borders and nonenhancing internal septae.[20]

6. Invasive Lobular Carcinoma

Invasive lobular carcinoma (ILC) accounts for less than 10% of breast cancers. Patients with ILC often present with more locally advanced disease than patients with invasive ductal carcinoma, as ILC can be difficult to detect on physical examination or imaging. The sensitivities in the detection of ILC have been reported as 57% to 81% for mammography and 68% for sonography.[28–30] Mammography may reveal a focal mass, architectural distortion, or subtle increased density. Suspicious microcalcifications are not a common feature of ILC. Ultrasound may show a mass in an area of palpable or mammographic abnormality.[28–30]

Histologically, tumor cells infiltrate the stroma in a single file arrangement without formation of a mass or development of associated fibrosis.[31] This leaves a considerable amount of intervening stroma that makes it difficult to detect the growth of this malignancy. Variants include a solid pattern, alveolar pattern, and mixed solid/alveolar pattern.[19] Studies have suggested that MRI is more accurate in the detection of ILC and in determining the extent of involvement when compared with conventional methods.[32,33]

On MRI, the morphologic appearance of ILC is variable. A focal enhancing mass is the most common finding and the easiest to detect[32,34,35] (Figure 10.4). In the absence of a mass with or without rim enhancement, diffuse enhancement patterns resembling normal glandular patterns may be visualized.[22,35] Variability in gadolinium uptake and morphology of ILC reflects the tumor histology. Yeh and coworkers[35] used a quantitative measure of gadolinium uptake over time (the extraction flow product)

and concluded that some ILCs may infiltrate and grow without significant angiogenesis and/or neovascularity. This may be the reason why MRI has been reported to be falsely negative on occasion when ILC is present. Because enhancement of the tumor is variable, interpretation of MRI should take place with the simultaneous review of all available imaging studies.

Magnetic resonance imaging may detect additional sites of cancer in the ipsilateral breast or contralateral breast in women with ILC (Figure 10.5). In a study of women with percutaneously proven cancer at MSKCC, MRI found additional sites of cancer in the ipsilateral breast in 27% of women; the likelihood of additional sites of cancer was higher in women with ILC as opposed to other histologies (55% vs. 19%, $P < 0.06$).[36] In another study of women with proven cancer at MSKCC, MRI found an otherwise unsuspected cancer in the contralateral breast in 5% of women;

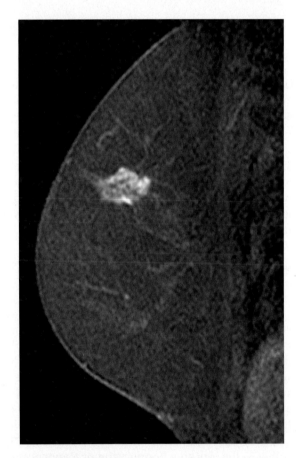

FIGURE 10.4. This 60-year-old patient presented with a palpable, mammographically occult lump in the right breast that yielded invasive lobular carcinoma at biopsy. Sagittal, T1-weighted, contrast-enhanced MRI of the right breast demonstrates this irregular, inhomogeneously enhancing mass, corresponding to the biopsy-proven invasive lobular carcinoma.

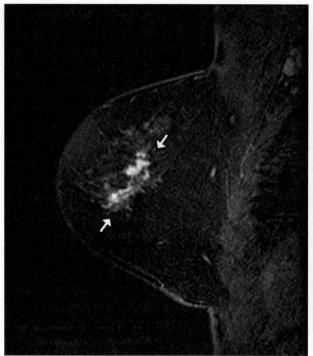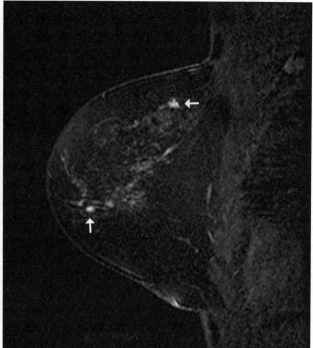

A   B

FIGURE 10.5. A 78-year-old woman with spiculated mass right upper outer quadrant on mammogram for which ultrasound-guided core biopsy yielded invasive lobular carcinoma. (A) Sagittal, subtraction MRI of the right breast shows an irregular, spiculated enhancing mass in the right upper outer quadrant (arrows) consistent with biopsy-proven invasive lobular carcinoma. (B) Image from a more lateral plane from sagittal, subtraction MRI of the right breast shows additional enhancing masses (arrows). Multicentric invasive lobular carcinoma was found at surgery.

the likelihood of finding an additional site of cancer was higher in women with ILC as opposed to other histologies (13% vs. 4%, $P < 0.07$).[37] Women with ILC may be among those most likely to benefit from use of MRI for assessment of extent of disease.

7. Other Breast Malignancies

7.1. Lymphoma

Breast lymphoma is infrequent, accounting for approximately 0.15% of malignant breast tumors.[38] Less than 0.5% of all malignant lymphomas and approximately 2% of extranodal lymphomas involve the breast. Patients are usually women with a mean age of approximately 55 years. Histologically, the tumor is almost always of non-Hodgkin's lymphoma (NHL) type. In breast, diffuse large cell (histiocytic) lymphoma is the most common NHL type according to the Working Formulation or Rappaport classifications.[39] In a study from our institution,[40] mammographic patterns of non-Hodgkin's lymphoma were a solitary uncalcified mass in 21 of 32 cases (69%), multiple masses in 3 cases (9%), and diffuse increased opacity with skin thickening in 3 cases (9%). Four cases had normal findings.

The MRI appearance of breast lymphoma has been described as ill-defined, nonspiculated, hypointense masses in T1-weighted images, which showed rapid and strong enhancement in dynamic sequences.[41] Rim enhancement may also be observed[42] (Figure 10.6).

7.2. Phyllodes Tumors

Phyllodes tumors are structurally similar to fibroadenomas, but are distinguished histologically by large leaf-like projections of stroma with increased stromal cellularity.[43,44] These tumors are initially seen as discrete, palpable masses. The disease is a common occurrence among women between 30 and 70 years of age, an average of 15 to 20 years older than patients with fibroadenoma.[45] Phyllodes tumors account for 2% to 3% of fibroepithelial breast neoplasms and less than 1% of mammary tumors.[46]

The gross appearance of the phyllodes tumor may vary according to the size. Smaller tumors may resemble a fibroadenoma with a gray-white fibrous appearance. However, large tumors appear fleshy and resemble sarcomas in their gross appearance. Cystic spaces, necrosis, and hemorrhage can be seen in large tumors.[47] Approximately 25% of phyllodes tumors are malignant, with the capacity to spread hematogenously; both benign and malignant

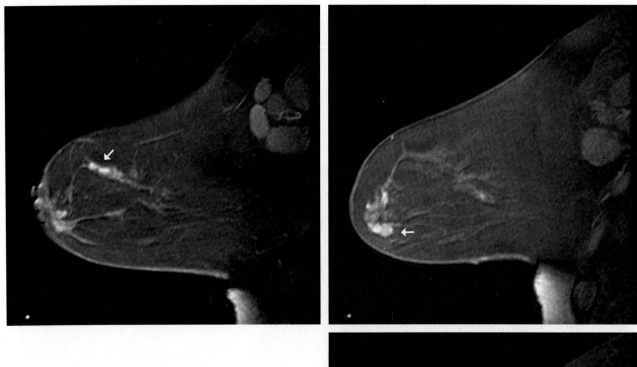

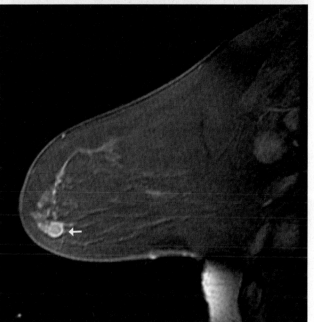

FIGURE 10.6. A 56-year-old woman with history of lymphoma. Mammogram (not shown) showed bilateral axillary adenopathy but no suspicious findings in the breast parenchyma. (A) Sagittal, T1-weighted, contrast-enhanced MRI of the left breast shows markedly enlarged lymph nodes in the left axilla. There is also focal clumped enhancement in the left upper outer quadrant (arrow). (B) Image from a more medial plane from sagittal, T1-weighted, contrast-enhanced MRI of the left breast shows left axillary adenopathy and clumped enhancement in the retroareolar region (arrow). (C) Image from even more medial plane from sagittal, T1-weighted, contrast-enhanced MRI of the left breast shows a rim enhancing mass in the 6:00 axis (arrow). Magnetic resonance imaging guided needle localization was performed of the three suspicious enhancing breast lesions shown in A, B, and C. All three sites yielded lymphoma, low-grade B cell type, involving breast tissue.

phyllodes tumors also have the capacity to be locally aggressive, growing to large sizes. Tumors more than 3cm are more likely to be malignant.[46]

Magnetic resonance imaging has demonstrated a multilobulated lesion rapidly and markedly enhanced on dynamic studies of contrast-enhanced T1-weighted imaging without washout. A morphology similar to fibroadenomas with internal septations has also been reported, as well as a more specific leafy appearance best seen on subtraction images with enhancing solid foci within cystic blood-filled spaces.[48,49]

7.3. Breast Sarcomas

Breast sarcomas are rare tumors, accounting for less than 1% of breast malignancies.[50,51] Breast sarcomas are classified histologically as low-, intermediate-, and high-grade lesions.

7.3.1. Angiosarcoma

Primary angiosarcomas account for less than 0.04% of primary tumors of the breast.[52] Among the most rare and the most lethal breast malignancies, angiosarcoma arises in the breast more often than in any other organ. Angiosarcoma in the upper extremity can occur after radical mastectomy or breast-conserving treatment with lymphedema of the extremity. Angiosarcomas have also been reported arising in mastectomy scars after chest wall irradiation.[53] On MRI, angiosarcoma has been described as having low signal intensity on T1-weighted images, and higher signal intensity on T2-weighted images.[54] However, others have described higher signal intensity of T1-weighted images with relatively lower intensity in the central area of the tumor.[55] These tumors are very vascular and show marked enhancement (Figure 10.7).

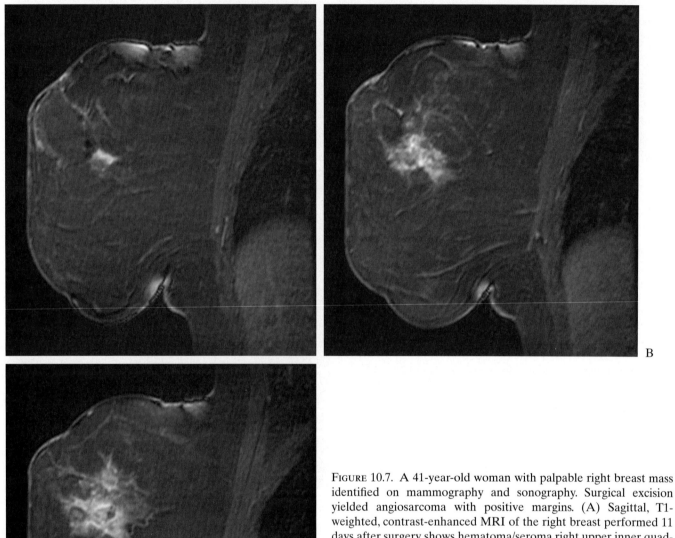

FIGURE 10.7. A 41-year-old woman with palpable right breast mass identified on mammography and sonography. Surgical excision yielded angiosarcoma with positive margins. (A) Sagittal, T1-weighted, contrast-enhanced MRI of the right breast performed 11 days after surgery shows hematoma/seroma right upper inner quadrant. Focal enhancement is present at the inferior/posterior aspect of the lumpectomy site, suspicious for residual disease. (B) MRI from more lateral plane of the right breast obtained in the same study shown in part A shows irregularly shaped, irregularly marginated, heterogeneously enhancing right breast mass contiguous with the enhancement shown in part A, suspicious for residual disease. (C) MRI from even more lateral plane of the right breast obtained in the same study shows irregularly shaped, irregularly marginated, heterogeneously enhancing mass in the central right breast, suspicious for residual tumor, contiguous with the enhancement shown in parts A and B. Subsequent surgery showed residual angiosarcoma.

7.4. Metastases to the Breast

Metastatic disease to the breast accounts for 0.5% to 6.6% of all breast malignancies.[56] Aside from metastasis arising from the opposite breast, the most common primary tumor sources in order of decreasing frequency are lymphoma, melanoma, rhabdomyosarcoma, lung tumors, ovarian tumors, renal-cell carcinoma, leukemia, thyroid and cervix carcinomas, intestinal carcinoid, epidermoid carcinoma of the head and neck, and leiomyosarcoma.[56] Interestingly, rhabdomyosarcoma was found to be the most frequent origin of breast metastases in adolescent girls.[56] In approximately 25% of patients who have metastatic disease to the breast, the breast lesion is the initial manifestation of a nonmammary malignant neoplasm.[57]

To date only a few cases of MRI in metastases to the breast have been reported. These were well-defined or lobulated lesions with early enhancement.[58] Magnetic resonance imaging may detect breast metastases in young patients with dense breast parenchyma.[59] In a case of metastatic rhabdomyosarcoma, a pattern of early rim enhancement raised the suspicion of malignancy in an otherwise innocent-appearing smooth, round mass.[59] In metastatic melanoma, high signal with T1 weighting and low T2-weighted signal has been useful to suggest a melanin-containing tumor,[60] although other patterns may be seen.

8. Ductal Carcinoma In Situ Versus Invasive Carcinoma

It has been suggested that the MRI sensitivity for the detection of ductal carcinoma in situ (DCIS) is less than for invasive ductal cancer.[61,62] There is no doubt that it can be difficult to differentiate invasive cancers and DCIS on MRI. Because invasive ductal carcinoma is most likely to present as a mass lesion, whereas DCIS usually presents as a nonmass lesion with linear/ductal enhancement, the differentiation between these two can be suggested based on this difference.[6,63] However, morphologic and kinetic patterns of enhancement are variable, requiring biopsy confirmation of findings before a definitive determination can be made.[64]

References

1. Heywang SH, Wolf A, Pruss E, et al. MR imaging of the breast with Gd-DTPA: use and limitations. *Radiology* 1989;171: 95–103.
2. Harms SE, Flamig DP, Hesley KL, et al. MR imaging of the breast with rotating delivery of excitation off resonance: clinical experience with pathologic correlation. *Radiology* 1993;187:493–501.
3. Gilles R, Guinebretiere J, Lucidarme O, et al. Nonpalpable breast tumors: diagnosis with contrast-enhanced subtraction dynamic MR imaging. *Radiology* 1994;191:625–631.
4. Kaiser WA, Zeitler E. MR imaging of the breast: fast imaging sequences with and without Gd-DTPA—preliminary observations. *Radiology* 1989;170:681–686.
5. Kuhl CK, Mielcareck P, Klaschik S, et al. Dynamic breast MR imaging: are signal intensity time course data useful for differential diagnosis of enhancing lesions? *Radiology* 1999; 211:101–110.
6. Liberman L, Morris EA, Lee MJY, et al. Breast lesions detected by MR imaging: features and positive predictive value. *AJR Am J Roentgenol.* 2002;179:171–178.
7. Rak J, Filmus J, Kerbel RS. Reciprocal paracrine interaction between tumour cells and endothelial cells: the "angiogenesis progression" hypothesis. *Eur J Cancer.* 1996;32A:2438–2450.
8. Folkman J. What is the evidence that tumors are angiogenesis dependent? *J Natl Cancer Inst.* 1990;82:4–6.
9. Heywang SH, Hahn D, Schmidt H, et al. MR imaging of the breast using gadolinium DTPA. *J Comput Assist Tomogr.* 1986;10:199–204.
10. Buadu LD, Murakami J, Murayama S, et al. Breast lesions: correlation of contrast medium enhancement patterns on MR images with histopathologic findings and tumor angiogenesis. *Radiology* 1996;200:639–649.
11. Buckley DL, Drew PJ, Mussurakis S, et al. Microvessel density of invasive breast cancer assessed by dynamic Gd-DPTA enhanced MRI. *J Magn Reson Imaging.* 1997;7: 461–464.
12. Furman-Haran E, Margalit R, Maretzek AF. Angiogenic response of MCF7 human breast cancer to hormonal treatment: assessment by dynamic Gd-DTPA-enhanced MRI at high spatial resolution. *J Magn Reson Imaging.* 1996;6:195–202.
13. Leach MO. Application of magnetic resonance imaging to angiogenesis in breast cancer. *Breast Cancer Res.* 2001;3: 22–27.
14. Carriero A, Ambrossini R, Mattei PA, et al. Magnetic resonance of the breast: correlation between enhancement patterns and microvessel density in malignant tumors. *J Exp Clin Cancer Res.* 2002;21(Suppl 3):83–87.
15. American College of Radiology (ACR). Magnetic Resonance Imaging. In: *ACR Breast Imaging Reporting and Data System, Breast Imaging Atlas.* Reston, VA: American College of Radiology, 2003.
16. Fisher ER, Gregorio RM, Fisher B, et al. The pathology of invasive breast cancer. A syllabus derived from findings of the National Surgical Adjuvant Breast Project (protocol no. 4). *Cancer* 1975;36:1–85.
17. Rosen PP. Invasive duct carcinoma and morphological prognostic markers. In: Rosen PP, ed. *Rosen's Breast Pathology.* Philadelphia: Lippincott-Raven; 1997:275–293.
18. Allred DC, Mohsin SK, Fuqua SAW. Histological and biological evolution of human premalignant breast disease. *Endocr Rel Cancer.* 2001;8:46–61.
19. World Health Organization. Histological typing of breast tumors. *Tumori* 1982;68:181–198.
20. Nunes LW, Schnall MD, Orel SG. Update of breast MR imaging architectural interpretation model. *Radiology* 2001; 219:484–494.

21. Rosen PP. Mucinous carcinoma. In: Rosen PP, ed. *Rosen's Breast Pathology*. Philadelphia: Lippincott-Raven; 1997: 405–420.

22. Kuhl CK. MRI of breast tumors. *Eur Radiol*. 2000;10:46–58.

23. Nunes LW, Schnall MD, Orel SG, et al. Correlation of lesion appearance and histologic findings for the nodes of a breast MR imaging interpretation model. *Radiographics* 1999;19: 79–92.

24. Rosen PP. Tubular carcinoma. In: Rosen PP, ed. *Rosen's Breast Pathology*. Philadelphia: Lippincott-Raven; 1997:321–334.

25. Rosen PP. Medullary carcinoma. In: Rosen PP, ed. *Rosen's Breast Pathology*. Philadelphia: Lippincott-Raven; 1997:355–374.

26. Liberman L, LaTrenta LR, Samli B, et al. Overdiagnosis of medullary carcinoma: a mammographic-pathologic correlative study. *Radiology* 1996;201:443–446.

27. Rosen PP. Papillary carcinoma. In: Rosen PP, ed. *Rosen's Breast Pathology*. Philadelphia: Lippincott-Raven; 1997:335–354.

28. Paramagul CP, Helvie MA, Adler DD. Invasive lobular carcinoma: sonographic appearance and role of sonography in improving diagnostic sensitivity. *Radiology* 1995;195: 231–234.

29. Butler RS, Venta LA, Wiley EL, et al. Sonographic evaluation of infiltrating lobular carcinoma. *AJR Am J Roentgenol*. 1999;172:325–330.

30. Skaane P, Skjorten F. Ultrasonographic evaluation of invasive lobular carcinoma. *Acta Radiol Diagn*. 1999;40:369–375.

31. Rosen PP. Invasive lobular carcinoma. In: Rosen PP, ed. *Rosen's Breast Pathology*. Philadelphia: Lippincott-Raven; 1997:545–565.

32. Rodenko GN, Harms SE, Pruneda JM, et al. MR imaging in the management before surgery of lobular carcinoma of the breast: correlation with pathology. *AJR Am J Roentgenol*. 1996;167:1415–1419.

33. Weinstein SP, Orel SG, Heller R, et al. MR imaging of the breast in patients with invasive lobular carcinoma. *AJR Am J Roentgenol*. 2001;176:399–406.

34. Qayyum A, Birdwell RL, Daniel BL, et al. MR imaging features of infiltrating lobular carcinoma of the breast: histopathologic correlation. *AJR Am J Roentgenol*. 2002;178: 1227–1232.

35. Yeh ED, Slanetz PJ, Edmister WB, et al. Invasive lobular carcinoma: spectrum of enhancement and morphology on magnetic resonance imaging. *Breast J*. 2003;9:13–18.

36. Liberman L, Morris EA, Dershaw DD, et al. MR imaging of the ipsilateral breast in women with percutaneously proven breast cancer. *AJR Am J Roentgenol*. 2003;180:901–910.

37. Liberman L, Morris EA, Kim CM, et al. MR imaging findings in the contralateral breast in women with recently diagnosed breast cancer. *AJR Am J Roentgenol*. 2003;180: 333–341.

38. Rosen PP. Lymphoid and hematopoietic tumors. In: Rosen PP, ed. *Rosen's Breast Pathology*. Philadelphia: Lippincott-Raven; 1997:757–778.

39. Mattia AR, Ferry JA, Harris NL. Breast lymphoma: a B-cell spectrum including the low-grade B-cell lympoma of mucosa associated lymphoid tissue. *Am J Surg Pathol*. 1993;17: 574–587.

40. Liberman L, Giess CS, Dershaw DD, et al. Non-Hodgkin's lymphoma of the breast: imaging characteristics and correlation with histopathology. *Radiology* 1994;192:157–160.

41. Mussurakis S, Carleton PJ, Turnbull LW. MR imaging of primary non-Hodgkin's breast lymphoma: a case report. *Acta Radiol*. 1997;38:104–107.

42. Buadu LD, Murakami J, Murayama S, et al. Patterns of peripheral enhancement in breast masses: correlation of findings on contrast medium enhanced MRI with histologic features and tumor angiogenesis. *J Comput Assist Tomogr*. 1997; 21:421–430.

43. Dyer NH, Bridges EI, Taylor RS. Cystosarcoma phyllodes. *Br J Surg*. 1966;53:450–455.

44. Rosen PP. Fibroepithelial neoplasms. In: Rosen PP, ed. *Rosen's Breast Pathology*. Philadelphia: Lippincott-Raven; 1997:143–176.

45. Pandey M, Mathew A, Kattoor J, et al. Malignant phyllodes tumor. *Breast J*. 2001;7:411–416.

46. Liberman L, Bonaccio E, Hamele-Bena D, et al. Benign and malignant phyllodes tumors: mammographic and sonographic findings. *Radiology* 1996;198:121–124.

47. Sahin AA, Sneige N, Singletary SE. Phyllodes tumors of the breast. *Cancer Bull*. 1995;47:392–395.

48. Ogawa Y, Nishioka A, Tsuboi N, et al. Dynamic MR appearance of benign phyllodes tumor of the breast in a 20-year-old woman. *Radiat Med*. 1997;15:247–250.

49. Farria DM, Gorczyca DP, Barsky SH, et al. Benign phyllodes tumors of the breast: MR imaging features. *AJR Am J Roentgenol*. 1996;167:187–189.

50. Kennedy T, Biggart JD. Sarcoma of the breast. *Br J Cancer*. 1967;21:635–644.

51. Pollard SG, Marks PV, Temple LN, Thompson HH. Breast sarcoma: a clinicopathologic review of 25 cases. *Cancer* 1990; 66:941–944.

52. Chen KTK, Kirkegaard DD, Bocian JJ. Angiosarcoma of the breast. *Cancer* 1980;46:368–371.

53. Marchal C, Weber B, de Lafontan B, et al. Nine breast angiosarcomas after conservative treatment for breast carcinoma: a survey from French comprehensive cancer centers. *Int J Radiat Oncol Biol Phys*. 1999;44:113–119.

54. Liberman L, Dershaw DD, Kaufman R, Rosen PP. Angiosarcoma of the breast. *Radiology* 1992;183:649–654.

55. Murakam S, Nagano H, Okubo K, et al. Angiosarcoma of the breast: report of a case and its findings on MRI. *Breast Cancer* 2001;8:254–258.

56. Vizcaino I, Torregrosa A, Higueras V, et al. Metastases to the breast from extramammary malignancies: a report of four cases and a review of literature. *Eur Radiol*. 2001;11:1659–1665.

57. Rosen PP. Metastases in the breast from non-mammary malignant neoplasms. In: Rosen PP, ed. *Rosen's Breast Pathology*. Philadelphia: Lippincott-Raven; 1997:597–608.

58. Heywang-Kobrunner SH, Beck R. *Contrast-enhanced MRI of the Breast*. 2nd ed. Berlin: Springer; 1996.

59. Perlet C, Sittek H, Forstpointer R, et al. Metastases to the breast from rhabdomyosarcoma: appearances on MRI. *Eur Radiol*. 1999;9:1113–1116.

60. Ho LWC, Wong KP, Chan JHM, et al. MR appearances of metastatic melanotic melanoma in the breast. *Clin Radiol*. 2000;55:572–573.

61. Orel SG, Schnall MD. MR imaging of the breast for the detection, diagnosis, and staging of breast cancer. *Radiology* 2001; 220:13–30.

62. Zuiani C, Francescutti GE, Londero V, et al. Ductal carcinoma in situ: is there a role for MRI? *J Exp Clin Cancer Res.* 2002;21(Suppl 3):89–95.

63. Menell JH, Morris EA, Dershaw DD, et al. Determination of presence and extent of pure ductal carcinoma in situ by mammography and MR imaging. *AJR Am J Roentgenol.* 2003; 180(Suppl 3):52–53.

64. Viehweg P, Lampe D, Buchmann J, Heywang-Kobrunner SH. In situ and minimally invasive breast cancer: morphologic and kinetic features on contrast-enhanced MR imaging. *MAGMA* 2000;11:129–137.

11
The High-Risk Patient and Magnetic Resonance Imaging

Laura Liberman

A woman's average lifetime risk for developing breast cancer in the United States is one in eight, but some women are at higher risk.[1] The highest risk of breast cancer is among women with an inherited predisposition to breast cancer due to genetic mutations of *BRCA1* or *BRCA2*; among these women, the cumulative lifetime risk of breast cancer is 50 to 85%.[1a] Other risk factors for breast cancer include personal or family history of breast cancer, prior breast biopsy yielding lobular carcinoma in situ, atypia, or radial scar, and prior chest radiation for Hodgkin's disease.[2–8] For high-risk women, management options include close mammographic surveillance, chemoprevention, and prophylactic bilateral mastectomies.[1,9]

Breast magnetic resonance imaging (MRI) has high sensitivity in breast cancer detection, but lower specificity. In prior reports, the sensitivity of breast MRI has ranged from 88% to 100% with reported specificities of 37% to 97%.[10,11] The low specificity is a problem, because it could lead to benign biopsies, which cost money, take time, cause anxiety, and may lead to deformity.[12] Some investigators have evaluated the use of breast MRI as a screening test in high-risk women.[13–19] This chapter examines the results of breast MRI screening in women at high risk of developing breast cancer in the literature and at Memorial Sloan-Kettering Cancer Center (MSKCC).

1. Models for Predicting Breast Cancer Risk

High risk for developing breast cancer can be defined in terms of the presence of specific risk factors or can be estimated by one of four currently available models.[1] The most commonly used model, developed by Gail and coworkers,[20] predicts the cumulative risk of breast cancer by decade up to age 90. Factors considered in the Gail model include the number of first-degree relatives with breast cancer, age at menarche, age at first live birth, and the number of breast biopsies. The Gail model is the basis of the internet-based tool from the National Cancer Institute that enables calculation of a woman's individualized estimate of risk for invasive breast cancer over a 5-year period and over a lifetime.[21]

Another prediction model, developed by Claus and coworkers,[22] relies more on family history. The Claus model predicts individual estimates of breast cancer risk according to decade from age 29 to 79, based on knowledge of first- and second-degree relatives with breast cancer and their age at diagnosis. For women with at least one first- or second-degree relative with breast cancer (for whom the Claus model is applicable), the risk assessments based on the Gail and Claus model may differ.[1] Two other models are available for breast cancer risk prediction,[23,24] but are infrequently used.

2. Screening Mammography: Guidelines and Limitations

Mammography remains the standard of care for breast cancer screening. Although most women should begin annual screening mammography at age 40, some women with specific risk factors may benefit from beginning annual mammographic screening at an age younger than 40 years.[2,3] An expert panel recommended that women with mutations of *BRCA1* or *BRCA2* should begin annual screening mammography between the ages of 25 and 35.[4] It has been suggested that women who have had prior breast cancer, atypia, or lobular carcinoma in situ should begin annual screening mammography after diagnosis; that women with a family history of premenopausal breast cancer in a first-degree relative should begin annual screening mammography at an age that is 10 years younger than the relative was when she got her breast cancer, but not before age 25; and that women who have received mantle radiation for Hodgkin's disease should begin annual screening mammography 8 years after radiation is completed.[2,3]

Although screening mammography can detect breast cancers in high-risk women, it has limitations, particularly in dense breasts.[25,26] According to Kopans,[27] if 100 women with breast cancer are screened with mammography and physical examination, 80 of the cancers will be detected: by mammography in 68 of 80 (85%) women and by physical examination in 12 of 80 (15%) women. Another 20 *interval* cancers (which tend to be aggressive) will become palpable and diagnosed during the next year. Nonmammographic screening modalities, as a supplement to mammography, have the potential to detect at least some of these interval cancers early, which could in theory reduce breast cancer mortality.[27] These supplemental screening modalities also could have false-positive results, generating benign biopsies with their attendant costs.[12]

The American Cancer Society Guidelines for 2003[28] suggest that patients be given the following information:

Women who have a higher than average risk of developing breast cancer may benefit from starting early detection practices at a younger age or having additional tests or more frequent examinations. Factors that help determine if a woman is at high risk include: a strong family history of breast cancer (especially if their mother, sister, or daughter developed breast cancer at a young age or if several close relatives have breast or ovarian cancer), genetic tests that showed changes in the *BRCA1* or *BRCA2* breast cancer genes, a breast cancer treated in the past, or radiation therapy in the chest area for another type of cancer. There is not enough research yet on the value of screening women younger than 40 with mammograms or with other tests such as magnetic resonance imaging and ultrasound. Some doctors may recommend these tests for women with the above risk factors. If you think are at higher risk based on the factors above, talk to your doctor about what is known about these tests and their potential benefits, limitations, and harms. Then make a decision together about the testing that is best for you.

Data regarding breast MRI screening in high-risk women are discussed below.

3. Breast Magnetic Resonance Imaging Screening: Published Results

3.1. Meta-analysis

Breast MRI can detect cancers that are mammographically and clinically occult[13-19] (Table 11.1). Investigators have studied use of breast MRI to screen women at high risk, defined by the presence of specific risk factors or by quantitative models.

In published series of breast MRI screening through 2003, which included 1305 women, a biopsy was recommended based on MRI findings in 14% (range, 7%–18%). Cancer was found by MRI (but not mammography) in 34% (range, 24%–89%) of women who had biopsy and in 4% (range, 2%–7%) of high-risk women who had MRI screening. The 34% positive predictive value of biopsy based on MRI-detected lesions in high-risk women is within the 20% to 40% range of positive predictive values of mammographically detected lesions in the general population.[29] Among cancers detected by MRI screening, histology was invasive in 67% (range, 43%–100%) and ductal carcinoma in situ (DCIS) in 33% (range, 0%–57%). A biopsy that did not yield cancer was performed in 9% (range, 1%–15%) of women who had breast MRI screening (Table 11.1).[13-19] Examples of mammographically occult, nonpalpable cancers detected by breast MRI screening at our institution are shown in Figures 11.1 through 11.6.

TABLE 11.1. High-Risk Screening with Breast MRI: Published Results

Investigator	No. of Women	Age Mean (Range)	Biopsy (%)[a]	PPV of Biopsy (%)[b]	No. of Cancer (%)[c]	No. of DCIS (%)
Kuhl et al.[13]	192	39 (18–65)	14 (7)	9/14 (64)	6/192 (3)	1/6 (17)
Tilanus-Linthorst et al.[14]	109	43 (20–74)	9 (8)	3/9 (33)	3/109 (3)	0/3 (0)
Lo et al.[15]	157	43 (26–77)	28 (18)	5/28 (18)	5/157 (3)	Not stated
Warner et al.[16]	196	43 (26–59)	23 (12)	6/23 (26)	4/196 (2)	0/4 (0)
Stoutjesdijk et al.[17d]	179	Not stated	30 (17)	13/30 (43)	8/179 (4)	2/8 (25)
Podo et al.[18]	105	46 (25–77)	9 (9)	8/9 (89)	7/105 (7)	3/7 (43)
Morris[19]	367	50 (23–82)	64 (17)	14/59 (24)	14/367 (4)	8/14 (57)
Total	1305	45 (18–82)	177 (14)	58/172 (34)	47/1305 (4)	14/42 (33)

Source: Adapted from Morris EA et al.[19] with permission. *Abbreviations*: PPV, positive predictive value of biopsy; DCIS, ductal carcinoma in situ.
[a] Refers to biopsies recommended for MRI-detected lesions that were or were not seen by mammography.
[b] Refers to MRI-detected cancers that were or were not seen by mammography.
[c] Refers to mammographically occult, MRI-detected cancers. Percentage refers to prevalence of mammographically occult, MRI-detected cancers in all women who had breast MRI screening.
[d] In this study of 179 women, 40 had only mammography, 49 had only MRI, 15 had both mammography and MRI but in different years, and 75 had both mammography and MRI within 4 months. Some women who had MRI on the basis of abnormal mammograms were included. Eight MRI-detected malignant lesions include one DCIS in woman who did not have mammography and one lymphoma.

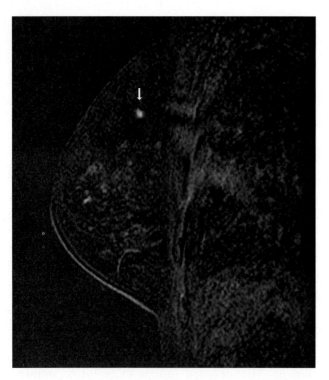

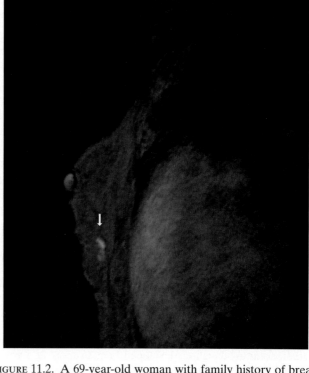

FIGURE 11.1. A 42-year-old woman with family history of breast cancer who had a prior right lumpectomy 1 year previously. Sagittal, T1-weighted, fat-suppressed, contrast-enhanced, subtraction MRI of the left breast shows irregular, indistinct 0.5-cm mass with peripheral enhancement in 12:00 axis (arrow), not seen on mammography or ultrasound. Magnetic resonance imaging guided needle localization and surgical excision revealed invasive ductal carcinoma, pure tubular type, measuring 0.3cm, and ductal carcinoma in situ, with negative sentinel nodes. The patient was treated with breast-conserving surgery.

FIGURE 11.2. A 69-year-old woman with family history of breast cancer, in whom prior biopsy showed radial scar. Sagittal, T1-weighted, fat-suppressed, contrast-enhanced MRI of the left breast showed irregular, spiculated, heterogeneously enhancing 1.2-cm mass deep in the left lower inner quadrant (arrow), not seen on mammography or ultrasound. Magnetic resonance imaging guided needle localization and surgical excision showed invasive ductal carcinoma, histologic and nuclear grade I, with negative sentinel lymph nodes.

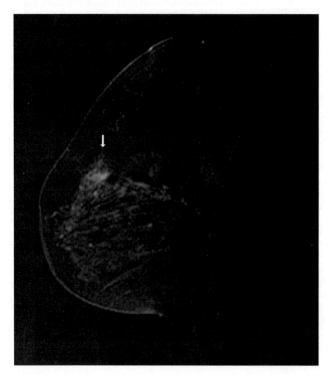

FIGURE 11.3. A 54-year-old woman with family history of breast cancer and history of LCIS. Sagittal, T1-weighted, fat-suppressed, contrast-enhanced MRI of the left breast shows irregularly shaped, irregularly marginated, heterogeneously enhancing mass measuring 1.3cm in upper outer quadrant (arrow), not evident on mammography or ultrasound. Magnetic resonance imaging guided needle localization revealed invasive lobular cancer measuring 0.2cm and LCIS, with positive sentinel nodes. The patient was treated with mastectomy, which showed extensive LCIS and a microscopic (0.1cm) focus of invasive lobular carcinoma in the lower inner quadrant.

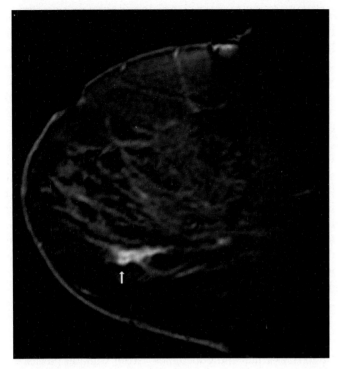

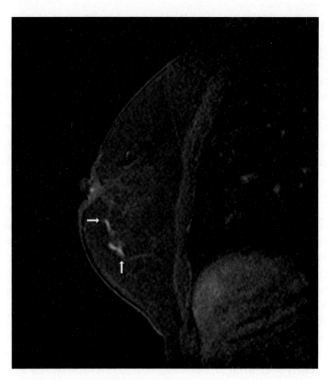

FIGURE 11.4. A 61-year-old woman with history of prior left mastectomy 19 months previously. Sagittal, T1-weighted, fat-suppressed, contrast-enhanced MRI of the right breast shows heterogeneous ductal enhancement in the right lower inner quadrant spanning 2.2 cm (arrow), without mammographic correlate. Magnetic resonance imaging guided needle localization yielded DCIS, cribriform and micropapillary types with apocrine cytology, low nuclear grade with minimal necrosis, involving complex sclerosing adenosis. The patient had subsequent mastectomy, which showed no residual cancer.

FIGURE 11.5. A 50-year-old woman with history of prior right lumpectomy 5 years previously. Collimated sagittal, T1-weighted, fat-suppressed, contrast-enhanced MRI of the right breast showed heterogeneous ductal enhancement in right 6:00 axis spanning 2.3 cm (arrows), without mammographic correlate. Magnetic resonance imaging guided needle localization showed DCIS, cribriform type with apocrine features, intermediate nuclear grade. The patient had mastectomy, which showed one residual microscopic focus of DCIS.

FIGURE 11.6. A 56-year-old woman who had prior left lumpectomy 9 years previously. Sagittal, T1-weighted, fat-suppressed, contrast-enhanced MRI of the left breast shows somewhat bilobed, irregularly shaped, irregularly marginated, heterogeneously enhancing mass left breast 12:00 axis (arrow), without mammographic or ultrasound correlate. Magnetic resonance imaging guided needle localization and surgical excision revealed DCIS, solid type, intermediate nuclear grade with moderate necrosis.

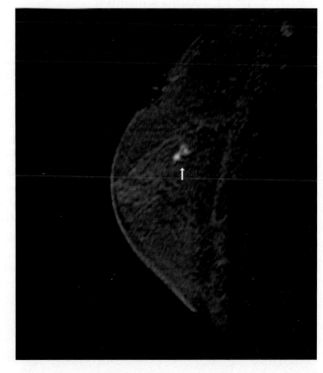

3.2. Results by Kuhl and Colleagues

In 2000, Kuhl and colleagues[13] from Germany published results of a study comparing MRI with conventional mammography in screening women at high risk of developing breast cancer. This prospective trial included 192 asymptomatic and 6 symptomatic women who were suspected or known to carry a breast cancer susceptibility gene of the 192 asymptomatic women, 35 were proven to have mutations in *BRCA1* or *BRAC2*. The study protocol included physical examination, high-frequency breast ultrasound, mammography, and breast MRI.

Among the 192 asymptomatic women, 9 breast cancers were found (6 in the first screening round and 3 in the second round). The mammogram was interpreted as normal (n = 2), benign (n = 3), or "probably benign" (n = 1) in six of these nine cancers, including five T1 node-negative invasive ductal cancers and one DCIS. Based on a combination of mammography and ultrasound, four of the nine breast cancers were detected and correctly classified; another two were well-circumscribed masses and thought to be fibroadenomas. Seven of the nine cancers occurred in women who had *BRCA* mutations. All nine cancers were detected and correctly classified by MRI. In 105 asymptomatic women with follow-up data, the sensitivities of the different imaging modalities were 33% for mammography, 33% for ultrasound, 44% for the combination of ultrasound and mammography, and 100% for MRI; the positive predictive values were 30% for mammography, 12% for ultrasound, and 64% for MRI.[13]

3.3. Results by Tilanus-Linthorst and Colleagues

In 2000, Tilanus-Linthorst and colleagues[14] from the Netherlands published the results of first experiences in screening women at high risk for breast cancer with MRI. Their population included 109 women with over 25% risk of breast cancer and more than 50% dense breast tissue with no suspicious findings at mammography; twelve (11%) women were *BRCA* mutation carriers. Magnetic resonance imaging detected three T1 invasive nodenegative breast cancers. Magnetic resonance imaging gave false-positive results in six women, leading to benign biopsies. During subsequent follow up of patients with a familial risk in whom the first breast cancer was detected at MRI, follow-up MRI revealed two T1 invasive node-negative recurrent cancers in the ipsilateral breast and one T1 invasive node-negative cancer in the contralateral breast.[14]

3.4. Results by Lo and Colleagues

In 2001, Lo and colleagues[15] from the Hospital of the University of Pennsylvania presented the results of a pilot study of breast MRI screening in a high-risk cohort. Risk factors included personal history of breast cancer or lobular carcinoma in situ (LCIS), family history of breast cancer, or genetic tendency to breast cancer. During a 6-year period, 170 patients had contrast-enhanced MRI; 13 patients were excluded due to mammographic or clinical abnormalities prior to MRI. The remaining 157 patients constituted the study population.

Abnormalities were found in 43 of 157 (27%) patients. Of these 43 patients, 13 of 43 (30%) had follow-up MRI showing resolution or stability of the MRI finding over at least 2 years. An additional 28 of 43 (65%) patients had interventional procedures based on MRI findings, yielding benign results in 21, LCIS in 2, and cancer in 5. Four of the five patients with cancer had normal mammograms; the fifth patient had an abnormality that was difficult to see with mammography. Two of the 43 patients with abnormalities did not have a follow-up study.[15]

3.5. Results by Warner and Colleagues

In 2001, Warner and colleagues[16] from Canada published results of a comparison of breast MRI, mammography, and ultrasound for surveillance of women at high risk for hereditary breast cancer. The patient population included 196 women aged 26 to 59 years with proven *BRCA1* or *BRCA2* mutations or strong family histories of breast or ovarian cancer. The protocol included mammography, ultrasound, MRI, and clinical breast examination on a single day. Biopsy was performed if any of the four studies was considered suspicious.

In the 196 high-risk women in the study, 7 cancers were detected, including 6 invasive cancers and one DCIS. Five of the invasive cancers were in mutation carriers and the sixth was in a woman with a personal history of breast cancer. Among 96 mutation carriers, the prevalence of breast cancer was 6.2%. All six invasive cancers had negative lymph nodes, measured 1 cm or less, and were detected by MRI. Of the six invasive cancers detected by MRI, two were also detected by both mammography and ultrasound, one by physical examination and ultrasound, and one by physical examination. The DCIS lesion was detected only by mammography in a woman who was BRCA2 positive.[16]

3.6. Results by Stoutjesdijk and Colleagues

In 2001, Stoutjesdijk and colleagues[17] from the Netherlands published results of a retrospective study of MRI and mammography in women with a hereditary risk of breast cancer. Patients included had a lifetime risk of breast cancer greater than 15% based on family history of breast or ovarian cancer or the presence of *BRCA1* or *BRCA2* mutations. Patients had no personal history of breast cancer and had to have either biopsy or minimum of 2 years MRI follow up. Although all women received biannual physical examination and annual imaging by MRI, mammography, or both, the imaging protocol was variable: among 179 women, 40 received only mammography, 49 had received only MRI, 75 received mammography and MRI within a 4-month period at least once, and 15 received mammography and MRI a year or more apart.

Thirteen malignant lesions were detected by MRI in 179 women, including 9 invasive cancers, 3 DCIS lesions, and 1 lymphoma. Two of the 13 malignant lesions occurred in women with *BRCA1* mutations. Among the nine invasive cancers, two were T1 node-negative cancers and seven were T2 lesions, including four with positive nodes. Six cancers and one lymphoma were not detected by mammography, and one DCIS lesion was found in a woman who did not undergo mammography. For the entire cohort, the area under the curve (AUC) for mammography was 0.74 [95% confidence interval (CI), 0.68–0.79] and the AUC for MRI was 0.99 (95% CI, 0.98–1.0). For women who had both examinations, the AUC for mammography was 0.70 (95% CI, 0.60–0.80) and the AUC for MRI was 0.98 (95% CI, 0.95–1.0).

3.7. Results by Sardanelli and Colleagues

In 2002, Sardanelli and colleagues[18] from Italy presented preliminary results of a prospective, nonrandomized, multicenter trial of MRI screening in women at genetic high risk of breast cancer. The patient population included BRCA1/2 mutation carriers or first-degree relative of BRCA1/2 mutation carriers, including women with personal history of unilateral breast cancer. Among 105 women enrolled, 91 had the first round of screening and 14 had first and second rounds; 40 (38%) had a previous personal history of breast cancer.

Breast cancer was identified in 8 of 105 patients, in the first round in 7 and in the second round in 1. Five (63%) of these eight patients had a personal history of breast cancer. Histologic findings in these eight cancers were invasive in five (ductal in two, lobular in two, and mixed in one) and DCIS in three. Among the eight cancers, seven were detected only by MRI; one was also detected by mammography and ultrasound. Magnetic resonance imaging had one false-positive case; mammography and ultrasound had no false-positive results.[18]

3.8. Morris and Colleagues: Results at Memorial Sloan-Kettering Cancer Center

3.8.1. Patient Population

In 2003, Morris and colleagues[19] reported results of the first round of breast MRI screening in women at high risk of developing breast cancer at MSKCC. Risk factors included personal history of breast cancer, lobular carcinoma in situ or atypia, or family history of breast cancer. The patient population included 367 asymptomatic high-risk women of median age 50 years (range, 23–82 years) with normal mammogram results, who had their first breast MRI screening examinations during a 2-year period. Magnetic resonance imaging technique, interpretation, and biopsy methods are described elsewhere.[30,31]

3.8.2. Biopsy Rate and Method

Biopsy was recommended for a nonpalpable, mamographically occult, MRI-detected lesion in 64 women (17% of the 367 women who had breast MRI screening) and performed in 59 women. Sonography, which was performed in 44 women who had subsequent biopsy, revealed sonographic correlates to the MRI-detected lesions in 11 (25%).

In 59 women who had biopsy, biopsy method was MRI-guided localization in 50 women and sonographically guided biopsy in 9 women (core biopsy in 5, needle localization in 3, and fine needle aspiration in 1). Of the five women who did not have the recommended biopsy, two declined biopsy, two were scheduled for MRI-guided needle localization but the enhancing lesions were no longer seen, and one went elsewhere for her care.

3.8.3. Biopsy Results: Patients

Biopsy showed cancer that was nonpalpable and mammographically occult in 14 women, constituting 24% of women who had biopsy and 4% of women who had breast MRI screening (Table 11.2). Biopsy revealed high-risk lesions in 13 women, constituting 22% of women who had biopsy and 4% of women who had MRI screening (Table 11.2). Biopsy revealed benign results in 32 women, constituting 54% of women who had biopsy and 9% of women who had MRI screening (Table 11.2).[19]

Among 14 women with cancer detected by MRI, histologic findings DCIS in 8 (57%) and invasive cancer in 6 (43%). The higher prevalence of DCIS in this study as compared with others (Table 11.1) may reflect an emphasis on morphology over kinetic information for interpretation. The median size of invasive cancer was 0.4 cm (range, 0.1–1.2 cm); two had axillary metastases. The stage of cancer detected by breast MRI was known in 13 women, and was stage 0 in 8 (62%), I in 3 (23%), and II in 2 (15%). The treatment of cancer detected by MRI was known in 13 women: 7 (54%) had mastectomy and 6 (46%) had breast conservation.

3.8.4. Biopsy Results: Magnetic Resonance Imaging Findings

Seventy-nine MRI-detected lesions in 64 women had biopsy (average, 1.2 lesions per woman; range, 1–3 lesions

TABLE 11.2. Biopsy Histology in 367 High-Risk Women Who Had Breast MRI Screening

Histology	Biopsied Women (%)	All Women (%)
Benign[a]	32/59 (54)	32/367 (9)
High risk[b]	13/59 (22)	13/367 (4)
Malignant	14/59 (24)	14/367 (4)
DCIS[c]	8/59 (14)	8/367 (2)
Invasive[d]	6/59 (10)	6/367 (2)

Source: Adapted from Morris EA et al.[19] with permission. Abbreviations: DCIS, ductal carcinoma in situ.

[a] Dominant findings in these benign biopsies were fibrocystic change (n = 6), fibrosis (n = 6), duct hyperplasia (n = 5), fibroadenomatoid changes (n = 4), fibroadenoma (n = 2), benign lymph node (n = 2), benign breast tissue (n = 2), sclerosing adenosis (n = 1), pseudoangiomatous stromal hyperplasia (n = 1), papilloma (n = 1), chronic inflammation (n = 1), and adenomyoepithelioma (n = 1).

[b] High-risk lesions included atypical ductal hyperplasia (n = 5), lobular carcinoma in situ (n = 4), atypical lobular hyperplasia (n = 2), and radial scar (n = 2).

[c] Among eight women with DCIS, nuclear grade was low in three, low to intermediate in two, and high in three; histologic subtype was cribriform (n = 2), cribriform and micropapillary (n = 1), cribriform and papillary (n = 1), cribriform and solid (n = 1), clinging (n = 1), clinging and micropapillary (n = 1), or solid (n = 1).

[d] Histologic findings in six women with infiltrating carcinoma were infiltrating ductal carcinoma (n = 4), infiltrating ductal and infiltrating lobular carcinoma (n = 1), and infiltrating lobular carcinoma (n = 1).

per woman). The median size of MRI lesion that had biopsy was 1.0cm (range, 0.4–5.9cm). The median MRI lesion size was 0.9cm (range, 0.4–4.9cm) for benign lesions and 1.3cm (range, 0.5–5.9cm) for cancers. Of these 79 lesions, 51 (65%) were masses and 38 (35%) were nonmass lesions.

Cancer was found in 16 lesions, constituting 20% of 79 lesions that had biopsy. Among these 16 cancers, 10 (63%) were DCIS and 6 (38%) were invasive. These 16 cancers occurred in 14 women, including 1 with multifocal cancer and 1 with synchronous bilateral cancers detected by MRI. The features with highest positive predictive value were ductal enhancement for nonmass lesions and spiculated margins for masses. Cancer was frequent in lesions classified as highly suggestive of malignancy rather than suspicious (50% vs. 18%, $P = 0.09$). Visually assessed kinetic features and signal intensity on T2-weighted images were not significant predictors of cancer.[19]

3.8.5. Statistics

The positive predictive value of biopsy was significantly higher in women with rather than without a family history of breast cancer (32% vs. 6%, $P < 0.05$) and in women with rather than without both a personal and a family history of breast cancer (50% vs. 12%, $P = 0.006$). The prevalence of MRI-detected cancer was significantly higher in women

with rather than without a family history of breast cancer (6% vs. < 1%, $P = 0.02$), in women who had prior breast conservation rather than prior mastectomy (7% vs. 2%, $P < 0.05$), and in women with rather than without both a personal and family history of breast cancer (8% vs. 2%, $p < 0.02$).[19]

4. Ductal Carcinoma In Situ

Among breast cancers detected at high-risk screening breast MRI in the literature, an average of 33% (range, 0%–57%) have been DCIS (see Table 11.1). The proportion of cancers that were DCIS was higher at MSKCC (57%) as compared with other studies (0%–43%; see Table 11.1). The high proportion of DCIS encountered in our study may reflect our high-resolution technique and emphasis on morphology for interpretation. Some investigators have suggested that detection of DCIS may in fact be disadvantageous, leading to overtreatment of an innocuous disease;[32] however, published data refute this contention. Long-term follow-up studies of women with untreated DCIS show that approximately 30% of them develop invasive cancer in the ipsilateral breast; of those, half develop distant metastases.[33–35] These follow-up studies demonstrate the potential for DCIS to progressive to invasive cancer with its associated morbidity and mortality, and reinforce the importance of detecting and treating DCIS.

5. False-positive Results

Among high-risk women reported in studies of breast MRI screening, a biopsy was performed that did not yield cancer in 9% (range, 1%–15%). These biopsies are usually considered false-positive results, and a disadvantage of MRI screening due to costs in money, time, anxiety, and scarring.[12] In fact, some of these biopsies result in removal of *high-risk* lesions such as atypical hyperplasia, lobular carcinoma in situ, and radial scar. In our study of screening breast MRI,[19] high-risk lesions were identified in 22% of women who had biopsy and in 4% of women who had breast MRI screening (Figures 11.7 through 11.9).

Diagnosing these high-risk lesions, which have high prevalence in women at hereditary risk for breast cancer (particularly those over the age of 40 years),[36] could be advantageous for two reasons. First, identification of high-risk lesions may assist in making management decisions regarding chemoprevention or prophylactic mastectomy. Secondly, because some of these lesions (e.g., atypical ductal hyperplasia) may be premalignant, their removal could lower a woman's risk of subsequent cancer.[36]

It is important for the patient and referring physician to be aware of the 14% chance that screening breast MRI

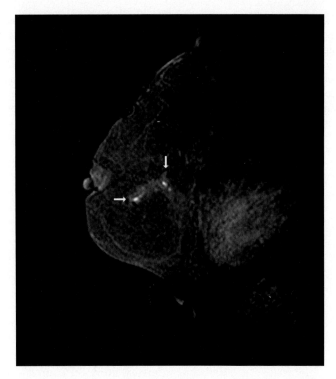

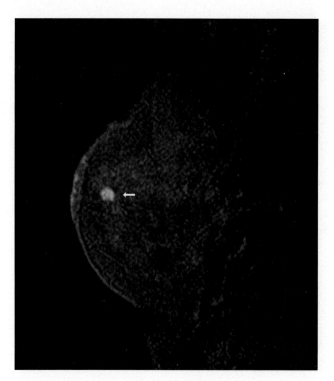

FIGURE 11.7. A 58-year-old woman with family history of breast cancer. Sagittal, T1-weighted, fat-suppressed, contrast-enhanced MRI of the left breast shows clumped enhancement in a vaguely ductal distribution spanning 2.7cm in central breast, mid to posterior third (arrows), not identified at mammography or ultrasound. Magnetic resonance imaging guided needle localization for surgical excision revealed atypical ductal hyperplasia, cystic hypersecretory type.

FIGURE 11.8. A 53-year-old woman with history of LCIS. Sagittal, T1-weighted, fat-suppressed, contrast-enhanced image of left breast shows irregularly marginated, lobulated, heterogeneously enhancing mass measuring 0.8cm in retroareolar region, lower outer quadrant (arrow), not seen at mammography or ultrasound. Magnetic resonance imaging guided needle localization yielded LCIS involving sclerosing adenosis and intraductal papilloma, as well as a 0.8cm focus of apocrine adenosis.

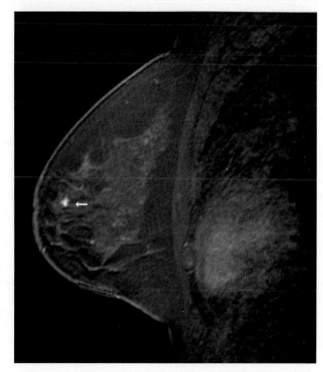

FIGURE 11.9. A 48-year-old woman with family history of breast cancer. Sagittal, T1-weighted, fat-suppressed, contrast-enhanced image of left breast shows spiculated, irregularly shaped, heterogeneously enhancing mass measuring 0.8cm in left retroareolar region (arrow), without mammographic or ultrasound correlate. Magnetic resonance imaging guided needle localization for surgical excision revealed radial scar and benign findings including duct hyperplasia, fibrocystic change, and stromal fibrosis.

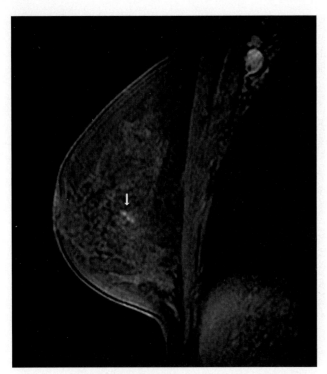

FIGURE 11.10. A 39-year-old woman with family history of breast cancer. Sagittal, T1-weighted, fat-suppressed, contrast-enhanced MRI of the right breast shows clumped ductal enhancement spanning 0.9 cm in upper outer quadrant/retroareolar region (arrow), without mammographic or ultrasound correlate. Magnetic resonance imaging guided needle localization yielded fibrocystic change, stromal fibrosis, and apocrine cysts. Fibrocystic change is one of the most common benign findings encountered at MRI-guided needle localization.

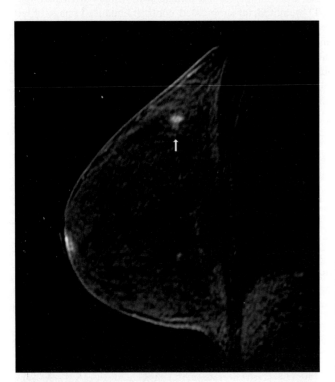

FIGURE 11.11. A 39-year-old women with family history of breast cancer. Sagittal, T1-weighted, fat-suppressed, contrast-enhanced MRI of the right breast shows irregularly shaped, irregularly marginated, heterogeneously enhancing 0.7-cm mass right upper outer quadrant (arrow), not seen on mammography. Ultrasound-guided core biopsy yielded fibrosis. Magnetic resonance imaging guided needle localization confirmed the diagnosis of benign breast tissue with dense stromal fibrosis.

will lead to a biopsy, and of the 66% chance that the biopsy will be benign (see Table 11.1; Figures 11.10 and 11.11). Experience and use of the breast MRI lexicon[37] should refine criteria for interpretation, decreasing the number of benign biopsies. Further refinement and dissemination of technology for MRI-guided breast needle biopsy will enable biopsies, when necessary, to be performed in a minimally invasive manner with lower cost, less anxiety, and no deformity.

Attention to the timing of the breast MRI study with respect to the menstrual cycle may reduce false-positive interpretations. Kuhl and coworkers[38] have demonstrated a higher prevalence of contrast-enhancing lesions during week 1 and week 4 of the menstrual cycle, with diminution in contrast-enhancing lesions during weeks 2 and 3 (midcycle). For premenopausal women, scheduling the high-risk screening breast MRI study at midcycle (if feasible) may decrease the likelihood of encountering enhancing lesions that may raise concern. In addition, if an enhancing area is identified on MRI in a premenopausal woman during week 1 or 4 of her cycle, repeating the study at midcycle (a very short-interval follow up) may distinguish benign hormonal enhancement from a lesion that warrants biopsy.

6. False-negative Results

The high reported sensitivities of breast MRI, ranging from 88% to 100%,[10,11] are primarily derived from studies of diagnostic MRI. Few data address the sensitivity of breast MRI in the screening setting. Some investigators have suggested that breast MRI may have higher sensitivity in depicting invasive cancer rather than DCIS,[39] but more recent data indicate that MRI may have higher sensitivity than mammography in DCIS detection (89% vs. 30%, $P < 0.001$).[40] It has also been suggested that MRI may be less sensitive in depicting invasive lobular rather than invasive ductal cancer, although MRI still provides better assessment of extent of disease for invasive lobular carcinoma than does mammography.[41–44]

In one study of breast MRI at 1.0 Tesla (T) performed for clinical indications, MRI imaging failed to depict 41 (12%) of 354 malignant tumors, including 28 (8%) of 334 invasive cancers and 13 (65%) of 20 DCIS lesions.[11] The low sensitivity, particularly for DCIS, may reflect the low field strength of the magnet. Reasons for failing to diagnose cancers in this study included diffuse growth patterns or lesions measuring 5 mm or less (n = 33), masking of tumor by enhancing glandular tissue (n = 3), tumor near or beyond the boundary of the field of view (n = 3), motion artifacts (n = 1), or inadequate contrast (n = 1).[11] Other potential reasons for failure to diagnose breast cancer at MRI include suboptimal fat suppression, delay in acquisition of the first images after contrast injection, and inter-

pretive error. Further study in the screening setting, including long-term follow-up of women with breast MRI studies interpreted as normal, is necessary to determine the true false-negative rate of screening breast MRI.

7. Probably Benign Lesions at High-risk Screening Magnetic Resonance Imaging

Short-term follow up is widely accepted for nonpalpable mammographic lesions that are *probably benign*.[45–56] Short-term follow up for probably benign lesions has several advantages over biopsy: It is not invasive, it is less expensive, and it causes less anxiety for the patient.[48] In prior studies, nonpalpable probably benign lesions were reported in 3% to 11% of mammograms.[49–52,54–56] Subsequent cancer was found in 0.5% to 2% of probably benign mammographic lesions, with most cancers identified due to interval change at short-term follow-up mammography when they were small and early stage, with excellent prognosis.[49–52,54,55] Few data address the findings and outcome of MRI-detected lesions interpreted as probably benign: Even the lexicon states that regarding probably benign lesions, "most approaches are intuitive."[37]

7.1. Probably Benign Lesions at Memorial Sloan-Kettering Cancer Center

Among first high-risk screening MRI examinations performed in 367 women at our institution, 24% (89 of 367) were interpreted as "probably benign."[57] Among these 89 MRI studies, probably benign findings were solitary in 34 (38%), multiple and unilateral in 22 (25%), and multiple and bilateral in 33 (37%); probably benign lesion type was nonmass in 58 (65% and mass in 31 (35%). Factors associated with a higher likelihood of a probably benign interpretation included no personal history of breast cancer (39% vs. 21%, $P < 0.001$), family history of breast cancer in a first-degree relative (31% vs. 21%, $P = 0.05$), premenopausal status (29% vs. 20%, $P = 0.07$), and dense or heterogeneously dense mammographic parenchymal patterns (27% vs. 16%, $P = 0.08$). Follow-up MRI was performed in 70 of 89 (79%) women in whom it was recommended, with median follow-up 11 months (range, 1–24 months).

Twenty women had subsequent biopsy at a median of nine (range, 1–18) months after MRI, due to progression on follow-up MRI in 14 and other reasons in 6. Cancer was found in nine women, constituting 45% (9 of 20) women who had biopsy and 10% (9 of 89) women with probably benign lesions. In six of nine women who developed cancer, constituting 7% (6 of 89) of women in the study, cancer was detected by follow-up MRI in an area previously interpreted as probably benign. In three remaining women who developed cancer, MRI showed stable findings (n = 1) or was not performed prior to biopsy (n = 2). In these nine cancers, histology was DCIS in five and invasive ductal cancer in four. Median histologic size of invasive cancer was 0.6cm (range, 0.2–0.9cm); two women had sentinel lymph node micrometastases. Our data did not enable reliable identification of a subgroup of lesions with a less than 2% chance of being malignant.

In summary, short-term follow up was recommended on the basis of 24% of first high-risk screening MRI examinations. Subsequent cancer developed in an area interpretated as probably benign in 7% to 10%; among these cancers, over half were DCIS and half were detected by MRI only. The frequency of follow up and the proportion of lesions followed that proved to be cancer in this MRI study are higher than those reported in studies of probably benign nonpalpable mammographically detected lesions.[49–52,54,55] This may reflect the difference between MRI (which detects solid hypervascular lesions) and mammography, as well as our high-risk population and learning curve. These findings indicate the need to establish evidence-based criteria for probably benign lesions at breast MRI studies.

8. Ultrasound Versus Magnetic Resonance Imaging for High-risk Screening

Breast ultrasound is fast, comfortable, and readily available; it does not require the use of ionizing radiation, provides ready access for biopsy procedures, and is relatively inexpensive. A multicenter trial to evaluate ultrasound for screening high-risk women with dense breasts could provide important information.[58] The rationale for this trial is supported by promising results from investigations performed at single institutions.[59–65]

In published studies of screening breast ultrasound, which have included women at normal and high risk, biopsy was recommended in 3% to 4% of women; cancer was found in 9% to 18% of biopsies, or in 0.3% to 0.5% of women who had screening breast ultrasound.[62–65] These results should be interpreted in the context of screening mammography data, which show the prevalence of cancer in the general population to be 0.5% to 0.7% on the initial screening mammogram, decreasing to 0.2% to 0.3% in women undergoing regular mammographic screening.[58,66–68]

Some studies of screening breast ultrasound specifically reported results in the subpopulation of women at high risk of developing breast cancer as compared with women at normal risk. In these studies, the prevalence of cancer detected by screening breast ultrasound was 0.5% to 1.0% in high-risk women versus 0.2% to 0.3% in normal-risk women.[62,64,65] Furthermore, the positive predictive value of biopsy based on a sonographically detected lesion is higher in high-risk as compared with normal-risk women. Crystal and colleagues[65] reported that the positive predictive value of biopsy of sonographically detected lesions was 40% in high-risk women versus 11% in normal-risk women. In comparing results of MRI screening to breast ultrasound screening, it is necessary to compare the results in the relevant population: women at high risk of developing breast cancer.

Breast MRI has several advantages compared with ultrasound for screening high-risk women. The prevalence of cancer in high-risk women who undergo screening MRI is 2% to 7% (see Table 11.1), higher than the 0.5% to 1.0% prevalence of cancer in high-risk women who undergo screening breast ultrasound.[62,64,65] Among high-risk women who had ultrasound and MRI in addition to mammography,[13,16,18] the 86% to 100% sensitivity of MRI was higher than the 13% to 43% sensitivity of ultrasound. Magnetic resonance imaging is more sensitive than ultrasound in detecting DCIS.[69] DCIS, which constituted one-third of cancers detected in published studies of high-risk screening MRI, accounted for only 0% to 17% of cancers detected at screening ultrasound.[13,60–65] Breast MRI does have some disadvantages, however: It is more expensive and less widely available than ultrasound, and the technology for MRI-guided biopsy is not yet widely disseminated. Further study of supplementing mammography with breast MRI, ultrasound, or both for screening high-risk women is needed.

9. Second Look Ultrasound

Whether or not breast ultrasound will be proven to be beneficial as a screening test, it is useful as an adjunct to breast MRI. *Second look* or directed ultrasound may identify an ultrasound correlate for an MRI-detected lesion, even if ultrasound examination before MRI showed no abnormalities. For MRI-detected lesions warranting biopsy, identification of an ultrasound correlate enables the biopsy to be performed under ultrasound guidance (Figure 11.12). In prior reports, the frequency of identifying an ultrasound correlate for MRI-detected lesions referred for biopsy has ranged from 23% to 100%.[70–72]

In a study by LaTrenta and colleagues[72] from our institution, an ultrasound correlate was found for 23% of MRI-detected lesions referred for biopsy. An ultrasound correlate was identified in 25% of masses versus 11% of nonmass lesions ($P = 0.34$) and in 58% of invasive cancers versus 29% of DCIS lesions ($P = 0.35$). The frequency of cancer was higher among MRI-detected lesions with rather than without ultrasound correlates (43% vs. 14%, $P = 0.01$), but even among the lesions that lacked ultrasound correlates, 14% were malignant. These data reinforce the

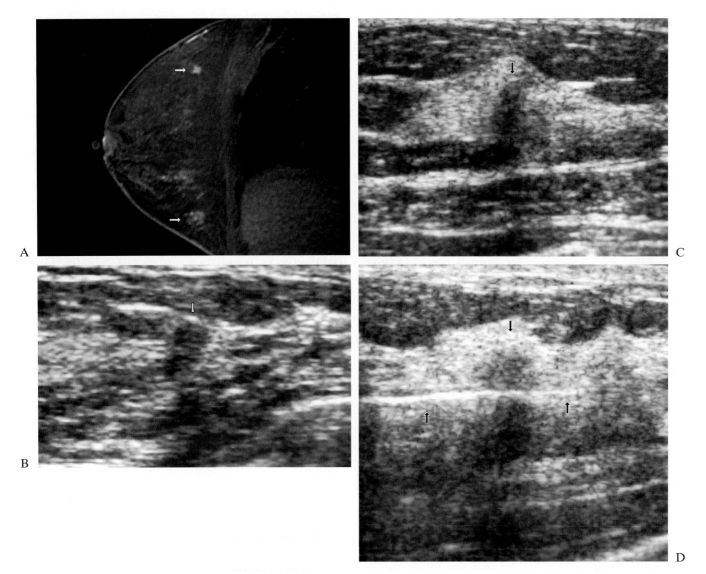

FIGURE 11.12. A 47-year-old woman status post bilateral lumpectomies 1 year ago. (A) Sagittal, T1-weighted, fat-suppressed, contrast-enhanced MRI of the right breast shows a 0.6-cm mass with spiculated margins, irregular shape, and heterogeneous enhancement in right 12:00 axis (upper arrow) and irregularly shaped, irregularly marginated, heterogeneously enhancing 1.2-cm mass right 6:00 axis (lower arrow). Mammogram (not shown) revealed moderately dense breast tissue, without suspicious findings. (B) Ultrasound of right 12:00 axis shows 0.6-cm hypoechoic mass that is taller than wide (arrow), corresponding to the superior MRI lesion. (C) Ultrasound of right 6:00 axis shows 0.6-cm hypoechoic mass that is taller than wide (arrow), corresponding to the inferior MRI lesion. (D) Ultrasound image obtained during ultrasound-guided core biopsy of the 12:00 axis mass demonstrates the needle (lower arrows) traversing the lesion (upper arrow). Ultrasound-guided core biopsy was also performed of the 6:00 axis lesion (not shown). Histologic analysis of core biopsy material yielded invasive ductal carcinoma with tubulolobular features at 12:00 and a microscopic focus of invasive ductal carcinoma at 6:00. The patient was treated with mastectomy, which revealed foci of residual invasive ductal carcinoma measuring 0.1–0.5 cm and ductal carcinoma in situ.

fact that MRI screening requires the capability to perform biopsies for lesions detected solely by MRI.

10. Breast MRI in Women with *BRCA* Mutations

Women with genetic predisposition to breast cancer due to mutations of *BRCA1* or *BRCA2* account for approximately 5–10% of women with breast cancer.[1a] Among women with *BRCA1* mutations, the cumulative risk of breast cancer is 3% by age 30, 19% by age 40, 51% by age 50, 54% by age 60, and 85% by age 70. Women with *BRCA* mutations, whose cumulative lifetime risk of breast cancer is 50–85%, are also at risk for ovarian cancer. Annual mammograms detect less than half of the breast cancers in *BRCA* mutation carriers, perhaps due to dense breast tissue in young women, pathologic features of the tumors (including rapid growth rate) and sometimes benign mammographic features.[13] Half of the breast cancers in mutation carriers appear in the interval between mammograms; among these interval cancers, the median size is 1.7 cm and half have axillary metastases. Previous management strategies for these women have included prophylactic bilateral mastectomy and/or oophorectomy, chemoprevention, and close surveillance.[1a] Recent studies have addressed the use of breast MRI in addition to mammography to screen mutation carriers.

Kriege et al.[75] reported a prospective, nonrandomized study of clinical breast exam (CBE), mammography, and MRI in 1,909 women who had a genetic or familial predisposition to breast cancer (lifetime risk, ≥15%) in the Netherlands; among these women, 358 (19%) had *BRCA* mutations. Kriege et al.[75] found that the breast cancer detection rate was 9.5 per 1,000 women-years of follow-up overall: 7.8 per 1,000 for women whose lifetime risk was 15–29%, 5.4 per 1,000 for women whose lifetime risk was 30–49%, and 26.5 per 1,000 for *BRCA1* or *BRCA2* mutation carriers. Method of identification of 45 cancers was MRI but not mammography in 22 (49%), MRI and mammography in 10 (22%), and mammography but not MRI in 8 (18%); four were interval cancers and one was detected only by physical examination. Only 17% of cancers in mutation carriers were interval cancers. MRI had higher sensitivity (particularly for invasive breast cancer) but lower specificity than mammography. Using BI-RADS Category 3 or higher as the cut-off for an abnormal test, MRI had 71.1% sensitivity and 89.8% specificity; mammography had 40.0% sensitivity and 95.0% specificity. Using BI-RADS Category 4 or higher as the cut-off for an abnormal test, MRI had sensitivity of 46.6% and specificity of 98.9%; mammography had a sensitivity of 24.4% and specificity of 99.7%. Limitations of the study include primary analysis based on using BI-RADS Category 3 as the cut-off for an abnormal result, and relatively low sensitivity of both mammography and MRI.

Warner et al.[76] reported a prospective, nonrandomized study of 236 women age 25 to 65 with *BRCA1* or *BRCA2* mutations in Canada. These women had one to three annual screening examinations that included MRI, mammography, and ultrasound on the same day. Of the 236 women, all completed at least one round of screening, 136 had at least two rounds, and 85 had all three rounds. Clinical breast examination (CBE) was performed on the day of imaging and at six-month intervals. Each radiologist reported the level of suspicion as per the BI-RADS scale, where lesions interpreted as 4 (suspicious) or 5 (highly suggestive of malignancy) had biopsy.[37] An abnormal test was defined as one for which a biopsy was suggested (ie BI-RADS 4 or 5). Twenty-two cancers were identified in 21 women; histologies of these 22 cancers were invasive in 16 (73%) and DCIS in six (27%). Among these 22 cancers, 17 (77%) were identified by MRI, eight (36%) were identified by mammography, seven (33%) were identified by ultrasound, and two (9%) were identified by CBE. Only two (9%) cancers had axillary nodal metastases; there was one interval cancer. MRI was significantly more sensitive than either mammography (p = 0.014) or ultrasound (p = 0.006). The sensitivities were 45% for mammography and CBE, 64% for mammography, CBE, and ultrasound, 86% for mammography, CBE, and MRI, and 95% for mammography, CBE, and MRI combined with ultrasound.

Warner et al.[76] calculated that for mammography, the sensitivities in the first, second, and third screening rounds were 38%, 43%, and 0%, with specificities of 99.6%, 100%, and 100%, respectively. For ultrasound, the sensitivities in the first, second, and third screening rounds were 25%, 57%, and 0%, with specificities of 95%, 96%, and 98%, respectively. For MRI, the sensitivities for the first, second, and third screening rounds were 85%, 71%, and 50%, with specificities 93%, 97%, and 99%. Positive predictive values ranged from 85–100% for mammography, 0–44% for ultrasound, and 42–56% for MRI. Negative predictive values ranged from 97–98% for mammography, 96–98% for ultrasound, and 98–99% for MRI. In an accompanying editorial, Robson and Offit[77] suggested that an optimal screening strategy in mutation carriers may include alternating mammography and MRI (with or without ultrasound) at 6 month intervals, to enable detection of rapidly growing cancers ("kinetic failures of detection") that would otherwise develop in the interval between screening examinations.

Published data support the utility of supplementing mammography with breast MRI to screen *BRCA* mutation carriers. Kopans[27] has suggested that only a randomized controlled trial with death as the endpoint can provide definitive proof of benefit of breast cancer screening. Such data do not exist for breast MRI. In the absence of a randomized controlled trial, management recommendations may be appropriately based on other information, such as data extrapolation, observational studies, and expert opinion.[1a] In women with an extremely high likelihood of developing breast cancer, the benefit of high sensitivity of breast MRI screening may outweigh the disadvantage of suboptimal specificity. In a 2003 report, the Blue Cross Blue Shield Association's Technology Evaluation Center[78] concluded that breast MRI to screen women at high genetic risk improved the net health outcome. The 2004 studies of Kriege et al.[75] and Warner et al.[76] provide further evidence of benefit in women with inherited *BRCA* mutations.

11. Caveats

Although breast MRI screening can detect early breast cancers in high-risk women, it is important to remember several caveats. Magnetic resonance imaging is an expensive test that has a high likelihood of leading to other tests: in our experience, 41% of women were referred either for biopsy (17%) or short-term follow up (24%) on the basis of their first MRI screening examinations. Although a lexicon has been created to standardize reporting,[37] there is variability in technique and interpretation.[73] Some women (e.g., those with pacemakers, aneurysm clips, or claustrophobia) are not candidates for MRI.[74] Breast MRI screening requires the capability to perform biopsy of lesions detected only by MRI; biopsy systems are commercially available but not in widespread use.[30] False-positive results can occur with breast MRI, with their associated costs.[12] The results reported in this chapter refer to women at high risk; MRI screening in women at lower risk would have more false-positive results and detect fewer cancers. Finally, no studies have evaluated the impact of breast MRI screening on survival.

12. Conclusion

High-risk screening breast MRI is of most benefit to women at the highest risk. Increasing data support supplementing mammography with MRI to screen women with *BRCA* mutations. MRI may be useful as a supplement to mammography in screening women at high risk due to other factors such as previous breast cancer, but more study is needed. The optimal timing of MRI with respect to mammography and the potential role of adding ultrasound in addition to MRI to the screening regimen are issues that require further investigation. A randomized controlled trial of breast MRI in women at high risk for breast cancer could provide mortality data but accrual to such a study may be difficult. Institutions that perform breast MRI as a high-risk screening examination should have the capability to perform biopsy of lesions detected

only by MRI. No data support the use of breast MRI to screen women at normal risk of developing breast cancer.

Women at high risk for breast cancer should discuss the use of breast MRI as a supplement to mammography with their doctors, and institutions that perform breast MRI should track their results. At our center, for example, the first high-risk screening breast MRI examination led to a biopsy recommendation in 17%; cancer was found in 24% of women who had biopsy and in 4% of women who had breast MRI screening. Among the cancers found, more than half were DCIS.[19] Awareness of MRI outcomes should help patients and referring clinicians make an informed decision about supplementing mammography with breast MRI for high-risk screening. Additional study is needed to develop evidence-based recommendations for screening that are suitable for women with specific risk factors and quantified levels of breast cancer risk.

References

1. Armstrong K, Eisen A, Weber B. Assessing the risk of breast cancer. *N Engl J Med*. 2000;342:564–571.
1a. Liberman L. Breast cancer screening with MRI—what are the data for patients at high risk? *N Engl J Med*. 2004;351: 497–500.
2. Dershaw DD. Indications for screening asymptomatic women less than 40 years old. *AJR Am J Roentgenol*. 1999; 172:1136.
3. Dershaw DD. Mammographic screening of the high-risk woman. *Am J Surg*. 2000;180:288–289.
4. Burke W, Daly M, Garber J, et al. Recommendations for follow-up care of individuals with an inherited predisposition to cancer II. BCRA1 and BRCA2. *JAMA*. 1997;277: 997–1003.
5. Page DL, Dupont WD, Rogers LW, Rados MS. Atypical hyperplastic lesions of the female breast: a long-term follow-up study. *Cancer* 1985;55:2698–2708.
6. Frykberg ER. Lobular carcinoma in situ of the breast. *Breast J*. 1999;5:296–302.
7. Jacobs TW, Byrne C, Colditz G, et al. Radial scars in benign breast biopsy specimens and the risk of cancer. *N Engl J Med*. 1999;340:430–436.
8. Dershaw DD, Yahalom J, Petrek JA. Breast carcinoma in women previously treated for Hodgkin disease: mammographic evaluation. *Radiology* 1992;184:421–423.
9. Fisher B, Costantino JP, Wickerham DL, et al. Tamoxifen for prevention of breast cancer: report of the National Surgical Adjuvant Breast and Bowel Project P-1 Study. *J Natl Cancer Inst*. 1998;90:1371–1388.
10. Orel SG, Schnall MD. MR imaging of the breast for the detection, diagnosis, and staging of breast cancer. *Radiology* 2001; 220:13–30.
11. Teifke A, Hlawatsch A, Beier T, et al. Undetected malignancies of the breast: dynamic contrast-enhanced MR imaging at 1.0 T. *Radiology* 2002;224:881–888.
12. Elmore JG, Barton MB, Moceri VM, et al. Ten year risk of false positive screening mammograms and clinical breast examinations. *N Engl J Med*. 1998;338:1089–1096.

13. Kuhl CK, Schmutzler RK, Leutner CC, et al. Breast MR imaging screening in 192 women proved or suspected to be carriers of a breast cancer susceptibility gene: preliminary results. *Radiology* 2000;215:267–279.

14. Tilanus-Linthorst MMA, Obdeijn IMM, Bartels KCM, et al. First experiences in screening women at high risk for breast cancer with MR imaging. *Breast Cancer Res Treat.* 2000;63: 53–60.

15. Lo LD, Rosen MA, Schnall MD, et al. Pilot study of breast MR screening of a high-risk cohort [abstr]. *Radiology* 2001; 221:432.

16. Warner E, Plewes DB, Shumak RS, et al. Comparison of breast magnetic resonance imaging, mammography, and ultrasound for surveillance of women at high risk for hereditary breast cancer. *J Clin Oncol.* 2001;19:3524–3531.

17. Stoutjesdijk MJ, Boetes C, Jager GJ, et al. Magnetic resonance imaging and mammography in women with a hereditary risk of breast cancer. *J Natl Cancer Inst.* 2001;93:1095–1102.

18. Podo F, Sardanelli F, Canese R, et al. The Italian multi-centre project on evaluation of MRI and other imaging modalities in early detection of breast cancer in subjects at high genetic risk. *J Exp Clin Cancer Res.* 2002;21: Suppl:115–124.

19. Morris EA, Liberman L, Ballon DJ, et al. MRI of occult breast carcinoma in a high risk population. *AJR Am J Roentgenol.* 2003;181:619–626.

20. Gail MH, Brinton LA, Byar DP, et al. Projecting individualized probabilities of developing breast cancer for white females who are being examined annually. *J Natl Cancer Inst.* 1989;81:1879–1886.

21. National Cancer Institute. Breast cancer risk assessment tool. Available at: http://bcra.nci.nih.gov/brc/. Accessed 9/1/03.

22. Claus EB, Risch N, Thompson WD. Autosomal dominant inheritance of early-onset breast cancer: implications for risk prediction. *Cancer* 1994;73:643–651.

23. Anderson DE, Badzioch MD. Risk of familial breast cancer. *Cancer* 1985;56:383–387.

24. Ottman R, Pike MC, King MC, Henderson BE. Practical guide for estimating risk for familial breast cancer. *Lancet* 1983;2:558.

25. Brekelmans CTM, Seynaeve C, Bartels CCMM, et al. Effectiveness of breast cancer surveillance in BRCA1/2 gene mutation carriers and women with high familial risk. *J Clin Oncol.* 2001;19:924–930.

26. Armstrong K, Weber BL. Breast cancer screening for high-risk women: too little, too late? *J Clin Oncol.* 2001;19: 919–920.

27. Kopans DB. Breast cancer screening with ultrasonography (commentary). *Lancet* 1999;354:2096–2097.

28. Smith RA, Saslow D, Sawyer KA, et al. American Cancer Society guidelines for breast cancer screening: update 2003. *CA Cancer J Clin.* 2003;53:141–169.

29. Jackman RJ, Marzoni FA. Needle-localized breast biopsy: why do we fail? *Radiology* 1997;204:677–684.

30. Morris EA, Liberman L, Dershaw DD, et al. Preoperative MR imaging-guided needle localization of breast lesions. *AJR Am J Roentgenol.* 2002;178:1211–1220.

31. Liberman L, Morris EA, Lee MJY, et al. Breast lesions detected by MR imaging: features and positive predictive value. *AJR AM J Roentgenol.* 2002;179:171–178.

32. Ernster V, Barclay J, Kerlikowske K, et al. Incidence of and treatment for ductal carcinoma in situ. *JAMA.* 1996;275: 913–918.

33. Betsill WL, Rosen PP, Lieberman PH, Robbins GF. Intraductal carcinoma. Long-term follow-up after treatment by biopsy alone. *JAMA.* 1978;239:1863–1867.

34. Page DL, Dupont WD, Rogers LW, Landenberger M. Intraductal carcinoma of the breast: follow-up after biopsy only. *Cancer* 1982;49:751–758.

35. Page DL, Dupont WD, Rogers LW, et al. Continued local recurrence of carcinoma 15–25 years after a diagnosis of low-grade ductal carcinoma in situ of the breast treated only by biopsy. *Cancer* 1995;76:1197–1200.

36. Hoogterbrugge N, Bult P, de Widt-Levert LM, et al. High prevalence of premalignant lesions in prophylactically removed breasts from women at hereditary risk for breast cancer. *J Clin Oncol.* 2003;21:41–45.

37. American College of Radiology (ACR). ACR BI-RADS®—Magnetic Resonance Imaging. In: ACR Breast Imaging Reporting and Data System, Breast Imaging Atlas. Reston, VA. American College of Radiology; 2003.

38. Kuhl CK, Bieling HB, Gieseke J, et al. Healthy premenopausal breast parenchyma in dynamic contrast-enhanced MR imaging of the breast: normal contrast medium enhancement and cyclical-phase dependency. *Radiology* 1997;203:137–144.

39. Orel SG, Mendonca MH, Reynolds C, et al. MR imaging of ductal carcinoma in situ. *Radiology* 1997;202:413–420.

40. Menell JH, Morris EA, Dershaw DD, et al. Determination of presence and extent of pure ductal carcinoma in situ by mammography and MR imaging. *AJR Am J Roentgenol.* 2003;180(Suppl):52–53.

41. Rodenko GN, Harms SE, Pruneda JM, et al. MR imaging in the management before surgery of lobular carcinoma of the breast: correlation with pathology. *AJR AM J Roentgenol.* 1996;167:1415–1419.

42. Weinstein SP, Orel SG, Heller R, et al. MR imaging of the breast in patients with invasive lobular carcinoma. *AJR Am J Roentgenol.* 2001;176:399–406.

43. Qayyum A, Birdwell RL, Daniel BL, et al. MR imaging features of infiltrating lobular carcinoma of the breast: histopathologic correlation. *AJR Am J Roentgenol.* 2002;178: 1227–1232.

44. Quan ML, Sclafani L, Heerdt A, et al. Magnetic resonance imaging (MRI) detects unsuspected disease in patients with invasive lobular cancer. *Ann Surg Oncol.* 2003;10:1048–1053.

45. Homer MJ. Nonpalpable mammographic abnormalities: timing the follow-up studies. *AJR Am J Roentgenol.* 1981;136: 923–926.

46. Moskowitz M. The predictive value of certain mammographic signs in screening for breast cancer. *Cancer* 1983;51: 1007–1011.

47. Homer MJ. Imaging features and management of characteristically benign and probably benign breast lesions. *Radiol Clin N Am.* 1987;25:939–951.

48. Brenner RJ, Sickles EA. Acceptability of periodic follow-up as an alternative to biopsy for mammographically detected lesions interpreted as probably benign. *Radiology* 1989;17: 645–646.

49. Wolfe JN, Buck KA, Salane M, Parekh NJ. Xeroradiography of the breast: overview of 21,057 consecutive cases. *Radiology* 1987;165:305–311.

50. Helvie MA, Pennes DR, Rebner M, Adler DD. Mammographic follow-up of low-suspicion lesions: compliance rate and diagnostic yield. *Radiology* 1991;178:155–158.

51. Sickles EA. Periodic mammographic follow-up of probably benign lesions: results of 3,184 consecutive cases. *Radiology* 1991;179:463–468.

52. Varas X, Leborgne F, Leborgne JH. Nonpalpable, probably benign lesions: role of follow-up mammography. *Radiology* 1992;184:409–414.

53. Sickles EA. Management of probably benign breast lesions. In: Jackson VP, ed. Breast *Imaging*. 33rd ed. Philadelphia: Saunders; 1995:1123–1130.

54. Vizcaino I, Gadea L, Andreo L, et al. Short-term follow-up results in 795 nonpalpable probably benign lesions detected at screening mammography. *Radiology* 2001;219: 475–483.

55. Varas X, Leborgne JH, Leborgne F, et al. Revisiting the mammographic follow-up of BI-RADS Category 3 lesions. *AJR Am J Roentgenol.* 2002;179:691–695.

56. Taplin SH, Ichikawa LE, Kerlikowske K, et al. Concordance of breast imaging reporting and data system assessments and management recommendations in screening mammography. *Radiology* 2002;222:529–535.

57. Liberman L, Morris EA, Benton CL, et al. Probably benign lesions at breast MR imaging: preliminary experience in high-risk women. *Cancer.* 2003;87:377–388.

58. Berg WA. Rationale for a trial of screening breast ultrasound: American College of Radiology Imaging Network (ACRIN) 6666. *AJR Am J Roentgenol.* 2003;180:1225–1228.

59. Gordon PB, Goldenberg SL. Malignant breast masses detected only by ultrasound: a retrospective review. *Cancer* 1995;76:626–630.

60. Kolb TM, Lichy J, Newhouse JH. Occult cancer in women with dense breasts: detection with screening US—diagnostic yield and tumor characteristics. *Radiology* 1998;207:191–199.

61. Buchberger W, DeKoekkoek-Doll P, Springer P, et al. Incidental findings on sonography of the breast: clinical significance and diagnostic workup. *AJR Am J Roentgenol.* 1999;173:921–927.

62. Buchberger W, Niehoff A, Obrist P, et al. Clinically and mammographically occult breast lesions: detection and classification with high-resolution sonography. *Semin Ultrasound CT MR.* 2000;21:325–336.

63. Kaplan SS. Clinical utility of bilateral whole-breast US in the evaluation of women with dense breast tissue. *Radiology* 2001;221:641–649.

64. Kolb TM, Lichy J, Newhouse JH. Comparison of the performance of screening mammography, physical examination, and breast US and evaluation of the factors that influence them: an analysis of 27,825 patient examinations. *Radiology* 2002;225:165–175.

65. Crystal P, Strano SD, Shcharynski S, Koretz MJ. Using sonography to screen women with mammographically dense breasts. *AJR Am J Roentgenol.* 2003;181:177–182.

66. Thurfjell EL, Lindgren JA. Population-based mammography screening in Swedish clinical practice: prevalence and incidence screening in Uppsala County. *Radiology* 1994;193: 351–357.

67. Kan L, Olivotto IA, Burhenne LJW, et al. Standardized abnormal interpretation and cancer detection ratios to assess reading volume and reader performance in a breast screening program. *Radiology* 2000;215:563–567.

68. Sohlich RE, Sickles EA, Burnside ES, Dee KE. Interpreting data from audits when screening and diagnostic mammography outcomes are combined. *AJR AM J Roentgenol.* 2002; 178:681–686.

69. Berg WA, Gilbreath PL. Multicentric and multifocal cancer: whole-breast US in preoperative evaluation. *Radiology* 2000; 214:59–66.

70. Panizza P, De Gaspari A, Vanzulli A, et al. Accuracy of post-MR imaging second-look-sonography in previously undetected breast lesions [abstract]. *Radiology* 1997;205:489.

71. Dhamanaskar KP, Muradall D, Kulkarni SR, et al. MRI directed ultrasound: a cost effective method for diagnosis and intervention in breast imaging [abstract]. *Radiology* 2002;225:653.

72. LaTrenta LR, Menell JH, Morris EA, et al. Breast lesions detected with MR imaging: utility and histopathologic importance of identification with US. *Radiology* 2003;227:856–861.

73. Ikeda DM, Hylton NM, Kinkel K, et al. Development, standardization, and testing of a lexicon for reporting contrast-enhanced breast magnetic resonance imaging studies. *J Magn Reson Imaging.* 2001;13:889–895.

74. Kanal E, Borgstede JP, Barkovich AJ, et al. American College of Radiology White Paper on MR Safety. *AJR Am J Roentgenol.* 2002;178:1335–1347.

75. Kriege M, Brekelmans CTM, Boetes C, et al. Efficacy of MRI and mammography for breast-cancer screening in women with a familial or genetic predisposition. *N Engl J Med.* 2004;351:427–437.

76. Warner E, Plewes D, Hill K, et al. Surveillance of *BRCA1* and *BRCA2* mutation carriers with magnetic resonance imaging, ultrasound, mammography, and clinical breast examination. *JAMA* 2004;292:1317–1325.

77. Robson ME, Offit K. Breast MRI for women with hereditary cancer risk. *JAMA* 2004;292:1368–1370.

78. Blue Cross Blue Shield. Magnetic resonance imaging of the breast in screening women considered to be at high genetic risk of breast cancer, December 2003. (Accessed July 9, 2004, at http://www.bluecares.com/tec/vol18/18_15.html.)

12
Assessment of Extent of Disease Using Magnetic Resonance Imaging

Laura Liberman

Accurate assessment of extent of disease is essential for planning appropriate treatment for women with breast cancer. The presence of cancer in more than one quadrant (*multicentric* disease) usually indicates the need for mastectomy rather than breast conservation. The presence of multiple sites of cancer in one quadrant (*multifocal* disease) indicates the need for wider excision and may preclude breast conservation. Involvement of the pectoral muscle, chest wall, and/or skin may indicate the need for surgical excision to include the involved areas. Finally, identification of cancer in the contralateral breast indicates the need for contralateral surgery. This chapter discusses the use of magnetic resonance imaging (MRI) in women with breast cancer to determine tumor size; detect additional sites of disease in the ipsilateral breast; assess for involvement of the pectoral muscle, chest wall, and skin; and evaluate the contralateral breast.

1. Ipsilateral Breast

1.1. Tumor Size

Breast MRI may provide more accurate assessment of tumor size than mammography or sonography. Gribbestad and colleagues[1] found excellent correlation between MRI measurement and size determined at histology for 29 patients with known breast tumors. Boetes and coworkers[2] correlated mammography, ultrasound, and MRI in 61 breast cancers. The index cancer was identified by ultrasound in 85%, by mammography in 90%, and by MRI in 98% of women. On mammogram and ultrasound images, tumor size was underestimated significantly ($P < 0.005$) by 14% and 18%, respectively, while MRI showed no significant difference in size compared with pathologic examination. In another study correlating MRI, ultrasound, and mammographic measurements with histologic measurements in 14 breast cancers, Davis and colleagues[3] found that MRI measurements had the highest correlation coef-

ficient ($r = 0.98$), compared with lower correlation coefficients for ultrasound ($r = 0.45$) and mammography ($r = 0.46$). Magnetic resonance imaging measurements also had the smallest standard error (0.34), compared with higher standard errors for ultrasound (0.78) and mammography (1.04).

Although in many cases the size assessment by MRI is more accurate than that of other imaging modalities, MRI size does not always correlate with histologic size of the cancer. Merchant and colleagues[4] performed preoperative MRI in 40 patients, including 32 with malignant tumors. Magnetic resonance imaging estimated the tumor size to be larger than mammography in 71% of cases and larger than histologic measurement in 84%. Magnetic resonance imaging would have upstaged 22% of evaluated cases from T1 to T2 and 10% of cases from T2 to T3. In spite of the high accuracy of MRI in assessing tumor size, it is important to remember that not all enhancement in the region of the tumor represents malignancy; enhancement could represent fibrosis, atypia, or other benign findings.

1.2. Additional Sites of Cancer: Pathologic Considerations

Women with one area of proven breast cancer may harbor additional sites of cancer in the ipsilateral breast.[5] Pathologic analyses of mastectomy specimens have shown sites of cancer other than the index lesion in 20% to 63%[6–13] (Table 12.1). Of these additional sites of cancer, 19% to 67% were invasive. In 20% to 47% of mastectomy specimens, additional sites of cancer were present in quadrants other than that of the index tumor. Among women who had mastectomy for ductal carcinoma in situ (DCIS), a multifocal distribution with gaps larger than 1 cm was present in 8%[14] and DCIS involved more than one quadrant in 23% to 47%[14,15]; the likelihood of cancer outside the index quadrant was higher in women with DCIS measuring 2.5 cm or larger.[8]

TABLE 12.1. Pathologic Analysis of the Ipsilateral Breast in Mastectomy Studies

Investigator	No. of Mastectomy Specimens	No. with Additional Sites of Ipsilateral Cancer (%)[a]	No. Same Quadrant (%)[b]	No. Different Quadrant (%)[b]
Qualheim[6c]	157	85 (54)	27 (17)	58 (37)
Rosen[7d]	203	65 (32)	NA	65 (32)
Lagios[8e]	84	17 (20)	NA	17 (20)
Schwartz[9f]	43	16 (37)	NA	16 (37)
Egan[10g]	116	71 (61)	NS	NS
Holland[11h]	282	177 (63)	56 (20)	121 (43)
Anastassiades[12i]	365	169 (46)	NA	169 (46)
Vaidya[13j]	30	19 (63)	5 (17)	14 (47)

Source: Adapted from Liberman et al.[5] with permission.

Abbreviations: NA, not applicable: study focused on quadrants other than index cancer; NS, not stated.

Note: Many of these pathology studies included cases of lobular carcinoma in situ (LCIS) among index lesions, additional sites of cancer, or both. Currently, LCIS is not considered cancer, but rather a risk factor for subsequent development of cancer. Therefore, in calculating proportion of mastectomies in which additional sites of cancer were found for this table, an attempt was made to remove cases in which index cancer was LCIS from denominator and cases in which additional sites were LCIS from numerator.

[a] Number of mastectomies in which cancer was found in areas other than index cancer, expressed as percent of all mastectomies.

[b] Number of mastectomies with additional sites of cancer in quadrant indicated, expressed as percent of all mastectomies.

[c] Number of cases of LCIS not stated but authors state that "The few examples of lobular carcinoma in situ appearing in this series were obviously manifestations of independency of origin."

[d] All index cancers were invasive. Number of additional sites that were LCIS was not stated. Additional sites of cancer were found in 26% (26 of 100) mastectomies with index cancers <2cm and in 38% (39/103) mastectomies with index cancers ≤2cm.

[e] Excludes one case in which index cancer was LCIS and one case in which additional site was LCIS.

[f] Excludes one case in which index cancer was LCIS and three cases in which additional sites were LCIS.

[g] Excludes one case in which index cancer was unicentric LCIS and one case in which index lesion and additional sites were LCIS.

[h] All index cancers were invasive. Number of additional sites that were LCIS was not stated. Analysis was with respect to distance from index cancer rather than quadrant: of 177 additional sites of cancer, distance from index cancer was ≤2cm in 56 and >2cm in 121.

[i] Excludes one case in which index cancer and additional sites were LCIS and 17 cases in which additional sites were LCIS.

[j] All index cancers were invasive. Includes one case in which index cancer was infiltrating lobular and additional site was LCIS.

1.3. Local Recurrences

In previous studies of women with invasive breast cancer who had breast conservation, local recurrence rates at 15-year follow up were 36% for women who did not receive radiation and 12% for women who received radiation.[16] In previous studies of women with DCIS who had breast conservation, local recurrence rates at 8-year follow up were 31% for women who did not receive radiation and 13% for women who received radiation.[17] The greater than 30% local recurrence rates in women who did not receive radiation are within the 20% to 63% range expected on the basis of the frequency of cancer at additional sites in the breast in the pathology studies.[5] That the local recurrence rates are lower in women who receive radiation therapy indicates that radiation destroys or retards growth of some of these sites of disease.

One could hypothesize that preoperative identification of additional sites of cancer may allow their removal and could lower the frequency of local recurrence. It is also possible that MRI-guided resection of these additional sites could reduce the need for postoperative radiation therapy. Further work is needed to validate these hypotheses.

1.4. Additional Sites of Cancer at Magnetic Resonance Imaging

In published studies, MRI identified additional sites of ipsilateral cancer that were not identified on mammography or physical examination in 6% to 34% of women with breast cancer[5,18–25] (Table 12.2). Additional sites of cancer in the same quadrant as the index cancer were found in 1% to 20% of women, and additional sites of cancer in different quadrants from the index cancer were found in 2% to 24% of women[5,18–25] (Table 12.2).

1.5. Magnetic Resonance Imaging of the Ipsilateral Breast at Memorial Sloan-Kettering Cancer Center

In a study of 70 women with percutaneously diagnosed breast cancer who were considering breast conservation at our hospital, MRI identified additional sites of cancer in the ipsilateral breast in 19 (27%)[5] (Figures 12.1 and 12.2). Additional sites of cancer in 19 women were infiltrating in 11 (16%) and ductal carcinoma in situ in 8 (11%) women. These additional sites of cancer were in the same quadrant

TABLE 12.2. MRI of the Ipsilateral Breast in Women with Breast Cancer

Investigator	No. of Women	No. of Women with Additional Ipsilateral MRI-Detected Cancer (%)[a]	No. of Same Quadrant (%)[b]	No. of Different Quadrant (%)[b]
Harms[18]	29[c]	10 (34)	3 (10)	7 (24)
Orel[19]	64	13 (20)	NS[d]	NS[d]
Boetes[20]	61[c]	9 (15)	8 (13)	1 (2)
Mumtaz[21]	92[c]	10 (11)	1 (1)	9 (10)
Fischer[22]	336	54 (16)	30 (9)	24 (7)
Drew[23]	178	41 (23)	15 (8)	26 (15)
Esserman[24]	58[c]	6 (10)	NS	NS
Bedrosian[25]	231	14 (6)	6 (3)	8 (3)
Liberman[5]	70	19 (27)	14 (20)	5 (7)[e]

Source: Adapted from Liberman et al.[5] with permission. *Abbreviation*: NS, not stated.

[a] Number of women with MRI-detected sites of cancer other than index lesion, as percent of all women in study.

[b] Number of women with MRI-detected sites of cancer in quadrant indicated, as percentage of all women in study.

[c] Expressed as number of breasts rather than number of women.

[d] Quadrant of additional sites of MRI-detected cancer, given for 11 of 13 women, was same as index cancer in 7 and different in 4. Among 13 women with additional sites of cancer detected at MRI, 9 were considered to have multifocal disease (defined in study as distinct at gross examination or demonstrating separate, dispersed, microscopic foci) and 4 were considered to have diffuse disease (defined in study as several lesions that were ill-defined at gross examination with large areas of dispersed intraductal and infiltrating carcinoma).

[e] Includes two women with additional MRI-detected sites of cancer in both same quadrant and different quadrant.

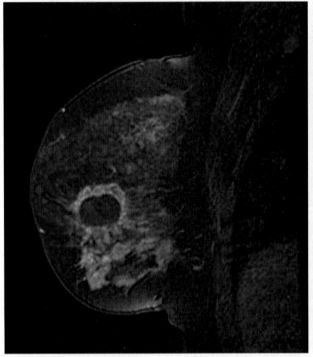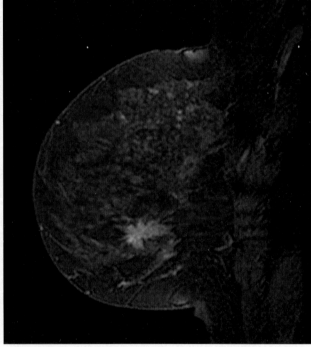

A   B

FIGURE 12.1. A 39-year-old woman 1 month status post excision of a palpable, uncalcified, spiculated mass in the right breast retroareolar region, lower inner quadrant. Surgical pathology yielded invasive ductal carcinoma, measuring 0.1–0.4cm, and DCIS, with positive margins. (A) Sagittal, T1-weighted, contrast-enhanced MRI of right breast shows 3-cm seroma right lower inner quadrant with extensive surrounding clumped enhancement, suspicious for residual disease. (B) Sagittal, T1-weighted, contrast-enhanced MRI of right breast shows separate spicu-lated, heterogeneously enhancing, 1.8-cm mass right lower outer quadrant, not seen on mammography or ultrasound. Magnetic resonance imaging guided needle localization of this mass yielded invasive ductal carcinoma, 1.7cm, and DCIS (i.e., multicentric disease). Mastectomy, performed during the same procedure, revealed residual invasive ductal carcinoma and DCIS at and extending away from the lumpectomy site. Sentinel nodes were free of tumor.

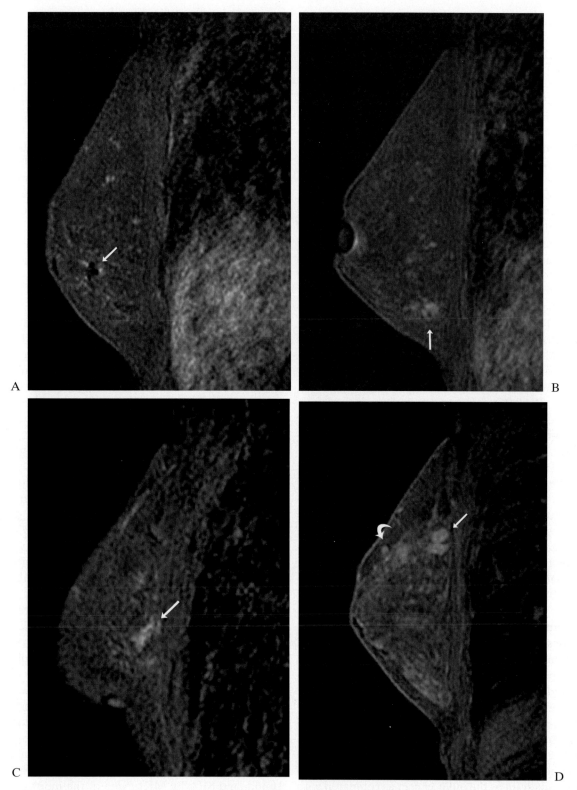

FIGURE 12.2. A 47-year-old woman who had stereotactic biopsy of a subcentimeter cluster of calcifications in the left breast 1 month previously, yielding DCIS. (A) Sagittal, contrast-enhanced, T1-weighted MRI of left breast shows stereotactic clip in the left lower inner quadrant evident as 3 mm focus of low signal intensity (arrow), with subtle surrounding clumped enhancement. (B) Sagittal, contrast-enhanced, T1-weighted MRI of left breast shows additional irregular, heterogeneously enhancing mass left breast 6:00 axis (arrow). (C) Sagittal, contrast-enhanced, T1-weighted MRI of left breast shows ductal, heterogeneous enhancement left lower outer quadrant (arrow). All three of these areas underwent MRI-guided needle localization, yielding DCIS. (D) Sagittal, contrast-enhanced, T1-weighted MRI of right (contralateral) breast shows irregularly shaped, irregularly marginated, heterogeneously enhancing mass posteriorly (straight arrow) and clumped enhancement anteriorly (curved arrow). Magnetic resonance imaging guided needle localization with bracketing wires yielded ductal carcinoma in situ, with a small focus of microinvasion at the site of the posterior lesion. The patient had bilateral mastectomies. Sentinel nodes were negative.

as the index cancer in 14 (20%) women, in a different quadrant in 3 (4%) women, and in the same and different quadrants in 2 (3%) women. In 17 (24%) women, MRI detected ipsilateral lesions that were benign. Changes caused by prior percutaneous biopsy were infrequent on MRI examination and included a clip in 12 (17%) women and small hematoma in two (3%) women. No skin thickening or skin enhancement were observed, and no needle tract could be identified. Postbiopsy change did not interfere with MRI interpretation.

The 27% frequency of finding additional sites of cancer by MRI is within the 20% to 63% range of frequencies of additional sites of cancer reported in previous pathologic analyses of mastectomy specimens (Table 12.1), as well as within the 6% to 34% range of ipsilateral MRI-detected cancers in previously published literature[5] (Table 12.2). The proportion of women in whom MRI depicted additional sites of ipsilateral cancer was higher in women with a family history of breast cancer than in women without this history (14/33 = 42% vs. 5/37 = 14%, P < 0.02), and in women in whom the index tumor was infiltrating lobular carcinoma rather than other histologies (6/11 = 55% vs. 13/70 = 19%, P < 0.06).

Among women with additional ipsilateral sites of cancer detected by MRI in the study from our hospital, approximately three fourths (74%) had additional sites only in the quadrant of the index cancer and one fourth (26%) had additional sites of cancer in other quadrants.[5] This distribution mirrors the distribution of local recurrences at 15-year follow up of women with invasive breast cancer who had breast conservation, in which 75% were found within the same quadrant as the index lesion and 25% in different quadrants.[16] In other studies of MRI, the distribution of MRI-detected additional sites of cancer has been variable, with 10% to 89% in the same quadrant as the index tumor.[5]

In our study of women with percutaneously proven cancer, biopsy was recommended for MRI-detected ipsilateral lesions in 51% of women; the positive predictive value of biopsy for these lesions was high (52%).[5] This 52% positive predictive value is within the 18% to 88% range of positive predictive values for biopsy based on MRI findings in high-risk women[26-32] and higher than the 20% to 40% range of PPVs for mammographically guided needle localization and surgical excision in the general population.[33] The positive predictive value was higher in lesions in the same quadrant as the index cancer as compared with lesions in different quadrants (18/28 = 64% vs. 5/16 = 31%, P = 0.07.)

1.6. Detection of Ductal Carcinoma In Situ in the Ipsilateral Breast

In published studies, the sensitivity of MRI in DCIS detection has ranged from 40% to 100%.[34] Recent data,

however, suggest that MRI may be more sensitive than mammography in detection of DCIS. In a retrospective study of 37 breasts in 35 women with pure DCIS who had preoperative breast MRI, Menell and colleagues[35] found that the sensitivity for DCIS detection was higher for MRI than for mammography (89% vs. 30%, P < 0.001). Magnetic resonance imaging was the only study to find DCIS in 24 (65%) breasts; in 2 (5%) breasts, DCIS was found only with mammography. Magnetic resonance imaging detection of additional sites of DCIS, if confirmed by biopsy, may assist in treatment planning (Figure 12.2).

1.7. Ultrasound Versus Magnetic Resonance Imaging to Detect Additional Disease in the Ipsilateral Breast

Breast ultrasound can detect additional ipsilateral disease in women with breast cancer,[2,36-39] but breast MRI may be more sensitive in this regard. Boetes and colleagues[2] compared accuracy of MRI, mammography, and ultrasound in 61 cancers in 60 women undergoing mastectomy for cancer. They found that mammography depicted 31% of additional invasive cancers, while ultrasound showed showed 38% and MRI showed 100%.

Berg and colleagues[38] compared mammography, ultrasound, and MRI in 77 women with recently diagnosed breast cancer. Pathologic examination yielded 110 foci of cancer, of which 89 were invasive and 21 were DCIS. Of 89 foci of invasive cancer, mammography depicted 56 (63%), ultrasound 85 (96%), and MRI 84 (94%). Of 21 foci of DCIS, mammography depicted 14 (67%), ultrasound 13 (62%), and MRI 15 (71%). Either MRI or ultrasound depicted additional mammographically occult malignant foci in approximately one third of women with breast cancer. Size and extent of tumor was more accurately depicted with MRI than ultrasound, with 12% of patients undergoing more extensive surgery on the basis of MRI even after combined ultrasound, mammography, and clinical breast examination.

Hlawatsch and colleagues[39] compared whole breast ultrasound and MRI as adjuncts to mammography in 101 women with breast cancer. Twenty-seven tumors showed multifocal or multicentric invasive cancer at pathology. Of these 27, 48% were correctly diagnosed by mammography alone, 63% by a combination of mammography and ultrasound, and 81% by MRI. Nine of the index cancers were not seen at mammography but were visible at ultrasound. Use of ultrasound benefited 13 women and yielded false-positive studies in 2. Use of MRI benefited seven women and produced false-positive studies in eight.

Data regarding extent of disease assessment in the ipsilateral breast should be interpreted in conjunction with other published data comparing breast ultrasound and MRI. Studies of high-risk women who were screened with mammography, ultrasound, and MRI reported sensitivities of 86% to 100% for MRI versus 33% to 43% for ultrasound.[26,29] Magnetic resonance imaging is more sensitive than ultrasound in the detection of DCIS.[36] The 18% to 88% positive predictive value (PPV) of biopsy in studies of MRI screening[26–32] is significantly higher than the 7% to 14% PPV of biopsy in studies of screening breast ultrasound.[26,40–42]

Both ultrasound and MRI may detect additional sites of ipsilateral cancer, potentially impacting on treatment. Magnetic resonance imaging has the advantage of higher sensitivity, particularly for detecting DCIS. Breast ultrasound has the advantages of speed, lower cost, wider availability, and ready access for biopsy procedures. Both examinations have the disadvantage of false-positive results, with the proportion of false-positives depending on operator experience and technique. Further study comparing MRI and ultrasound in assessment of extent of disease would be helpful. At our institution if the decision is made to supplement mammography with another imaging test to assess extent of disease, we generally start with MRI; if suspicious lesions are identified on MRI, we often perform directed ultrasound examination to determine if there is an ultrasound correlate that would be amenable to ultrasound-guided biopsy.

1.8. Involvement of Pectoral Muscle, Chest Wall, and Skin

Masses that are posterior in location can be difficult to evaluate with mammograms and physical examination.[43] Involvement of the pectoral muscle may require specific surgical treatment, such as excision of a portion of the muscle if the tumor superficially invades it, radical mastectomy if the tumor involves the full thickness of the muscle, or chest wall resection for a tumor that extends to involve chest wall (ribs, intercostal muscles, serratus anterior muscle).[44] Preoperative knowledge of involvement of pectoral muscle and/or chest wall therefore impacts on treatment planning.

Breast MRI may be useful in assessing involvement of the pectoral muscle and chest wall. Morris and colleagues[43] reported 19 patients with posterior breast masses who had preoperative breast MRI. Enhancing masses were identified at breast MRI in all 19 patients. Five (26%) had masses that abutted the muscles, with obliteration of the fat plane and muscle enhancement. All five had muscle involvement at surgery. In the remaining 14 (74%) patients, no enhancement of muscle was seen; none of these had invasion of the muscle at surgery. The authors concluded that extension of tumor into underlying muscle or chest wall was indicated by abnormal enhancement within these deep structures (Figure 12.3); violation of the fat plane without other findings did not indicate muscle or chest wall involvement.[43]

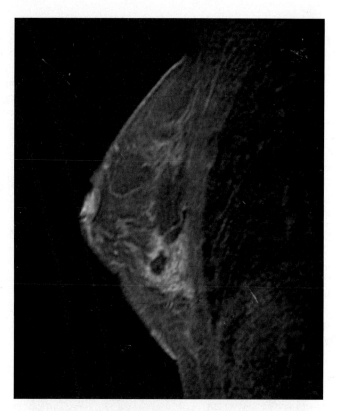

FIGURE 12.3. A 39-year-old woman with palpable, mammographically evident mass left lower inner quadrant, for which core biopsy yielded invasive ductal carcinoma and ductal carcinoma in situ. Sagittal, contrast-enhanced, T1-weighted MRI of the left breast shows an irregularly shaped, irregularly marginated, heterogeneously enhancing mass in the left lower inner quadrant corresponding to the palpable cancer. Enhancement extends into the chest wall, consistent with chest wall invasion.

Skin involvement can also be assessed with breast MRI (Figure 12.4). The identification of skin enhancement may help to identify a site for biopsy, may guide the surgeon toward excision to include the suspect area, and may serve as a baseline for follow up after treatment for locally advanced breast cancer.[44] Inflammatory carcinoma is characterized by tumor involvement of the dermal lymphatics and produces skin induration. In inflammatory carcinoma, MRI may show focal or diffuse enhancement of the thickened skin, a pattern similar to that of mastitis[44] (Figure 12.5). Rieber and colleagues[45] reported skin thickening that was bright on T2-weighted images and medium intensity on T1-weighted images in 90% of patients with inflammatory carcinoma versus 55% of patients with mastitis. Further study is needed to define the sensitivity and specificity of breast MRI in the assessment of skin involvement.

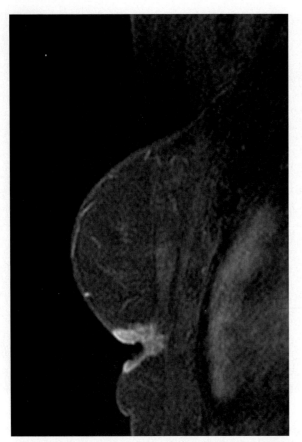

FIGURE 12.4. A 65-year-old woman with palpable lump breast mass lower inner quadrant, for which core biopsy yielded invasive ductal carcinoma. Sagittal, contrast-enhanced, T1-weighted MRI of the left breast shows minimally spiculated, irregular, heterogeneously enhancing mass left lower inner quadrant, corresponding to biopsy proven cancer. Contiguous with the lesion is thickening and irregular, heterogeneous, mass enhancement involving the overlying skin. The mass abuts the pectoral muscle, but there is no enhancement in the muscle; therefore, no evidence of pectoral invasion. Mastectomy, performed after chemotherapy, revealed invasive ductal carcinoma and DCIS. Invasive cancer involved the skin dermis by direct extension. No pectoral muscle involvement was found at surgery.

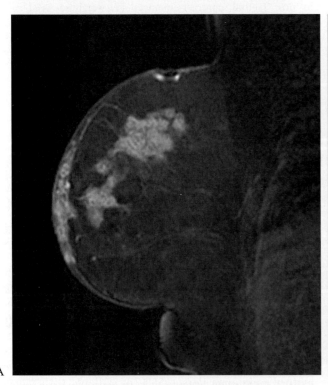

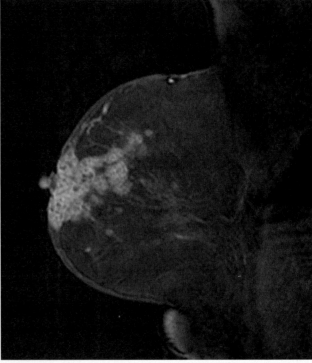

A   B

FIGURE 12.5. A 59-year-old woman who presented with inflammatory right breast cancer. (A) Sagittal, post-contrast, T1-weighted MRI of the medial right breast shows multiple conglomerate heterogeneously enhancing masses, as well as nodular enhancement in the skin. (B) Sagittal, post-contrast, T1-weighted MRI of the right breast at the plane of the nipple shows extensive heterogeneous mass enhancement within the breast, with heterogeneous nodular enhancement involving the nipple. Mastectomy, performed after chemotherapy, yielded invasive ductal carcinoma, histologic and nuclear grade III, measuring 0.1 to 3.5 cm, and DCIS. Skin and dermal lymphatics were involved with invasive cancer. No tumor was found in the axillary nodes.

2. Contralateral Breast

2.1. Synchronous Bilateral Breast Cancer

For women with breast cancer, the contralateral breast is at high risk. A synchronous contralateral cancer, variably defined as occurring within 3 months, 6 months, or 1 year after diagnosis of the index cancer, is found by mammography, physical examination, or both in approximately 2% of women with breast cancer. Women with synchronous bilateral breast cancer are more likely to have a genetic predisposition to breast cancer, multicentric disease in the index cancer, and a trend toward decreased local control and overall survival.[46]

2.2. Metachronous Contralateral Cancer

For women with unilateral breast cancer, a subsequent (metachronous) contralateral cancer develops in 0.5% to 1.0% per year, with a cumulative risk of 15%. Sixteen percent of metachronous contralateral cancers metastasize and 7% are fatal. Management options for the asymptomatic contralateral breast have included close observation, blind contralateral biopsy, chemoprevention, and prophylactic mastectomy.[46]

2.3. Magnetic Resonance Imaging Detection of Contralateral Cancer

In published reports of women with breast cancer, MRI detected an otherwise occult cancer in the contralateral breast in 3% to 24%[22,46–50] (Table 12.3; Figures 12.6 and 12.7). These results should be interpreted in the context of high-risk screening MRI investigations, in which MRI identified a cancer occult to mammography and physical examination in 2% to 7%.[26–32]

2.4. Magnetic Resonance Imaging of the Contralateral Breast at Memorial Sloan-Kettering Cancer Center

Among 223 women with breast cancer who had contralateral breast MRI at our institution, contralateral breast biopsy was recommended in 72 (32%) women and performed in 61 women.[46] Cancer occult to mammography and physical examination was detected by MRI in 12 women, constituting 20% (12 of 61) women who had contralateral biopsy and 5% (12 of 223) women who had contralateral breast MRI. Among these 12 cancers, 6 (50%) were DCIS and 6 (50%) were invasive cancer (median size, 0.5cm; range, 0.1–1.0cm). Contralateral biopsy revealed

TABLE 12.3. MRI of the Contralateral Breast in Women with Breast Cancer

Investigator	No. of Women	No. of Biopsies (%)[a]	PPV of Biopsy (%)[b]	No. MRI-only Cancer (%)[c]
Rieber[47]	34	NS	NS	3/34 (9)
Fischer[22]	336	NS	NS	15/363 (4)
Kuhl[48]	710[d]	91 (13)	45/91 (49)	45/710 (6)
Slanetz[49]	17	5 (29)[e]	4/5 (80)[e]	4/17 (24)
Liberman[46]	223	72 (32)	12/61 (20)	12/223 (5)
Lee[50]	182	15 (8)	7/15 (47)	6/182 (3)[f]

Source: Adapted from Liberman et al.[46] with permission. *Abbreviations*: PPV, positive predictive value; NS, not stated.

[a] Refers to number of women in whom contralateral biopsy was recommended.

[b] Refers to number of women in whom contralateral biopsy showed cancer divided by number of women who had contralateral biopsy.

[c] Refers to number of women with mammographically occult, nonpalpable cancers detected by MRI divided by number of women in study.

[d] Includes women with synchronous and prior cancer in contralateral breast.

[e] Ten contralateral lesions were identified in five women; nine lesions in four women were malignant.

[f] One additional cancer (invasive ductal carcinoma and DCIS) was identified on mammography performed after MRI.

benign (n = 31) or high-risk (n = 18) lesions in 49 women, constituting 80% (49 of 61) women who had contralateral biopsy and in 22% (49 of 223) women who had contralateral MRI.

Magnetic resonance imaging depicted an otherwise unsuspected contralateral cancer in 5% of women with breast cancer in our study. A contralateral cancer was more often found in women with rather than without a family history of breast cancer in a first-degree relative (13% vs. 3%, $P = 0.02$) and in women whose index tumor was invasive lobular cancer rather than other histologies (13% vs. 4%, $P < 0.07$). The frequency of identifying a contralateral cancer was higher in postmenopausal as compared with premenopausal women, but this difference did not achieve statistical significance (9% vs. 3%, $P = 0.13$). No significant difference was observed in the frequency of finding contralateral cancer as a function of mammographic parenchymal density, but most (87%) women had either heterogeneously dense or dense breasts.

The 5% frequency of detecting contralateral breast cancer by MRI in our study does not differ significantly ($P = 0.12$) from the 3% (26 of 871) prevalence of cancer at blind contralateral upper outer quadrant surgical biopsy reported by Cody.[51] However, all of the patients in Cody's study had contralateral breast biopsy[51]; in our study, MRI enabled diagnosis of these contralateral cancers while only requiring biopsy in one third (32%) of women.

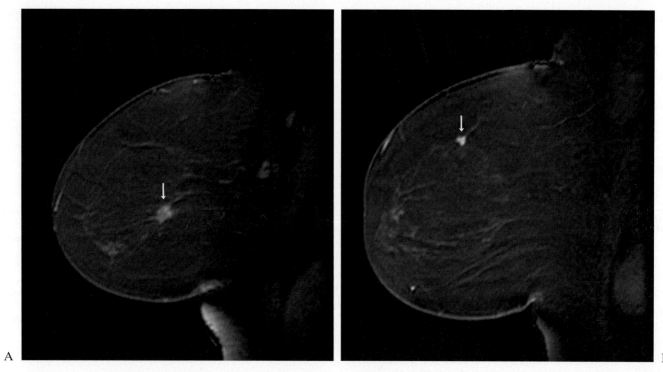

FIGURE 12.6. A 74-year-old woman with mammographic and sonographically evident right breast mass, for which ultrasound-guided core biopsy yielded invasive lobular carcinoma. (A) Sagittal, T1-weighted, contrast-enhanced MRI of the right breast shows irregular, spiculated, heterogeneously enhancing 1-cm mass in the right lower outer quadrant, corresponding to the biopsy-proven cancer. (B) Sagittal, T1-weighted, contrast-enhanced MRI of the left breast shows lobulated, minimally irregular, mildly heterogeneously enhancing mass left upper outer quadrant, without mammographic or sonographic correlate. Magnetic resonance imaging guided needle localization yielded invasive ductal carcinoma, 0.6 cm.

In our study, cancer was found in 20% of women who had contralateral breast biopsy based on MRI findings.[46] This positive predictive value is lower than the 47% to 80% range of positive predictive values previously reported for biopsy based on MRI findings in the contralateral breast in women with known breast cancer[48–50] and on the low end of the 18% to 64% range of positive predictive values reported for biopsy based on MRI findings in women at high risk for developing breast cancer.[26–30] The 20% positive predictive value is also at the low end of

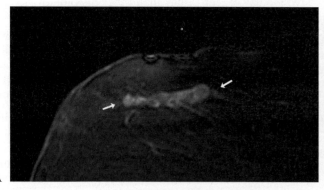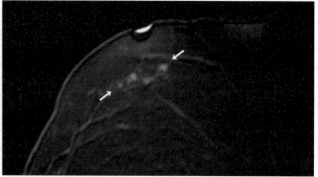

FIGURE 12.7. A 61-year-old woman 5 years status post excision of DCIS from the right breast, with abnormal right mammogram showing dilated duct. Ultrasound-guided core biopsy yielded invasive ductal carcinoma and DCIS. (A) Collimated photograph of sagittal, contrast-enhanced, T1-weighted MRI of the right breast shows heterogeneous ductal enhancement spanning 4.6 cm in right upper outer quadrant (arrows), corresponding to biopsy-proven cancer. (B) Collimated photograph of sagittal, contrast-enhanced, T1-weighted MRI of the left (contralateral) breast shows clumped ductal enhancement spanning 2.8 cm (arrows). Magnetic resonance imaging guided needle localization yielded invasive ductal carcinoma measuring 0.3 cm and DCIS.

the 20% to 40% range of positive predictive values for mammographically guided needle localization and surgical excision in the general population.[33]

Our data suggest a potentially disturbing consequence of MRI of the contralateral breast. Prophylactic contralateral mastectomy was performed in 5% of our women. The frequency of prophylactic mastectomy was higher in women in whom a biopsy was recommended based on MRI findings than among women who were not referred for biopsy, although this difference did not achieve statistical significance (9% vs. 3%, $P = 0.11$). Identification of an abnormality on MRI may have contributed to the decision to perform prophylactic contralateral mastectomy. Prophylactic mastectomy can be a rational choice, but women and their physicians should be aware of the limited specificity of MRI to make an informed decision[52]: In our practice, 80% of breast biopsies for MRI-detected contralateral lesions were benign.

3. Invasive Lobular Cancer

Invasive lobular cancer accounts for approximately 10% to 14% of invasive breast carcinomas.[53] The mammogram is more often falsely negative in invasive lobular than in invasive ductal cancer, due to the tendency of the cells to grow in a single file arrangement, usually without calcification.[54] Invasive lobular cancer also may have a higher frequency of multicentricity and bilaterality than invasive ductal cancer.[53] Breast MRI may be particularly helpful in assessing extent of disease in women with invasive lobular cancer (Figure 12.8).

Rodenko and colleagues[55] correlated MRI and mammography with pathology in the ipsilateral breast in 20 women with invasive lobular cancer. Correlation between imaging and pathologic extent of disease was 85% for breast MRI versus 32% for mammography ($P < 0.0001$). Interobserver agreement regarding lesion morphology and extent of disease was higher for MRI (91% and 100%, respectively) than for mammography (64% and 91%, respectively). Magnetic resonance imaging correctly classified all nine pathologically confirmed multicentric cases (100%) and overestimated 2 of 11 unicentric cases (18%). In comparison, mammography incorrectly classified all seven pathologically confirmed multicentric cases as unicentric disease; one woman classified as having multicentric disease by mammography had unicentric disease at pathology.[55]

Weinstein and colleagues[56] reviewed MRI and pathology findings in the ipsilateral breast in 32 women with invasive lobular cancer. Overall, MRI showed more extensive tumor than conventional imaging and impacted on clinical management in half (16 of 32) of the women. Among 18 women who did not have excisional biopsy before MRI, MRI was equal to mammography and sonography in predicting extent of disease in 10 (56%) and superior to mammography and sonography in 8 (44%). Patterns of invasive lobular cancer on MRI in these 18 women were spiculated or irregular mass (n = 10), regional or multifocal contrast enhancement (n = 7), or regional enhancement and architectural distortion (n = 1).

Qayyum and colleagues[57] reviewed MRI findings in 13 women with invasive lobular cancer. They reported three patterns: a solitary mass with irregular margins (n = 4), correlating with the same pattern at pathologic analysis; multiple lesions, either connected by enhancing strands (n = 6) or separated by nonenhancing intervening tissue (n = 2), that correlated with the pathologic appearance of noncontiguous tumor foci, with malignant cells in single-file arrangement; and enhancing septa (n = 1), correlated at pathology with tumor cells streaming in breast stroma. Comparison of MRI findings with mammography and sonography was not provided in this study.

Yeh and colleagues[58] reviewed the preoperative MRI findings of 19 women with invasive lobular cancer and found focal heterogeneously enhancing mass in 8 (42%) cases, regional enhancement in 5 (26%), and other patterns in 6 (32%), including segmental enhancement (n = 1), segmental enhancement with multiple small nodules (n = 1), a mixture of focal mass and regional enhancement (n = 1), diffuse enhancement (n = 1), multiple small nodules (n = 1), and bilateral disease (n = 1). Among eight focal masses, shape was irregular in seven and round in one; margins were ill-defined in six and spiculated in two. The extraction flow (EF) product, a quantitative measure of gadolinium uptake over time, was assessed in 15 cases. In these 15 invasive lobular cancers, peak EFs ranged from 25 to 120 (with normal tissue threshold EF level 25 or less); most tumors had EFs in the 30s. Four cases had multifocal disease and one had unsuspected contralateral disease detected by MRI.

Quan and colleagues[59] evaluated the impact of breast MRI on surgical management in 62 women with invasive lobular carcinoma at our institution. Among 51 women who had ipsilateral breast MRI, biopsy was recommended in 19 (37%) and yielded a cancer separate from the index lesion in 11 women, constituting 58% (11 of 19) women who had ipsilateral biopsy and 22% (11 of 51) women who had ipsilateral breast MRI. Histology of these 11 ipsilateral cancers was invasive lobular in 10 and DCIS in 1. Among 53 women who had contralateral breast MRI, biopsy was recommended in 20 (38%) and led to detection of cancer in 5 women, constituting 25% (5 of 20) women who had contralateral biopsy and 9% (5 of 53) women who had contralateral breast MRI. Of the five contralateral cancers, three were invasive (ductal in two and lobular in one) and two were DCIS.

These studies show the variable MRI patterns of invasive lobular cancer and indicate that breast MRI has a high likelihood of detecting more than one site of cancer in

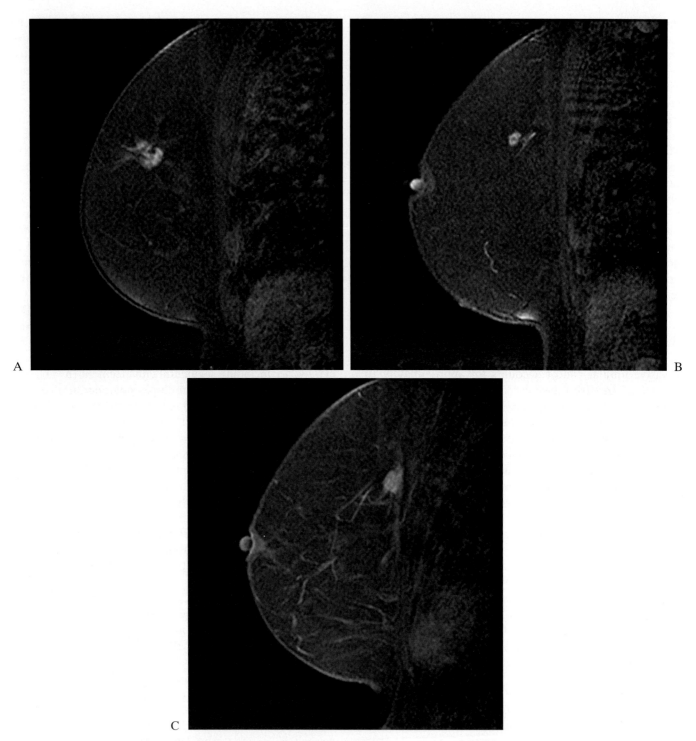

FIGURE 12.8. A 60-year-old woman with palpable right breast mass, for which core biopsy yielded invasive lobular carcinoma. (A) Sagittal, contrast-enhanced, T1-weighted MRI of right breast shows irregular, spiculated, heterogeneously enhancing 2.4-cm mass in the 12:00 axis corresponding to biopsy-proven invasive lobular cancer. (B) Sagittal, contrast-enhanced, T1-weighted MRI of the right (ipsilateral) breast more laterally shows lobulated, minimally irregular, heterogeneously enhancing 0.8-cm mass right breast upper outer quadrant, just anterior to a vessel. Magnetic resonance imaging guided needle localization of this mass showed infiltrating lobular carcinoma, metastatic to an intra-mammary lymph node. (C) Sagittal, contrast-enhanced, T1-weighted MRI of the left (contralateral) breast shows irregularly shaped, irregularly marginated, heterogeneously enhancing mass in the 12:00 axis abutting the pectoral muscle, not seen on mammography or ultrasound. Magnetic resonance imaging guided needle localization yielded multifocal invasive mammary carcinoma with mixed ductal and lobular features, 1.0 cm at maximal diameter, and lobular carcinoma in situ.

women with invasive lobular cancer. The frequency of recommending biopsy and the likelihood of detecting cancer are higher in the ipsilateral breast than in the contralateral breast. Even in women with invasive lobular cancer, a substantial proportion of biopsies based on MRI findings prove to be benign. Therefore, we do not recommend mastectomy based on MRI findings; if a woman with cancer desires breast conservation, and MRI depicts additional suspicious areas, biopsy is necessary.

4. Conclusion

Accurate assessment of extent of disease is necessary to plan optimal surgical treatment for women with breast cancer. Magnetic resonance imaging can detect breast cancer that is not palpable and not evident at mammography or ultrasound and may provide more accurate assessment of tumor size than these other modalities. In studies of women with breast cancer who had breast MRI for assessment of extent of disease, MRI detected an otherwise unsuspected cancer in the ipsilateral breast in 6% to 34% of women and in the contralateral breast in 3% to 24%. Magnetic resonance imaging can also assess for involvement of the pectoral muscle, chest wall, and skin, information that affects surgical planning. The American College of Radiology states that indications for breast MRI include (but are not limited to) assessment for extent of disease in women with infiltrating cancer, evaluation of the contralateral breast in women with breast cancer, and defining the relationship of a breast cancer to the pectoral muscle or chest wall.[60] Magnetic resonance imaging for extent of disease assessment may be most valuable for women with a strong family history of breast cancer and invasive lobular histology in the index cancer.

Although MRI can detect additional sites of cancer in women with proven breast cancer, a few caveats should be remembered. No data address the impact of MRI detection of additional sites of breast cancer on survival. Furthermore, the benefit of detecting these additional sites of cancer must be weighed against the added time, expense, and consequences of MRI and downstream examinations. Breast MRI may benefit from new sequences that allow rapid, high-resolution, simultaneous imaging of both breasts. Further work, including refinement of criteria and methods for performing of biopsy for MRI-detected lesions, analysis of cost effectiveness, and long-term follow up, is necessary to optimize the use of MRI for assessment of extent of disease in women with breast cancer.

References

1. Gribbestad IS, Nilsen G, Fiosene H, et al. Contrast-enhanced magnetic resonance imaging of the breast. *Oncologica* 1992; 31:833–842.
2. Boetes C, Mus RDM, Holland R, et al. Breast tumors: comparative accuracy of MR imaging relative to mammography and US for demonstrating extent. *Radiology* 1995;197: 743–737.
3. Davis PL, Staiger MJ, Harris KB, et al. Breast cancer measurements with magnetic resonance imaging, ultrasonography, and mammography. *Breast Cancer Res Treat.* 1996;37: 1–9.
4. Merchant TE, Obertop H, de Graaf PW. Advantages of magnetic resonance imaging in breast surgery treatment planning. *Breast Cancer Res Treat.* 1993;25:257–264.
5. Liberman L, Morris EA, Dershaw DD, et al. MR imaging of the ipsilateral breast in women with percutaneously proven breast cancer. *AJR Am J Roentgenol.* 2003;180:901–910.
6. Qualheim RE, Gall EA. Breast carcinoma with multiple sites of origin. *Cancer* 1957;10:460–408.
7. Rosen PP, Fracchia AA, Urban JA, et al. "Residual" mammary carcinoma following simulated partial mastectomy. *Cancer* 1975;35:739–747.
8. Lagios MD. Multicentricity of breast carcinoma demonstrated by routine correlated serial subgross and radiographic examination. *Cancer* 1977;40:1726–1734.
9. Schwartz GF, Patchefsky AS, Feig SA, et al. Multicentricity of non-palpable breast cancer. *Cancer* 1980;45:2916.
10. Egan RL. Multicentric breast carcinomas: clinical-radiolographic-pathologic whole organ studies and 10-year survival. *Cancer* 1982;49:1123–1130.
11. Holland R, Veling SH, Mravunac M, Hendriks JH. Histologic multifocality of Tis, T1-2 breast carcinomas: implications for clinical trials of breast-conserving surgery. *Cancer* 1985;56: 979–990.
12. Anastassiades O, Iakovou E, Stavridou N, et al. Multicentricity in breast cancer. A study of 366 cases. *Am J Clin Pathol.* 1993;99:238–243.
13. Vaidya J, Vyas J, Chinoy R, et al. Multicentricity of breast cancer: whole-organ analysis and clinical implications. *Br J Cancer* 1996;74:820–824.
14. Faverly DRG, Burgers L, Bult P, Holland R. Three-dimensional imaging of mammary ductal carcinoma in situ: clinical implications. *Semin Diagn Pathol.* 1994;11:193–198.
15. Holland R, Hendriks JH, Verbeek AL, et al. Extent, distribution, and mammographic/histological correlations of breast ductal carcinoma in situ. *Lancet* 1990;335:519–522.
16. Fisher ER, Anderson S, Tan-Chiu E, et al. Fifteen-year prognostic discriminants for invasive breast carcinoma: National Surgical Adjuvant Breast and Bowel Project Protocol-06. *Cancer* 2001;91:1679–1687.
17. Fisher ER, Dignam J, Tan-Chiu E, et al. Pathologic findings from the National Surgical Adjuvant Breast Project (NSABP) eight-year update of Protocol B-17: intraductal carcinoma. *Cancer* 1999;86:429–438.
18. Harms SE, Flamig DP, Hesley KL, et al. MR imaging of the breast with rotating delivery of excitation off resonance: clinical experience with pathologic correlation. *Radiology* 1993;187.493–501.
19. Orel SG, Schnall MD, Powell CM, et al. Staging of suspected breast cancer: effect of MR imaging and MR-guided biopsy. *Radiology* 1995;196:115–122.
20. Boetes C, Mus RDM, Holland R, et al. Breast tumors: comparative accuracy of MR imaging relative to mammography

and US for demonstrating extent. *Radiology* 1995;197: 743–747.

21. Mumtaz H, Hall-Craggs MA, Davidson T, et al. Staging of symptomatic primary breast cancer with MR imaging. *AJR Am J Roentgenol.* 1997;169:417–424.

22. Fischer U, Kopka L, Grabbe E. Breast carcinoma: effect of preoperative contrast-enhanced MR imaging on the therapeutic approach. *Radiology* 1999;213:881–888.

23. Drew P, Chatterjee S, Turnbull L, et al. Dynamic contrast-enhanced magnetic resonance imaging of the breast is superior to triple assessment for the pre-operative detection of multifocal breast cancer. *Ann Surg Oncol.* 1999;5: 599–603.

24. Esserman L, Hylton NM, Yassa L, et al. Utility of magnetic resonance imaging in the management of breast cancer: evidence for improved preoperative staging. *J Clin Oncol.* 1999;17:110–119.

25. Bedrosian I, Schlencker J, Spitz FR, et al. Magnetic resonance imaging-guided biopsy of mammographically and clinically occult breast lesions. *Ann Surg Oncol.* 2002;9:457–461.

26. Kuhl CK, Schmutzler RK, Leutner CC, et al. Breast MR imaging screening in 192 women proved or suspected to be carriers of a breast cancer susceptibility gene: preliminary results. *Radiology* 2000;215:267–279.

27. Tilanus-Linthorst MMA, Obdeijn IMM, Bartels KCM, et al. First experiences in screening women at high risk for breast cancer with MR imaging. *Breast Cancer Res Treat.* 2000;63: 53–60.

28. Lo LD, Rosen MA, Schnall MD, et al. Pilot study of breast MR screening of a high-risk cohort. *Radiology* 2001; 221:432.

29. Warner E, Plewes DB, Shumak RS, et al. Comparison of breast magnetic resonance imaging, mammography, and ultrasound for surveillance of women at high risk for hereditary breast cancer. *J Clin Oncol.* 2001;19:3524–3531.

30. Stoutjesdijk MJ, Boetes C, Jager GJ, et al. Magnetic resonance imaging and mammography in women with a hereditary risk of breast cancer. *J Natl Cancer Inst.* 2001;93:1095–1102.

31. Sardanelli F, Trecate G, Morassut S, et al. Gd-enhanced MR screening in women at genetic high risk of breast cancer: preliminary results of a prospective non-randomized multicenter trial [abstract]. *Radiology* 2002;225:326.

32. Morris EA, Liberman L, Ballon DJ, et al. MRI of occult breast carcinoma in a high risk population. *AJR Am J Roentgenol.* 2003;181:619–626.

33. Jackman RJ, Marzoni FA. Needle-localized breast biopsy: why do we fail? *Radiology* 1997;204:677–684.

34. Orel SG, Mendonca MH, Reynolds C, et al. MR imaging of ductal carcinoma in situ. *Radiology* 1997;202:413–420.

35. Menell JH, Morris EA, Dershaw DD, et al. Determination of presence and extent of pure ductal carcinoma in situ by mammography and MR imaging [abstract]. *AJR Am J Roentgenol.* 2003;180(Suppl):52–53.

36. Berg WA, Gilbreath PL. Multicentric and multifocal cancer: whole-breast US in preoperative evaluation. *Radiology* 2000; 214:59–66.

37. Kolb TM, Lichy J, Newhouse JH. The impact of bilateral whole breast ultrasound in women with dense breasts and recently diagnosed breast cancer [abstr]. *Radiology* 2000;217: 318.

38. Berg WA, Nguyen TK, Gutierrez L, Segers A. Local extent of disease: preoperative evaluation of the breast cancer patient with mammography, ultrasound, and MRI [abstr]. *Radiology* 2001;221:230.

39. Hlawatsch A, Teifke A, Schmidt M, Thelen M. Preoperative assessment of breast cancer: sonography versus MR imaging. *AJR Am J Roentgenol.* 2002;179:1493–1501.

40. Kolb TM, Lichy J, Newhouse JH. Occult cancer in women with dense breasts: detection with screening US–diagnostic yield and tumor characteristics. *Radiology* 1998; 207:191–199.

41. Buchberger W, DeKoekkoek-Doll P, Springer P, et al. Incidental findings on sonography of the breast: clinical significance and diagnostic workup. *AJR Am J Roentgenol.* 1999;173:921–927.

42. Kaplan SS. Clinical utility of bilateral whole-breast US in the evaluation of women with dense breast tissue. *Radiology* 2001;221:641–649.

43. Morris EA, Schwartz LH, Drotman MB, et al. Evaluation of pectoralis major muscle in patients with posterior breast tumors on breast MRI: early experience. *Radiology* 2000;214: 67–72.

44. Morris EA. Cancer staging with breast MR imaging. In: Schnall MD, Orel SG, eds. *Breast MR Imaging.* Philadelphia: Saunders; 2001:333–344.

45. Rieber A, Tomczak RJ, Mergo PJ, et al. MRI of the breast in the differential diagnosis of mastitis versus inflammatory carcinoma and follow-up. *J Comput Assist Tomogr.* 1997;21: 128–132.

46. Liberman L, Morris EA, Kim CM, et al. MR imaging findings in the contralateral breast in women with recently diagnosed breast cancer. *AJR Am J Roentgenol.* 2003;180: 333–341.

47. Rieber A, Tomczak R, Merkle E, et al. MRI of histologically confirmed mammary carcinoma: clinical relevance of diagnostic procedures for detection of multifocal or contralateral secondary carcinoma [abstract]. *AJR Am J Roentgenol.* 1998; 170(Suppl):48–49.

48. Kuhl CK, Schmiedel A, Morakkabati N, et al. Breast MR imaging of the asymptomatic contralateral breast in the work-up or follow-up of patients with unilateral breast cancer [abstract]. *Radiology* 2000;217:268.

49. Slanetz PJ, Edmister WB, Yeh ED, et al. Occult contralateral breast carcinoma incidentally detected by breast magnetic resonance imaging. *Breast J.* 2002;8:145–148.

50. Lee SG, Orel SG, Woo IJ, et al. MR imaging screening of the contralateral breast in patients with newly diagnosed breast cancer: preliminary results. *Radiology* 2003;226: 773–778.

51. Cody HS. Routine contralateral breast biopsy: helpful or irrelevant? *Ann Surg.* 1997;225:370–376.

52. Montgomery LL, Tran KN, Heelan MC, et al. Issues of regret in women with contralateral prophylactic mastectomies. *Ann Surg Oncol.* 1999;6:546–552.

53. Rosen PP. Invasive lobular carcinoma. In: Rosen PP, ed. *Rosen's Breast Pathology.* Philadelphia: Lippincott-Raven; 1997:545–565.

54. Dershaw DD. False negative mammograms. *Contemp Diagn Radiol.* 1995;18:1–5.

55. Rodenko GN, Harms SE, Pruneda JM, et al. MR imaging in the management before surgery of lobular carcinoma of the breast: correlation with pathology. *AJR Am J Roentgenol.* 1996;167:1415–1419.

56. Weinstein SP, Orel SG, Heller R, et al. MR imaging of the breast in patients with invasive lobular carcinoma. *AJR Am J Roentgenol.* 2001;176:399–406.

57. Qayyum A, Birdwell RL, Daniel BL, et al. MR imaging features of infiltrating lobular carcinoma of the breast: histopathologic correlation. *AJR Am J Roentgenol.* 2002;178: 1227–1232.

58. Yeh ED, Slanetz PJ, Edmister WB, et al. Invasive lobular carcinoma: spectrum of enhancement and morphology on magnetic resonance imaging. *Breast J.* 2003;9:13–8.

59. Quan ML, Sclafani L, Heerdt A, et al. Magnetic resonance imaging detects unsuspected disease in patients with invasive lobular cancer. *Ann Surg Oncol.* 2003;10:1048–1053.

60. American College of Radiology. ACR practice guideline for the performance of magnetic imaging (MRI) of the breast. In: Practice Guidelines and Technical Standards 2004. Reston, VA: American College of Radiology, 2004:269–274.

13
Assessment of Residual Disease

Elizabeth A. Morris

Breast-conserving therapy followed by radiation therapy and chemotherapy is the treatment of choice for early stage breast carcinoma. Negative margin status has become a prerequisite for breast conservation therapy, recognizing that positive margins impact negatively on local recurrence rates. Residual disease following initial attempt at breast conservation is estimated to be between up to 70%.[1] Even with accurate preoperative needle localization, the negative margin rate is high because there is often incomplete knowledge of the true extent of the tumor before the operation, despite our best attempts with physical examination, magnification mammography, and ultrasound. Gwin and colleagues[2] demonstrated that 45% of women undergoing re-excision had residual tumor and that the majority (62%) had residual invasive carcinoma. This is the basis for re-excision in the patient with questionable or inadequate margin status.

Re-excision or mastectomy is performed when initial margins of resection are positive or close for tumor. The extent of margin positivity correlates with risk of residual tumor and recurrent disease. Schnitt and colleagues[3] noted the relationship between microscopic margins of resection and the risk of local recurrence in patients with breast cancer treated with breast-conserving surgery and radiation therapy. No recurrences were found at a minimum of 5-year follow up in patients with negative margins, 4% recurrence rate with close margins (<1mm), 6% recurrence with focally positive margins (≥3 high power fields), and 21% with more than focally positive margins. Additional factors such as young patient age and extensive intraductal component (EIC) have been associated with a higher risk of recurrence.[4] Further, when initial margins are positive, younger women have been shown in one series to be more likely to have residual tumor at re-excision despite radiation therapy.[5,6]

It is known in the pathology literature that unifocal carcinoma diagnosed on mammography and clinical examination can have residual disease following surgery not only at the lumpectomy site but also in a separate quadrant.

Holland and colleagues[7] have examined mastectomy specimens for clinically and mammographically suspected unifocal disease and found that 37% of women have no additional disease, 20% have disease within 2cm of the lumpectomy site, 43% had disease greater than 2cm away from the lumpectomy site, and 7% had disease greater than 4cm away from the lumpectomy site. Difficult histologies, such as invasive lobular carcinoma and EIC tumors, are notoriously difficult to predict tumor extent and are more likely to have associated positive margins (Figure 13.1). But unsuspected residual disease can occur with all breast cancer histologies (Figure 13.2).

1. The Preoperative Work-Up

The traditional work-up of suspect lesions involves mammography and ultrasound, even though there is compelling data in some specific cases that MRI may add significant information (Figure 13.3). The preoperative extent of disease is better assessed with magnetic resonance imaging (MRI) than with conventional imaging such as mammography and ultrasound in multiple studies.[8] This is particularly true with specific tumor histology of invasive lobular carcinoma[9] but also applies to invasive ductal carcinoma, which is much more prevalent. In addition to invasive carcinomas, there is emerging data that MRI may also better stage patients who are diagnosed preoperatively with pre-invasive ductal carcinoma in situ (DCIS)[10] (Figure 13.4).

2. Relationship Between Residual and Recurrent Disease

Residual disease following lumpectomy is not the same as recurrence. However, there is a distinct relationship between these two entities. Residual carcinoma is suspected when the initial attempt at surgical resection is incomplete (Figure 13.5). Pathologic analysis of the

FIGURE 13.1. Residual invasive lobular carcinoma (thin arrow) posterior to the lumpectomy site (thick arrow). This and all following examinations are performed several weeks following initial lumpectomy. Images are performed on a 1.5 Tesla (T) system using a fat-suppressed three-dimensional (3D) fast spoiled gradient echo (FSPGR) sequence in the sagittal plane unless otherwise indicated.

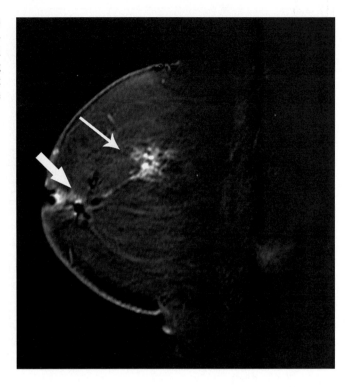

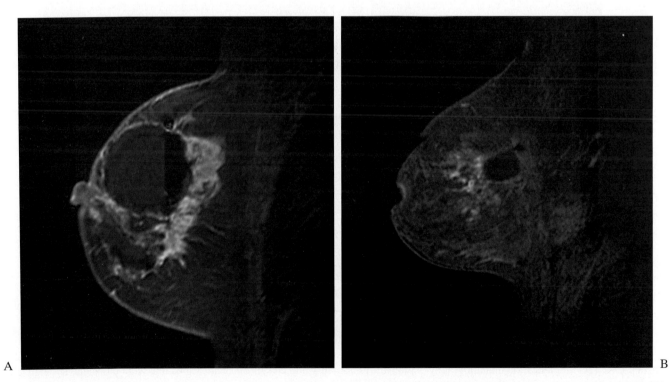

A   B

FIGURE 13.2. Two patients with positive margins. (A) Residual invasive ductal carcinoma posterior to the seroma cavity. (B) Residual DCIS anterior to the seroma cavity.

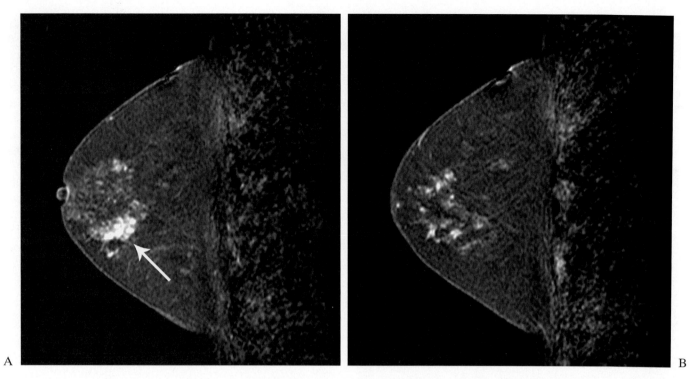

FIGURE 13.3. (A) Biopsy proven invasive ductal carcinoma (arrow) was identified on mammography but is much larger on MRI (arrow). (B) What was not appreciated on mammography was the extensive intraductal component (EIC) seen on this image.

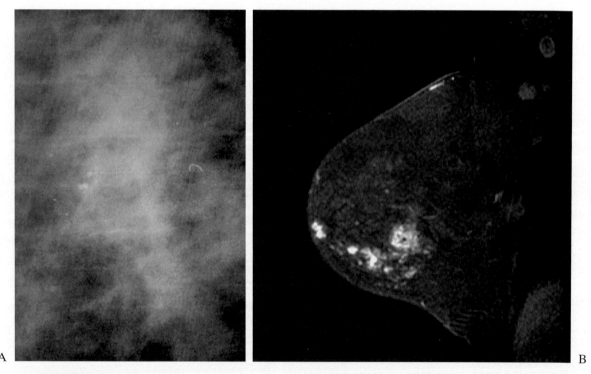

FIGURE 13.4. (A) Magnification mammography demonstrates a small 4-mm cluster of calcifications that were biopsied yielding DCIS. (B) Preoperative staging MRI demonstrates more extensive DCIS involving an entire segment.

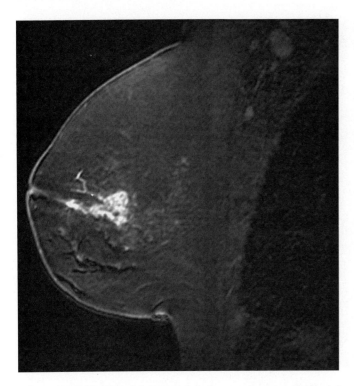

FIGURE 13.5. Residual invasive lobular carcinoma adjacent to seroma cavity (not shown).

lumpectomy specimen and the inked surgical margins may indicate that the carcinoma is at or close to the margins of resection. Specimen radiography is useful to determine lesion retrieval.[11] If the initial carcinoma contained calcification, then magnification mammography can be performed to assess whether residual suspicious calcifications are remaining.[12] If present, these can be localized under mammographic guidance, which, it is to be hoped, can direct the surgeon to area of residual disease. Problems arise if the original tumor did not contain calcifications. Radiographically, the ability to detect residual masses at the lumpectomy site is limited as postoperative distortion obscures evaluation for residual masses.[13] (Figure 13.6). Additionally, if the in situ component is not associated with calcifications, then assessment of residual disease is very limited (Figure 13.7). In these cases the surgeon usually returns to the operating room and blindly excises the edge of the lumpectomy cavity.

There is strong emerging evidence that breast MRI can offer important information regarding the presence of residual carcinoma[14] (Figure 13.8), particularly in difficult histologies such as invasive lobular carcinoma and carcinomas associated with an extensive intraductal component (Figure 13.9). Additionally, in patients with difficult-to-evaluate dense breasts there may be a role for MRI following resection with positive or close margins (Figure 13.10). Carcinomas without associated calcifications may also benefit from the use of MRI if margins are close or positive (Figure 13.11).

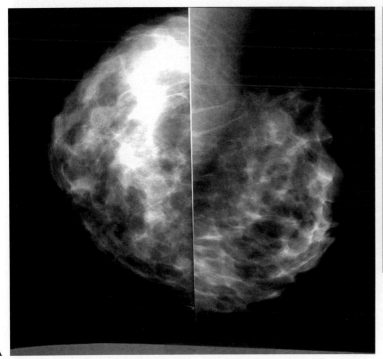

A

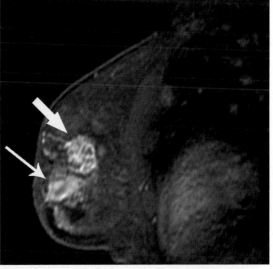

B

FIGURE 13.6. (A) Postoperative mammogram limited due to breast density and distortion; no suspicious findings are identified. (B) MRI demonstrated seroma cavity (thin arrow) and large residual mass posterior to the seroma cavity (thick arrow) that represented residual invasive ductal carcinoma.

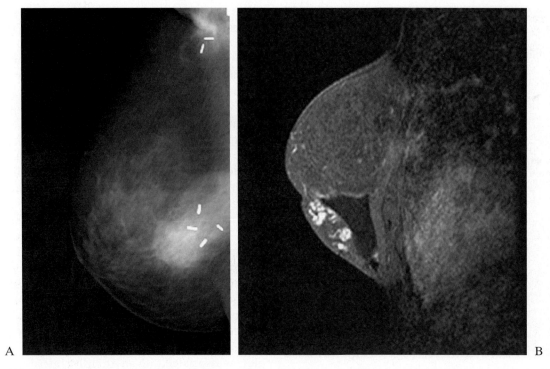

FIGURE 13.7. (A) Postoperative mammography performed for positive margins in a patient with invasive ductal carcinoma and associated DCIS. The original tumor had no associated calcifica- tions. Posterior biopsy cavity identified associated with clips. (B) Postoperative MRI demonstrated residual foci of uncalcified DCIS surrounding the biopsy cavity.

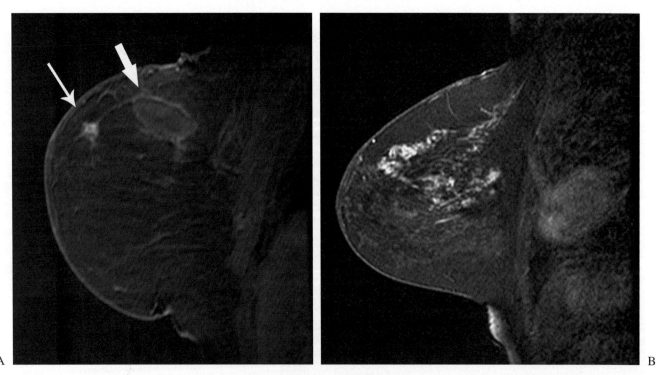

FIGURE 13.8. (A) Residual invasive ductal carcinoma (thin arrow) in same quadrant as lumpectomy site (thick arrow). Patient was treated with needle localization and re-excision with ultimately negative margins. (B) Residual DCIS in multiple quadrants from the lumpectomy site (not shown) necessitating mastectomy.

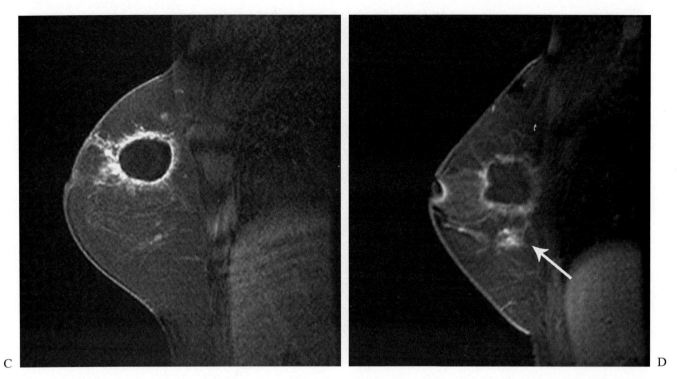

C

D

FIGURE 13.8. (*Continued*) (C) Invasive lobular carcinoma with positive margins. Nodular enhancement along the anterior seroma cavity represented residual invasive disease. Contrast this to thin enhancement along the posterior cavity where no residual disease found at surgery. Note that MRI cannot diagnose residual microscopic disease as the granulation tissue at the margin will enhance. (D) Residual invasive ductal carcinoma (arrow) in the same quadrant (multifocal) as the initial lumpectomy. Although the patient had positive margins, no residual disease was found at the lumpectomy site (seen with thin rim enhancement). Patient received breast conservation.

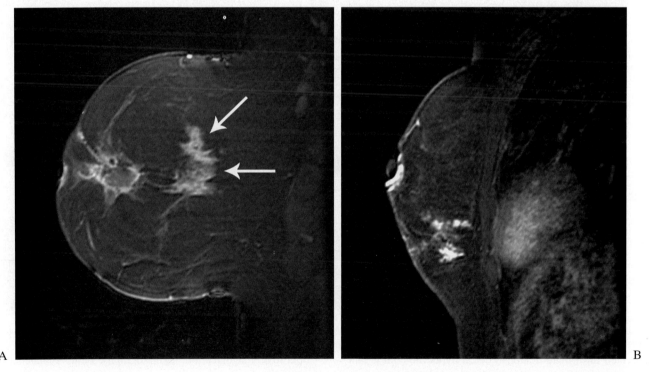

A

B

FIGURE 13.9. (A) Residual invasive lobular carcinoma (arrows) posterior to seroma cavity. (B) Residual DCIS in a patient with EIC (lumpectomy site not imaged on this section).

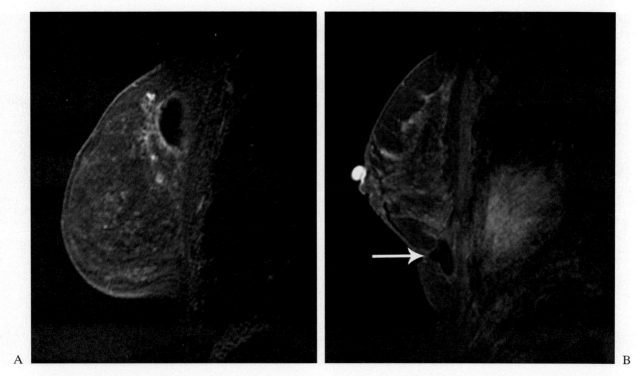

A   B

FIGURE 13.10. (A) Clumped enhancement anterior to the lumpectomy site in the upper outer quadrant in a patient with extremely dense breasts represents residual DCIS. (B) Post-operative seroma (arrow) in a heterogeneously dense breast does not disclose any suspicious abnormalities. At re-excision no residual disease was found.

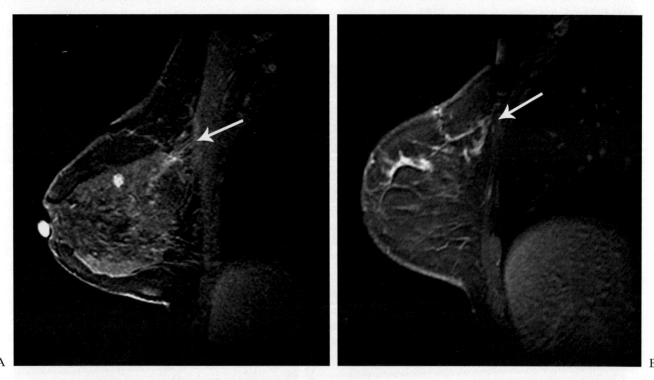

A   B

FIGURE 13.11. (A) Residual mass in same quadrant as lumpectomy (arrow) performed for DCIS with positive margins. Directed ultrasound demonstrated a hypoechoic mass that was biopsied percutaneously yielding invasive ductal carcinoma. The patient elected to undergo mastectomy. (B) Residual linear clumped enhancement represented residual DCIS anterior to the lumpectomy site (arrow). No calcifications were noted on post-operative magnification mammography. Note enhancing scar extending from skin to site of surgery.

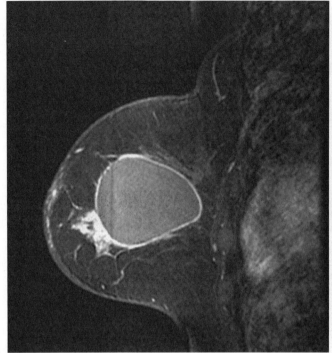

A   B

FIGURE 13.12. (A) Bulky residual disease anterior to the lumpectomy site. (B) Postoperative seroma without evidence of bulky disease. Margins enhance irregularly though uniformly. On the basis of the MRI findings, small microscopic disease cannot be excluded.

The role of MRI in the case of close or positive margins is to evaluate for the presence of bulky residual disease (Figure 13.12). Residual microscopic disease at the surgical margin will not be well evaluated with MRI; however, this is likely not the role of MRI in the immediate postoperative patient (Figure 13.13). Uniformly, if the patient has close or positive margins the surgeon will re-excise the seroma cavity margin. Microscopic residual disease will usually be successfully excised with the re-excision, regardless of the imaging results. The role of MRI, therefore, is in the assessment of bulky residual disease at the margin of resection that can direct the surgeon to a particular margin and the assessment of residual disease distant from the lumpectomy site that would indicate the patient be best served by mastectomy (Figure 13.14).

Recurrence occurs in a treated breast following lumpectomy (with negative margins) and usually chemotherapy and radiation therapy (Figure 13.15). It occurs after treatment has been initiated or terminated and is thought to be either due to undetected tumor that was not adequately treated at the time of detection of the index tumor or due to de novo development of cancer. Recurrence may develop despite the presence of negative margins at the time of surgery and despite the administration of whole breast radiation. The undetected carcinoma that causes recurrence likely is residual multifocal or multicentric tumor that is not detected by means of conventional imaging at the time of diagnosis. Rates of recurrence vary and are increased in patients with positive margins, in young patients, and in tumors with an extensive intraductal component.

The clinical experience with recurrence occurred in the days before the use of breast MRI for preoperative staging. There is some hope that by using preoperative breast MRI the incidence of recurrence can be decreased. Breast MRI has been shown to detect 13% to 33% more disease preoperatively than mammography.[15–17] Therefore, it would be assumed that breast MRI in the preoperative setting is detecting some of the undetected yet present tumor at the time of surgery that is unsuspected by the treating physicians. However, a discrepancy arises, as the recurrence rate (1%–2% per year) is not identical to the undetected disease rate shown with MRI (13%–33%). This is likely due to the fact that the chemotherapy and/or radiation therapy directed to the breast are extremely efficacious and that some, if not the majority, of this residual disease is successfully treated. At this writing, disease that is susceptible to treatment by additional therapy such as

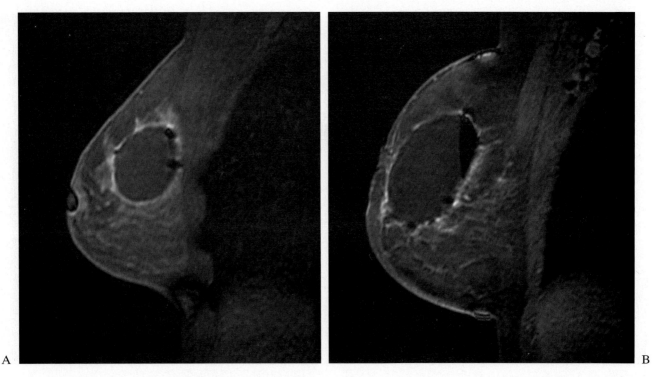

FIGURE 13.13. (A) Postoperative seroma demonstrates clip artifact and thin enhancement around the cavity due to granulation
tissue. No nodules or masses or asymmetric areas of enhancement are identified to suggest residual disease. Pathologically, no
residual was found on re-excision. (B) False-negative MRI. Postoperative seroma with tiny focus (2 mm) of DCIS at re-excision.
Small foci of residual disease may not be seen with MRI. A negative MRI does not preclude re-excision.

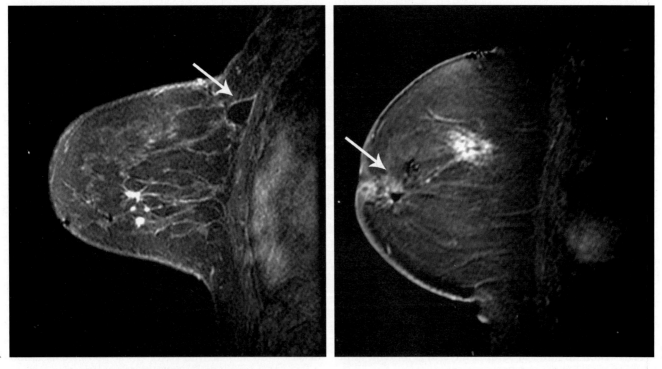

FIGURE 13.14. (A) Additional clumped enhancement representing DCIS in a separate quadrant from the lumpectomy site
(arrow). Patient received mastectomy. (B) Several months following lumpectomy patient presents for radiation. Surgery performed for mammographic calcifications elsewhere yielded DCIS
with close margins. Magnetic resonance imaging performed to
evaluate adequate excision. Lumpectomy site is demonstrated by
clips (arrow). Note the postoperative seroma has resolved. An
irregular heterogeneously enhancing mass is seen posteriorly in
the breast and was biopsied yielding invasive ductal carcinoma.
The patient subsequently received mastectomy.

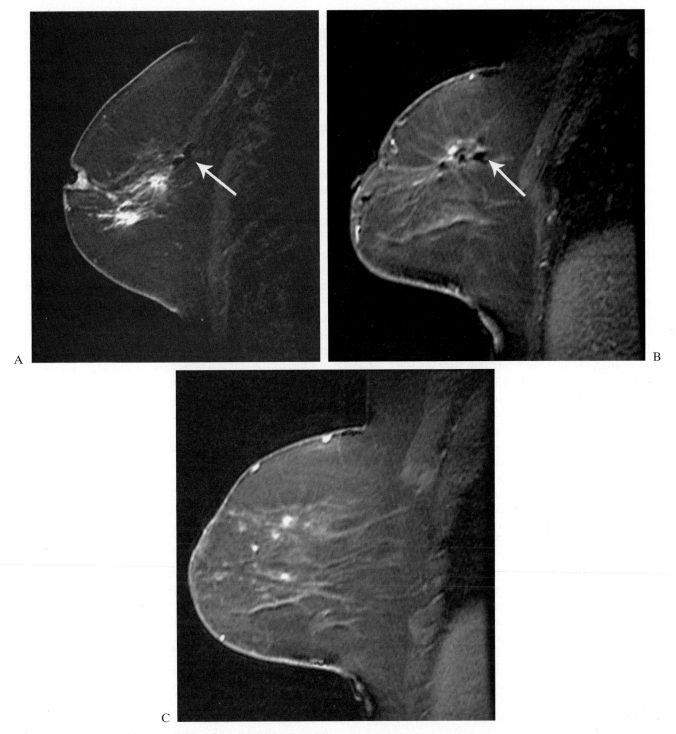

FIGURE 13.15. One year following breast-conserving therapy for invasive ductal carcinoma followed by chemotherapy and radiation, a patient presents with fullness at her lumpectomy site. Mammography was unrevealing and on ultrasound there was a suggestion of a mass. Magnetic resonance imaging performed to evaluate for possible recurrence. (A) On MRI the lumpectomy site is marked by clips causing artifact (arrow). In the breast there are two irregular heterogeneously enhancing masses that represent recurrence. (B) MRI perfomed in a patient as a baseline following treatment with chemotherapy and radiation therapy. Margins were negative. Lumpectomy site demonstrates clip artifact (arrow) and associated clumped enhancement as well as (C) additional small masses in a separate quadrant, all of which represented DCIS with invasion. The patient underwent mastectomy.

chemotherapy and radiation therapy is unable to be differentiated from disease that is resistant to treatment. It may be useful in the future to use MRI to identify those patients in whom adjuvant radiation may not be helpful as the course of radiation is not without associated morbidity, not to mention cost and time savings.

3. Pathology Issues

Breast cancer growth is not always predictable and not always in the same pattern. Certain histologies have classic growth patterns, but in general all breast histologies can demonstrate overlapping appearances, particularly on MRI. Similarly, overlapping kinetic parameters are also seen. However, preoperative MRI may give an indication whether the tumor is truly unifocal, multifocal, or multicentric. In general, invasive ductal carcinomas generally present as a mass and can be entirely removed at surgery. However, if the tumor is associated with satellite lesions representing multifocal disease or if it is associated with an extensive intraductal component, then the likelihood of positive margins increases significantly. Invasive lobular carcinomas are notoriously difficult to detect and have a specific characteristic growth pattern of single file growth, allowing the tumor to attain a large overall size without amassing great cellular density so that even large tumors in fatty or mildly dense breasts are difficult to perceive. Ductal carcinoma in situ is perhaps the easier of all to detect because it can manifest as calcifications and can be detected on mammography. The problem arises that not all DCIS is calcified and even significant grades of DCIS may not produce necrosis and, therefore, calcifications may be absent and the tumor may evade detection on the mammogram. Use of preoperative MRI in these patients may also significantly impact the presence of residual DCIS.

When localizing nonpalpable lesions for surgical removal, it is known that despite efforts to bracket lesions and add additional wires under mammographic or ultrasound guidance, the chance for complete surgical removal is not altered and the chance of obtaining negative margins is not increased.[18] Therefore, despite our best attempts at defining tumor extent with conventional imaging, we are not always successful. It remains to be seen whether localization under MRI can achieve an improved negative margin rate.

4. Postoperative Work–Up

Mammographic assessment is currently the gold standard for preoperative assessment of disease extent and for the postoperative assessment of residual disease and has been discussed previously. Coned magnification views are helpful in detecting additional suspicious calcifications before surgery to plan for adequate excision and are useful for detecting residual calcifications after surgery. The presence of residual calcifications regardless of morphology is highly predictive of residual disease.[12] Residual masses, suspicious for residual invasive carcinoma, however, are much less well assessed on mammography, as there has been a surgical procedure in the area with a postoperative hematoma/seroma that can easily obscure a residual mass.

Ultrasound assessment after surgery is not helpful for calcifications and therefore residual DCIS is not reliably detected. However, assessment by ultrasound may be valuable if there is a high suspicion for a residual mass and may be a follow-up test if the mammogram result is negative. Additionally, there is some evidence that postoperative ultrasound may be extremely helpful in assessing residual masses away from the lumpectomy site.[19]

Out of the modalities discussed so far, MRI has the clear advantage in the detection of residual disease following initial attempt at lumpectomy when close or positive margins are found. By virtue of the fact that MRI uses intravenous contrast and assesses areas of vascularity, significant residual disease can be reliably assessed.

One of the areas where MRI is not particularly helpful is directly at the margin of resection where there is normal granulation tissue that enhances due to the increased angiogenesis. Therefore, the strength of MRI is not at the margin of lumpectomy site for small microscopic disease. Magnetic resonance imaging is good at suggesting asymmetric residual bulky disease directly at the lumpectomy site. Magnetic resonance imaging is best used in the detection of residual disease at a distance from the lumpectomy site that was not suspected preoperatively.

5. Magnetic Resonance Imaging Experience

Orel and colleagues[20] evaluated postoperative patients with MRI to assess for residual disease and found a positive predictive value (PPV) of 82% and negative predictive value (NPV) of 61%. False-positive enhancement at the biopsy site was seen. In a study conducted by Hwang and colleagues[10] with 51 patients diagnosed with DCIS, it was found that MRI had an accuracy of 88% in predicting residual disease, 82% in predicting invasive disease, and 90% at predicting multicentricity. From this study the detection of additional disease that impacts on the patient's management (multicentricity) was the strength of MRI. A prior study from the same institution investigated the optimal timing between surgery and the performance of MRI.[14] Based on the analysis of 68 patients at varying days following surgery, it was found that the best time to image was approximately 1 month following surgery. Although it is very likely that the false-negative areas of enhancement are less the longer one waits after initial surgery, the trade-off is prolonging definitive surgical treatment for the patient. It is doubtful that most patients will elect to wait for the MRI for a modest benefit in PPV and NPV.

In a study at Memorial Sloan-Kettering Cancer Center (MSKCC), we evaluated 100 patients with positive or close margins following initial attempt at breast conservation. All patients were potential candidates for breast conservation before MRI. Lesions on MRI were classified as multicentric (different quadrant than operative site), multifocal (same quadrant, >2cm away from operative site), and unifocal (within 2cm of operative site). All patients underwent definitive surgery. Fifty-eight patients had residual disease at surgery: 20 multicentric, 15 multifocal, and 23 unifocal. Magnetic resonance imaging identified 18 of 20 (90%) cases of multicentric, 14 of 15 (93%) cases of multifocal, and 18 of 23 (78%) cases of unifocal residual disease. There were 13 false-positive findings, including 5 cases of high-risk lesions [lobular carcinoma in situ (LCIS), atypia], 6 suspicious lesions at the lumpectomy site, and 2 lesions elsewhere in the breast. Eight false-negative findings included two cases of multicentric DCIS occult to MRI and six cases of residual disease (four invasive and two microscopic DCIS) immediately at or near the lumpectomy site. Overall PPV was 82% and NPV was 84%. Magnetic resonance imaging was most successful at identifying unsuspected multicentric and multifocal disease.

6. Goals of Breast Cancer Treatment

Clearly, the goal in breast cancer treatment is the surgical removal of all foci of carcinoma. In addition to surgical removal, traditional treatment involves the administration of whole breast radiation and boost radiation to the lumpectomy site in the thought that there are undetected residual islands of tumor that have not been removed surgically and can benefit from treatment by external beam radiation. With improvements in the ability to detect these previously unknown sites of additional carcinoma, modifications in the algorithm of treatment following successful lumpectomy may be feasible.

7. Treatment Issues

Residual disease and recurrence are related. Residual disease that is untreated may eventually manifest itself as a recurrence, either early (within the first 2 years) or late (following 2 years). One of the issues is that some residual disease is treated by radiation therapy that is currently routinely given and/or adjunctive chemotherapy. Radiation therapy treats a significant portion of residual disease, but not all. The disease that is not treated presents as recurrence. It is currently not known which disease can be safely left behind in the breast following surgery as it will be treated adequately by radiation and which disease will not. Therefore, at this time it is surgically necessary to remove all detected tumor.

As MRI detects more tumor than what we have been able to detect with conventional imaging, there has been much more extensive surgery in the efforts to remove all tumor. Some critics have suggested that the extra surgery may be unnecessary. The question can be turned around and posed whether radiation therapy is necessary in all cases. It may be that there is a role for careful MRI monitoring in the patient with complete MRI excision of a tumor and no appreciable undetected disease. These patients may be able to forego radiation therapy. Additionally, careful MRI evaluation may be able to better identify those patients who may benefit from radiation and those who may need more extensive surgery based on size of residual tumor. Faverly and colleagues[21] have estimated that approximately 50% of invasive ductal carcinomas are of limited extent and may be treated well with limited resection and may not need additional radiation therapy. Magnetic resonance imaging may be helpful in identifying those patients.

8. Conclusion

For the sometime perplexing problem of positive margins, MRI can be a suitable alternative to blind re-excision. The results can direct appropriate surgery so that the entire carcinoma extent can be excised. Alternatively, the results may indicate which patients would be better served with mastectomy rather than breast conservation. As MRI may identify benign disease, patients should not be recommended for mastectomy without histologic proof of additional disease. The real benefit of MRI in patients with close or positive margins is not to evaluate the immediate postoperative margin for microscopic residual disease, as the surgeon is planning on re-excision regardless of the MRI result. Rather, the benefit lies in the detection of bulky additional disease or disease entirely separate from the lumpectomy site. As MRI is used more and more preoperatively to stage patients, the issue of residual disease following initial attempt at lumpectomy may be less of a problem in the future than is currently found in clinical practice.

References

1. Jardines L, Fowble B, Schultz D, et al. Factors associated with a positive reexcision after excisional biopsy for invasive breast cancer. *Surgery* 1995;118:803–809.

2. Gwin JL, Eisenberg BL, Hoffman JP, et al. Incidence of gross and microscopic carcinoma in specimens from patients with breast cancer after re-excision lumpectomy. *Ann Surg.* 1993; 218:729–734.

3. Schnitt SJ, Abner A, Gelman R, et al. The relationship between microscopic margins of resection and the risk of local recurrence in patients with breast cancer treated with breast-conserving surgery and radiation therapy. *Cancer* 1994;74:1746–1751.

4. Kini VR, Vincini FA, Frazier R, et al. Mammographic, pathologic and treatment-related factors associated with local recurrence in patients with early-stage breast cancer treated with breast conserving therapy. *Int J Radiat Oncol Biol Phys.* 1999;43:341–346.

5. Neuschatz AC, DiPetrillo T, Safaii H, et al. Long-term follow-up of a prospective policy of margin-directed radiation dose escalation in breast-conserving therapy. *Cancer* 2003;97: 30–39.

6. Wazer DE, Schmidt-Ullrich RK, Ruthazer, et al. The influence of age and extensive intraductal component histology upon breast lumpectomy margin assessment as a predictor of residual tumor. *Int J Radiat Oncol Biol Phys.* 1999;45: 885–891.

7. Holland R, Veling SH, Mravunac M, Hendriks JH. Histologic multifocality of Tis, T1-2 breast carcinomas. Implications for clinical trials of breast-conserving surgery. *Cancer* 1985;56: 979–990.

8. Berg WA. Imaging the local extent of disease. *Semin Breast Dis.* 2001;4:153–173.

9. Quan ML, Sclafani L, Heerdt AS, et al. Magnetic resonance imaging detects unsuspected disease in patients with invasive lobular cancer. *Ann Surg Oncol.* 2003;10:1048–1053.

10. Hwang ES, Kinkel K, Esserman LJ, et al. Magnetic resonance imaging in patients diagnosed with ductal carcinoma-in-situ: Value in the diagnosis of residual disease, occult invasion and multicentricity. *Ann Surg Oncol.* 2003;10:381–388.

11. Lee C, Carter D. Detecting residual tumor after excisional biopsy of impalpable breast carcinoma: efficacy of comparing preoperative mammograms with radiographs of the biopsy specimen. *AJR Am J Roentgenol.* 1995;164:81–85.

12. Gluck BS, Dershaw DD, Liberman L, Deutch BM. Micro-calcifications on postoperative mammograms as an indicator of adequacy of tumor excision. *Radiology* 1993;188:469–472.

13. Dershaw DD. Mammography in patients with breast cancer treated by breast conservation (lumpectomy with or without radiation). *AJR Am J Roentgenol.* 1995;164:309–316.

14. Frei K, Kinkel K, Bonel HM, et al. MR imaging of the breast in patients with positive margins after lumpectomy: influence of the time interval between lumpectomy and MR imaging. *AJR Am J Roentgenol.* 2000;175:1577–1584.

15. Harms SE, Flamig DP, Hesley KL, et al. MR imaging of the breast with rotating delivery of excitation off resonance: clinical experience with pathologic correlation. *Radiology* 1993;187:493–501.

16. Orel SG, Schnall MD, Powell CM, et al. Staging of suspected breast cancer: effect of MR imaging and MR-guided biopsy. *Radiology* 1995;196:115–122.

17. Fischer U, Kopka L, Grabbe E. Breast carcinoma: effect of preoperative contrast-enhanced MR imaging on the therapeutic approach. *Radiology* 1999;213:881–888.

18. Liberman L, Kaplan J, Van Zee KJ, et al. Bracketing wires for preoperative breast needle localization. *AJR Am J Roentgenol.* 2001;177:565–572.

19. Berg WA. Rationale for a trial of screening breast ultrasound: American College of Radiology Imaging Network (ACRIN) 6666. *AJR Am J Roentgenol.* 2003;180:1225–1228.

20. Orel SG, Reynolds C, Schnall MD, et al. Breast carcinoma: MR imaging before re-excisional biopsy. *Radiology* 1997;205: 429–436.

21. Faverly DR, Hendriks JH, Holland R. Breast carcinomas of limited extent: frequency, radiologic-pathologic characteristics, and surgical margin requirements. *Cancer* 2001; 91: 647–59.

14
Posttherapeutic Magnetic Resonance Imaging

Jennifer B. Kaplan and D. David Dershaw

In addition to its usefulness in evaluating the breast for the diagnosis and staging of breast cancer, magnetic resonance imaging (MRI) can be useful in examining the breast after treatment. Specifically, MRI can be used to monitor the effects of preoperative (neoadjuvant) chemotherapy. It is also useful in assessing breasts after conservation therapy, including lumpectomy and radiation. Information that is important for treatment planning can be obtained about the activity and extent of breast carcinoma using MRI. Therefore, it can be a useful addition to mammography, physical examination, and sonography for these clinical situations.

1. Neoadjuvant Therapy

Physicians are increasingly using multimodality treatments for locally advanced breast cancer, including inflammatory carcinoma. These regimens include preoperative chemotherapy, followed by surgery, postoperative chemotherapy, and possibly radiation therapy. Neoadjuvant therapy is used to shrink or eliminate the tumor, and tumor regression from that therapy correlates with successful cancer treatment.

Monitoring the effects of neoadjuvant therapy is important to assess effectiveness of chemotherapy after initial doses, thereby determining if a specific treatment should be continued, and to evaluate the extent of disease within the breast after chemotherapy to decide on the extent of surgery required for successful tumor excision. While clinical examination, mammography, and ultrasound are of some utility, studies have found that each of them can lead to incorrect conclusions. Data suggest that MRI is a more effective means to monitor the results of neoadjuvant therapy than these traditional techniques.

Patients with extensive tumor within the breast typically do poorly. It has been difficult to achieve locoregional control using either radiation therapy or surgery alone; 5-year survival rates are less than 10% with single therapies,

while patients with combined surgery and radiation therapy have a 20% 5-year survival rate. In contrast, multimodality therapy, including preoperative chemotherapy, followed by surgery, postoperative chemotherapy, and possibly radiation therapy, improves both the disease-free interval and overall survival, with 5-year survival rates reported at 35% to 50%.[1]

In multimodality treatment, neoadjuvant therapy is used to reduce the size of the tumor or involved lymph nodes, and any residual disease is then treated by surgery and other therapies. The extent or absence of residual tumor in the breast or lymph nodes after neoadjuvant therapy is an excellent predictor of patient outcome.[2-6] Complete response is defined as total disappearance of the lesion, and partial response is defined as the reduction of a lesion by 50% or more of its volume.[7] Limited microscopic residual cancer does not play a significant role and is found on pathology in 95% of cases thought to have complete response.[7] In a study by Feldman and colleagues,[1] patients without gross residual tumor after chemotherapy had 6-year survival increase from 34% to 93%. That study identified a 17% complete pathologic response after neoadjuvant therapy.

1.1. Monitoring Neoadjuvant Therapy

The clinical implications of accurate monitoring of neoadjuvant therapeutic response are substantial and include the following points:

1. Identification of complete response or reduction of tumor volume to less than 1 cm, as well as nodal response to therapy, indicates an improvement in the patient's long-term prognosis.[3]

2. Determination of failure of tumor to respond to therapy makes it possible to alter management, reducing suffering from unsuccessful therapy and saving costs.

3. With partial or complete response to therapy, surgery is warranted, and the extent or required breast resection

can be accurately gauged. In some cases, conservation is possible. In one study, 59% of patients were eligible for breast conservation after neoadjuvant treatment of large, primary tumors.[8]

Conventional modalities for monitoring response to neoadjuvant therapy include clinical examination, mammography, and ultrasound. Many studies have correlated therapy response based on these modalities with pathologic findings and have demonstrated that all three can underestimate or overestimate residual tumor size, leading to incorrect decisions as to surgery and other subsequent treatment. The studies differ as to which method is more accurate. Balu-Maestro and colleagues[7] found that physical examination, mammography, and ultrasound correlated with histopathology in 52%, 38%, and 43% of cases, respectively. In a study by Dershaw and colleagues[9] mammography was more reliable than physical examination. Although mammography and physical examination often had concordant results in that study, the mammogram sometimes showed disease that was not detected clinically.

The determination of posttreatment residual tumor by physical examintion can be extremely difficult and can result in both over- and underestimation of residual tumor size. On palpation, chemotherapy-induced fibrotic and necrotic mass can mimic residual tumor and cause overestimation.[7] In contrast, apparent clinical regression is sometimes identified by the physician as a result of the resolution of adjacent inflammatory changes, even when there is little change in the underlying tumor mass. Clinical palpation is also dependent on the clinician's expertise, the breast size, and the lesion type.[10] Feldman and coworkers[1] showed that 45% of patients who had a complete response in clinical examination had macroscopic tumor on histology and that 60% of patients who had no gross residual tumor on histology had incomplete clinical response. Mumtaz and colleagues[11] showed that patients who had a complete clinical response had residual tumor measuring up to 6.5cm on histology. In a study by Partridge and coworkers,[10] five of eight complete clinical responders were found to have residual disease on pathology, with a mean size of 4.7cm.

Although mammography and ultrasound have been used conventionally for monitoring response to neoadjuvant therapy, each is seriously limited in this setting and can yield incorrect data.

1.1.1. Mammography

Chemotherapy leads to necrosis and fibrosis, which appear as persistent density on a mammogram. Similarly, calcifications associated with a carcinoma can persist even when viable tumor cells are no longer present. Both persistent density and calcification can be incorrectly identified as a site of carcinoma on a mammogram, resulting in falsepositive results.[12] False-negative cases or underestimation can occur when chemotherapy decreases calcifications although residual disease persists, or when focal tumor mass is obscured by posttreatment density or by dense, adjacent parenchyma. Vinnicombe and coworkers[13] found that of eight patients with complete response on mammography, five had residual disease on pathology, and of eight patients with complete response on pathology, only three had complete response on mammography. Gilles and colleagues[14] studied 14 women with residual disease on pathology who had preoperative mammograms; only 9 demonstrated residual disease on mammography.

1.1.2. Ultrasound

Ultrasound has been shown to be the most accurate of the conventional modalities for evaluating lymph node response and is useful for assessing edematous infiltration.[15] However, it is less reliable for large lesions, particularly if the lesions are poorly defined, fragmented, or multifocal, all of which are difficult to identify by ultrasound and result in false-negative results.[7] Although histology confirmed complete response in 5% of cases, a complete response was predicted by ultrasound in 13% of cases in a study by Minckwitz and coworkers.[8] False-negative results were seen in breasts with as much as 0.8cm of residual tumor. Because ultrasound is also user-dependent, an exact comparison may be difficult on follow-up examinations.[16] Color Doppler ultrasound, like MRI, may have an additional role because it can better evaluate tumor size and can also monitor vascularity, but this requires further study.[7]

1.2. Role of Magnetic Resonance Imaging in Monitoring Response

In the untreated breast, MRI has a high sensitivity for detection of breast cancer as small as 1cm (95%–97%) with variable specificity of 30% to 97%. Magnetic resonance imaging detects lesions not only based on morphological pattern, but also based on characteristics of contrast enhancement. Early contrast enhancement in MRI generally identifies untreated breast cancer due to hypervascularity and increased vascular permeability. Fibrotic tissue is responsible for some of the false-positive results in conventional imaging. Because fibrosis generally does not demonstrate early enhancement, fibrosis should not result in frequent false-positive MRI studies.[7]

Magnetic resonance imaging also has other advantages. Abraham and colleagues[17] demonstrated 100% agreement among three independent readers using MRI, whereas two independent clinical examiners only agreed in 75% of cases. In determining size of residual tumor after treatment, Partridge and coworkers[10] showed variation on MRI measurement of tumor size between two radiologists in only 11% of the cases.

Magnetic resonance imaging is also useful in evaluating multifocal and multicentric disease. Of the 32 patients who had mastectomy in one study, MRI correctly identified multifocal tumor in 9 of 12 and all 3 cases of multicentric disease.[7] In this same study, mammography and ultrasound identified multifocal lesions in only 6 of 12. These results are supported by a study by Abraham and colleagues[17] in which MRI detected 23 of 24 cases of multicentric disease. Magnetic resonance imaging may also play a role in evaluating lymph nodes, chest wall, nipple, and skin involvement and their response to neoadjuvant therapy.

Magnetic resonance imaging is also useful in evaluation of the contralateral breast, which is especially helpful in these preoperative patients. Studies have shown that MRI detects contralateral cancer in 4% to 24% of patients with recently diagnosed breast cancer.[18–21]

While MRI should work better than conventional modalities, it does have limits, as described in the following discussion. In addition, cytotoxic agents used in neoadjuvant therapy reduce vascularization, requiring the reader to adjust parameters for reading magnetic resonance (MR) in the postneoadjuvant therapy breast.

Studies agree that MRI can accurately determine a response to neoadjuvant therapy, but there have been mixed results in the determination of whether MRI can accurately evaluate the extent of residual disease. Early studies were promising and demonstrated that MRI accurately identified response to therapy and extent of residual disease. In a study of 18 cases of residual tumor, Gilles and colleagues[14] showed dynamic MRI to correctly assess 17, and MRI correlated well with histologic size in 15 of 18 cases (83%). Only one false-negative case was found in which a 2-mm cluster of invasive tumor cells was not detected. Different techniques, including thinner slices, may have identified this cluster. Thirty-nine women were reported by Abraham and colleagues[17]; tumors studied were stages 2 to 4. It was found that MRI findings correlated with the extent of residual tumor seen on histology in 97% of cases (30 of 31 cases), and MRI more accurately defined response than conventional methods. Among these patients, MRI and mammography accurately agreed in their evaluation of the complete and partial response groups; however, in 12 patients thought to have no response by mammography, MRI accurately showed a response in 8 cases, and in 4 cases viewed by mammography as indeterminate, MRI showed them to have either a partial or complete response. In the study by Partridge and colleagues,[10] MRI accurately identified all 44 cases of residual disease, and accurately identified 3 of 8 complete responses seen on histology. Balu-Maestro and coworkers[7] correctly identified the extent of residual disease in 63% of patients evaluated with MRI. MRI identified all 5

tumors with complete response and 45 of 55 with partial or no response. The series included 10 false-negative MRI assessments of response: MRI indicated no residual tumor but cancer was found at pathology (invasive ductal carcinoma in 8 and ductal carcinoma in situ in 2). In another study of 58 women, MRI was qualitatively accurate for identifying response to therapy with a specificity of 96.3% and negative predictive value of 89.7%.[22]

More recent studies have been less encouraging about the ability of MRI to evaluate extent of residual disease. Rieber and colleagues[22] evaluated whether MRI could accurately determine the quantitative response to neoadjuvant therapy. Patients were assigned to the no response, partial response, or complete response group. Magnetic resonance imaging was relatively reliable in determining those with any response, with a positive predictive value of 83.3%. Only two patients with pathologic partial response were assigned to the nonresponder group based on MRI findings. The accuracy of MRI in this study suggests that it is a useful tool to determine those who would benefit from change in therapy. The usefulness of MRI in determining a complete response was less encouraging: 66.7% of cases were false-negatives including studies of breasts containing invasive tumor nodules up to 1 cm as well as disseminated disease. Residual tumor was underestimated in seven of nine cases of invasive lobular carcinoma. This may be due to differences in contrast medium uptake in lobular cancers that more often leads to false-negative results.[22] The reliability of MRI in those with a partial response seemed to depend on the degree of response to chemotherapy. Magnetic resonance imaging size determination was more reliable in tumors with a modest response than with tumors with a more significant response. Magnetic resonance imaging overestimated residual tumor in more than half (56%) of the partial response group by an average of 1.1 cm. Two patients with no response on histologic analysis were incorrectly placed in the partial response group based on MRI findings. This may be due to compromise in vascularity occurring in response to chemotherapy that appears as size reduction on MRI.[22] In still another series it was demonstrated that the size of residual disease after chemotherapy was often over- or underestimated on MRI. However, MRI was of value in predicting tumor size when there was no response or a complete response. In those with no response to treatment, MRI was highly accurate, correlating with pathology within a few millimeters, except in those three cases that were infiltrating lobular carcinoma.[16]

1.2.1. Explanation for Magnetic Resonance Imaging False-Positive and False-Negative Results

The inaccuracy of MRI determination of tumor volume after neoadjuvant therapy can be due to a variety of factors. These include (1) therapy-induced changes causing decrease in tumor enhancement that is independent of response to treatment resulting in overestimation of chemotherapy effect; (2) increased contrast enhancement that occurs due to therapy-induced noncancerous alterations within the tumor, including reactive changes in tumor such as fibrosis, necrosis, and inflammation—these can simulate tumor enhancement and lead to overestimation; and (3) loss of tumor contiguity in a previously continuous tumor can lead to underestimation of residual tumor size.[16] Additionally, there is controversy about the ability of MRI to accurately detect and stage the extent of ductal carcinoma in situ (DCIS). Unlike mammography, MRI is unable to detect microcalcifications and therefore, may fail to identify foci of DCIS that are readily appreciated on a mammogram. False-negative MRI can also be due to variation in technique and the speed image acquisition. With technological advances, sequences and speed of scanning have improved. Improved spatial resolution and smaller slice thickness have also decreased the false-negative rate. However, further studies are needed to determine if sequences that maximize spatial or temporal resolution are of the greatest value when evaluating the postneoadjuvant therapy breast.

1.3. Magnetic Resonance Imaging Procedures for Monitoring Neoadjuvant Therapy

1.3.1. Determining Residual Disease on Magnetic Resonance Imaging

To evaluate residual disease using MRI, physicians should determine the number and size of tumors as well as the dynamics of contrast enhancement (Figures 14.1 through 14.3). Cytotoxic agents affect tumor vascularization and vascular wall permeability, which causes a decrease or delayed enhancement observed in tumors after neoadjuvant therapy. One should still be able to differentiate residual tumor enhancement from fibrotic tissue, which generally does not demonstrate early enhancement.

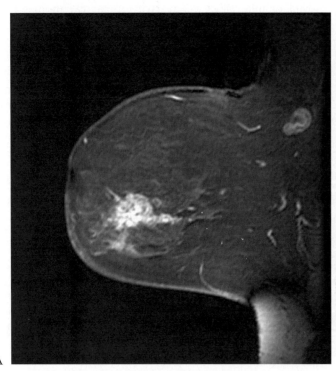

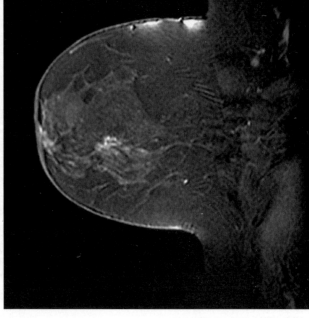

A   B

FIGURE 14.1. This 57-year-old woman with a palpable mass underwent core biopsy yielding invasive ductal carcinoma. Magnetic resonance imaging was performed during the patient's course of preoperative neoadjuvant chemotherapy. (A) Sagittal fat-suppressed T1-weighted image postcontrast revealed an irregular heterogeneously enhancing mass with associated spiculations spanning approximately 5.5cm in the lower outer quadrant. An abnormal enlarged axillary lymph node is also seen. (B) Approximately 5 weeks after initiation of chemotherapy, repeat MRI demonstrated decrease in enhancement consistent with response to chemotherapy of the tumor and axillary nodes. Pathologic analysis showed invasive carcinoma in the form of multiple tumor emboli in lymphatic vessels and scattered microscopic foci of DCIS, with tumor in 2 of 13 lymph nodes.

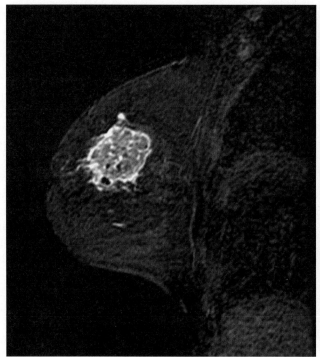
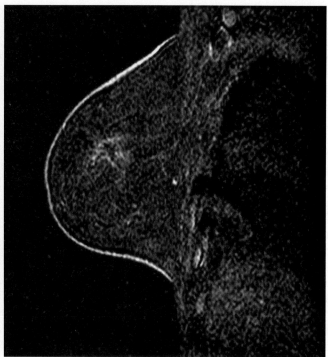

FIGURE 14.2. This 39-year-old woman with a palpable mass underwent core biopsy yielding invasive ductal carcinoma. Magnetic resonance imaging was performed before and after preoperative neoadjuvant therapy. (A) Sagittal subtraction image obtained before chemotherapy revealed an irregular rim-enhancing mass in the upper outer quadrant measuring 4.0 cm. (B) Postchemotherapy, preoperative MRI subtraction image demonstrated interval decrease in enhancement that was concordant with the physical examination. Mastectomy was performed and showed no residual carcinoma.

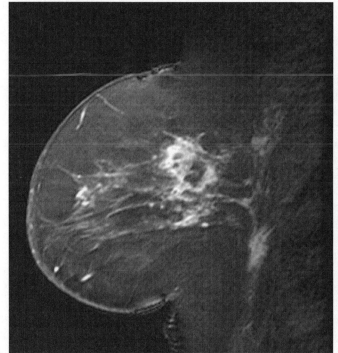
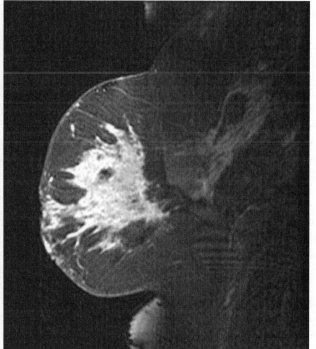

FIGURE 14.3. This 53-year-old woman with a palpable mass underwent core biopsy yielding invasive ductal carcinoma and DCIS. Magnetic resonance imaging was obtained before and after chemotherapy. (A) Sagittal fat-suppressed contrast-enhanced T1-weighted image before chemotherapy revealed an irregular heterogeneously enhancing mass spanning 6 cm in the upper outer quadrant with enhancement extending to the chest wall. (B) MRI taken approximately 7 weeks after the initiation of chemotherapy demonstrated an increase in the abnormal enhancement of the tumor, with progressive involvement of the chest wall and skin, consistent with progression of disease. Surgery was not performed due to disease progression, but medical therapy was subsequently altered to a different chemotherapeutic regimen.

Residual disease was determined differently in the various studies. Residual disease was identified as any early contrast enhancement (less than 1 min, 34 s) in the study by Gilles and colleagues[14] Partridge and colleagues[10] identified any notable enhancement in the tumor bed in the posttreatment MRI as suspicious, attempting to compensate for the decreased contrast uptake of tumor after chemotherapy. Magnetic resonance imaging evaluation was performed before and after neoadjuvant therapy, and changes in contrast enhancement uptake and washout were studied by looking at decreases in peak percentage of enhancement and peak signal enhancement ratio. Partridge and colleagues[10] also used maximum intensity projections to visualize the extent of the lesion in three dimensions. Esserman and coworkers[3] measured changes in the longest diameter of the tumor to determine treatment response. Further study is needed to determine if volumetric changes in tumor are a better way to evaluate the response to therapy than unidimensional changes.

The appropriate timing of MRI to optimize accuracy of assessment of tumor response is as yet unestablished. Rieber[22] suggested that MRI should be performed no sooner than 6 weeks after initiation of neoadjuvant therapy if it is to reliably monitor the response to therapy. However, preliminary studies by Partridge and colleagues[10] suggested that MRI accurately assesses change in tumor volume after only one cycle of chemotherapy.

1.4. Areas of Future Study

A multiinstitutional study has been set up (American College of Radiology Imaging Network [ACRIN] Study 6657) to further evaluate breast MRI usage for patients undergoing neoadjuvant therapy, to quantify early responses to therapy using MRI measurements of tumor volume and contrast kinetics, and to assess the various MRI patterns of disease and their response to therapy and impact on survival.

Positron emission tomography (PET) may have a role in monitoring response to neoadjuvant therapy by evaluating changes in glucose metabolism. Further studies are needed to compare the accuracy of PET with MRI and other modalities in this clinical setting.[23]

With the increasing use of neoadjuvant therapy, accuracy of monitoring response to this therapy is needed. Conventional methods have been studied and shown to be inaccurate. Magnetic resonance imaging will increasingly play a role due to its capability to evaluate changes in enhancement before and after therapy. Although studies have demonstrated mixed results as to the accuracy of MRI in evaluating extent of residual disease, clear evidence suggests that MRI can be used to predict tumor response within 6 weeks of therapy, perhaps as soon as the completion of the first cycle of chemotherapy.

2. Magnetic Resonance Imaging and Breast Conservation Therapy

Breast conservation, including wide local excision with radiation, is increasingly being used for early breast carcinoma, as overall survival and recurrence rates are not significantly different than total mastectomy.[24] When the breast is completely removed, the issue of recurrence of tumor in residual breast tissue does not arise. However, with increasing breast conservation, detection of tumor recurrence in the treated breast is an increasingly common clinical issue. As with the postneoadjuvant therapy breast, conventional monitoring methods have limitations, and MRI offers some advantages when monitoring for recurrence.

Local recurrence after breast conservation occurs at a rate of 1% to 2% a year, with the majority occurring within the first 5 years. However, recurrence is rare within the first 18 months after treatment.[25-28] Recurrences in the first decade after treatment are usually due to failure to cure the originally diagnosed cancer. Therefore, these usually occur at or near the lumpectomy site. Cancers developing in the treated breast 7 or more years after treatment are usually due to growth of new carcinoma in the breast and are often at a distance from the lumpectomy site.[25] As with the original tumor, earlier detection and treatment of the local recurrence can improve the long-term survival.[25,29] According to Kurtz and colleagues,[25] a significant correlation exists between survival after local recurrence and extent of recurrence. Local recurrence that is <2 cm and confined to the breast had a 74% overall 5-year survival. Additionally, compared with the average-risk woman, these patients have a six-fold risk of a second primary in the contralateral breast.[30]

2.1. Local Recurrence: Detection with Conventional Methods

Conventional methods for detection of local tumor recurrence include physical examination and mammography; less frequently ultrasound can be used. On mammography, local recurrence is usually detected as a focal mass, distortion, increased density at the scar, or calcifications. On physical examination, a mass may be palpated.[31]

Detection of local tumor recurrence, as well as evaluation of the remainder of the breast, by conventional methods can be difficult due to posttreatment alteration, especially within dense breasts. On physical examination, it is often difficult to differentiate recurrence from the postsurgical scar and postradiation changes. On mammography posttreatment changes such as edema, stromal coarsening, architectural distortion, increased density, focal mass, skin thickening, and fat necrosis calcifications can mimic or obscure recurrent disease. Mammography can also be technically problematic due to difficulty in positioning the entire lumpectomy bed on the mammogram and decreased compressibility of the breast.[32] Diagnostic problems can be compounded in women receiving chemotherapy as well as radiation. In these women, skin thickening and parenchymal changes such as stromal coarsening and increased breast density are more severe.[33] Ultrasound is also limited for the detection of recurrence, as it is operator dependent. Also, hypoechogenicity and shadowing at the site of scarring can limit evaluation due to their similarity to patterns seen with recurrent tumor. There is also the problem of diminished reliability of sonography for detection of small and noninvasive cancers, even in the untreated breast.[32,34]

In addition to the problem of detecting recurrent tumors, diagnosis with mammography and physical examination is hampered by the inability to differentiate recurrent tumor from scarring and fat necrosis.[32] Repeated biopsy to make this differentiation can compromise the cosmetic result of breast conservation. Therefore, it is desirable to differentiate scar from tumor by noninvasive techniques, if possible.

2.2. Posttreatment Findings on Magnetic Resonance Imaging

Because MRIs show areas of increased blood flow rather than tissue density and because clinical issues with recurrence versus scar arise 18 months or more after therapy, MRI offers some advantages over conventional methods in assessing some clinical issues in this patient population. This is illustrated in results from a study by Heywang-Kobrunner and coworkers[32] of 62 patients who had breast conservation who presented with suspicious findings on conventional methods or had dense breasts in which it was difficult to evaluate changes in the breast tissue after radiation and surgery. During the first 9 months, irradiated normal tissue demonstrated patchy or diffuse enhancement. Enhancement appeared early in a least one third of these cases. Between 10 and 18 months, the amount and rate of enhancement decreased on a variable basis. At 18 months after therapy, enhancement was insignificant in 93% of cases. The enhancement pattern of the scar after radiation showed a similar pattern as the radiated normal breast tissue, with early strong enhancement postradiation that decreased with time. Even without radiation, the postsurgical scar tended to enhance within the first 6 months.

This study by Heywang-Kobrunner and colleagues[32] demonstrated that within the first 18 months, contrast-enhanced MRI was limited but could exclude a recurrence if no suspicious enhancement was identified. The utility of MRI was limited by the discovery of many false-positive results. After 18 months, MRI was able to exclude malig-

nancy, confirm suspected local recurrence, and detect unsuspected malignancy as small as 3 mm with 100% positive and negative predictive values. Benign results for women who did not undergo biopsy were confirmed by at least 24 months of clinical, mammographic follow up or pathologic correlation.[32]

Although scar generally does not enhance more than 18 months after treatment, enhancement has been reported several years after excision. Solomon and coworkers[35] described a case of delayed development of enhancement in fat necrosis that developed 32 months after breast-conserving surgery and noted that this is a potential pitfall of breast MRI. Late enhancement of scar tissue is a relatively infrequent occurrence, but the possibility of a benign etiology for enhancement at the lumpectomy site years after surgery reinforces the importance of biopsy to determine histology for suspicious areas of enhancement detected at breast MRI.

Other studies have proven MRI to be highly sensitive as well as specific in detecting local tumor recurrence compared with mammography and clinical examination. Lewis-Jones and cowokers[36] reported that MRI detected all 11 recurrent tumors (100% sensitivity) with only 2 false-positive cases (94% specificity). One case of false-positive enhancement on histology revealed atypical lobular hyperplasia, and the other was fat necrosis and fibrous tissue. Of nine cases suspected on mammography, only two demonstrated tumor recurrence on histology. On clinical examination, only five of the proven recurrences were considered highly suspicious, and seven lesions considered highly suspicious on clinical examination were benign. Kerslake and coworkers[37] reported a series in which MRI detected all four recurrences, whereas mammography detected two. Of the 16 benign scars detected on MRI, mammography demonstrated suspicious lesions in 8. In another series, this one by Gilles and coworkers,[31] MRI detected all 14 cases of local recurrence. The one false-positive case of strong early enhancement on histology was fat necrosis. Of the other 11 suspected lesions, MRI showed no early enhancement; benignity was demonstrated either with biopsy or follow up. Supporting these data is the experience of Dao and coworkers,[38] who reported that all 10 reported recurrences were detected on MRI, while mammography detected only 6 of these. In a series by Murray and coworkers[30] of 37 patient examinations suspected for carcinoma, 5 patients showed six lesions that demonstrated rapid enhancement, all of which were biopsy proven carcinomas. Six patients with lesser degrees of enhancement had benign biopsy or follow up, and the other 25 patients had no enhancement.

Still others have reported a high sensitivity and specificity for MRI in the diagnosis of recurrence after breast conservation. In one study of 105 patients with 9 local recurrences who had clinical examination, mammography, and MRI, the sensitivities for clinical examination alone, mammography alone, clinical examination and mammography together, and MRI alone were 89%, 67%, 100%, and 100%, respectively. However, the specificities were 76%, 85%, 67%, and 93%, respectively.[27] In a study by Hickman and colleagues,[39] MRI detected all 4 recurrences in 24 women. There was one false-positive result that on histology was a myxoid fibroadenoma, which can enhance in a similar pattern as carcinoma.[39]

Magnetic resonance imaging also is advantageous due to its ability to detect multifocal and contralateral lesions within treated and dense breasts. In the study of Gilles and coworkers,[31] MRI detected all cases of multifocal disease except one case in which the lesion was not imaged and two other foci measuring 1 mm each. In the study by Dao and coworkers,[38] the one case of multifocal disease that was evident on MRI could not be seen on mammography, even in retrospect. In the study of Murray and coworkers,[30] one of five patients had unexpected contralateral carcinoma discovered on MRI.

2.3. Imaging Findings on Magnetic Resonance Imaging to Detect or Exclude Local Recurrence

Magnetic resonance imaging findings in recurrences are identical to those seen in cancers developing in the untreated breast. Recurrences demonstrate early strong enhancement (Figures 14.4 and 14.5). It has been suggested that quantitative evaluation of signal intensity may be helpful in this situation with strong enhancement reported at 1.5 to 3.0 min after injection.[30–32,37] Fibrous postoperative scar is often identified as a mass with less marked and slower enhancement; cysts or seroma/hematoma can confidently be identified by signal characteristics on MRI.[36] Early studies suggested that the T2-weighted sequences are useful to differentiate tumor from scar, with tumor being of higher signal on T2-weighted images; however, this is not consistently demonstrated in the literature.[36,38]

Secondary signs of malignancy such as skin thickening, retraction, and nipple inversion are less useful in the treated breast because these findings could be due to the initial therapy as well as due to recurrence.[36,37] Additionally, early skin enhancement can be caused by recurrence and by radiation. Therefore, this sign may not enable distinction of recurrence from postradiation change in the treated breast.

There are some situations in which other imaging modalities may have advantages over MRI in detection of recurrence. It should be remembered that microcalcifications associated with carcinoma can be readily appreciated on mammography in a tumor that is not identified on MRI. The evolution of fibrosis into an avascular, nonenhancing lesion may take up to 18 months. Earlier than this, it can be difficult to differentiate posttreatment inflammation

from carcinoma in enhancing lesions. This is particularly true in the first 9 months after treatment. It should also be noted that the size of tumor recurrence detectable with magnetic resonance (MR) depends on scanning parameters. The lower limit of recurrence size detectable with MRI is yet to be determined.

There is little doubt that MRI in the treated breast is very sensitive as well as specific, unlike in the untreated breast where MRI has higher sensitivity than specificity. Although radiation changes may decrease MRI detection of benign entities, MR is useful in differentiating tumor recurrence from scar, particularly 18 months after radiation therapy when treatment-induced alterations are generally no longer enhancing and the clinical need to differentiate these two entities is most important.

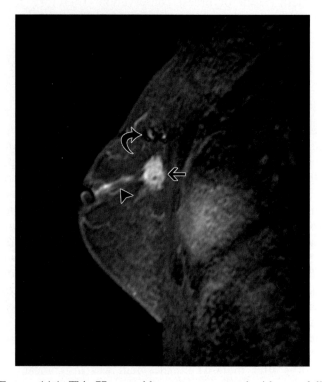

FIGURE 14.4. This 77-year-old woman presented with new fullness at the lumpectomy site. She was 6 years postlumpectomy and axillary dissection for node positive invasive carcinoma. Mammography failed to demonstrate suspicious findings. Sagittal fat-suppressed contrast-enhanced T1-weighted image of the treated breast demonstrated a 2.5-cm irregular heterogeneously enhancing mass (straight arrow) in the 12:00 axis with ductal extension into the nipple (arrowhead) just inferior to the prior lumpectomy site, identified by susceptibility artifact from the surgical clips (curved arrow). Cytology confirmed adenocarcinoma. At mastectomy, a 2.5-cm invasive carcinoma with associated DCIS was found.

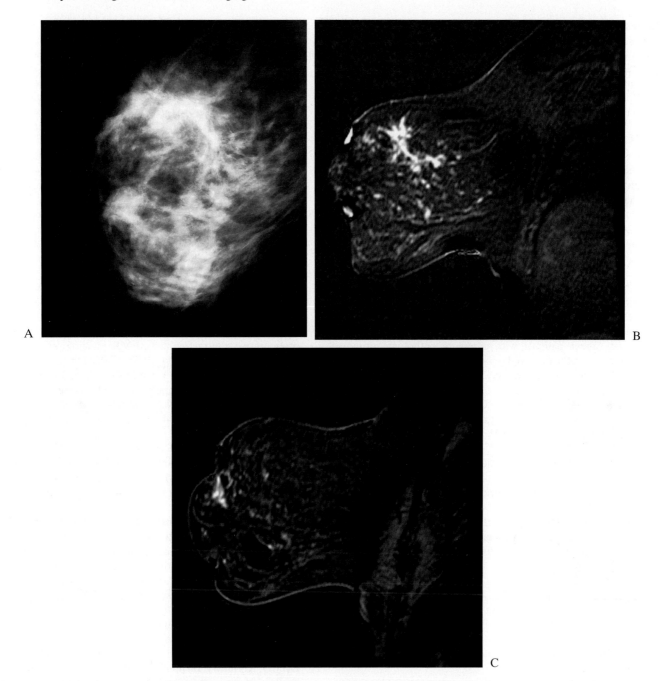

FIGURE 14.5. This 52-year-old woman had a history of right breast DCIS 6 years ago. (A) Collimated mediolateral oblique mammographic view of the right breast demonstrated possible increased distortion in the superior right breast at the lumpectomy site. (B) On sagittal subtraction MRI of the right breast, distortion and irregular nodular enhancement extended from the lumpectomy site laterally with a greater extent than seen on mammography. Histologic analysis yielded multiple foci of invasive and in situ ductal and lobular carcinoma, treated with mastectomy. (C) Sagittal subtraction image of the contralateral (left) breast demonstrates an irregular retroareolar mass. Surgery revealed a 1.1-cm invasive cancer, treated with mastectomy.

References

1. Feldman L, Hortobagyi GN, Buzdar AU, et al. Pathological assessment of response to induction chemotherapy in breast cancer. *Cancer Res.* 1986;46:2578–2581.

2. Bonadonna G, Valagussa P, Brambilla C, et al. Primary chemotherapy in operable breast cancer: eight-year experience at the Milan Cancer Institute. *J Clin Oncol.* 1998;16: 93–100.

3. Esserman L, Kaplan E, Partridge S, et al. MRI phenotype is associated with response to doxorubicin and cyclophosphamide neoadjuvant chemotherapy in Stage III breast cancer. *Ann Surg Oncol.* 2001;8:549–559.

4. Hortobagyi G, Ames FC, Buzdar AU, et al. Management of stage III primary breast cancer with chemotherapy, surgery, and radiation therapy. *Cancer* 1988;62:2507–2516.

5. Kuerer HM, Newman LA, Buzdar AU, et al. Residual metastatic axillary lymph nodes following neoadjuvant cxhemotherapy predict disease-free survival in patients with locally advanced breast cancer. *Am J Surg.* 1998;176: 502–509.

6. Kuerer HM, Newman LA, Smith TL, et al. Clinical course of breast cancer patients with complete pathologic primary tumor and axillary lymph node response to doxorubicin-based neoadjuvant therapy. *J Clin Oncol.* 1999;17: 460–469.

7. Balu-Maestro C, Chapellier C, Bleuse A, et al. Imaging in evaluation of response to neoadjuvant breast cancer treatment benefits of MRI. *Breast Cancer Res Treat.* 2002;72:145–152.

8. Minckwitz GV, Costa SD, Eiermann W, et al. Maximized reduction of primary breast tumor size using preoperative chemotherapy with doxorubicin and docetaxel. *J Clin Oncol.* 1999;17:1999–2005.

9. Dershaw DD, Drossman S, Liberman L, Abramson AF. Assessment of response to therapy of primary breast cancer by mammography and physical examination. *Cancer* 1995;75:2093–2098.

10. Partridge SC, Gibbs JE, Lu Y, et al. Accuracy of MR imaging for revealing residual breast cancer in patients who have undergone neoadjuvant chemotherapy. *AJR Am J Roentgenol.* 2002;179:1193–1199.

11. Mumtaz H, Davidson T, Spittle M, et al. Breast surgery after neoadjuvant treatment. Is it necessary? *Eur J Surg Oncol.* 1996;22:335–341.

12. Segel MC, Paulus DD, Hortobagyi GN. Advanced primary breast cancer: assessment at mammography of respose to induction chemotherapy. *Radiology* 1988;169:49–54.

13. Vinnicombe SJ, Macvicar AD, Guy RL, et al. Primary breast cancer: mammographic changes after neoadjuvant chemotherapy, with pathologic correlation. *Radiology* 1996;198: 333–340.

14. Gilles R, Guinebretiere JM, Toussaint C, et al. Locally advanced breast cancer: contrast-enhanced subtraction MR imaging of response to preoperative chemotherapy. *Radiology* 1994;191:633–638.

15. Herrada J, Iyer RB, Atkinson EN, et al. Relative value of physical examination, mammography, and breast sonography in evaluating the size of the primary tumor and regional lymph node metastases in women receiving neoadjiuvant

chemotherapy for locally advanced breast carcinoma. *Clin Cancer Res.* 1997;3:1565–1569.

16. Wasser K, Sinn HP, Fink C, et al. Accuracy of tumor size measurement in breast cancer using MRI is influenced by histological regression induced by neoadjuvant chemotherapy. *Eur Radiol* [serial online]., 2002;13:1213–1223. Available at: http://link.springer.de/link/service/journals/00330/contents/02/01730/paper/s00330-002-1730. Accessed 09/05/2004.

17. Abraham DC, Jones RC, Jones SE, et al. Evaluation of neoadjuvant chemotherapeutic response of locally advanced breast cancer by magnetic resonance imaging. *Cancer* 1996;78:91–100.

18. Lee SG, Orel SG, Woo IJ, et al. MR imaging screening of the contralateral breast in patients with newly diagnosed breast cancer: preliminary results. *Radiology* 2003;226: 773–778.

19. Liberman L, Morris EA, Kim CM, et al. MR imaging findings in the contralateral breast in women with recently diagnosed breast cancer. *AJR Am J Roentgenol.* 2003;180: 333–341.

20. Fischer U, Kopka L, Grabbe E. Breast carcinoma: effect of preoperative contrast-enhanced MR imaging on the therapeutic approach. *Radiology* 1999;213:881–888.

21. Slanetz PJ, Edmister WB, Yeh ED, et al. Occult contralateral breast carcinoma incidentally detected by breast magnetic resonance imaging. *Breast J.* 2002;8:145–148.

22. Rieber A, Brambs HJ, Gabelmann A, et al. Breast MRI for monitoring response of primary breast cancer to neoadjuvant chemotherapy. *Eur Radiol.* 2002;12:1711–1719.

23. Schelling M, Avril N, Nahrig J, et al. Positron emission tomography using [18F] fluorodeoxyglucose for monitoring primary chemotherapy in breast cancer. *J Clin Oncol.* 2000; 18:1689–1695.

24. Fisher B, Redmond C, Poisson R, et al. Eight-year results of a randomized clinical trial comparing total mastectomy and lumpectomy with or without irradiation in the treatment of breast cancer. *N Engl J Med.* 1989;320:822–828.

25. Kurtz JM, Amalric R, Brandone H, et al. Local recurrence after breast conserving surgery and radiotherapy. *Cancer* 1989;63:1912–1917.

26. Rieber A, Merkle E, Zeitler H, et al. Value of MR mammography in the detection and exclusion of recurrent breast carcinoma. *J Comput Assist Tomogr.* 1997;21:780–784.

27. Drew P, Kerin MJ, Turnbull LW, et al. Routine screening for local recurrence following breast-conserving therapy for cancer with dynamic contrast-enhanced magnetic resonance imaging of the breast. *Ann Surg Oncol.* 1998;5:265–270.

28. Dershaw DD. Mammography in patients with breast cancer treated by breast conservation (lumpectomy with or without radiation). *AJR Am J Roentgenol.* 1995;164:309–316.

29. Davis PL, McCarty KS. Sensitivity of enhanced MRI for the detection of breast cancer: new, multicentric, residual, and recurrent. *Eur Radiol.* 1977;7 (Suppl 5):S289–S298.

30. Murray AD, Redpath TW, Needham G, et al. Dynamic magnetic resonance mammography of both breasts following local excision and radiotherapy for breast carcinoma. *Br J Radiol.* 1996;69:594–600.

31. Gilles R, Guinebretiere J, Shapeero LG, et al. Assessment of breast cancer recurrence with contrast-enhanced subtraction

MR imaging: preliminary results in 26 patients. *Radiology* 1993;188:473–478.

32. Heywang-Kobrunner SH, Schlegel A, Beck R, et al. Contrast-enhanced MRI of the breast after limited surgery and radiation therapy. *J Comput Assist Tomogr.* 1993;17:891–900.

33. Dershaw DD, Shank B, Reisinger S. Mammographic findings after breast cancer treatment with local excision and definitive irradiation. *Radiology* 1987;164:455–461.

34. Sickles EA, Filly RA, Callen PW. Breast cancer detection with sonography and mammography: comparison using state-of-the-art equipment. *AJR Am J Roentgenol.* 1983;140:843–845.

35. Solomon B, Orel S, Reynolds C, Schnall MD. Delayed development of enhancement in fat necrosis after breast conservation therapy: a potential pitfall of MR imaging of the breast. *AJR Am J Roentgenol.* 1998;170:966–968.

36. Lewis-Jones HG, Whitehouse GH, Leinster SJ. The role of magnetic resonance imaging in the assessment of local recurrent breast carcinoma. *Clin Radiol.* 1991;43:197–204.

37. Kerslake RW, Fox JN, Carleton PJ, et al. Dynamic contrast-enhanced and fat suppressed magnetic resonance imaging in suspected recurrent carcinoma of the breast: preliminary experience. *Br J Radiol.* 1994;67:1158–1168.

38. Dao TH, Rahmouni A, Campana F, et al. Tumor recurrence versus fibrosis in the irradiated breast: differentiation with dynamic gadolinium-enhanced MR imaging. *Radiology* 1993;187:751–755.

39. Hickman PF, Moore NR, Shepstone BJ. The indeterminate breast mass: assessment using contrast enhanced magnetic resonance imaging. *Br J Radiol.* 1994;67:14–20.

15
Magnetic Resonance Imaging in Women with Breast Implants

Laura Liberman and Wendie A. Berg

Approximately 1 to 2 million women in the United States have breast implants, placed for cosmetic augmentation in approximately 80% of these women and for reconstruction after breast cancer surgery in approximately 20%.[1] There are two primary purposes for performing magnetic resonance imaging (MRI) after implant placement: evaluation for silicone implant rupture and detection of breast cancer. Magnetic resonance imaging to evaluate for silicone implant rupture is a noncontrast examination, using specific sequences optimized for evaluation of the internal structure of the implant and for identification of free silicone. Magnetic resonance imaging for detection of breast cancer involves both precontrast and postcontrast images, ideally with fat suppression and subtraction. This chapter discusses the use of breast MRI in women with implants, both for identification of silicone implant rupture and breast cancer detection.

1. Implants: Types and Terms

Implants are defined in terms of their location and their composition.[2–4] Breast implants may be placed behind the glandular tissue but in front of the pectoral muscle, in a position that has been called *subglandular, retroglandular,* or *retromammary*. This position maximizes the augmentation effect of the implant, but obscures more tissue on the mammogram. The second possible position of breast implants is behind the pectoral muscle, in a position that has been termed *subpectoral* or *retropectoral*. Placing the implant behind the muscle is a more involved surgery and has less of a cosmetic augmentation effect, but may decrease the risk of capsular contracture and enables better visualization of the tissue for subsequent mammography. For women who have implants placed after mastectomy, the implant is always placed behind the muscle.

Implants may be composed of saline, silicone, or a combination of these materials. The silicone gel within silicone implants is a lightly crosslinked polymer of polydimethyl-siloxane (PDMS).[5] Some implants contain a single lumen; others may contain two or three lumens. Implants with multiple lumens may have one lumen within another (e.g., silicone within saline), or the implants may be *stacked*, one behind the other. A standard double lumen (silicone within saline implant) can be recognized at mammography because the outer saline lumen is more lucent than the inner silicone lumen; identification of the concentric lucent outer saline lumen at mammography demonstrates that the implant is intact.[6] Expander type implants can be gradually filled through a subcutaneous port and tubing. Expanders can be entirely saline or have an inner saline and outer silicone lumen.

Implants also differ in the composition of the outer envelope, with one example being a silicone elastomer shell.[5] Textured surfaces and a layer of polyurethane coating the surface were developed to decrease the likelihood of contracture and can sometimes be identified on mammography as a fuzzy border to the implant. The polyurethane-textured implant is no longer available due to concern about release of a by-product [2,4-diamino-toluene (TDA)] that may be carcinogenic in laboratory animals.[7] Knowledge of the specific type of implant used is helpful in interpretation of the MRI, because the MRI pattern will vary depending on the type of implant.[8] Correlation with the mammogram and specific clinical history regarding the type of implant are useful in this regard.

In 1992, the Food and Drug Administration (FDA) reviewed existing data regarding silicone gel implants and concluded that there was insufficient evidence of safety to support their widespread use.[9] On the basis of that decision, the FDA restricted the placement of new silicone implants to women with temporary breast-tissue expanders who were awaiting permanent reconstructive surgery, patients who had reconstruction at the time of mastectomy; patients who required the device for urgent medical reasons, such as rupture of a device already in place; and patients who participated in extended availability protocols or carefully controlled clinical trials.[9]

In January 2004, three months after an advisory committee from the FDA voted 9 to 6 to recommend approval of silicone gel implants for cosmetic use, the FDA decided to defer its decision on this issue.[10] The FDA notified the Inamed Corporation, a California company that sells implants for breast reconstruction, that more studies were necessary. The FDA indicated the need for more information regarding implant safety and failure rate, reasons for and sequelae of leakage or ruture, how women can recognize implant failure, and long-term consequences of breast implants.[10] At the time of this writing, the 1992 ban on placing silicone implants for cosmetic breast augmentation persists.

When an implant is placed, a fibrous capsule forms around it, essentially representing the layer of scar tissue that forms around any device implanted in the body.[11] The capsule may become firm to palpation, a process known as *capsular contracture*.[12] Calcifications may develop within this fibrous capsule that can be detected by mammography.[13] In addition to capsular contracture and calcification, potential complications of implants include breast pain, hematoma, and infection.[12] A possible link between silicone implants and connective tissue diseases has been suggested; studies have excluded a significant increased risk of these disorders, but do not exclude a small association or connection with atypical syndromes.[1,7,12,14] Another possible complication of any implant is implant failure.[1,7,12]

2. Implant Failure

When saline implants develop a tear in the silicone polymer shell, there is rapid loss of the saline. Failure of saline implants is a clinical diagnosis and imaging is not necessary. Saline implants nearly always have a textured surface. A small amount of fluid can be seen around saline implants as a normal finding. Similarly, Ahn and colleagues[15] reported intracapsular fluid with 15% of silicone implants and noted a trend that fluid was more common when implant shells were textured or covered in polyurethane. Positive microbial cultures were identified in 39% of implants with fluid and 43% of those without fluid.[15]

Many terms have been used to describe implant failure.[6,11] *Gel bleed* is the normal transudation of microscopic amounts of low-molecular-weight silicone gel through an intact shell. *Gel leak* or *uncollapsed rupture* has been variably defined. Dowden[11] considered a leak to be an abnormal condition in which a small amount of silicone gel passes through a detectable small hole in the shell, resulting in a thin coating of gel, usually less than 0.5mm thick, on the external surface of the shell; Berg and colleagues[6] defined an implant to be leaking at surgery if it appeared sticky but grossly intact. There are two types of rupture: *intracapsular rupture*, in which a tear or disruption

of the shell occurs such that a significant portion of the silicone gel lies outside the shell, but within the capsule, and the shell collapses into the gel to varying degrees; and *extracapsular rupture*, when there is displacement of silicone gel from a ruptured implant through the fibrous scar or *capsule* into the adjacent tissues, often caused by a strong external force.

Berg and colleagues[6] suggested that implant rupture be thought of as a spectrum of loss of integrity of the implant shell, from microscopic gel bleed to gross extracapsular rupture. The FDA advisory panel's review suggested that in 4% to 6% of asymptomatic women with implants, the implants have ruptured.[9]

Implants can rupture from a variety of traumatic stresses, including manual compression to break up a painful capsule (*closed capsulotomy*), motor vehicle accidents, insertion of pleural tubes, or gunshot wounds.[1] Cases have been reported in which implant rupture was attributed to breast compression during mammography,[16,17] although the relationship between mammographic compression and implant rupture remains unproven.[1] Most implant ruptures have no specific identifiable cause.

The most important factor predisposing to rupture is age of the implant. Berg and colleagues[3] found that the mean duration of implantation of ruptured implants was 13.4 years (range, 1–22y), as compared with mean duration of 7.7 years (range, 6mo to 24y) for intact implants. Robinson and colleagues[18] found that 64% of implants that had been placed for 1 to 25 years were ruptured or leaking. The number of women who had two intact implants decreased with age, from 89% after 8 years to 51% after 12 years to 5% after 20 years.[18] The clinical observation that older implants are more likely to rupture is consistent with results of mechanical studies, which suggest a weakening of the implant shell with increasing time after implantation.[19-21]

Among implant ruptures, 77% to 89% are intracapsular and 11% to 23% are extracapsular.[1] When the rupture is extracapsular, silicone can migrate within the breast parenchyma, rarely even in an intraductal fashion, through the ducts and out through the nipple, and even transcutaneously through the skin. Silicone may also migrate to axillary lymph nodes as well as to more distant sites, including pleura, chest, ribs, extremities, abdominal wall, inguinal region, and liver. Silicone granulomas occur in response to silicone migration. This may be particularly problematic in the region of the brachial plexus. Silicone migration and resulting scarring may yield sequelae such as lumps, pain, swelling, and skin tightening.

The diagnosis of implant rupture can be challenging. History and physical findings may be helpful but are often nonspecific. A history of trauma may or may not be present: Among 18 patients with ruptured implants treated by Anderson and colleagues,[16] 3 (17%) gave a history of recent trauma, 7 (39%) gave a history of trauma more than

1 year before any sign or symptom, and 8 (44%) gave no history of trauma. Symptoms can include pain; palpable masses in the axilla, breast, or chest wall; or change in size, shape, or texture of the breast. The presence of symptoms is not a reliable predictor of rupture: Robinson and colleagues[18] found the frequency of rupture was 72% among women with symptoms versus 71% among women without symptoms.

Treatment of implant rupture is somewhat variable. The FDA has recommended removal of breast implants known to be ruptured.[9] Although most would agree that extracapsular rupture warrants explantation, there is difference of opinion regarding the need for explantation in women with intracapsular rupture. Some surgeons have suggested that routine *prophylactic* explantation be performed at 8 years, to prevent potential future rupture.[18] Whether the benefit of removing an intact implant outweighs the potential risks associated with the surgery remains to be determined.

3. Imaging Implant Rupture

Imaging studies can be useful in diagnosing implant rupture. The FDA has not advocated the use of imaging studies specifically to screen asymptomatic women for implant rupture.[9] However, for women who are of an appropriate age to undergo screening mammography, the mammographic findings may demonstrate or suggest the possibility of implant rupture and may prompt further evaluation.[3] In addition, women with signs or symptoms of implant rupture may come to imaging. This section describes the use of mammography, sonography, and MRI in women with breast implants, concentrating specifically on findings associated with silicone implant rupture.

3.1. Mammography

The primary indication for performing mammography in women with implants is the same as that for women without implants—to detect breast cancer. Mammographic evaluation of the augmented breast should include, when possible, standard craniocaudal and mediolateral oblique views as well as two additional views of each breast, which have been called "implant displaced," "push-back," or "Eklund" views.[22,23] In these implant displaced craniocaudal and mediolateral oblique views, the implant is pushed back and the breast tissue is pulled forward. The conventional views encompass as much of the breast tissue as possible; the implant displaced views exclude the most posterior tissues, but provide better separation of parenchymal densities in the more anterior portion of the breast.[24]

In one study of mammography in 350 asymptomatic women with implants, mammography identified dense silicone globules in the breast parenchyma in 16 (5%) women, consistent with extracapsular rupture (Figure 15.1); 2 of these women had bilateral ruptures.[13] Fibrous

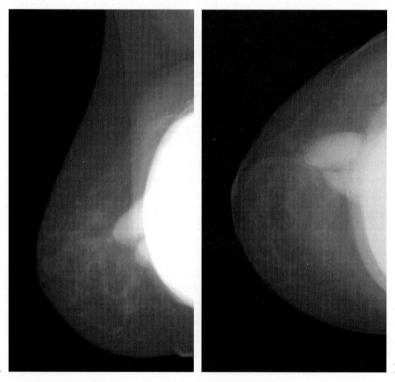

A   B

FIGURE 15.1. Extracapsular silicone imaged by mammography in a 60-year-old asymptomatic women who had silicone implants that ruptured and were replaced 3 years previously. (A) Mediolateral oblique view from digital left mammogram shows a mildly dense breast with a subpectoral silicone augmentation prosthesis. Dense collections anterior and smaller dense foci superior to the implant represent extracapsular silicone from prior implant rupture. (B) Craniocaudal view from the same left digital mammogram confirms the presence of extracapsular silicone.

FIGURE 15.2. Ruptured saline implants imaged by mammography. A 62-year-old woman with bilateral retroglandular saline implants placed 25 years ago, who felt that her left implant deflated during chiropractic manipulation 2 weeks prior to mammography. (A) Mediolateral oblique view of the left breast from digital mammogram shows the deflated left retroglandular saline implant. (B) Mediolateral oblique view of the right breast from digital mammogram shows that the right retroglandular saline implant remains intact.

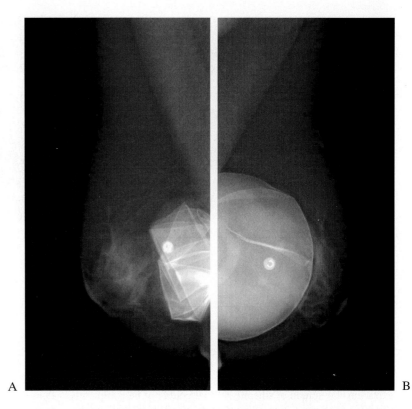

A

B

encapsulation of breast implants was seen in 257 (73%) of 350 women. Periprosthetic calcification was seen in 90 (26%) women, and 60 (17%) women had implant herniations, a focal bulge or contour deformity that may be due to focal weakening of a still-intact capsule. In a study by Berg and colleagues,[3] a contour bulge at mammography was associated with a higher likelihood of implant rupture. For women known to have a double lumen implant (silicone within saline), nonvisualization of the outer lucent saline lumen at mammography is suggestive of outer lumen rupture.[6]

These studies indicate that some extracapsular ruptures can be detected on mammograms. However, because the dense silicone can obscure much of the breast tissue at mammography and because mammography does not show the internal structure of the silicone implant, film-screen mammography cannot detect intracapsular silicone implant rupture. Postprocessing of digital mammograms can demonstrate additional detail within the implant, though its accuracy in depicting rupture has not been reported. Ruptured saline implants can be seen as an incidental finding at mammography (Figure 15.2).

3.2. Sonography

Unlike mammography, sonography is capable of delineating some of the internal structure of the implant, particularly in its anterior aspect, and therefore can depict both extracapsular and intracapsular ruptures. Extracapsular silicone can result in a mass characterized by a highly echogenic pattern of scattered and reverberating echoes with loss of detail posterior to the echogenic area, which has been variably described as *snowstorm*, echodense noise, echodense shadowing, or echogenic confusion[25] (Figure 15.3).[26] This finding is sensitive in diagnosing extracapsular rupture: Harris and colleagues[25] found that the snowstorm sonographic appearance was present in 19 (95%) of 20 surgically confirmed sites of extracapsular rupture, as compared with mammography, which only depicted 14 (70%).

Free (extracapsular) silicone may also have a hypoechoic appearance in the breast parenchyma. In a study of 19 ruptured implants evaluated with sonography, Rosculet and colleagues[26] found the snowstorm pattern and hypoechoic masses of silicone in 10 (53%), the snowstorm pattern alone in 7 (37%), and hypoechoic masses of silicone only in 2 (11%). These authors suggested that the snowstorm pattern is caused by phase aberration related to the speed of sound being slower in silicone than in soft tissue. The hypoechoic pattern of silicone may occur when the beam encounters a mass of silicone that is large compared with the wavelength.[26]

The implant shell is visible sonographically as a set of parallel echogenic lines. When intracapsular rupture has occurred with substantial collapse of the elastomer shell, sonography may demonstrate the collapsed shell as a

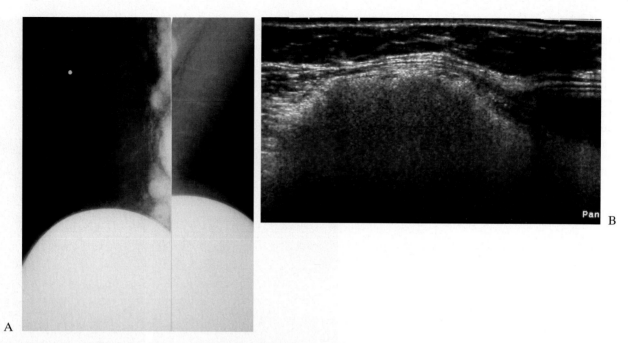

FIGURE 15.3. Extracapsular silicone imaged by mammography and sonography in a patient who had rupture of her original silicone implants, which had been in place for 13 years, with extracapsular spread of silicone gel that could not be completely removed at surgery. New silicone implants were placed and are presumed intact. (A) Collimated mediolateral oblique views from film-screen mammogram of left and right breast shows dense foci of extracapsular silicone superior to the left breast implant, consistent with extracapsular silicone. (B) Ultrasound demonstrates the snowstorm pattern of echodense noise consistent with extracapsular silicone.

series of sets of discontinuous parallel echogenic lines, termed the *stepladder sign* (Figure 15.4), seen in 32% to 70% of ruptured implants.[27,28] The collapsed shell can only be well seen sonographically when it collects anteriorly. The deeper aspect of the implant is not well evaluated due to the slower speed of sound within the gel. Normal infoldings of the implant shell, called *radial folds*, may cause confusion in assessment of the stepladder sign, particularly in double lumen implants and those with textured coatings. Central internal echoes in the implant have been reported in 41% to 55% of ruptured implants, but may also be seen in normal implants related to reverberation artifact or mixing of gel with fluid injected into the implant at the time of insertion.[1,28]

Venta and colleagues[29] evaluated 236 implants with sonography; surgical confirmation was available in 78, of which 22 (28%) were ruptured. Whether the ruptures were intracapsular or extracapsular was not stated. These investigators found the snowstorm pattern, multiple discontinuous parallel linear echoes, and echodense aggregates in the implant lumen to be statistically associated with rupture. They found that sonography had a sensitivity of 50% and a specificity of 55%.

Although intracapsular rupture may be seen on sonography, the sonographic diagnosis of intracapsular rupture is not reliable. Among ruptured implants examined sonographically, 41% to 55% appear normal.[1,28] Uncollapsed

rupture with minimal separation of the elastomer shell from the fibrous capsule may not be detected by sonography. Furthermore, the interpretation of breast sonography for the purpose of detecting implant rupture has a learning curve.[29]

3.3. Magnetic Resonance Imaging

3.3.1. Magnetic Resonance Imaging Technique

Magnetic resonance imaging has high sensitivity in the diagnosis of intracapsular and extracapsular silicone implant rupture.[3,6,30–34] Magnetic resonance imaging in women with silicone implants is best performed using a dedicated breast coil, with high-resolution techniques.[35] Respiratory motion artifact is minimized by imaging in the prone position, and by phase-encoding in the superoinferior rather than anteroposterior direction.

A variety of sequences have been used in MRI to evaluate silicone gel implant integrity (Table 15.1). High-resolution fast spin echo (FSE) T2-weighted imaging [retention time (TR) 5,700; echo time (TE) 120; slice thickness 3–4 mm; field of view (FOV) 18 cm; 2 number of excitations (NEX)] has been described as fast and accurate in detecting implant rupture, with sensitivities of 95% to 98%.[6,34] Uncollapsed rupture can be subtle even on MRI, with only 50% of leaking implants identified prospectively

FIGURE 15.4. Intracapsular rupture on ultrasound and MRI. This polyurethane-covered silicone implant had been placed 5 years earlier. (A) Ultrasound demonstrates multiple layers of collapsed shell anteriorly (the stepladder sign). (B) Axial fast spin echo (FSE) T2-weighted MRI (TR 5700, TE 126, 5mm slice thickness, 18cm FOV, 2 NEX, 256 × 256 matrix) demonstrates collapsed shell anteriorly (linguine sign). (C) Axial inversion recovery MRI (TR 5700, TE 43, TI 160, 5mm slice thickness, 18cm FOV, 2 NEX, 256 × 128 matrix) also shows the linguine sign of intracapsular rupture. Compared to the FSE T2-weighted image shown in B, this inversion recovery image has lower resolution for the implant's internal structure.

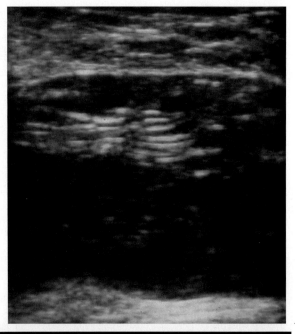

A

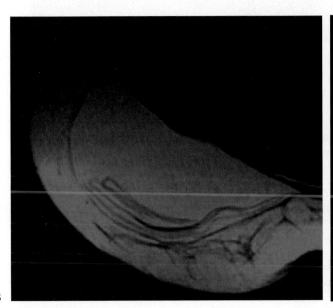

B

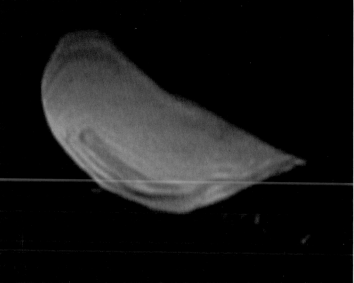

C

on MRI in one series.[34] Some special sequences designed to make the silicone look bright (such as three-point Dixon method or silicone-selective techniques) have diminished spatial resolution, but have also been used in the evaluation of breast implants.[31,36,37]

We suggest that MRI to evaluate for implant rupture should include a localizing sequence and at least three additional sequences (Table 15.2). The high-resolution T2-weighted axial and sagittal sequences, in which the silicone looks bright (isointense to fat) and water looks brighter, provide excellent evaluation of the internal structure of the implant; each of these sequences can be performed in approximately 3 to 4 minutes per breast. The axial inversion recovery (IR) sequence with water saturation is a

"silicone only" sequence in which silicone is bright but fat and water are dark. The IR images provide excellent evaluation for extracapsular silicone, and can be performed in approximately 5 minutes per breast. Hence with this technique, both breasts can be imaged in a total of 25 to 30 minutes at 1.5 Tesla (T).

3.3.2. Magnetic Resonance Imaging of the Normal Implant

On T2-weighted fast-spin echo images, the normal single lumen silicone implant shows high signal internally and is surrounded by a hypointense line that represents the elastomer shell and surrounding fibrous capsule.[8] Radial folds,

TABLE 15.1. MRI Sequences and Resulting Signal Intensities of Silicone, Fat, and Water

Pulse Sequence	Signal Intensity		
	Silicone	Fat	Water
Sagittal T2-weighted FSE (TR 4,000/TE 170)	Medium	Medium	High
Axial T2-weighted FSE with water suppression (TR 5,000/TE 300)	High[a]	Medium	Low
Axial T1-weighted SE with silicone suppression (TR 600/TE 15)[b]	Very low	Low	Medium
Axial IR with water suppression (TR 5700/TE 30/TI 160)	High	Low	Low

Source: Adapted from Gorczyca et al.[30] with permission.
Abbreviations: FSE, fast spin echo; IR, inversion recovery; SE, spin echo; TE, echo time (msec); TI, inversion time (msec); TR, repetition time (msec). TR, TE, and TI at 1.5 T.
[a] Longer echo times, up to 300 msec, will result in higher signal of silicone relative to fat, as in Figure 15.8(A).
[b] In manual prescan mode, the silicone peak can be observed 96 Hz upfield from fat (at 1.5 T). To achieve silicone suppression, the 100 Hz "fat" saturation pulse is applied 150 Hz upfield of the fat peak to avoid overlap with the fat peak and inadvertent suppression of the fat signal.

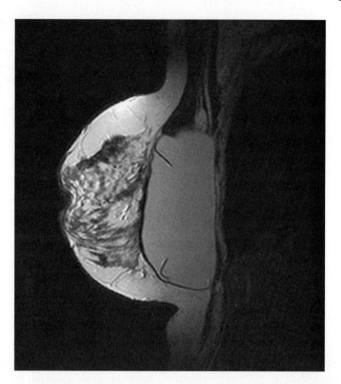

FIGURE 15.5. Magnetic resonance imaging of radial folds. Sagittal T2-weighted image (TR 4000, TE 102.64, slice thickness 3 mm, FOV 24 cm) from MRI in this 61-year-old woman with subpectoral silicone implants demonstrates radial folds, evident as hypointense lines contiguous with the hypointense line surrounding the implant, indicating their connection to the outer shell.

or invaginations of the implant shell, are evident as curvilinear hypointense lines within the implant; paging through sequential slices should demonstrate that these folds are contiguous with the hypointense line surrounding the implant, indicating the connection of these folds to the outer shell (Figure 15.5). Fluid droplets may be seen within the silicone of a single lumen implant, due to injection of saline, betadine, antibiotics, or steroids.[8] A single lumen silicone implant with surrounding reactive fluid can resemble an intact double lumen implant in which the inner lumen is silicone and the outer lumen is saline.[8] Intracapsular fluid tends to be seen more often with textured surface implants, including saline implants.[15]

TABLE 15.2. Sample Protocol to Evaluate Silicone Implants for Possible Rupture

Sequence Name	3-Plane Localizer	Sagittal T2	Axial T2	Axial IR with Water Suppression
Sequence	2D FSPGR	2D FSE	2D FSE	IR
TE (msec)	1.4	120	120	34
TR (msec)	113	5000	5000	5000
TI (msec)	—	—	—	160
Flip angle (degrees)	30	90	90	90
Bandwidth (kHz)	32	16	16	15
Field of view (cm)	48	16–22	16–22	16–22
Slice thickness (mm)	10	4	4	4
Gap (mm)	2.5	1	1	1
Phase encoding steps	128	256	256	192
Frequency steps	256	256	256	256
NEX	1	2	2	2
Frequency direction	Variable	Anterior/posterior	Right/left	Right/left

Abbreviations: FSE, fast spin echo; FSPRG, fast spoiled gradient echo; IR, inversion recovery; NEX, number of excitations; TE, echo time; TI, inversion time; TR, repetition time.

3.3.3. Magnetic Resonance Imaging Signs of Implant Rupture

Several signs may suggest implant rupture on MRI. In the earliest stages of gel leakage, tiny amounts of gel may be seen outside the implant, trapped within folds of the shell. This can create the *inverted teardrop*, *keyhole*, or *noose sign* of uncollapsed rupture[38] (Figure 15.6).[8] With further leakage, a thin layer of gel may be interposed between the shell and the fibrous capsule, evident as the *subcapsular line sign* of minimally collapsed rupture[39] (Figure 15.6). With increasing violation of implant integrity but with the capsule intact, the shell collapses and folds on itself, generating the appearance of stacked hypointense lines within the bright silicone, which has been termed the *linguine sign* of intracapsular rupture[30] (Figure 15.7).

Gross extracapsular rupture is evident as free silicone, separate from the implant, which has extended beyond the implant capsule into the breast or axilla, and may be best seen with silicone-only sequences [such as water-

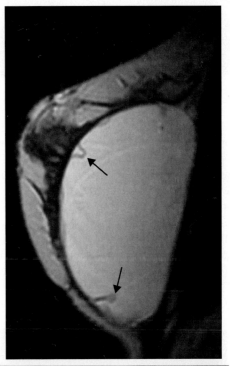

FIGURE 15.6. Leakage/minimally collapsed rupture imaged by MRI in a woman with silicone implants placed 10 years previously. (A) Sagittal fast spin echo T2-weighted MRI (TR 5700, TE 199, 4mm slice thickness) shows the noose sign (arrows). (B) Axial FSE T2-weighted MRI (TR 5700, TE 119, 4mm slice thickness) shows the subcapsular line (curved arrows) and noose (straight arrow) signs. (C) Intraoperative photograph demonstrates the sticky contour of the leaking implant. No gross violation of the implant shell was found at surgery. (From Brown et al.,[1] with permission.)

A

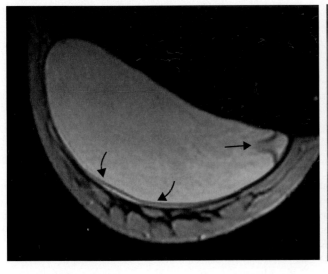

B

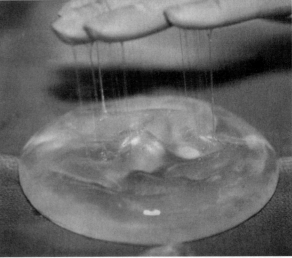

C

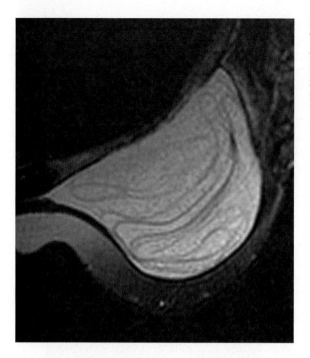

FIGURE 15.7. Magnetic resonance imaging of intracapsular rupture. Axial T2-weighted image with water saturation (TR 4000, TE 117, slice thickness 4mm, FOV 20cm) from MRI in a 60-year-old woman with a history of right mastectomy and reconstruction shows a subpectoral double lumen implant with multiple curvilinear hypointense lines, the linguine sign of intracapsular rupture.

suppressed inversion recovery images with inversion time (TI) = 150–180][40] (Figures 15.8 through 15.10). In a study of implants imaged by MRI and sonography before removal, Berg and colleagues[6] quantified the performance of specific MRI and sonographic criteria for implant rupture (Table 15.3).

Although the MRI signs of implant failure have been defined and illustrated in the literature, their differential diagnosis can be challenging. Normal radial folds, infold-

ings of the elastomer shell, may be mistaken for the linguine sign of intracapsular rupture. The distinction between radial folds and collapsed implant shell can be facilitated by imaging multiple planes and following the course of the hypointense lines in question. Radial folds always connect to the periphery of the implant, while linguine does not. Complex radial folds may present diagnostic dilemmas (Figure 15.11) and are a source of disagreement in MRI interpretation.[39,41]

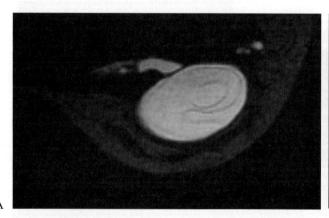

A

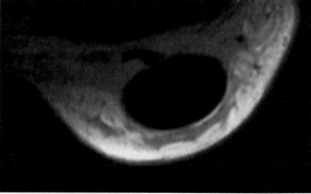

B

FIGURE 15.8. Magnetic resonance imaging of intracapsular and extracapsular rupture. (A) Axial water-suppressed fast spin echo T2-weighted MRI (TR 5200, TE 304, 4mm slice thickness, FOV 20cm) demonstrates collapsed shell and extensive extracapsular silicone. (B) Axial, silicone suppressed T1-weighted MRI (TR 950, TE 11, 4mm slice thickness, FOV 20cm) also demonstrates

the extracapsular silicone. Silicone appears dark on silicone-suppressed images, as does fibrosis. Note that the internal structure of the implant, with its collapsed shell, is better evaluated on the water-suppressed fast spin echo T2-weighted image (A) than on this silicone-suppressed image.

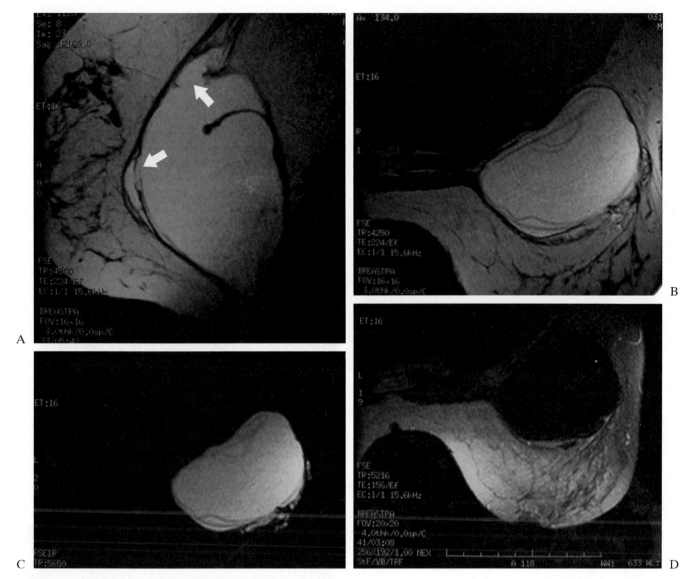

FIGURE 15.9. Magnetic resonance imaging of intracapsular and extracapsular rupture: comparing different sequences. (A) Sagittal, fast spin echo T2-weighted MRI with water saturation (TR 4500, TE 224) shows a subpectoral silicone implant with a radial fold posteriorly. Subtle discontinuities of the capsule are present anteriorly and superiorly (arrows), with silicone extending beyond the capsule at these sites, consistent with extracapsular rupture. (B) Axial, fast spin echo T2-weighted MRI with water saturation (TR 4250, TE 224) shows multiple hypointense lines within the implant, consistent with the "linguine" sign of intracapsular rupture. Subtle hyperintensity is seen anteriorly, representing extracapsular spread of silicone. (C) Axial, fast spin echo inversion recovery MRI with water saturation (TR 5650, TE 156, TI 180) gives an image in which only the silicone is bright. Compared to the FSE T2-weighted image in B, this lower resolution inversion recovery image provides somewhat less optimal depiction of the internal structure of the implant (with the collapsed shell), but better delineation of the extracapsular silicone anterior to the implant. (D) Axial, T2-weighted MRI with silicone saturation (TR 5216, TE 156) shows the hypointense silicone implant and extracapsular silicone. Compared to the sequences illustrated in A through C, this sequence is probably the least helpful in assessing for either intracapsular or extracapsular rupture.

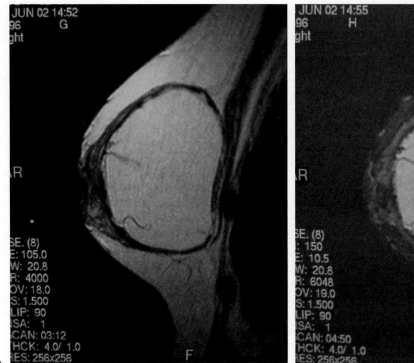

FIGURE 15.10. Magnetic resonance imaging of intracapsular and extracapsular rupture: comparing fast spin echo T2-weighted and inversion recovery images. (A) Sagittal, fast spin echo T2-weighted image (TR 4000, TE 105, FOV 18cm) shows a retroglandular silicone implant, which is approximately isointense to surrounding fat. Note the "noose" sign of intracapsular leakage at the anteroinferior aspect of the implant. (B) Sagittal inversion recovery image (TR 6048, TE 10.5, TI 150) from the same patient shown in A. The noose sign of intracapsular leakage is again - identified. In addition, subtle hyperintensity is noted outside the capsule superiorly and posteriorly, consistent with extracapsular rupture. The extracapsular rupture is better depicted on this sequence (in which the fat is dark) than on the fast spin echo T2 sequence (in which the fat is bright). Extracapsular rupture was found at surgery.

TABLE 15.3. MRI and Ultrasound Criteria for Rupture Versus Surgical Findings

Criteria	Rupture[a] (n = 40) [No. (%)]	Leakage[a] (n = 28) [No. (%)]	Intact[a] (n = 54) [No. (%)]
MRI			
Linguine	29 (72)	4 (14)	2 (4)
Noose	10 (25)	10 (36)	3 (6)
Intact	1 (2)	14 (50)	49 (91)
Extracapsular spread	2 (5)	1 (4)	0 (0)
Fluid in the gel	15 (38)	4 (14)	9 (17)
Ultrasound			
Stepladder	17 (42)	4 (14)	1 (2)
Moderate low-level echoes	9 (22)	3 (11)	9 (17)
Stepladder + moderate low-level echoes	12 (30)	1 (4)	1 (2)
Minimal low-level echoes	9 (22)	8 (28)	11 (20)
Intact	4 (10)	9 (32)	30 (56)
Snowstorm	4 (10)	3 (11)	2 (4)

Source: Adapted from Berg et al.[6] with permission.
[a] At surgery, implants were considered ruptured if there was obvious disruption of the implant shell; leaking if the implant appeared sticky but grossly intact; and intact if there was no evidence of rupture or leak.

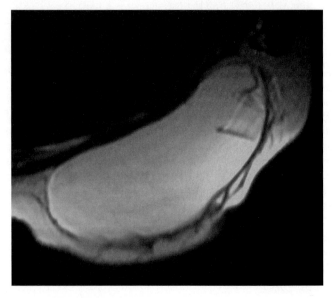

FIGURE 15.11. Magnetic resonance imaging of complex radial fold. Axial, T2-weighted MRI (TR 5700, TE 102, 4mm slice thickness) shows a complex hypointense curvilinear line that was falsely interpreted as the noose sign of leakage. The implant was intact at explantation.

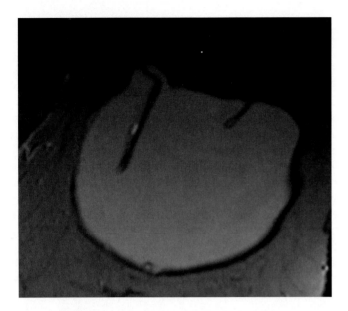

FIGURE 15.12. Magnetic resonance imaging of double lumen implant, minimally collapsed rupture. This axial T2-weighted MRI (TR 5700, TE 126, 4mm slice thickness) demonstrates the noose sign and fluid within the gel.

When there is failure of both lumens of double lumen or expander implants, the shell will be visualized in varying degrees of collapse (Figure 15.12). Provided the saline lumen was intact at the time of rupture, there will be fluid mixing with the gel. Isolated failure of the shell separating lumens will result in fluid mixing with the gel in what has been termed the *salad oil sign* (Figure 15.13), which mimics a single lumen implant that has been injected with saline, betadine, steroids, or antibiotics; there is no known clinical significance to this finding. For standard double lumen implants, isolated outer saline lumen failure mimics an intact silicone implant; this too has no known clinical significance.

3.3.4. Magnetic Resonace Imaging: Results of Prior Studies

In pioneering work, Gorczyca and colleagues[30] evaluated pulse sequences and patient positioning for MRI of silicone breast implants. They evaluated 143 patients with 281 silicone implants using a combination of T2-weighted fast spin echo method, T2-weighted fast spin echo with water suppression, and T1-weighted spin echo with silicone suppression (see Table 15.1). Seventy patients had 140 implants removed; among these 140 implants, surgery showed intracapsular rupture in 19 (14%), extracapsular rupture in 2 (1%), and no rupture in 119 (85%). These authors found that MRI had a sensitivity of 76% and a specificity of 97% in detecting silicone implant rupture and

found that prone positioning improved image quality.[30] The relatively low sensitivity in this early study probably reflects the learning curve.

In a later study, Gorczyca and colleagues[31] compared two different techniques for MRI of breast implants: three-point Dixon and fast spin echo imaging. Eighty-two symptomatic women with silicone implants were examined with both techniques, and 41 had subsequent surgery to remove their implants. Four radiologists reviewed MRI studies from the patients who had surgery and graded the likelihood of rupture on a scale of 1 to 5. Of 81 implants removed, 18 (22%) were ruptured, intracapsular in 16 (20%) and extracapsular in 2 (2%). Ruptures were better identified on the fast spin echo sequence as compared with the three-point Dixon sequence, with areas under the receiver-operator-characteristic (ROC) curve of 0.95 and 0.84, respectively. The sensitivity for detecting silicone implant rupture was 89% for fast spin echo versus 61% for three-point Dixon, although this difference did not achieve statistical significance.

Monticciolo and colleagues[37] evaluated the use of a silicone-selective pulse sequence in detecting implant rupture on MRI, using a 24-cm diameter circular surface coil used for lumbar, shoulder, and cardiac imaging. Twenty-eight patients with 38 implants had silicone selective MRI and surgical removal of the studied implant. All but four also had mammography. Silicone selective MRI, interpreted by two radiologists (individually and then by consensus), showed an intact implant in 21 cases, of which 20 (95%) were intact at surgery. Silicone selective MRI showed leakage in 17 implants, all of which showed leakage at surgery. The sensitivity for detection of leakage

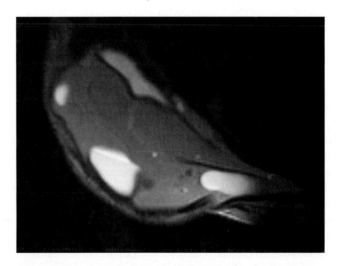

FIGURE 15.13. Salad oil sign of failed inner lumen only of double lumen implant. This axial MRI (fast spin echo T2-weighted sequence, TR 5900, TE 196, 4mm slice thickness, FOV 18cm) shows hyperintense fluid admixed with the silicone gel.

was 94% and the specificity was 100%. In 30 of 34 (88%) cases in which both mammography and MRI were performed, the findings of both studies were in agreement. In the four cases of disagreement, surgical findings agreed with MRI in three and with mammography in one. These authors concluded that the silicone selective sequence was useful for detecting leakage from silicone breast implants.

Brown and colleagues[42] evaluated the prevalence of rupture of silicone gel implants at MRI in a population of unreferred women in Birmingham, Alabama, without regard to the presence or absence of symptoms. A total of 344 women with 687 silicone gel breast implants had MRI. Surgical correlation of implant status is not provided in this study. Rupture was reported by at least two of the three radiologists for 387 (55%) of the 687 implants. Another 50 (7%) implants were rated as indeterminate or suspicious for rupture. Of 344 women in the study, 265 (77%) women had at least one implant considered indeterminate or suspicious for rupture. Radiologists found silicone gel outside the fibrous capsule in 85 of 687 (12%) implants, or in 73 of 344 (21%) women. Rupture was reported more frequently in older implants: The median age of implants reported to be ruptured was 10.8 years [95% confidence interval (CI), 8.4–13.9 y]. Rupture was more common with subpectoral placement, reported in 270 of 408 (66%) subpectoral implants versus 108 of 279 (39%) subglandular implants.

There is interobserver variability in the MRI diagnosis of extracapsular rupture. In a study by Berg and colleagues,[40] three experienced observers reviewed MRI studies from the same population of unreferred women in Birmingham, Alabama,[42] a group of 359 women with current (n = 320), prior (n = 15), or both current and prior (n = 24) silicone gel implants. Axial fast spin echo T2-weighted images with water suppression, axial inversion-recovery T2-weighted images with water suppression, and axial T2-weighted images with silicone suppression were obtained on a 1.5 T magnet with a dedicated phased array breast coil. Surgical correlation of implant status was not available.

In that study, as stated previously, rupture was identified in 265 (77%) women with current silicone implants and in 378 (55%) of 687 implants. Observers agreed in describing extracapsular silicone in 85 (12%) of 687 breasts with current silicone gel implants, of which 81 (95%) showed definite MRI evidence of rupture. One observer reported extracapsular silicone in another 79 breasts. Sources of disagreement included distinction of fibrous capsule bulge from herniation through the capsule (42% of disagreements); poor conspicuity of extracapsular silicone on fast spin echo T2-weighted images with some observer failure to review inversion recovery images (25% of disagreements); subtle findings (22% of disagreements); and technical issues such as ghosting artifacts and failed water suppression of pleural effusion or cysts (11% of disagreements).[40]

A different approach to the evaluation of women with breast implants involves the use of spectroscopy. Pfleiderer and colleagues[43] described spectroscopic evaluation of the liver in 55 women, including 39 with silicone gel implants, 7 women whose implants had been removed, and 9 control subjects without silicone implants. Twenty of 39 (51%) women with implants had ruptured prostheses, as determined by MRI. These investigators found resonances associated with the presence of silicone and partially hydrolyzed silicone in the liver in 27 (69%) women with ruptured implants. The relative signal intensities of silicone species in the liver varied and did not correlate with the status of the implants ($P > 0.7$). Silicone resonances were not detected in the livers of nine control subjects. These data suggest the proton MRI spectra in the liver of women with silicone implants does not correlate with implant status as determined by MRI, but may help measure systemic silicone exposure.

3.4. Implant Rupture: Comparing Imaging Methods

In an animal study, Gorczyca and colleagues[32] at UCLA placed 40 single-lumen silicone implants into 20 rabbits. Each rabbit received one intact and one ruptured implant and was examined with mammography, MRI, ultrasound, and computed tomography (CT). Magnetic resonance imaging was performed with a 1.5 T magnet (Signa, GE Medical Systems, Milwaukee, WI) with a knee coil to image both implants simultaneously. Protocol included axial T1-weighted scout view with Fourier-acquired steady-state technique and gradient recalled acquisition in the steady state (FAST GRASS, GE Medical Systems) (repetition time msec/echo time msec = 9/3) and a flip angle of 30 degrees. A coronal T2-weighted fast spin echo (FSE) sequence (4,000/170; matrix, 256×256; two signals averaged; section thickness, 5 mm) and axial T2-weighted FSE (4,000/170) sequence with water suppression (matrix, 256×256; two signals averaged; section thickness, 5 mm) were used. Five radiologists reviewed all images, and receiver operating characteristic (ROC) analysis was performed. Magnetic resonance imaging and CT were the most accurate modalities in detecting implant ruptures, with areas under the ROC curves of .95 and .91. Mammography and ultrasound were significantly ($P < 0.05$) inferior, with areas under the ROC curves of .77 for each.

Several studies have compared different imaging modalities in the detection of silicone implant rupture in women (Table 15.4).[1,6,33,34,44,45] In these studies of imaging evaluation for implant rupture, mammography had a sensitivity of 11% to 69% and specificity of 82% to 98%; sonography had a sensitivity of 47% to 70% for single lumen implants (as low as 20% for double lumen implants) and specificity of 20% to 92% (with lowest values for double lumen

TABLE 15.4. Studies Comparing Imaging Methods in Detecting Implant Rupture

Study/Year	Mammography			Sonography			MRI		
	N	Sens (%)	Spec (%)	N	Sens (%)	Spec (%)	N	Sens (%)	Spec (%)
Ahn/1994[33a]	51	11	89	57	70	92	55	81	92
Everson/1994[34b]	63	23	98	61	59	79	59	95	93
Reynolds/1994[44c]	24	69	82	24	54	64	24	69	55
Weizer/1995[45d]	NA	NA	NA	143	47	83	160	46	88
Berg/1995[6e]									
Single lumen	NA	NA	NA	122	65	57	122	98	91
Double lumen	NA	NA	NA	22	20	20	22	80	90

Source: Adapted from Brown et al.[1] with permission.
Abbreviations: N, number of implants; NA, not applicable. Sens, sensitivity; Spec, specificity.
[a] MRI technique: body coil, T1- and T2-weighted imaging with fat suppression.
[b] MRI technique: breast coil, T1- and T2-weighted imaging with fat suppression.
[c] MRI technique: shoulder and breast coils, T1-weighted imaging.
[d] MRI technique: body coil compared to breast coil.
[e] MRI technique: breast coil/general purpose coils, some T1 weighting with silicone suppression.

implants); MRI had a sensitivity of 46% to 98% and specificity of 55% to 92% (Table 15.5). The reported time to perform MRI examination to rule out implant rupture ranged from 45 minutes[34] to 2 hours.[44]

Although the studies show varying outcomes, several conclusions can be drawn. First, interpretation of breast MRI studies for the evaluation of implant rupture can be complex and has a learning curve. Second, better results may be obtained with a dedicated breast coil rather than a body coil. Third, because most ruptures are intracapsular, attention should be paid to the specific criteria for intracapsular rupture including the linguine sign, as well as

TABLE 15.5. Cancers in Augmented Breasts: Published Experience

Study/Year	No. Cancers	No. Seen by Mammography	No. Palpable (%)	Histology			Node+ (%)
				Invasive (%)	DCIS (%)	LCIS (%)	
Leibman/ 1990[55]	11	9 (82)[a]	6 (55)	8 (73)	2 (18)	1 (9)	4 (36)
Grace/1990[56]	6	5 (83)[b]	5 (83)	5 (83)	1 (17)	0 (0)	3 (50)
Silverstein/ 1992[49]	42	27 (64)[c]	40 (95)	38 (90)	3 (7)	1 (2)	19 (45)
Carlson/1993[57]	37	17/31 (55)[d]	35 (95)	34 (92)	3 (8)	0 (0)	16 (43)
Birdsell/1993[53]	41	NS[b]	34/36 (94)[e]	34 (83)	7 (17)	0 (0)	16 (39)
Clark/1993[58]	33	23 (70)[f]	23 (70)	29 (88)	4 (12)	0 (0)	6 (18)
Fajardo/1995[59]	18	6 (33)[g]	16 (89)	16 (89)	2 (2)	0 (0)	7 (39)
Cahan/1995[60]	23	NS[h]	19 (83)	19 (83)	4 (17)	0 (0)	7 (30)

Abbreviations: DCIS, ductal carcinoma in situ; LCIS, lobular carcinoma in situ; NS, not stated.
[a] Implant displaced views were performed in 2/11 (18%) cases.
[b] The number of cases in which implant displaced views were performed was not stated.
[c] Implant displaced views were performed in 7/42 (17%) cases. Among these seven cases, the cancer was identified by both implant displaced and standard views in five, by neither in five, and only by standard views in one.
[d] Mammography was performed in 31 cases using standard views only (xeromammography in 27 and film-screen mammography in four).
[e] Among 41 cases, the cancer was identified by routine mammography in 2, by physical examination by the physician in 4, and by the patient in 30. In five cases, there was no information available regarding the method of detection.
[f] Patients were accrued from 1982 to 1991; implant displaced views were used after 1988.
[g] Implant displaced views were used in 12/18 (67%) cases. Among these 12 cases, the cancer was identified on implant displaced views only in 3 and on both standard and implant displaced views in 1; in 2 patients, the cancer was identified only on tangential views to the palpable findings. Among the six patients who had standard views only, none of the cancers were seen by mammography.
[h] Four (17%) of 23 cancers presented as nonpalpable calcifications detected only by mammography.

the signs of uncollapsed rupture such as the subcapsular line sign and noose/keyhole/inverted teardrop appearance of gel outside the shell. Identification of these subtle signs of rupture requires evaluation of multiple images obtained in sagittal and axial planes. Fourth, the use of silicone-only sequences improves the visibility of extracapsular silicone. Finally, the comparative studies taken together suggest that MRI, although more expensive than the other imaging modalities, has higher sensitivity than mammography or sonography in depicting implant rupture (see Table 15.4).

4. Breast Cancer Detection in Women with Implants

Mammography is the primary imaging technique for detecting breast cancer in all women, including women with breast implants. For women with breast implants, as stated, the mammographic examination generally consists of four views of each breast: conventional craniocaudal and mediolateral oblique views, as well as additional Eklund (implant displaced or push-back) craniocaudal and mediolateral oblique views.[22,23] This doubles the radiation dose, and Monsees and Destouet[46] showed that average compression achieved in women with implants was only 7cm compared with 4.5cm in women without implants. Reduced compression increases scatter and radiation dose and decreases fine detail.

Data from phantom studies suggest that implants may impede lesion detection at mammography. Gumucio and colleagues[47] used "artifacts" of specks, fibers, and densities placed in the American College of Radiology (ACR) mammography phantom to simulate calcifications and masses. These authors found that placing the implant shell alone over the phantom minimally altered resolution. However, silicone shells filled with silicone gel, silicone gel and saline, saline alone, polyurethane-covered silicone gel, and gelatin completely obscured all artifacts.[47]

In vivo studies have shown that even with Eklund views, implants obscure some breast tissue. Investigators have found a decrease in the amount of measurable parenchyma on mammograms obtained after as compared with before augmentation, particularly for implants that are placed in front of the muscle. For subglandular implants, studies have shown a decrease in measurable parenchyma of 43% to 49% on standard views and 37% to 39% on Eklund views; for submuscular implants, studies have shown a decrease in measurable parenchyma of 26% to 28% on standard views and 9% to 15% on Eklund views.[48,49] When moderate-to-severe capsular contracture was present, the average decrease in measurable parenchyma was 50%, as compared with 30% in women without contracture.[50]

Breast implants have not been shown to increase the risk of developing breast cancer. Berkel and colleagues[51] studied a cohort of 11,676 women with breast implants. This cohort was compared with the cohort of all 13,557 women in Alberta in whom a first primary breast cancer was diagnosed. These authors found that 41 patients with implants subsequently had breast cancer, as compared with an expected number of 86.2. The standardized incidence ratio was 47.6%, significantly lower than expected ($P < 0.01$). A re-analysis of data from that study found that breast implants did not significantly increase or decrease the risk of breast cancer, regardless of whether an induction period of 0, 5, or 10 years was used for analysis.[52] Birdsell and colleagues[53] found no significant difference in the likelihood of positive lymph nodes, distant metastases, or survival in 41 women with breast cancer who had implants as compared with all other patients with breast cancer. In a retrospective cohort study of 3112 women with breast implants in Los Angeles, Deapen and Brody[54] found that the observed number of cases of breast cancer and of all other cancers combined did not differ significantly from expected numbers based on Los Angeles County Cancer Registry incidence data. These studies have limitations, including lack of subgroup analysis on the basis of risk factors such as family history.[12]

Several studies have specifically examined features of breast cancers detected in women with implants (Table 15.5).[49,53,55–60] In eight studies that included a total of 211 cancers in augmented breasts, the cancer was identified on the mammogram in 62% (range, 33%–83%) and was palpable at diagnosis in 86% (range, 55%–95%). Cancer histology was invasive in 89% (range, 73%–92%), and axillary metastases were present in 37% (range, 18%–50%; Table 15.5). Published studies suggest that there may be a higher false-negative rate for mammography in detecting breast cancer in women with implants as compared with women without implants, and indicate that most cancers in women with augmented breasts were palpable at diagnosis. Implant displaced views were not routinely performed in the studies to date, and these results likely underestimate the sensitivity of mammography in women with implants. Importantly, the stage distribution of cancers in women with implants is similar to screened populations. In limited series evaluating breast cancer survival, no significant difference has been shown between women with and without implants.[52]

Contrast-enhanced MRI may be helpful in depicting breast cancer in women with breast implants[61] (Figure 15.14). The use of intravenous gadolinium may enable MRI visualization of a cancer that is obscured by the implant on the mammogram. Furthermore, the ability to image the posterior tissues of MRI is also helpful. In situations in which abnormality is suspected but not confirmed by mammography, MRI may be useful in problem solving. Furthermore, in women with implants who have proven breast cancer, MRI may be helpful in preoperative assessment of extent of disease.

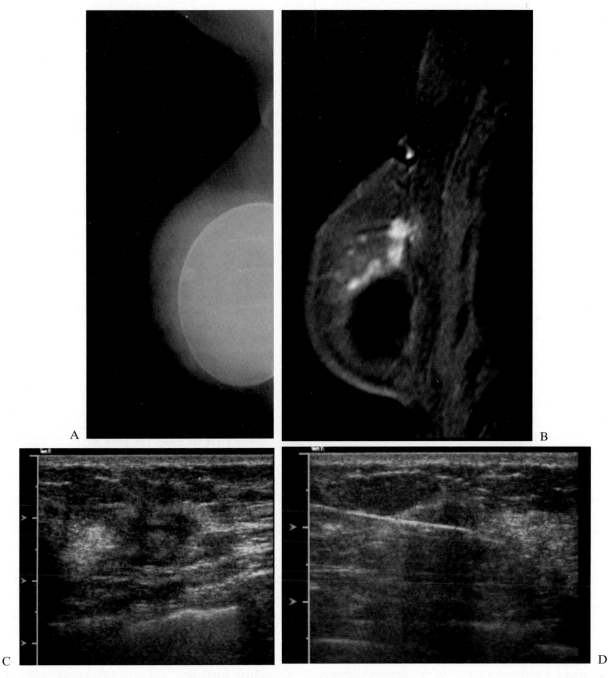

FIGURE 15.14. Magnetic resonance imaging of cancer in 59-year-old woman with breast implants who had a history of left lumpectomy and axillary dissection 5 years previously for invasive lobular carcinoma. (A) Mediolateral oblique view from digital mammogram shows that the left breast is moderately dense with a retroglandular saline implant. No suspicious findings are seen. (B) Sagittal, contrast-enhanced, fat-suppressed T1-weighted image from MRI of the left breast (TR 17, TE 2.276, slice thickness 3 mm, FOV 20 cm) shows extensive suspicious enhancement in the left breast upper outer quadrant, superolateral to the implant. (C) Correlative ultrasound performed after MRI shows an irregular, indistinct mass in the left breast upper outer quadrant. (D) Image from ultrasound-guided core biopsy shows the needle traversing the lesion. Histologic analysis yielded poorly differentiated invasive cancer. Multifocal invasive lobular carcinoma was found at mastectomy.

When planning the protocol for MRI in a woman with breast implants, knowledge of the clinical question is essential. If the MRI is being performed to assess silicone implant integrity, the appropriate examination is a non-contrast study, with use of axial and sagittal images and specific sequences described previously to evaluate the internal structure of the implant and to assess for extravasated silicone. If the MRI is being performed for cancer detection, the appropriate examination is a study optimized for parenchymal breast MRI as discussed in previous chapters, with precontrast and postcontrast images, ideally using fat suppression and subtraction. If the clinician desires both assessment of implant integrity and evaluation for possible cancer (e.g., a vague palpable finding that may or may not be related to the implant), and mammography and sonography are not definitive, it may be necessary to perform MRI sequences designed for implant evaluation as well as those for parenchymal assessment.

If an abnormality occult to mammography is identified at contrast-enhanced MRI in a woman with breast implants, further evaluation can be performed with sonography to determine if the lesion is amenable to sonographically guided localization or sonographically guided biopsy. For MRI-detected lesions that are not identified at sonography, MRI-guided localization or biopsy can be performed for histologic diagnosis. During localization, placement of the needle parallel to the chest wall minimizes the likelihood of puncturing the implant. In MRI-guided vacuum-assisted biopsy, the probe can be placed just posterior to the lesion, and suction applied in the anterior direction (away from the implant). Displacing the implant posteriorly during MRI-guided interventions may also be helpful.

5. Summary and Conclusions

Existing data support the utility of MRI in evaluating women with breast implants. Noncontrast MRI, using multiple planes and employing sequences designed to evaluate the internal structure of the implant and to assess for extracapsular silicone, is the most sensitive imaging modality available to assess for silicone implant rupture. Although mammography remains the standard of care for breast cancer detection, contrast-enhanced MRI may assist in depicting cancer in augmented breasts: the use of intravenous contrast and ability to image posterior tissues are particularly valuable in women in whom mammography is compromised by the presence of implants. Additional analysis of the cost-effectiveness of breast MRI in assessing implant integrity is necessary. Furthermore, the role of MRI in screening asymptomatic women with breast implants either for implant rupture or for breast cancer remains to be determined.

References

1. Brown SL, Silverman BG, Berg WA. Rupture of silicone-gel breast implants: causes, sequelae, and diagnosis. *Lancet* 1997; 350:1531–1537.
2. Ganott MA, Harris KM, Ilkhanipous ZS, Costa-Greco MA. Augmentation mammoplasty: normal and abnormal findings with mammography and US. *Radiographics* 1992;12:281–295.
3. Berg WA, Caskey CI, Hamper UM, et al. Diagnosing breast implant rupture with MR imaging, US, and mammography. *Radiographics* 1993;13:1323–1336.
4. Caskey CI, Berg WA, Hamper U, et al. Imaging spectrum of extracapsular silicone: correlation of US, MR imaging, mammographic, and histopathologic findings. *Radiographics* 1999;19:S39–S51.
5. LeVier RR, Harrison MC, Cook RR, Lane TH. What is silicone? *Plast Reconstr Surg*. 1993;92:163–167.
6. Berg WA, Caskey CI, Hamper UM, et al. Single- and double-lumen silicone breast implant integrity: prospective evaluation of MR and US criteria. *Radiology* 1995;197:45–52.
7. Brinton LA, Toniolo P, Pasternack BS. Epidemiologic follow-up studies of breast augmentation patients. *J Clin Epidemiol*. 1995;48:557–563.
8. Berg WA, Anderson ND, Zerhouni EA, et al. MR imaging of the breast in patients with silicone breast implants: normal postoperative variants and diagnostic pitfalls. *AJR Am J Roentgenol*. 1994;163:575–578.
9. Kessler DA. The basis of the FDA's decision on breast implants. *N Engl J Med*. 1992;326:1713–1715.
10. Kolata G. FDA defers final decision about implants. *The New York Times*. January 9, 2004:A1.
11. Dowden RV. Definition of terms for describing loss of gel from breast implants. *AJR Am J Roentgenol*. 1993;160: 1360.
12. Silverman BG, Brown SL, Bright RA, et al. Reported complications of silicone gel breast implants: an epidemiologic review. *Ann Intern Med*. 1996;124:744–756.
13. Destouet JM, Monsees BS, Oser RF, et al. Screening mammography in 350 women with breast implants: prevalence and findings of implant complications. *AJR Am J Roentgenol*. 1992;159:973–978.
14. Fenske NA. Silicone-associated connective-tissue disease: the debate rages. *Arch Dermatol*. 1993;129:97–98.
15. Ahn CY, Ko CY, Wagar EA, et al. Clinical significance of intracapsular fluid in patients' breast implants. *Ann Plast Surg*. 1995;35:455–457.
16. Anderson B, Hawtof D, Alani H, Kapetansky D. The diagnosis of ruptured breast implants. *Plast Reconstr Surg*. 1989;84:903–907.
17. de Camara DL, Sheridan JM, Kammer BA. Ruptures and aging of silicone gel breast implants. *Plast Reconstr Surg*. 1993;91:828–834.
18. Robinson OG, Bradley EL, Wilson DS. Analysis of explanted silicone implants: a report of 300 patients. *Ann Plast Surg*. 1995;34:1–7.
19. van Rappard JHA, Sonneveld GJ, van Twisk R, Borghouts JMHM. Pressure resistance of breast implants as a function of implantation time. *Ann Plast Surg*. 1988;21:566–569.
20. Phillips JW, de Camara DL, Lockwood MD, Grebner WCC. Strength of silicone breast implants. *Plast Reconstr Surg*. 1996;97:1215–1225.
21. Greenwald DP, Randolph M, May JW Jr. Mechanical analysis of explanted silicone breast implants. *Plast Reconstr Surg*. 1996;98:269–275.
22. Eklund GW, Busby RC, Miller SH, Job JS. Improved imaging of the augmented breast. *AJR Am J Roentgenol*. 1988;151: 469–473.
23. American College of Radiology. ACR practice guideline for the performance of diagnostic mammography. In: *Practice*

Guidelines and Technical Standards 2004. Reston, VA: American College of Radiology (ACR); 2004:257–261.

24. Dershaw DD, Chaglassian TA. Mammography after prosthesis placement for augmentation or reconstructive mammoplasty. *Radiology* 1989;170:69–74.

25. Harris KM, Ganott MA, Shestak KC, et al. Silicone implant rupture: detection with US. *Radiology* 1993;187:761–768.

26. Rosculet KA, Ikeda DM, Forrest ME, et al. Ruptured gel-filled silicone breast implants: sonographic findings in 19 cases. *AJR Am J Roentgenol.* 1992;159:711–716.

27. DeBruhl ND, Gorczyca D, Ahn CY, et al. Silicone breast implants: US evaluation. *Radiology* 1993;189:95–98.

28. Caskey CI, Berg WA, Anderson ND, et al. Breast implant rupture: diagnosis with US. *Radiology* 1994;190:819–823.

29. Venta LA, Salomon CG, Flisak ME, et al. Sonographic signs of breast implant rupture. *AJR Am J Roentgenol.* 1996;166: 1413–1419.

30. Gorczyca DP, Sinha S, Ahn CY, et al. Silicone breast implants in vivo: MR imaging. *Radiology* 1992;185:407–410.

31. Gorczyca DP, Schneider E, DeBruhl ND, et al. Silicone breast implant rupture: comparison between three-point Dixon and fast spin-echo MR imaging. *AJR Am J Roentgenol.* 1994; 162:305–310.

32. Gorczyca DP, DeBruhl ND, Ahn CY, et al. Silicone breast implant ruptures in an animal model: comparison of mammography, MR imaging, US and CT. *Radiology* 1994;190: 227–232.

33. Ahn CY, DeBruhl ND, Gorczyca DP, et al. Comparative silicone breast implant evaluation using mammography, sonography, and magnetic resonance imaging: experience with 59 implants. *Plast Reconstr Surg.* 1994;94:620–627.

34. Everson LI, Parantainen H, Detlie T, et al. Diagnosis of implant rupture: imaging findings and relative efficacies of imaging techniques. *AJR Am J Roentgenol.* 1994;163:57–60.

35. American College of Radiology. ACR practice guideline for the performance of magnetic resonance imaging (MRI) of the breast. In: *Practice Guidelines and Technical Standards 2004.* Reston, VA: American College of Radiology (ACR); 2004:269–274.

36. Glover GH, Schneider E. Three-point Dixon technique for true water/fat decomposition with Bo inhomogeneity correction. *Magn Reson Imaging Med.* 1991;18:371–393.

37. Monticciolo DL, Nelson RC, Dixon WT, et al. MR detection of leakage from silicone breast implants: value of a silicone-selective pulse sequence. *AJR Am J Roentgenol.* 1994;163: 51–56.

38. Mund DF, Farria DM, Gorczyca DP, et al. MR imaging of the breast in patients with silicone-gel implants: spectrum of findings. *AJR Am J Roentgenol.* 1993;161:773–778.

39. Soo MS, Kornguth PJ, Walsh R, et al. Complex radial folds versus subtle signs of intracapsular rupture of breast implants: MR findings with surgical correlation. *AJR Am J Roentgenol.* 1996;166:1421–1427.

40. Berg WA, Nguyen TK, Middleton MS, et al. MR imaging of extracapsular silicone from breast implants: diagnostic pitfalls. *AJR Am J Roentgenol.* 2002;178:465–472.

41. Soo MS, Kornguth PJ, Walsh R, et al. Intracapsular implant rupture: MR findings of incomplete shell collapse. *J Magn Reson Imaging.* 1997;7:724–730.

42. Brown SL, Middleton MS, Berg WA, et al. Prevalence of rupture of silicone gel breast implants revealed on MR imaging in a population of women in Birmingham, Alabama. *AJR Am J Roentgenol.* 2000;175:1057–1064.

43. Pfleiderer B, Campbell T, Hulka CA, et al. Silicone gel-filled breast implants in women: findings at H-1 MR spectroscopy. *Radiology* 1996;201:777–783.

44. Reynolds HE, Buckwalter KA, Jackson VP, et al. Comparison of mammography, sonography, and magnetic resonance imaging in the detection of silicone-gel breast implant rupture. *Ann Plast Surg.* 1994;33:247–257.

45. Weizer G, Malone RS, Netscher DT, et al. Utility of magnetic resonance imaging and ultrasonography in diagnosing breast implant rupture. *Ann Plast Surg.* 1995;34:352–361.

46. Monsees BS, Destouet JM. Mammography in aesthetic and reconstructive breast surgery. *Perspect Plast Surg.* 1991;5: 103–119.

47. Gumucio CA, Pin P, Young WL, et al. The effect of breast implants on the radiographic detection of microcalcification and soft-tissue masses. *Plast Reconstr Surg.* 1989;84:772–778.

48. Silverstein MJ, Handel N, Gamagami P, et al. Mammographic measurements before and after augmentation mammaplasty. *Plast Reconstr Surg.* 1990;86:1126–1130.

49. Silverstein MJ, Handel N, Gamagami P, et al. Breast cancer diagnosis and prognosis in women following augmentation with silicone gel-filled prostheses. *Eur J Cancer.* 1992;28:635–640.

50. Handel N, Silverstein MJ, Gamagami P, et al. Factors affecting mammographic visualization of the breast after augmentation mammaplasty. *JAMA.* 1992;268:1913–1917.

51. Berkel H, Birdsell DC, Jenkins H. Breast augmentation: a risk factor for breast cancer? *N Engl J Med.* 1992;326: 1649–1653.

52. Bryant H, Brasher P. Breast implants and breast cancer-reanalysis of a linkage study. *N Engl J Med.* 1995;332: 1535–1539.

53. Birdsell DC, Jenkins H, Berkel H. Breast cancer diagnosis and survival in women with and without breast implants. *Plast Reconstr Surg.* 1993;92:795–800.

54. Deapen DM, Brody GS. Augmentation mammoplasty and breast cancer: a 5-year update of the Los Angeles study. *Plast Reconstr Surg.* 1992;89:660–665.

55. Leibman AJ, Kruse B. Breast cancer: mammographic and sonographic findings after augmentation mammoplasty. *Radiology* 1990;174:195–198.

56. Grace GT, Roberts C, Cohen IK. The role of mammography in detecting breast cancer in augmented breasts. *Ann Plast Surg.* 1990;25:119–123.

57. Carlson GW, Curley SA, Martin JE, et al. The detection of breast cancer after augmentation mammoplasty. *Plast Reconstr Surg.* 1993;91:837–840.

58. Clark CPI, Peters GN, O'Brien KM. Cancer in the augmented breast: diagnosis and prognosis. *Cancer* 1993;72: 2170–2174.

59. Fajardo LL, Harvey JA, McAleese KA, et al. Breast cancer diagnosis in women with subglandular silicone gel-filled augmentation implants. *Radiology* 1995;194:859–862.

60. Cahan AC, Ashikari R, Pressman P, et al. Breast cancer after breast augmentation with silicone implants. *Ann Surg Oncol.* 1995;2:121–125.

61. Huch RA, Kunzi W, Debatin JF, et al. MR imaging of the augmented breast. *Eur Radiol.* 1998;8:371–376.

16
Magnetic Resonance Imaging as a Clinical Tool

D. David Dershaw

The use of breast magnetic resonance imaging (MRI) in clinical practice is evolving. With increasing clinical experience and equipment availability, clinical applications for breast MRI have increased. The usefulness of this technology in any individual practice depends on the comfort of breast imagers in interpreting these studies, the availability of magnet time and MRI-compatible biopsy equipment, clinical issues in the patient population, as well as the desire of referring physicians for MRI assessment of possible breast disease. The uses of MRI in a variety of clinical situations listed in this chapter are suggestions of the possible applications of MRI. The appropriateness of these suggested uses will vary with different practices and as clinical experience increases.

In many practices the use of MRI to address breast problems is limited by the lack of available technology. Without MRI-compatible equipment for localization and/or biopsy, more clinical issues can be raised by searching for nonpalpable disease than might be answered. Just as with mammographic and sonographic findings in breast imaging, the radiologist should always remember that MRI findings require histologic (or cytologic) diagnosis before they can be clinically applied. The detection of these lesions requires biopsy confirmation before they can be diagnosed as malignant. Therefore, the search for nonpalpable disease that cannot be localized should be approached with caution.

As with mammographic imaging, the comparison of patterns in the two breasts is often important in differentiating normal from abnormal patterns. Most importantly, diffuse enhancement can be due to normal parenchyma or extensive carcinoma. Comparison with the normal breast makes this differentiation easy; without the opposite breast for comparison, the diagnosis cannot be made. Because of this, facilities performing breast MRI need to be able to image both breasts. Because this is most conveniently done for the patient in a single examination, facilities should attempt to image both breasts during the same study. The need to return a second day for imaging the second breast should be eliminated from the scanning protocol, if possible.

With these considerations in mind, it should be easiest for breast imaging facilities to include MRI in situations in which there is a known site of disease in the breast. These situations include palpable lesions, residual disease at the lumpectomy site, further evaluation of abnormalities seen on other imaging studies, and response to treatment of known breast carcinoma. Magnetic resonance imaging can also be useful in the work up of women with a suspicious discharge from a single duct and those with Paget's disease of the nipple. Other potential uses of MRI include search for unknown primary in women with axillary nodal metastases, search for multicentric disease in women contemplating breast conservation, and breast cancer screening. Magnetic resonance imaging is also useful in the evaluation of silicone gel implants. This chapter provides an overview of clinical uses of breast MRI, with many of the specific scenarios discussed in more detail in other chapters.

1. The Augmented Breast

Evaluation of possible ruptured silicone implant is best done with MRI.[1-4] The implant is studied without the injection of contrast material, and sequences are used to image silicone separately from fat and water. Because of the higher sensitivity and specificity of MRI versus sonography or mammography in evaluating silicone implant complications, questionable cases of rupture should be confirmed with MRI before patients are sent for implant removal. In many facilities, MRI is used as the initial imaging technique for the work up of women with possible implant complication. The radiologist should be aware that false-positive and false-negative results with MRI of silicone implants do occur.[4] Also, although it can be diagnosed with MRI, the clinical importance of intracapsular rupture is controversial, as is the significance of silicone gel bleed. However, MRI is the best technology for diagnosing intracapsular rupture. Additionally, MRI has the advantage of routinely imaging behind the implant, an area that is blind to mammography and often not seen with sonography. In cases in which silicone is extravasated deep to the implant, this finding may only be seen with MRI.

The evaluation of silicone implant complication can be compromised by multilumen implants that can mimic rupture of single-lumen implants.[3] Before evaluation with MRI, it is often useful to determine the implant type and configuration using mammography, if this information is unknown.

Magnetic resonance imaging can be useful in the evaluation of parenchymal breast disease in augmented breasts when the mammogram is compromised by the implant. These studies require intravenous contrast and are performed in a fashion identical to MRI of nonaugmented breasts. The same principles apply in the interpretation of these studies as to those in nonaugmented breasts. Whether there is an advantage to MRI over sonography in the work up of possible breast carcinoma, especially invasive carcinoma, in women with augmented breasts is unknown. Certainly, palpable lesions in these women are more easily addressed with sonography.

Saline-filled implants do not require special study with MRI. Saline is physiologic, and when saline implants rupture, extravasated saline is absorbed by the body.

Women who have been augmented with the injection of free silicone into the breast may have parenchymal disease that is better imaged by MRI than mammography. However, there is limited experience for MRI in these women, and its role as an adjunct to mammography in this population has not been determined.

As with other breast interventions, MRI interventional procedures can be performed on women with breast augmentation. Displacement of the implant away from the site to be localized or biopsied may be helpful. In obtaining consent for these procedures, the patient should be advised of the possibility of implant rupture.

2. Lesion Characterization

Multiple authors have addressed the difficulties of lesion characterization using MRI findings.[6–15] Data suggest that MRI is more reliable in excluding carcinoma than in making a definitive diagnosis of malignancy. Because breast cancers and other malignant breast tumors usually stimulate the growth of tumor neovascularity that enhances with MRI contrast, absence of an enhancing lesion is highly reliable in excluding most cancers. However, the presence of enhancement is a nonspecific finding. It is also associated with normal breast tissue, fibrocystic disease, hormonal stimulation, hyperplasia, dysplasia, atypia, and inflammatory processes. Spatial and temporal patterns of enhancement have been suggested as being useful in differentiating enhancement due to different etiologies. The reliability of these patterns in diagnosis is somewhat controversial. As with other breast imaging techniques, definitive diagnosis usually requires tissue sampling.

The use of MRI for lesion characterization can be basically divided into two situations: lesions found with other techniques for which MRI is used to refine diagnostic considerations, and lesions initially found on MRI for which the MRI pattern is used to limit diagnostic considerations.

2.1. Magnetic Resonance Imaging Characterization of Mammographic and Sonographic Lesions

In some select situations, the addition of MRI to mammographic (or sonographic) imaging can add important information. Magnetic resonance imaging is generally not useful in differentiating benign from malignant disease at a solitary, suspicious site found on mammography. Not only is a definite diagnosis often not obtained, but the cost of MRI is comparable with that of core needle biopsy, which is often capable of making a definitive diagnosis.[5]

Using enhancement as a positive finding, Lee and colleagues[6] looked at 86 mammographic lesions with MRI. All enhancing lesions were biopsied, and 35% were malignant. All nonenhancing sites were benign on biopsy or follow up. Magnetic resonance imaging was found to be useful in localizing lesions that were seen only on a single mammographic view or were difficult to target during attempted biopsy. It was also useful in assessing whether ambiguous mammographic lesions were real and in differentiating scar from recurrent tumor after breast conservation. Sonographic assessment of 47 of these lesions showed a solid, hypoechoic mass in six. Among these six, MRI showed enhancement in one; all six were benign on biopsy.

In using MRI time-intensity curves to try to further characterize mammographically discovered lesions, Stomper and colleagues[7] reported that a two-fold or greater increase in signal intensity above the preenhanced signal intensity of the lesion was found in all 22 invasive cancers studied, but this had a specificity of only 65% in this patient population. They also found that time-intensity curves were not useful in differentiating benign from malignant lesions. Among these women, one had a 4-cm comedo ductal carcinoma in situ (DCIS) with microinvasion and another had a 6 cm pure comedo DCIS, both of which did not enhance on MRI; both of these presented mammographically as microcalcifications. The geometric pattern of enhancement had some correlation with histology among these patients. All with well-defined lesions on mammography and MRI that showed uniform enhancement were benign. Poorly defined, nonuniform, or peripheral enhancement was usually associated with carcinomas. However, in this study only one third of studied lesions were benign, limiting the experience in this study with benign patterns.

The characterization of benign lesions has been difficult with MRI. This may be particularly true for fibroadenomas. In one study 20% of 19 fibroadenomas had features that overlapped with those of invasive cancers on MRI.[8] In another study, there was no difference in the time-intensity enhancement patterns of fibroadenomas versus carcinomas.[9] Rim enhancement, a pattern considered highly suspicious for carcinoma, has been reported in fibrocystic disease, intraductal papilloma, ductal adenoma, and benign and malignant phyllodes tumors.[10] Confusing MRI patterns that could not be differentiated from malignancy have also been reported with lymph nodes and normal breast tissue, resulting in a specificity for breast MRI comparable with that for mammography.[11] Similar experience has been reported by others.[12,13]

As suggested previously, the use of MRI for the determination of the significance of mammographically evident microcalcifications is not of great value. As previously noted, some areas of DCIS with or without microinvasion that are clearly evident on mammography as microcalcifications may not enhance on MRI.[7] In a study of MRI findings in 62 women with microcalcifications, of which 38 were associated with malignancy and 24 with benign processes, MRI had an overall accuracy of 56%.[14] Other groups of women have also been reported to present problems in differentiating benign from malignant tissue at MRI. Fibrocystic alteration, for example, may have suspicious patterns on MRI, requiring biopsy to make the distinction from carcinoma.[14,15]

In adding MRI to the work up of a woman with an abnormal mammogram, sonogram, or physical examination, the following should be kept in mind. Magnetic resonance imaging is not reliable in differentiating benign from malignant suspicious calcifications seen on mammography. Lack of enhancement of an area of microcalcifications that is mammographically suspicious does not exclude carcinoma. Magnetic resonance imaging is not accurate in differentiating benign from malignant enhancing lesions. Therefore, biopsy is necessary if this differentiation needs to be made. When lesions are questionable or only evident on one mammographic view, MRI can be useful to localize the lesion or determine if it is due to a possible carcinoma. Solid, sonographic masses that do not enhance on MRI are rarely malignant. However, there are not adequate data to permit these lesions to be ignored; short-term follow up may be an alternative to biopsy for these lesions, but further study addressing this issue is needed. Finally, MRI is not cost effective in replacing core biopsy for definitive analysis of mammographic or sonographic lesions. If a definitive diagnosis of a lesion is required, MRI should not be used to replace core biopsy.

2.2. Management of Lesions Initially Discovered on Magnetic Resonance Imaging

Lesions are commonly found on MRI that are not evident on other imaging studies or on physical examination. Those who perform MRI must be prepared to determine the clinical significance of these findings. The frequency of the discovery of these lesions is demonstrated in data from one study in which 12 incidental enhancing lesions were found during the MRI assessment of 26 mammographic lesions.[6] In another study, 100 lesions found on MRI that required biopsy were discovered on scans done for evaluation of high-risk patients in 41 cases, extent of disease in patients with synchronous cancer in 38 cases, and incidental findings on women being assessed for other breast problems in 21 cases.[16] Still another study reported the discovery of suspicious lesions in the contralateral breast in 29% of 17 women being scanned to assess a known breast carcinoma.[17] Yet another study also reported incidental enhancing lesion in 29% of 103 women.[18] Based on the experience of multiple investigators, it is reasonable to assume that the discovery of these lesions will not be unusual when performing breast MRI. Approaches to MRI-detected lesions include mammographic review, short-term follow up MRI, sonography, and biopsy.

Because of limited experience, data comparable with that available for mammographic lesions are not available to support algorithms including short-term follow up for MRI-detected lesions. One can hypothesize that lesions that are well defined, round or oval, multiple, and bilateral may be dismissed as innocent or followed with a 6-month follow-up MRI, but further study is needed to validate this approach. Lesions having classic patterns of fibroadenomas or lymph nodes can be dealt with in a similar fashion. Some lesions that are solitary and unilateral warrant tissue diagnosis. Findings of irregular shape, spiculation, or rim enhancement in mass lesions, and findings of segmental or clumped linear and ductal enhancement in nonmass lesions are suspicious and may require biopsy.[16,19,20] Some would also include time-enhancement curve patterns in defining lesions requiring biopsy, but this is less widely accepted.

For those lesions requiring biopsy, preoperative localization or imaging-guided tissue sampling frequently must performed. Facilities with the capability to perform MRI-guided breast intervention can perform biopsy using these procedures, if the lesion is not evident by any other technique. Facilities without this capability should ponder how these women will be managed before they initiate a breast MRI program.

The ability to correlate an MRI lesion with a lesion on mammography or sonography obviates the need for MRI-guided intervention. It will frequently be possible to find these lesions with other imaging techniques. In a series from Yale, 12 sites were found unexpectedly on MRI for assessment of other lesions.[6] Of these 12, correlation with the mammogram showed mass in 2 and no mammographic correlate in 10. Of the two with mammographic correlates, one mass was stable and consistent with fibroadenoma; the second was a missed neodensity that was malignant on biopsy. Sonography, performed in 8 of the 10 not mammographically evident, showed a solid mass in 1 that was benign on biopsy. Another seven were thought to be probably benign; follow up for 6 to 21 months has shown no change in any of these. Two lesions needed biopsy and could not be found with sonography or mammography; MRI-guided biopsy was required. In the Massachusetts General Hospital series of women with contralateral breast cancers, lesions that could not be found with mammography or sonography were all identified with contrast-enhanced computed tomography (CT) and were localized under CT guidance.[17] In our own patients, among 93 lesions that were suspicious on MRI and assessed as possibly identifiable on sonography, only 21 (23%) could be identified on the MRI-directed sonogram.[21] Interestingly, of the 21 MRI lesions with sonographic correlates, 7 (43%) were malignant. In contrast, only 10 of 42 (14%) MRI lesions without a sonographic correlate were malignant, one third the malignancy rate of those seen sonographically.

When searching for the sonographic correlate of an MRI-detected lesion, several things must be kept in mind. First, the ability to identify a sonographic correlate for MRI-detected lesions has varied in the literature from 23% at our institution[21] to 80% to 100% in other reports.[22,23] Second, failure to identify a sonographic correlate does not spare the need for biopsy.[21] Third, patient positioning is different for sonography and breast MRI. Therefore, the quadrant in which the lesion is identified on MRI may differ from the quadrant in which the same lesion appears on ultrasound examination. Finally, caution must be taken in identifying the sonographic correlate. If a sonographic lesion is thought to correlate to the MRI finding, but results of ultrasound-guided biopsy do not seem sufficient to account for the MRI lesion, then biopsy under the guidance of MRI may be prudent.

The published experience with unexpected, enhancing foci found on breast MRI studies suggests that they can be managed in the following fashion. Those that are probably benign may be reassessed with short-term follow-up MRI. Of those thought to require biopsy, an attempt should be made to correlate them with a mammographic finding; if this is stable or obviously benign, biopsy can be avoided. Otherwise, stereotactic biopsy or mammographic preoperative wire localization can be performed. Directed sonography may be performed to determine if the lesion can be seen with sonography. If the lesion is sonographically evident, sonographically guided core biopsy or localization can be performed (Figure 16.1). Lesions requiring biopsy that are nonpalpable and neither mammographically nor sonographically evident would be best evaluated by biopsy (preoperative needle localization or needle biopsy) under MRI guidance.

3. Breast Conservation: Staging Tumor and Detecting Recurrence

The success of breast conservation is partially dependent on removal of as much cancer as possible. The larger the amount of cancer left in the breast after surgery, the more likely that tumor will recur after radiation. Preoperative staging of cancers can replace the use of multiple re-excisions to determine extent of cancer in the breast. For women with positive margins at the time of their original lumpectomy, staging the extent of residual disease can be useful in determining if residual tumor volume is too great to permit conservation and requires mastectomy. In those women for whom conservation is appropriate, it is useful in guiding the surgeon in complete removal of residual carcinoma.

Although mammography is an excellent tool at identifying breasts that contain carcinoma, it often underestimates the extent of disease within the breast. For women contemplating lumpectomy and in whom the mammogram and physical examination indicate that tumor is small enough for conservation to be used, further evaluation with additional imaging can demonstrate more extensive tumor than previously suspected. This can be helpful in accurately planning the amount of tissue to be included in the lumpectomy or in suggesting the need for mastectomy.

Among mammography, sonography, and MRI, MRI has been demonstrated to be the most sensitive in determining the extent of tumor in the breast. In 104 women with suspected breast cancer at Guttenberg University Hospital, 27 cancers were found to be multicentric or multifocal.[24] Among these, mammography correctly diagnosed 48%; sonography with mammography correctly diagnosed 63%, and MRI with mammography correctly diagnosed 81%. In another study done 7 years earlier,[25] 61 breast cancers were evaluated by all three modalities. The index lesion was missed by mammography in 10%, sonography in 15%, and MRI in 2%. The single cancer missed by MRI was DCIS. Tumor size was underestimated on mammography in 14%, sonography in 18%, and in no cases by MRI. Of additional invasive lesions present, mammography showed 31%, sonography showed 38%, and MRI showed 100% (Figure 16.2).

Invasive lobular carcinoma (ILC) is notoriously difficult to detect by either physical examination or mammography. Studies have suggested that when this diagnosis is made, staging of the extent of ILC by MRI preoperatively may be valuable. In a study at the University of Pennsylvania of 32 women with ILC, MRI showed more extensive tumor

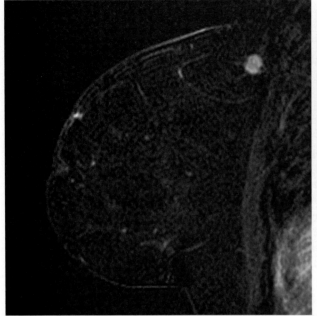

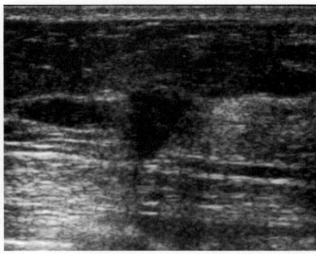

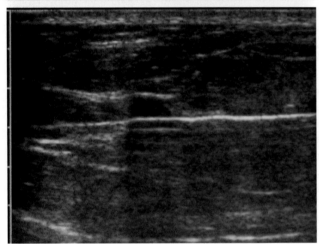

FIGURE 16.1. A 57-year-old woman 1 month status post left upper outer quadrant lumpectomy yielding moderately differentiated invasive ductal carcinoma, 1.1 cm, and ductal carcinoma in situ, with close margins. Postoperative mammogram (not shown) revealed moderately dense, nodular breasts with postoperative changes in the left upper outer quadrant from the recent lumpectomy. (A) Sagittal, T1-weighted, contrast-enhanced, subtraction MRI study shows 0.8 cm irregularly shaped, irregularly marginated, heterogeneously enhancing mass in the left upper inner quadrant posteriorly, suspicious for carcinoma. (B) Ultrasound of the left breast shows a 0.9 cm hypoechoic mass that is taller than wide in the left breast upper inner quadrant 11 o'clock axis, correlating with the MRI finding. (C) This image obtained during ultrasound-guided 14-gauge automated core biopsy shows the needle traversing the lesion. Histologic analysis yielded invasive ductal carcinoma and DCIS. This proved the presence of multicentric disease, for which the patient underwent mastectomy.

than mammography or sonography and altered the clinical management in 16 (50%).[26] In 13 cases of ILC examined by MRI at University of California San Francisco, only 4 were found to be a solitary mass.[27] Six had enhancing strands; two had multicentric or multifocal disease; and in one case enhancing septations in the breast on MRI were found to contain tumor cells on pathology.

The experience of MRI with DCIS is more confusing, and the utility of MRI in the diagnosis of DCIS is more controversial. When DCIS forms mammographically evident microcalcifications, mammography is the most reliable technique of detecting this disease. However, in some cases of DCIS and in some areas of those breasts in which DCIS has calcified, uncalcified DCIS can be present. This

may not be evident by sonography or mammography. Magnetic resonance imaging has been shown by some to be able to detect at least some of this disease. Whether MRI is a useful tool in the determination of the extent of DCIS in all cases is unclear. However, in women with positive lumpectomy margins and without residual tumor calcifications in their breast, MRI can be useful in determining the extent of residual disease.[28] This is true for invasive as well as in situ disease.

In women with possible recurrence of tumor in the treated breast after conservation, MRI can be helpful in differentiating avascular, nonenhancing scar, and fat necrosis from enhancing recurrent tumor.[29,30] Because the lumpectomy bed can contain vascular granulation tissue

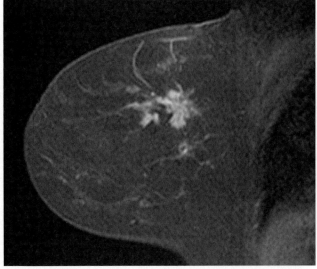
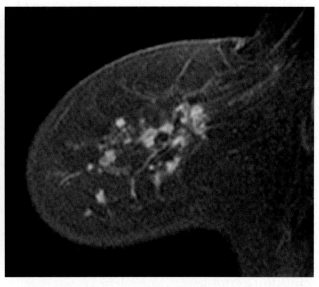

A

B

FIGURE 16.2. A 42-year-old woman with palpable mass in the right breast upper outer quadrant. Mammogram (not shown) revealed a spiculated mass at this site. Core biopsy showed invasive ductal carcinoma and DCIS. (A) Sagittal, T1-weighted, contrast-enhanced MRI shows spiculated, irregular, heterogeneously enhancing mass right upper outer quadrant consistent with biopsy-proven cancer. (B) Sagittal, T1-weighted, contrast-enhanced MRI shows segmental clumped enhancement extending from index cancer anteriorly and inferiorly toward nipple. Subsequent surgery showed invasive mammary carcinoma with mixed ductal and lobular features and ductal carcinoma in situ. The patient underwent mastectomy.

up to 9 to 18 months after treatment, MRI is only useful in these women after this time. However, recurrences are extremely rare earlier than 18 to 24 months posttreatment, so that this does not usually present a problem.[31] The reliability of MRI in differentiating recurrence from scar at the lumpectomy bed has been reported as approaching 100% with sensitivities of 93% to 100% and specificities reported at 88% to 100%.[32]

In the conservative treatment of breast cancer, MRI has been shown to be useful in several scenarios. Magnetic resonance imaging demonstrates the extent of invasive carcinoma, especially invasive lobular carcinoma, more accurately than mammography or sonography. Magnetic resonance imaging can show the extent of residual carcinoma in women with positive margins at lumpectomy. Finally, breast MRI assists in the differentiation of fibrosis from tumor recurrence in women with suspicion of recurrence at the lumpectomy site more than 9 to 18 months posttreatment.

4. Assessing Treatment Response

In women with large primary breast carcinomas, preoperative chemotherapy has been used to shrink tumor size to facilitate mastectomy or breast conservation. Increasingly, preoperative neoadjuvant chemotherapy is being used. Thus, the determination of tumor size after treatment is increasingly important to the surgeon to enable complete tumor removal without residual cancer left in the breast at the time of lumpectomy.

Early studies with MRI demonstrated that it was capable of identifying residual tumor enhancement in most women with partial reduction of tumor by preoperative chemotherapy.[33] In one study of 52 women treated with neoadjuvant chemotherapy, MRI was more accurate than physical examination in detecting residual tumor and was capable of identifying all breasts containing residual posttreatment tumor, whereas physical examination falsely identified five breasts as tumor free.[34] Another study found that when microcalcifications were associated with the primary carcinoma and were due to DCIS, mammography sometimes could detect posttreatment disease that was not appreciated on MRI.[35] Also, microscopic foci of residual disease could not be appreciated with mammography, sonography, or MRI.

Not all assessments of MRI in this setting have been optimistic about its utility. In a study of 58 women undergoing preoperative chemotherapy, MRI was not reliable in determining breast tumor size after treatment.[36] Magnetic resonance imaging was useful in determining within the first 6 weeks of chemotherapy if tumor response to treatment would occur. It had an 83% accuracy in determining which tumors would be nonresponsive, and a comparable accuracy in determining partial response. In complete responders, MRI was a reliable indicator of the extent of response in only two thirds of patients. Others have also reported reliability in assessment of tumor response using MRI only in those with no response.[37] This is due to changes due to therapy appearing identical to those of the primary breast carcinoma; when present, they compromised the ability to accurately assess response to treatment.

It appears that the ability of MRI to be useful in this setting is somewhat limited. As a predictor of tumor response or identifying complete failure of neoadjuvant chemotherapy, MRI can be of value. As in other situations in which it is used to identify DCIS seen as mammographic microcalcifications, MRI is not reliable in assessing treatment response when microcalcifications due to DCIS are mammographically present. Not suprisingly, as is the case with physical examination and other imaging techniques, MRI may be unable to detect microscopic residual tumor. Also, posttreatment changes can be mistaken for carcinoma.

5. Disease of the Nipple

Disease of the nipple is poorly evaluated using mammography and sonography. Sonographically, shadowing produced by the nipple makes it poorly assessed. Disease involving the nipple is also rarely imaged on mammography. If a discharge is present from a solitary duct, galactography can used to gain information about the underlying duct. However, this procedure is invasive, and sometimes the discharging duct cannot be catheterized.

Magnetic resonance imaging has been shown to be capable of imaging the source of nipple discharge in some women.[38] In 15 women with nipple discharge who were treated surgically, MRI was able to detect the underlying lesion in 73% (Figure 16.3). In this study all seven carcinomas were found with MRI. One fibroadenoma and two papillomas were found surgically and missed by MRI. In one patient, no focal lesion was found with surgery or MRI. In a case report of a woman with nipple discharge, MRI found the underlying microinvasive DCIS.[39] In this case, both intraductal and intravenous contrast were used.

The normal pattern of nipple enhancement with contrast can make its evaluation somewhat difficult. Comparison with the opposite nipple is needed to assess whether the pattern is abnormal. In the conserved breast, nodular enhancement of the nipple has been suggested to be evidence of tumor recurrence after conservation, while linear or diffuse enhancement is a normal postconservation pattern.[40] However, there is only limited experience with this observation.

It has been suggested that MRI may be of value in estimating the extent of disease in the breast in women who present with Paget's disease of the nipple.[41] This is due to the supposed superior imaging of the retroareolar region

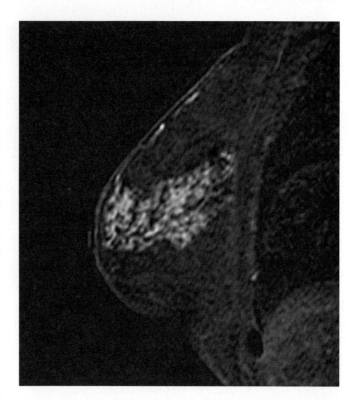

FIGURE 16.3. A 57-year-old woman who presented with bloody discharge of the right nipple and normal mammogram. Sagittal, T1-weighted, fat-suppressed, subtraction MRI of the right breast after injection of intravenous gadolinium shows extensive clumped segmental enhancement in the lateral right breast, 9–10:00 axis. Magnetic resonance imaging guided needle localization yielded invasive ductal carcinoma, not otherwise specified, and multifocal microinvasive carcinoma, ranging in size from 0.1 to 0.2 cm, and DCIS.

with MRI as compared with mammography and sonography. Early enhancement has been reported with Paget's disease.[42] This has also been seen with direct invasion from carcinoma and subareolar papilloma. However, the importance of MRI in this setting would be to demonstrate the extent of carcinoma when the clinical diagnosis of Paget's disease has been made. In this setting, over 40% of mammograms are normal, and disease is confined to the retroareolar region in only 25%.[43] Reliable assessment of the extent of tumor would assist with surgical planning.

6. Unknown Primary

Occult primary breast cancer presenting as isolated ipsilateral axillary metastases without evidence of tumor in the breast on mammography or physical examination accounts for approximately 0.3% to 0.8% of operable breast cancers.[44] Mastectomy, which had previously been the standard treatment for occult primary breast cancer without systemic disease, has yielded the primary cancer in approximately two thirds of patients. The other one third, in whom the primary is not found at mastectomy, presumably have a small breast lesion that is not detected at histologic analysis, or could possibly have a different primary tumor.[44] Breast conservation with radiation in women with occult breast cancer has high (19%–23%) rates of local recurrence, although overall survival is comparable with that of women treated with mastectomy.[45,46]

Magnetic resonance imaging can detect otherwise inapparent carcinoma in the breast. This has proven to be valuable in women who have axillary metastases consistent with a breast primary, but have no evidence of breast cancer on physical examination or mammography (Figure 16.4). Discovery of the primary lesion makes it possible to tailor therapy to breast cancer rather than unknown primary. For women without distant metastases who are surgical candidates, MRI may also make it possible to treat the primary tumor with breast conservation rather than mastectomy.

In a series of our patients at Memorial Sloan-Kettering Cancer Center, MRI was capable of finding the primary carcinoma in 75% of 12 women presenting with axillary

nodal disease consistent with metastatic breast cancer but no evident primary tumor on mammography or physical examination.[44] There were two true-negative and one false-positive MRI examinations in this series. In a study from the Hospital of the University of Pennsylvania, Orel and colleagues[47] reported that MRI detected the primary breast cancer in 86% of 22 women presenting with unknown primary and axillary nodal metastases.

In another study from our institution, Olson and colleagues[46] reported 40 women with biopsy-proven metastatic adenocarcinoma to an axillary lymph node and no evidence of primary tumor on mammography or physical examination. All patients had breast MRI examination. Magnetic resonance imaging identified the primary breast lesion in 28 of 40 women (70%). Of these 28 patients, 11 had modified radical mastectomy, 11 had lumpectomy and axillary dissection with radiotherapy, 2 had axillary dissection and radiation, and 4 had no local treatment due to distant metastases. Two women who initially had lumpectomy and axillary dissection underwent subsequent mastectomy for positive margins. Of the 22 women with positive MRI who had breast surgery, 21 (95%) of 22 had

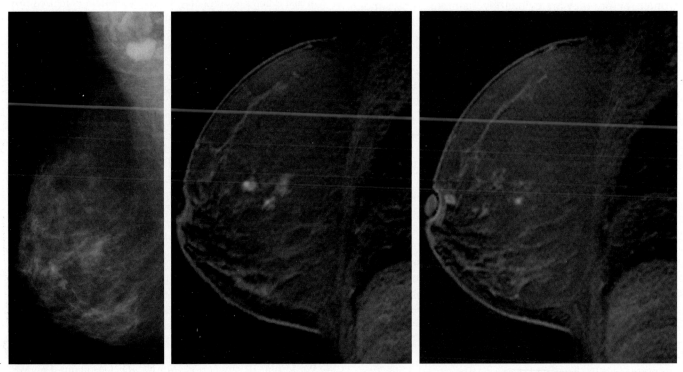

A   B, C

FIGURE 16.4. A 59-year-old woman who presented with adenocarcinoma in right axillary lymph nodes, compatible with breast primary. (A) Preoperative mammogram, right mediolateral oblique view, shows dense right axillary lymph node. The breast parenchyma is nodular without dominant mass or suspicious calcification. (B) Sagittal, T1-weighted, contrast-enhanced MRI of the right breast shows multiple irregularly shaped, irregularly marginated, heterogeneously enhancing masses in vaguely ductal orientation in the central right breast. (C) Sagittal, T1-weighted, contrast-enhanced MRI of the right breast shows additional clumped and mass enhancement extending from the central area to the retroareolar region, in the slice immediately contiguous to that shown in A. Magnetic resonance imaging guided needle localization yielded two foci of invasive ductal carcinoma (measuring 0.6 and 0.4 cm) and DCIS.

tumor in the surgical specimen. Twelve women had negative MRI; 5 of these 12 had mastectomy, of whom 4 had no tumor in the surgical specimen. The remaining seven patients had axillary dissection and whole breast irradiation (n = 5) or were observed (n = 2). Overall, 18 (53%) of 34 women surgically treated had mastectomy while 16 (47%) had breast conservation. Tumor yield for patients having breast surgery was 81%.

These studies suggest that MRI can identify the site of the primary tumor in most women who present with occult breast cancer metastatic to the axilla. Furthermore, one can hypothesize that a negative MRI may enable identification of a subset of women with occult carcinoma who can be managed with breast conservation rather than mastectomy.

7. Screening

The ability of MRI to identify otherwise inapparent breast cancer suggests that it might have a role to play in screening. Data addressing this issue are very preliminary. However, there is evidence of the ability of MRI to detect cancers in high-risk populations, such as *BRCA*-positive women, before they are evident by mammography, sonography, or physical examination. Although the expense, need for intravenous contrast, and lower positive predictive value than with mammography suggest that MRI may not be useful for general screening, its use in high-risk women may become accepted. Whether it is of value in women with mammographically dense breasts is unknown.

In screening women with very high risk of developing breast cancer, MRI has been shown to have some advantage over sonography when used in conjunction with mammography. Warner and colleagues[48] reported 196 women with strong family history or *BRCA* positivity who were screened with physical examination, MRI, sonography, and mammography. Among these women, six developed invasive cancer and one developed DCIS. All invasive tumors were detected by MRI. Mammography found three cancers, including the DCIS; sonography and physical examination each found two. Stoutjesdijk and colleagues[49] retrospectively reviewed the ability of mammography and MRI to detect 19 cancers in 179 high-risk women. The specificity and sensitivity were 93% and 100% for MRI, and 96% and 42% for mammography. Morris and colleagues[50] found that among 367 high risk women, MRI screening resulted in a biopsy recommendation in 17%, with cancer found in 24% of those biopsied. Increasingly, it appears that screening using MRI in addition to mammography may be accepted for those women who are *BRCA* positive.[51] These women have a risk as high as 80% of developing breast cancer in their lifetime. As risk decreases, the usefulness of this expensive tool for screening probably diminishes considerably. However, the role of MRI in breast cancer screening remains unestablished and is the subject of continuing study.

References

1. Gorczyca DP, Sinha S, Ahn CY, et al. Silicone breast implants in vivo: MR imaging. *Radiology* 1992;185:407–410.
2. Gorczyca DP, DeBruhl ND, Ahn CY, et al. Silicone breast implant ruptures in an animal model: comparison of mammography, MR imaging, US and CT. *Radiology* 1994; 190:227–232.
3. Berg WA, Caskey CI, Hamper UM, et al. Single- and double-lumen silicone breast implant integrity: prospective evaluation of MR and US criteria. *Radiology* 1995;197:45–52.
4. Berg WA, Nguyen TK, Middleton MS, et al. MR imaging of extracapsular silicone from breast implants: diagnostic pitfalls. *AJR Am J Roentgenol.* 2002;178:465–472.
5. Hrung JM, Langlotz CP, Orel SG, et al. Cost-effectiveness of MR imaging and core-needle biopsy in the preoperative work-up of suspicious breast lesions. *Radiology* 1999;213: 39–49.
6. Lee CH, Smith RC, Levine JA, et al. Clinical usefulness of MR imaging of the breast in the evaluation of the problematic mammogram. *AJR Am J Roentgenol.* 1999;173: 1323–1329.
7. Stomper PC, Herman S, Klippenstein DL, et al. Suspect breast lesions: findings at dynamic gadolinium-enhanced MR imaging correlated with mammographic and pathologic features. *Radiology* 1995;196:387–395.
8. Brink U, Rischer U, Korabiowska M, et al. The variability of fibroadenoma in contrast-enhanced dynamic MR mammography. *AJR Am J Roentgenol.* 1997;168:1331–1334.
9. Orel SG, Schnall MD, LiVolsi VA, Troupin RH. Suspicious breast lesions: MR imaging with radiologic-pathologic correlation. *Radiology* 1994;190:485–493.
10. Matsubayashi R, Matsuo Y, Edakuni G, et al. Breast masses with peripheral rim enhancement on dynamic contrast-enhanced MR images: correlation of MR findings with histologic features and expression of growth factors. *Radiology* 2000;217:841–848.
11. Fobben ES, Rubin C, Kalisher L, et al. Breast MR imaging with commercially available techniques: radiology-pathologic correlation. *Radiology* 1995;196:143–152.
12. Harms SE, Flamig DP, Hesley KL, et al. MR imaging of the breast with rotating delivery of excitation off resonance: clinical experience with pathologic correlation. *Radiology* 1993;187:493–501.
13. Wedegaertner U, Bick U, Woertler K, et al. Differentiation between benign and malignant findings on MR-mammography: usefulness of morphological criteria. *Eur Radiol.* 2001;11:1645–1650.
14. Westerhof JP, Fischer U, Moritz JD, Oestmann JW. MR imaging of mammographically detected clustered microcalcifications: is there any value? *Radiology* 1998;207:675–681.
15. Gilles R, Guinebretiere J, Lucidarme O, et al. Nonpalpable breast tumors: diagnosis with contrast-enhanced subtraction dynamic MR imaging. *Radiology* 1994;191:625–631.
16. Liberman L, Morris EA, Lee MJY, et al. Breast lesions detected by MR imaging: features and positive predictive value. *AJR Am J Roentgenol.* 2002;179:171–178.

17. Slanetz PJ, Edmister WB, Yeh ED, et al. Occult contralateral breast carcinoma incidentally detected by breast magnetic resonance imaging. *Breast J.* 2002;8:145–148.

18. Brown J, Smith RC, Lee CH. Incidental enhancing lesions found on MR imaging of the breast. *AJR Am J Roentgenol.* 2001;176:1249–1254.

19. Nunes LW, Schnall MD, Orel SG, et al. Breast MR imaging: interpretation model. *Radiology* 1997;202:833–841.

20. Siegmann KC, Muller-Schimpfle M, Schick F, et al. MR imaging-detected breast lesions: histopathologic correlation of lesion characteristics and signal intensity data. *AJR Am J Roentgenol.* 2002;178:1403–1409.

21. LaTrenta LR, Menell JH, Morris EA, et al. Breast lesions detected with MR imaging: utility and histopathologic importance of identification with US. *Radiology* 2003;227:856–861.

22. Panizza P, De Gaspari A, Vanzulli A, et al. Accuracy of post-MR imaging second-look-sonography in previously undetected breast lesions [abstract]. *Radiology* 1997;205:489.

23. Dhamanaskar KP, Muradall D, Kulkarni SR, et al. MRI directed ultrasound: a cost effective method for diagnosis and intervention in breast imaging [abstract]. *Radiology* 2002;225:653.

24. Hlawatsch A, Teifke A, Schmidt M, Thelen M. Preoperative assessment of breast cancer: sonography versus MR imaging. *AJR Am J Roentgenol.* 2002;179:1493–1501.

25. Boetes C, Mus RDM, Holland R, et al. Breast tumors: comparative accuracy of MR imaging relative to mammography and US for demonstrating extent. *Radiology* 1995;197:743–737.

26. Weinstein SP, Orel SG, Heller R, et al. MR imaging of the breast in patients with invasive lobular carcinoma. *AJR Am J Roentgenol.* 2001;176:399–406.

27. Qayyum A, Birdwell RL, Daniel BL, et al. MR imaging features of infiltrating lobular carcinoma of the breast: histopathologic correlation. *AJR Am J Roentgenol.* 2002;178:1227–1232.

28. Frei KA, Kinkel K, Bonel HM, et al. MR imaging of the breast in patients with positive margins after lumpectomy: influence of the time interval between lumpectomy and MR imaging. *AJR Am J Roentgenol.* 2001;175:1577–1584.

29. Gilles R, Guinebretiere J, Shapeero LG, et al. Assessment of breast cancer recurrence with contrast-enhanced subtraction MR imaging: preliminary results in 26 patients. *Radiology* 1993;188:473–478.

30. Dao TH, Rahmouni A, Campana F, et al. Tumor recurrence versus fibrosis in the irradiated breast: differentiation with dynamic gadolinium-enhanced MR imaging. *Radiology* 1993;187:751–755.

31. Dershaw DD, McCormick B, Cox L, Osborne MP. Differentiation of benign and malignant local tumor recurrence after lumpectomy. *AJR Am J Roentgenol.* 1990;155:35–38.

32. Orel SG, Schnall MD. MR imaging of the breast for the detection, diagnosis, and staging of breast cancer. *Radiology* 2001;220:13 30.

33. Gilles R, Guinebretiere JM, Toussaint C, et al. Locally advanced breast cancer: contrast-enhanced subtraction MR imaging of response to preoperative chemotherapy. *Radiology* 1994;191:633–638.

34. Partridge SC, Gibbs JE, Lu Y, et al. Accuracy of MR imaging for revealing residual breast cancer in patients who have undergone neoadjuvant chemotherapy. *AJR Am J Roentgenol.* 2002;179:1193–1199.

35. Junkermann H, von Fournier D. Imaging procedures for assessment of the response of mamary carcinoma to preoperative chemotherapy. *Der Radiologe* 1997;37:726–732.

36. Rieber A, Brambs HJ, Gabelmann A, et al. Breast MRI for monitoring response of primary breast cancer to neo-adjuvant chemotherapy. *Eur Radiol.* 2002;12:1711–1719.

37. Wasser K, Sinn HP, Fink C, et al. Accuracy of tumor size measurement in breast cancer using MRI is influenced by histological regression induced by neoadjuvant chemotherapy. *Eur Radiol.* 2003;13:1213–1223.

38. Orel SG, Dougherty CS, Reynolds C, et al. MR imaging in patients with nipple discharge: initial experience. *Radiology* 2000;216:248–254.

39. Yoshimoto M, Kasumi F, Iwase T, et al. Magnetic resonance galactrography for a patient with nipple discharge. *Breast Cancer Res Treat.* 1997;42:87–90.

40. Ralleigh G, Walker AE, Hall-Craggs MA, et al. MR imaging of the skin and nipple of the breast: differentiation between tumour recurrence and post-treatment change. *Eur Radiol.* 2001;11:1651–1658.

41. Douek M, Hall-Craggs MA. Can the use of preoperative MR imaging reduce local recurrence rates in patients with retroareolar breast cancer who undergo breast-conservation surgery? [letter]. *Radiology* 1999;210:880–881.

42. Buadu AA, Buadu LD, Murakami J, et al. Enhancement of the nipple-areolar-complex on contrast-enhanced MR imaging of the breast. *Breast Cancer* 1998;5:285–289.

43. Kothari AD, Beechey-Newman N, Hamed H, et al. Paget disease of the nipple, a multifocal manifestation of higher-risk disease. *Cancer* 2002;95:1–7.

44. Morris EA, Schwartz LH, Dershaw DD, et al. MR imaging of the breast in patients with occult primary breast carcinoma. *Radiology* 1997;205:437–440.

45. Rosen PP. Unusual clinical presentations of carcinoma. In: Rosen PP, ed. *Rosen's Breast Pathology.* Philadelphia: Lippincott-Raven; 1997:567–595.

46. Olson JA Jr, Morris EA, Van Zee KJ, et al. Magnetic resonance imaging facilitates breast conservation for occult breast cancer. *Ann Surg Oncol.* 2000;7:411–415.

47. Orel SG, Weinstein SP, Schnall MD, et al. Breast MR imaging in patients with axillary node metastases and unknown primary malignancy. *Radiology* 1999;212:543–549.

48. Warner E, Plewes DB, Shumak RS, et al. Comparison of breast magnetic resonance imaging, mammography, and ultrasound for surveillance of women at high risk for hereditary breast cancer. *J Clin Oncol.* 2001;19:3524–3531.

49. Stoutjesdijk MJ, Boetes C, Jager GJ, et al. Magnetic resonance imaging and mammography in women with a hereditary risk of breast cancer. *J Natl Cancer Inst.* 2001;93:1095–1102.

50. Morris EA, Liberman L, Ballon DJ, et al. MRI of occult breast carcinoma in a high-risk population. *AJR Am J Roentgenol.* 2003;181:619–626.

51. Liberman L. Breast cancer screening with MRI—what are the data for patients at high risk? (editorial) *N Engl J Med* 2004;351:497–500.

17
Breast Magnetic Resonance Spectroscopy

Robert E. Lenkinski and Rachel Katz-Brull

Over the past five decades, nuclear magnetic resonance (NMR) spectroscopy has evolved from a technique used in chemistry to determine the structure of molecules to a method with which to probe the metabolism of cells, tissues, intact animals, and humans.[1–13] The early generations of NMR spectrometers employed room temperature ferromagnets and operated at fields between approximately 1 to 2 Tesla (T) and could accommodate samples that contained less than 1 mL of solutions. In the 1970s, the development of vertical bore superconducting magnets provided a newer generation of NMR spectrometers that operated at higher fields and could obtain spectra from slightly larger volumes of samples (1–10 mL). As more of these instruments became available, several research groups began to use multinuclear NMR spectroscopy to investigate the bioenergetics and metabolism of cellular suspensions (see, e.g., Refs. 14–16) and perfused tissue (see, e.g., Refs. 17 and 18). Phosphorus-31 (^{31}P) NMR spectroscopy was used to study cellular bioenergetics because several important compounds that are involved in cellular energetics, such as adenosine triphosphate (ATP), phosphocreatine (PCR), and inorganic phosphate (Pi), are readily detectable. Carbon-13 (^{13}C) NMR spectroscopy could probe metabolism by following isotopically labeled substrates through various metabolic pathways (see, e.g., Ref. 19). Although proton magnetic resonance spectroscopy (MRS) was used extensively in chemical applications, its use in biological systems in which the concentration of the compounds of interest is approximately 1 to 10 mM was hampered by the presence of a large background signal arising from water in the sample, which could have a concentration approaching 90 M in protons. This large difference in signal intensities led to the development of a variety of techniques that either did not excite the background water signal or suppressed it substantially (see, e.g., Refs. 20–22). One of the major motivations for employing proton MRS methods is the greater sensitivity of this nucleus as compared with both ^{31}P and ^{13}C. The relative sensitivities for each of these nuclei are given in Table 17.1. Typical voxel sizes for each nucleus are also given for comparison.

The availability of horizontal bore magnets led to the extension of these studies to intact animals (see Ref. 23 for a review). Since the early 1980s, there has also been an increasing availability of whole-body magnetic resonance imaging (MRI) scanners for use in diagnostic imaging. A large number of these MRI scanners operate at 1.5 T, a magnetic field that is similar to the magnetic fields employed in the early days of NMR spectroscopy. As MRI technology has advanced, there have been an increasing number of applications of MRI to image organs outside of the brain. This book deals with one of the major emerging areas of MRI, namely, the breast.

The development of spatially localized MRS[24–26] has created the opportunity for adding the metabolic information about a lesion visualized on MRI alone or dynamic contrast-enhanced MRI into the diagnostic work up of breast disease. In the best case possible, malignant lesions would present with a characteristic metabolic fingerprint that is distinct from that of benign lesions, leading to high *metabolic contrast* between the two kinds of breast lesions. This metabolic information could then be used in conjunction with the more conventional MRI-based anatomical and physiological parameters to arrive at a diagnosis based on the aggregate behavior of the lesion on MRI/MRS. In effect, the MRS could be viewed as an additional imaging sequence (such as fast spin echo or delayed contrast-enhanced images) in the overall MRI protocol.

We have recently reviewed the clinical studies that have been carried out to date using MRS of the breast in diagnostic studies.[27] In this chapter we discuss the biological rationale behind employing MRS in the breast. We also discuss the technical challenges in applying MRS in the breast. Finally, we discuss some of the potential developments that may improve the performance of MRS of the breast in the future.

TABLE 17.1. The Relative Sensitivities of the Nuclei Together with Some Typical Voxel Sizes for MRS

Nucleus	Spin	Natural Abundance (%)	Frequency at 1.5T (MHz)	Physiological Concentration	Relative Sensitivity[a]	Relative Detectability[b]	Typical Voxel Size[c]
^1H	1/2	100	63.89	80–90M	1.0	1.0	$0.625 \times 0.625 \times 3$
^1H	1/2	Metabolites	63.89	1–10mM	1.0	10^{-5}–10^{-6}	$10 \times 10 \times 10$
^{13}C	1/2	1.18	16.06	10mM	2.5×10^{-4}	2.5×10^{-8}	$50 \times 50 \times 50$
^{31}P	1/2	100	25.85	10mM	8.3×10^{-2}	8.3×10^{-6}	$30 \times 30 \times 30$

[a] The relative sensitivity based on NMR theory for the same concentration of each nucleus.

[b] The relative detectability calculated by taking into account the relative concentrations present. The first entry for protons is for MRI.

[c] The typical voxel size achievable in about 10 minutes of signal averaging for MRS with surface coils. For comparison, a typical MRI voxel obtained with a head coil at 1.5T obtained in about 10 seconds is given in the first entry for protons.

1. Magnetic Resonance Spectroscopy of the Breast

1.2. Rationale for Using Choline

The rationale for using MRS in the breast is based on the observations, made both in excised human breast tissue and in model systems, that the level of the choline and its metabolites are elevated in tumors as compared with benign disease (for a review in tumors see Ref. 28; for breast tumors see Refs 29–32). Early NMR spectroscopy studies of tissue extracts and later in vivo MRS studies using ^{31}P, found elevated levels of phosphomonoesters [phosphocholine (PC) and phosphoethanolamine (PE)] in malignancies. More recently, there has been a growing literature that indicates that levels of choline and its metabolites can be detected by proton MRS. Although it is difficult to distinguish the different choline metabolites using proton MRS, these proton MRS studies are easier to perform on clinical scanners for two reasons. First, the sensitivity of proton MRS is higher than ^{31}P or ^{13}C, and proton MRS studies can use the same radiofrequency hardware as MRI. Also, if lesions of approximately 1cm linear dimension are of interest, it is clear that proton MRS offers the best possibility for metabolic investigations.

Degani and colleagues[29] and Ronen and Leach[32] have reviewed the preclinical studies of breast cancer. Nuclear magnetic resonance data obtained from ^{31}P studies, carried out on different malignant cell lines and human mammary epithelial cells, indicate differences in the phospholipid metabolism of human breast cancer cells either in tissue culture or implanted in nude mice.[29] The malignant cells consistently exhibited elevated levels of phosphocholine (PC) and phosphoethanolamine (PE). This review also describes the results of ^{13}C NMR studies that compared glucose utilization rates in malignant cell lines with human mammary epithelial cells. These studies indicated that the malignant cells produced ATP almost exclusively by glycolysis (with concomitant production of lactate), whereas the human mammary epithelial cells had about 20% oxidative metabolism.

Degani and colleagues[29] also describe the results of ^{13}C studies aimed at determining the details of phospholipid metabolism in human breast cancer cells. These results, carried out in spheroids, showed that the rate of synthesis of phosphatidylcholine was greatest in cells that were proliferating, as compared with nonproliferating cells. These studies provide a rationale for entertaining the hypothesis that breast lesions that are malignant will exhibit altered metabolism and elevated choline when compared with benign lesions. Aboagye and Bhujwalla[33] showed that the progression of human mammary epithelial cells from normal to malignant phenotype is associated with altered membrane choline phospholipid metabolism. In particular, they found that phosphocholine levels and total choline-containing phospholipid metabolite levels increased with progression from normal to immortalized to oncogene-transformed to tumor-derived cells. These studies indicate that there should be increased choline-containing compounds present in malignant tissue as compared with both normal and benign tissues. The only potential complication in using choline as a marker from malignancy can be found in the report of Rohlfs and colleagues.[34] These authors found that in the lactating rat the mammary gland was able to synthesize the choline metabolites found in milk. They also established that the total choline concentration in rat milk is seven-fold higher than previously reported, with more than 80% present as glycerophosphocholine and phosphocholine. However, this elevated choline level should only be present during lactation.

2. Nuclear Magnetic Resonance Studies of Human Tissues and Tissue Extracts

Gribbestad and colleagues[35,36] have reported a one- and two-dimensional NMR study of perchloric acid extracts of human breast carcinomas. Among a number of interesting findings, these authors found elevated levels of phosphocholine at 3.2ppm. The phosphocholine/valine ratio in malignant tissue was 18.7 ± 12.5, as compared with 6.60 ± 2.60 for uninvolved tissue. These differences were found to be statistically significant ($P < 0.01$) on a Mann-Whitney test. It was pointed out that the increase in phosphocholine might be accompanied by a decrease in glycerophosphocholine. These authors also reported a higher level of lactate/glucose in extracts of tumors, as compared with uninvolved tissue. Some caution in the interpretation of lactate levels in extracts is probably warranted because it is often difficult to remove the tissue in a manner that guarantees that agonal metabolism does not produce lactate. The observation of glucose resonances in the extract provides some confidence that this may not have occurred in the study.

Von Speckter and colleagues[37] have also reported a high-resolution NMR study carried out on 56 cases with suspected mammary carcinoma. These authors found that three ratios of compounds detected by NMR (the creatine/fat, choline/fat, and carnitine/fat ratios) could distinguish between malignant and normal tissues at the 0.995 confidence level. The spectra shown in this report suggested that, of the three compounds, the level of choline should be easiest to determine in vivo.

MacKinnon and colleagues[31] have shown that it is possible to differentiate benign from malignant lesions based on a visual inspection of the Cho/Cr ratio observed in the *ex vivo* MR spectra of fine needle biopsy samples. This work was followed recently by a report of a statistical classification strategy for diagnosing breast cancer based on ex vivo MR spectra obtained from fine-needle aspirates.[38] The results discussed previously show that there are differences in the metabolism of breast cancer compared with normal tissue. Moreover, these differences can be observed by MRS methods in cellular suspensions, model tumors, and extracts of excised human tissue.

3. Phosphorus-31 Magnetic Resonance Spectroscopy Studies of Human Breast Disease

Sijens and colleagues[39] have reported changes in both ^{1}H and ^{31}P MRS in patients (n = 5) with breast cancer. The fat-to-water ratio was found to be 0.45 in the tumors, as compared with 3.3 in normal tissue. The malignant lesions showed elevated levels of phosphomonoesters (which are primarily PC and PE), phosphodiesters (which are primarily glycerophosphoethanolamine and glycerophosphocholine), and inorganic phosphate (Pi). The malignant lesions all showed little or no phosphocreatine (PCr/ATP < 0.2). Similar alterations in ^{31}P spectral parameters have subsequently been reported by others.[40–45]

4. Clinical Single Voxel Proton Magnetic Resonance Spectroscopy of the Breast

An example of the MRS results obtained from a single voxel examination of an infiltrating ductal carcinoma is shown in Figure 17.1. For comparison, an example of the results of a similar examination carried out on a fibroadenoma is shown in Figure 17.2. Note the presence of choline in the spectra shown in Figure 17.1. This difference is the basis for the discrimination between malignant and benign lesions.

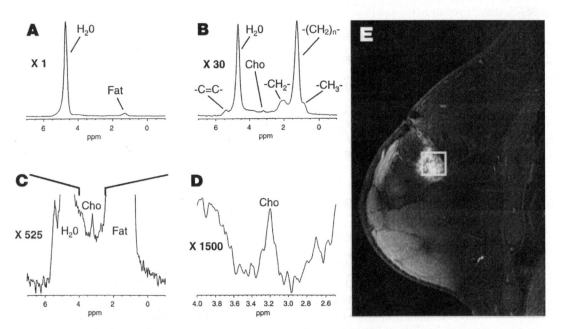

FIGURE 17.1. (A) Unsuppressed and (B–D) suppressed MR spectra (2000/31) of intraductal and infiltrating ductal carcinoma show resonance assignments for water, fat, and Cho. (E) Gadolinium-enhanced MRI (28/4) shows the tumor and the voxel (box) used for MR spectroscopy. In A–D, scale factors are relative to the unsuppressed spectrum. The horizontal axis units are expressed in ppm. The nominal voxel volume was 1.6 cm³. In A–D, X indicates the magnification.

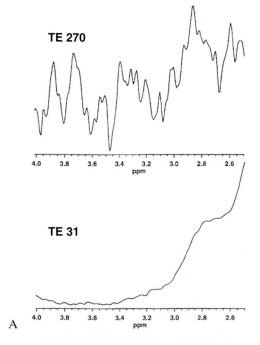

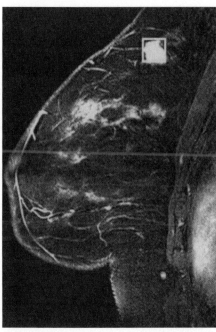

FIGURE 17.2. (A) MR spectra of a fibroadenoma obtained with a repetition time of 2000 msec and an echo time (TE) of 270 msec (TE 270) or a TE of 31 msec (TE 31). There is no detectable Cho present in these spectra. The horizontal axis units are expressed in ppm. (B) Gadolinium-enhanced MRI (28/4) shows the tumor and the voxel (box) used for MR spectroscopy. The nominal voxel volume was 1.2 cm³. Diffuse enhancement is demonstrated inferior to the fibroadenoma voxel location.

To date, six studies of in vivo ¹H MRS of breast cancer have been published that used choline as a marker for malignancy. Five of these studies (conducted by four different groups) have tested the diagnostic performance of ¹H MRS for distinguishing benign from malignant lesions of the breast based on the detection of a choline resonance.[46–50] The number of cancer and benign tumors included in each study, as well as the diagnostic results of these studies, are summarized in Table 17.2. The sixth study tested the capability of ¹H MRS to differentiate breast cancer from unaffected breast tissue.[51] The technical details of these studies are given in Table 17.3. Note that in spite of the different coils, pulse sequences, acquisition methods, and patient populations sampled, the results shown in Table 17.2 are surprisingly similar. The sensitivity ranges from 0.70 to 0.92, whereas the specificity ranges from 0.83 to 0.87. We suggest that these results indicate the robustness of using the presence of choline as an indicator of malignancy.

In our review,[27] we also noted that if the studies in which there were known technical problems were excluded from the pooled analysis, the sensitivity of MRS increased to 0.92 and the specificity increased to 0.92. We also pointed out that in women who were 40 years old and younger, MRS had a diagnostic accuracy of 100%. These encouraging results indicate that MRS might have an important role in distinguishing benign from malignant lesions in younger women who are at high risk for developing breast cancer.

5. Future Developments

The increasing availability of MRI scanners operating at 3 to 4 T could improve the performance of MRS of the breast. In our review,[27] we noted that one of the important factors limiting the diagnostic accuracy of breast MRS is the signal-to-noise (S/N) ratio of the examination. These higher field scanners offer potential significant S/N gains over 1.5 T scanners provided that magnetic field inhomogeneities can be *shimmed* out. The last column in Table 17.3 indicated the line-width of the choline resonance observed in vivo. This line-width was estimated from the spectra presented in each report and, thus, is a rough estimate only. Bakken and colleagues have reported a T2 for choline of 320 to 360 ms in two breast patients.[52] A T2 of 320 ms corresponds to a line-width of approximately 1 Hz. Because the experimental line-widths were as high as 8 Hz, it may be possible to gain a significant increase in S/N by reducing the contribution of static field inhomogeneity. One way to decrease the contribution of static field in homogeneities is by reducing the MRS voxel size. A smaller, but dramatic effect of reducing voxel size on S/N improvement was recently reported by Li and colleagues[53] in MRS studies of the brain. Thus, the combination of higher field and higher order shimming algorithms could provide significant increases in the S/N of the MRS examination.

TABLE 17.2. Clinical Breast ^{1}H MRS Studies and Results

Study No.	Author	Malignant Tumors	Benign Tumors	Mean Dimension (cm)*	Sensitivity %	Specificity %	TP	TN	FN	FP
1	Cecil et al.[50]	23	15	2.6	83	87	19	13	4	2
2	Yeung et al.[48]	24	6	4.9	92	83	22	5	2	1
3	Roebuck et al.[47]	10	7	2.0	70	86	7	6	3	1
4	Kvistad et al.[46]	11	11	3.2	82	82	9	9	2	2
5	Jagannathan et al.[49]	32	14	—	81	86	26	12	6	2
Sum		100	53		83	85	83	45	17	8

Abbreviations: TP, true positive; TN, true negative; FN, false negative; FP, false positive.

TABLE 17.3. Hardware, Methods, and Acquisition Parameters Used in Breast ^{1}H MRS Studies

Study No.	Author	Model and Make of 1.5-T Magnet	RF Coil	Pulse Sequence for Single Voxel Spectroscopy	Pulse Sequence for Water Suppression	TE	NEX	Line-Width of Cho
1	Cecil et al.[50]	Signa, GE Medical Systems, Milwaukee, WI	Custom build single-breast multi coil for receive-only, and body coil for transmit	STEAM	CHESS	31 270	128	5–7
2	Yeung et al.[48]	Gyroscan ACS-NT, Philips Medical Systems, Best, The Netherlands	Standard double-breast receive-only and body coil for transmit	PRESS	Not specified	38 135 270	64	8
3	Roebuck et al.[47]	Signa, GE Medical Systems, Milwaukee, WI	Custom build single-breast multi coil for receive-only, and body coil for transmit	STEAM	CHESS	31 270	128	5–7
4	Kvistad et al.[46]	Picker Edge EPI II, Picker, Cleveland, OH	Custom build single-breast receive-only, or a circular surface coil	PRESS	Frequency-selective inversion pulse at the water resonance	135 350 450	256	4
5	Jagannathan et al.[49]	Magnetom, Siemens	Standard bilateral surface coil for receive only, and body coil for transmit	STEAM	Not specified	135	32–64	5
6	Gribbestad et al.[51]	Gyroscan S15 HQ, Philips Medical Systems, Best, The Netherlands	Double breast coil, works as transmit and receive	PRESS	Frequency-selective inversion pulse at the water resonance	136	256	8

Abbreviations: CHESS, chemical shift selective pulses; NEX, number of excitation used in the acquisition of each spectrum; PRESS, point resolved spectroscopy; RF, radiofrequency; TE, echo time; STEAM, stimulated echo acquisition mode. The repetition time was 2000 msec in all the studies except study 5, in which 3000 msec were used.

The gain in S/N may also produce artifacts in the spectra. Recently, Bolan and colleagues[54] showed that at 4T there can be spurious peaks caused by modulations of the strong lipid signal by gradient vibrations. These authors showed an elegant solution to this problem called *TE-averaging*, which can readily be implemented for single voxel studies. An alternate approach is using radiofrequency excitation pulses that do not excite the lipid resonances. These lipid nonexcitation approaches have been employed in proton MRS of the prostate by the UCSF group.[55,56]

All of the clinical studies referenced to date have employed single voxel methods for spectral localization. There have been several groups pursuing the development of multivoxel MRS methods for proton studies of the breast. The rationale for employing a multivoxel MRS approach is based on the fact that there is usually more than one region of contrast enhancement observed on MRI. In clinical practice, the radiologist uses a combination of architectural features, as well as enhancement characteristics, to assess each of these regions. We visualize that the multivoxel MRS approach will enable radiologists to combine the choline level observed in each of these enhancing regions into their overall assessment of the probability for malignancy. The multivoxel approach is also time-efficient because the acquisition time for the whole breast sequence (2304 voxels) is equivalent to the time required for sampling three single voxels sequentially. An additional advantage of the multivoxel approach is that it permits retrospective review, whereas single voxel methods rely on accurate voxel choice and placement. The multivoxel methods also may avoid issues concerning the degradation of MRS by gadolinium-based contrast studies. Because the multivoxel MRS provides extensive coverage of the breast, it can be performed before the dynamic contrast enhancement. Also, multivoxel methods can be retrospectively voxel-shifted to optimally reposition the voxel over the lesion(s) identified on MRI. The large number of voxels examined, combined with the fact that these examinations are usually performed with phased array radiofrequency receiver coils, means that there can be several thousand spectra to process, display, and interpret. This points out the need for the development of robust, accurate, easy-to-use, automated, spectral processing algorithms.

6. Summary

Proton MRS of the breast can provide important diagnostic information that is based on the metabolic profile of malignant breast tissue, namely an elevated choline resonance. A potential complicating factor is that lactating women may also show elevated choline and should probably be excluded from MRS studies. Evidence suggests that MRS of the breast may be particularly useful for younger women. The advances in higher field magnets as well as multivoxel MRS methods should improve MRS studies in the future. There is a growing need for automated spectral analysis algorithms that can provide a means for integrating the metabolic information from MRS into the MRI examination.

References

1. Burt CT, Cohen SM, Barany M. Analysis with intact tissue with 31P NMR. Annu *Rev Biophys Bioeng.* 1979;8:1–25.
2. Burt CT, Wyrwicz AM. Nuclear magnetic resonance observations in biological systems. 1. Intact tissue. *Trends Biochem Sci.* 1979;4:244–246.
3. Kuchel PW. Nuclear magnetic-resonance of biological samples. *Crit Rev Analyt Chem.* 1981;12:155–231.
4. Roberts JKM, Jardetzky O. Monitoring of cellular metabolism by NMR. *Biochim Biophys Acta.* 1981;50:69–83.
5. Gadian DG, Radda GK. NMR studies of tissue metabolism. *Ann Rev Biochem.* 1981;50:69–83.
6. Iles RA, Stevens AN, Griffiths JR. NMR studies of metabolites in living tissue. *Prog Nucl Magn Resone Spectroscopy.* 1982;15:49–200.
7. Bernard M, Canioni P, Cozzone PJ. Nuclear magnetic resonance study of cellular metabolism in vivo. *Biochimie* 1983;65:449–470.
8. Radda GK, Taylor DJ. Applications of nuclear magnetic resonance spectroscopy in pathology. *Int Rev Exp Pathol.* 1985;27:1–58.
9. Avison MJ, Hetherington HP, Shulman RG. Applications of NMR to studies of tissue metabolism. *Annu Rev Biophys Biophys Chem.* 1986;15:377–402.
10. Bottomley PA. Human in vivo NMR spectroscopy in diagnostic medicine: clinical tool or research probe? *Radiology* 1989;170:1–15.
11. Cerdan S, Seelig J. NMR studies of human metabolism. *Annu Rev Biophys Biophys Chem.* 1990;19:43–47.
12. Allen PS. In vivo nuclear magnetic resonance spectroscopy applied to medicine. *J Can Assoc Radiol.* 1990;41:39–44.
13. Ruizcabello J, Cohen JS. NMR and the study of pathological state in cells and tissues. *Int Rev Cytol.* 1993;145:1–63.
14. Evans FE, Kaplan NO. 31P nuclear magnetic resonance studies of HeLa cells. *Proc Natl Acad Sci U S A.* 1977;74:4909–4913.
15. Navon G, Ogawa S, Shulman RG, Yamane T. High-resolution 31P nuclear magnetic resonance studies of metabolism in aerobic Escherichia coli cells. *Proc Natl Acad Sci U S A.* 1977;74:888–891.
16. Navon G, Ogawa S, Shulman RG, Yamane T. 31P nuclear magnetic resonance studies of Ehrlich ascites tumor cells. *Proc Natl Acad Sci U S A.* 1977;74:87–91.
17. Jelicks LA, Gupta RK. Multinuclear NMR studies of the Langendorff perfused rat heart. *J Biol Chem.* 1989;264:15230–15235.
18. Ackerman JJ, Bore PJ, Gadian DG, et al. NMR studies of metabolism in perfused organs, *Philos Trans R Soc Lond B Biol Sci.* 1980;289:425–436.
19. London RE. C-13 labeling in studies of metabolic regulation. *Prog Nucl Magn Reson Spectroscopy.* 1988;20:337–383.
20. Bottomley PA, Edelstein WA, Foster TH, Adams WA. In vivo solvent-suppressed localized hydrogen nuclear magnetic

resonance spectroscopy: a window to metabolism? *Proc Natl Acad Sci U S A*. 1985;82:2148–2152.

21. Frahm J, Michaelis T, Merboldt KD, et al. Localized NMR spectroscopy in vivo. Progress and problems. *Nucl Magn Reson Biomed*. 1989;2:188–195.

22. Frahm J, Bruhn H, Gyngell ML, et al. Localized high-resolution NMR spectroscopy using stimulated schoes: initial applications to human brain in vivo. *Magn Reson Med*. 1989;9:79–93.

23. Chatham JC, Blackband SJ. Nuclear magnetic resonance spectroscopy and imaging in animal research. *ILAR J*. 2001;42:189–208.

24. Bollinger L, Lenkinski RE. Localization in clinical MR spectroscopy. In: Berliner L, Reuben J, eds. *Biological Magnetic Resonance*. Vol. 11. New York: Plenum Press; 1992:1–65.

25. Narayana PA, DeLayre J. Localization methods in NMR. In: Partain CL, Price RR, Patton JA, et al, eds. *Magnetic Resonance Imaging: Physical Principles and Instrumentation*. Vol. 2. Philadelphia: Saunders; 1988:1609–1630.

26. Aue WP. Localization methods for in vivo nuclear magnetic resonance spectroscopy. *Rev Magn Reson Med*. 1986;1:21–72.

27. Katz-Brull R, Lavin PT, Lenkinski RE. Clinical utility of proton magnetic resonance spectroscopy in characterizing breast lesions. *J Natl Cancer Inst*. 2002;94:1197–1203.

28. Negedank W. Studies of human tumors by MRS: a review. *Nucl Magn Reson Biomed*. 1992;5:303–324.

29. Degani H, Ronen SM, Furman E. Breast cancer: spectroscopy and imaging of cells and tumors. In: Gilles R, ed. *Magnetic Resonance in Physiology and Medicine*. San Diego: Academic Press; 1994.

30. Gribbestad IS, Sitter B, Lundgren S, Krane J, Axelson D. Metabolite composition in breast tumors examined by proton nuclear magnetic resonance spectroscopy. *Anticancer Res*. 1999;19:1737–1746.

31. MacKinnon WB, Barry PA, Malycha PL, et al. Fine-needle biopsy specimens of benign breast lesions distinguished from invasive cancer ex vivo with proton MR spectroscopy. *Radiology* 1997;204:661–666.

32. Ronen SM, Leach MO. Imaging biochemistry: applications to breast cancer. *Breast Cancer Res*. 2001;3:36–40.

33. Aboagye EO, Bhujwalla ZM. Malignant transformation alters membrane choline phospholipid metabolism of human mammary epithelial cells. *Cancer Res*. 1999;59:80–84.

34. Rohlfs EM, Garner SC, Mar MH, Zeisel SH. Glycerophosphocholine and phosphocholine are the major choline metabolites in rat milk. *J Nutr*. 1993;123:1762–1768.

35. Gribbestad IS, Fjosne HE, Kvinnsland S. In vitro proton NMR spectroscopy of extracts from human breast tumours and non-involved breast tissue. *Anticancer Res*. 1993;13:1973–1980.

36. Gribbestad IS, Petersen SB, Fjosne HE, et al. 1H NMR spectroscopic characterization of perchloric acid extracts from breast carcinomas and non-involved breast tissue. *Nucl Magn Reson Biomed*. 1994;7:181–194.

37. Speckter H, Blumich B, Just M, et al. In vitro NMR spectroscopy of healthy, pathologically changed and carcinomatous breast tissue samples correlated with histological findings. *Rofo Fortschr Geb Rontenstr Neuen Bildgeb Verfahr*. 1994;161:147–153.

38. Mountford CE, Somorjai RL, Malycha P, et al. Diagnosis and prognosis of breast cancer by magnetic resonance spectroscopy of fine-needle aspirates analysed using a statistical classification strategy. *Br J Surg*. 2001;88:1234–1240.

39. Sijens PE, Wijredeman HK, Moerland MA, et al. Human breast cancer in vivo: H-1 and P-31 MR spectroscopy at 1.5 T. *Radiology* 1988;169:615–620.

40. Glaholm J, Leach MO, Collins DJ, et al. In vivo 31P magnetic spectroscopy for monitoring treatment response in breast cancer. *Lancet* 1989;1:1327.

41. Smith TAD, Glaholm J, Leach MO, et al. A comparison of in vivo and in vitro P-31 NMR spectra from human breast tumors: variations in phospholipid metabolism. *Br J Cancer*. 1991;63:514–516.

42. Redmond OM, Stack JP, O'Connor NG, et al. In vivo phosphorus-31 magnetic resonance spectroscopy of normal and pathological breast tissues. *Br J Radiol*. 1991;64:210–216.

43. Merchant TE, Gierke LW, Meneses P, Glonek T. 31P magnetic resonance spectroscopic profiles of neoplastic human breast tissues. *Cancer Res*. 1988;48:5112–5118.

44. Merchant TE, de Graaf PW, Nieuwenhuizen CW, et al. Fibroadenoma of the breast: in vivo magnetic resonance characterization. *Eur J Radiol*. 1991;13:91–95.

45. Merchant TE, Meneses P, Gierke LW, et al. 31P magnetic resonance phospholipid profiles of neoplastic human breast tissues. *Br J Cancer*. 1991;63:693–698.

46. Kvistad KA, Bakken IJ, Gribbestad IS, et al. Characterization of neoplastic and normal human breast tissues with in vivo 1H MR spectroscopy. *J Magn Reson Imaging*. 1999;10: 159–164.

47. Roebuck JR, Cecil KM, Schnall MD, Lenkinski RE. Human breast lesions: characterization with proton MR spectroscopy. *Radiology* 1998;209:269–275.

48. Yeung DKW, Cheung HS, Tse GMK. Human breast lesions: Characterization with contrast-enhanced in vivo proton MR spectroscopy—initial results. *Radiology* 2001;220:40–46.

49. Jagannathan NR, Kuman M, Seenu V, et al. Evaluation of total choline from in-vivo volume localized proton MR spectroscopy and its response to neoadjuvant chemotherapy in locally advanced breast cancer. *Br J Cancer*. 2001;84: 1016–1022.

50. Cecil KM, Schnall MD, Siegelman ES, Lenkinski RE. The evaluation of human breast lesions with magnetic resonance imaging and proton magnetic resonance spectroscopy. *Breast Cancer Res Treat*. 2001;68:45–54.

51. Gribbestad IS, Singstad TE, Nilsen G, et al. In vivo 1H MRS of normal breast and breast tumors using a dedicated double breast coil. *J Magn Reson Imaging*. 1998;8:1191–1197.

52. Bakken IJ, Gribbestad IS, Singstad TE, Kvistad KA. External standard method for the in vivo quantification of choline-containing compounds in breast tumors by proton MR spectroscopy at 1.5 Tesla. *Magn Reson Med*. 2001;46:189–192.

53. Li BSY, Regal J, Gonen O. SNR versus resolution in 3D H-1 MRS of the human brain at high magnetic fields. *Magn Reson Med*. 2001;46:1049–1053.

54. Bolan PJ, Delabarre L, Baker EH, et al. Eliminating spurious lipid sidebands in 1H MRS of breast lesions. *Magn Reson Med*. 2002;48:215–222.

55. Kurhanewicz J, Vigneron DB, Males RG, et al. The prostate: MR imaging and spectroscopy. Present and future. *Radiol Clin North Am*. 2000;38:115–138.

56. Schricker AA, Pauly JM, Kurhanewicz J, et al. Dualband spectral-spatial RF pulses for prostate MR spectroscopic imaging. *Magn Reson Med*. 2001;46:1079–1087.

18
The Surgeon's Perspective

Alexandra Heerdt

For most surgeons who care for patients with breast cancer, performing a surgical procedure for local control is only a small component of their involvement with this disease. In general, breast surgeons take an active role in both screening efforts and the evaluation of the abnormal mammogram. Subsequent to any diagnosis of breast cancer, it is the surgeon who must make the determination as to the appropriateness of breast conservation therapy versus mastectomy. Finally, after a cancer patient has undergone adjuvant therapy, the surgeon continues to participate in her care, evaluating her for any evidence of local recurrence or contralateral disease.

In many cases, all of these facets of the management of the breast patient are relatively uncomplicated. In such cases, there may be no need for imaging tests other than standard mammography. However, there are occasions on which either more intensive screening may be desired or a more thorough preoperative evaluation of the breast is desired in preparation for the definitive surgical procedure. In such situations, magnetic resonance imaging (MRI) is uniquely able to provide additional, important information. In order to best address its utility, it is helpful to discuss each of the tasks that a surgeon may face separately. Additionally, it is important to understand the technical keys to success when performing biopsy after MRI-guided localization.

1. Screening for and Diagnosis of Breast Cancer

As has been the case for many years, screening mammography remains the gold standard for evaluating the breast for cancer.[1-3] The increased use of screening mammography has almost solely led to an increase in the detection of breast cancer in the in situ stage of the disease.[4] Yet, despite its excellent ability to detect early breast cancers, mammography still has its limitations. Fully 10% to 15% of all palpable breast cancers are not detectable with mam-

mography, and its sensitivity decreases in younger women and those with increased breast density.[5,6] In general, because breast cancer is a rare disease in women under the age of 40, these limitations are not clinically significant. However, in a population of younger women at greater risk of developing breast cancer, the decrease in sensitivity of mammography in this setting could have important implications.

Women who either have a strong family history of breast and ovarian cancer or who are known to be carriers of a mutation of the *BRCA1* or *BRCA2* gene carry the greatest lifetime risk for development of breast cancer. Breast cancer screening efforts in this population are thwarted by the fact that over 50% of mutation carriers develop cancer before the age of 50,[7] the time at which screening sensitivity increases. It is in just such a population that a test such as MRI, which has been reported to have a sensitivity for breast cancer detection as high as 94% to 100%, would be ideal.[8] In this population, one might consider the use of MRI to evaluate the breast.

Several studies have addressed the use of MRI in a population of women either known or suspected to carry a breast cancer susceptibility gene.[9-11] Stoutjesdijk and colleagues[9] analyzed of a cohort of women at increased risk for breast cancer who were evaluated yearly by mammography alone, MRI alone, or both modalities. This group found that MRI was more accurate in the detection of breast cancer than mammography alone. A second group offered women with probable genetic susceptibility screening with physical examination, mammography, ultrasound examination, and MRI.[10] Of nine cancers found during the study period, mammography and ultrasound demonstrated three (33%) while MRI demonstrated all nine lesions. The positive predictive value for the tests was 30%, 14%, and 64% for mammography, ultrasound, and MRI, respectively. Similarly, in a study in which physical examination, mammography, ultrasound, and MRI were all performed on the same day, Warner and colleagues[11] found 6 cancers in 196 women. Of these cancers, mammography and/or ultrasound could detect only three, while MRI was able to detect all six. Based on these data, it would be appropriate to conclude that MRI may play a role in screening the population of women thought to carry a genetic susceptibility to breast cancer.

Other women are at increased risk for breast cancer development, including women who have a diagnosis of atypical hyperplasia or lobular carcinoma in situ (LCIS) and those who have had prior mantle radiation for the treatment of lymphoma.[12–14] Morris and colleagues[15] addressed these other populations in addition to that with an inherited susceptibility gene when they evaluated the first screening MRI of 367 high-risk women at Memorial Sloan-Kettering Cancer Center. Biopsy was recommended in 64 (17%) women and performed in 59 women. Biopsy revealed cancer occult to mammography and physical examination in 14 (24%) of 59 women who had biopsy and in 14 (4%) of 367 women who had breast MRI screening. Among these 14 women with MRI-detected cancer, histologic findings were ductal carcinoma in situ (DCIS) in 8 (57%) and invasive cancer in 6 (43%). Although MRI screening is not the standard of care, these data suggest that there may be a benefit to incorporating breast MRI into the screening protocol for women with genetic susceptibility to breast cancer as well as for other women at increased risk for the disease.

2. Local Therapy for Breast Cancer

Once a diagnosis of breast cancer has been made, the goal of every breast surgeon is to perform the appropriate surgical procedure for definitive management of the disease. While it would be ideal if all patients with breast cancer presented with a readily interpretable mammogram with a single site of microcalcifications or a small, spiculated mass, this presentation sometimes seems to be the exception to the rule. It is in the cases in which diagnostic dilemmas exist that MRI has its greatest utility for the breast surgeon.

One such diagnostic dilemma exists in the patient who presents with a highly suspicious breast mass and a negative mammogram. As indicated previously, mammographic examination of the breast is falsely negative in up to 15% of women who present with a palpable lesion subsequently determined to be a breast cancer.[5] Additionally, while a targeted ultrasound examination of the area of concern increases sensitivity, 2% to 3% of all palpable cancers are still undetectable by the combination of modalities.[16] In most of these cases, the patient will have extremely dense breast tissue, making the physical examination of the remainder of the breast more difficult. Because of the inability to adequately assess the breast for other possible sites of disease, the surgeon is often justifiably reluctant to perform breast conservation therapy. It is thought that

these patients will be at increased risk for local recurrence postlumpectomy. Additionally, the patient herself is often quite concerned about the contralateral breast and the ability to detect disease in that breast.

Magnetic resonance imaging can provide valuable information for both the surgeon and the patient in cases such as this. Not only may it highlight areas of potential concern elsewhere within the ipsilateral breast, it will also assist in evaluating the contralateral breast. Fischer and colleagues[17] studied the additional benefit of MRI over that of mammography and ultrasound alone in the preoperative evaluation of the patient with a known breast abnormality. In 50 patients found to have multicentric disease, MRI alone was able to detect it in 24 of 50 (48%). Thus, in a patient in whom a cancer has been diagnosed but mammography is negative, the additional information from MRI can be invaluable. A negative breast MRI suggests that breast conservation may be feasible, whereas mastectomy will be more appropriate if MRI leads to the diagnosis of multicentric disease.

Several studies have also investigated the ability of MRI to detect disease in the contralateral breast. In a small study of 17 patients with known breast cancers,[18] 4 of the 17 patients (24%) were found to have contralateral cancer. In a larger study of 182 patients with known breast cancers who had contralateral breast MRI, 15 patients had suspicious lesions; cancer was found in 47% (7 of 15) lesions, constituting 4% (7 of 182) patients who had contralateral breast MRI.[19] In a study from our institution of 223 women who had MRI of the contralateral breast, biopsy was recommended in 72 (32%) women and performed in 61 women. An otherwise unsuspected cancer was found in 20% of women who had biopsy, constituting 5% of women who had contralateral breast MRI.[20] Magnetic resonance imaging evaluation of the contralateral breast may be of particular benefit in patients in whom the index cancer was not visualized on conventional imaging modalities.

A clinical scenario similar to that of the patient with negative imaging and a known cancer is that of the patient in whom a cancer is incidentally found at the time of a biopsy for other benign pathology. While an even less common occurrence than that of the palpable cancer without imaging correlate, a breast surgeon is faced with this situation more frequently today because of the increased use of screening mammography. As increasing numbers of biopsies of microcalcifications and suspicious lesions are recommended, the likelihood of finding early, incidental cancers in the surrounding tissue will also increase. While the microcalcifications that were targeted for biopsy are known to be benign, the breast surgeon often feels that the remainder of the breast is unable to be adequately evaluated. In this situation, MRI again is ideal for further evaluation of the tissues in both the ipsilateral and the contralateral breast.

Even in clinical scenarios in which the cancer appears to be well visualized by conventional imaging studies, MRI can be of value. In a study of 70 women with percutaneously proven breast cancer who had preoperative ipsilateral breast MRI at our institution, a biopsy was recommended based on MRI findings in 51%; additional sites of ipsilateral cancer were found by MRI in 27%.[21] These ipsilateral MRI-detected cancers were in the same quadrant as the index cancer in 20% of women, in a different quadrant in 4% of women, and in both the same and a different quadrant in 3% of women.[21] These findings show that preoperative breast MRI can detect otherwise unsuspected additional sites of disease that impact on surgical treatment.

One of the more frustrating situations encountered by a breast surgeon is the presence of positive surgical margins in a patient who appears to have a focal lesion without other pathologic changes on mammogram or physical examination. While the presence of one positive margin does not discourage the surgeon from pursuing breast conservation therapy, the presence of multiple positive margins often discourages its use. Before relegating the patient to a mastectomy, it may be helpful to consider breast MRI in this setting. It has been shown to be quite effective in the evaluation of extent of disease within the breast.[22,23] In a study of 85 invasive cancers, MRI was statistically significantly better at determining lesion size with accuracy than mammography.[23] Thus, while MRI may not define the absolute extent of disease within the breast, it can certainly be an important adjunct to the management of the patient with positive surgical margins.

Similar to the patient just presented with multiple positive margins despite negative imaging examinations, the patient with an infiltrating lobular cancer (ILC) often confounds the efforts of even the most experienced breast surgeon. Because of its unique growth pattern, in which tumor cells grow in a linear rather than a radial fashion, ILC tends to present as an ill-defined thickening rather than a well-demarcated mass. This growth pattern often makes it difficult to adequately assess the extent of the tumor on clinical examination. Additionally, it leads to an increased incidence of false-negative mammographic examinations.[24] If these clinical concerns are not frustrating enough to the surgeon, he or she must also be concerned about the increased risk of contralateral disease in the patient with ILC. The combination of these clinical factors makes an additional imaging study such as MRI attractive in the management of ILC. One study of MRI in patients with ILC indicated that MRI showed more extensive disease in 16 of 32 (50%) women when compared with both mammography and breast ultrasound examination.[25] While it underestimated tumor in 1 of 32 patients and overestimated tumor in 1 of 32 patients studied, it provided important clinical information in the vast majority of patients in this study.

In another, larger study of MRI's clinical utility in the evaluation of ILC, the ability to detect unsuspected ipsilateral and contralateral disease was investigated.[26] In 62 patients who had MRI after the diagnosis of ILC was made, 38 (61%) had abnormal findings for which biopsy was recommended. Among these 62 women, MRI detected otherwise unsuspected sites of cancer in the ipsilateral breast in 22% and in the contralateral breast in 9%. Data such as these support the effectiveness of MRI in the evaluation of the patient with ILC. Thus, it is reasonable for the breast surgeon to consider its use in those patients in whom ILC is diagnosed.

While these clinical scenarios have all demonstrated the ability of MRI examination to enhance evaluation of the extent of disease in a breast already shown to contain a breast cancer, the surgeon may also be faced with a scenario in which the primary site of cancer within the breast is not yet known. Such *occult* primary breast cancers, in which an axillary metastasis is the first indication of disease, account for less than 1% of all breast cancers diagnosed.[27] However, its diagnosis and treatment can be particularly difficult for both the patient and the surgeon. The vast majority of patients who present with such disease undergo conventional imaging without identification of a lesion.[28] Because of this, surgical management of such cases has almost always entailed the performance of a modified radical mastectomy. Despite this, cancer was found in the breast in only two thirds of patients who underwent mastectomy. Additionally, while not all lesions found at the time of mastectomy would have been amenable to breast conservation therapy, some patients would clearly have been candidates for a lumpectomy.

With all of these issues with the occult breast cancer in mind, any form of imaging that could improve the ability to detect disease within the breast in such cases would be most valuable. Magnetic resonance imaging appears to be of significant benefit in such cases. Several studies have addressed the ability of MRI to detect disease in the patient with occult breast cancer. One report of 22 patients in whom the presentation of cancer was a positive axillary node demonstrated the ability of MRI to detect a primary lesion in 19 of 22 (86%) of patients.[29] While there were two false-negative examinations, the remaining studies revealed cancers ranging in size from 4 to 30mm.

A second study evaluated 40 patients presenting with occult primary breast cancers.[30] In this study, tumors were visualized in 28 of 40 (70%) women who had MRI. Tumors detected by MRI ranged in size from 2 to 30mm. Based on the information obtained from MRI in both these patient populations, some women were able to contemplate breast-conserving therapy for the treatment of their presumed occult breast cancer. Thus, performing MRI of the breast in women presenting with axillary metastases from breast cancer has the potential not only to detect disease but, in many cases, to obviate the need for a patient to undergo a mastectomy for treatment.

3. Continuing Surveillance of the Breast Cancer Patient

It is clear from the above information that MRI can have a significant impact on the decision-making process the surgeon faces in dealing with local control issues in the breast cancer patient. But what is the role of MRI in the continued surveillance of the breast patient? In most instances, the breast surgeon, in conjunction with the medical oncologist, is principally responsible for the continued evaluation of the breast. In many respects, the patient who has already been treated for a breast cancer is at the highest risk for development of a subsequent breast cancer. With the increasing frequency of breast-conserving therapy, screening for local recurrences, which occur in approximately 10% of patients, is extremely important. Additionally, the risk of subsequent contralateral disease varies from 15% to 20% in the breast cancer patient without a genetic abnormality to as high as 60% in those patients who have a genetically inherited predisposition for the development of breast cancer.[31,32] These statistics underscore the need for careful evaluation of the treated and the untreated breast posttreatment for breast cancer.

Even years after radiation therapy was administered as part of breast conservation therapy, the treated breast can develop fat necrosis, a condition that mimics a recurrence in that breast. Often, the patient presents with a tender mass at the site of prior lumpectomy. Mammographic and ultrasonographic findings in such situations may be equivocal. However, there appear to be several characteristics features of this condition that may be visible on MRI.[33,34] Alternatively, MRI may show findings suspicious for recurrence, and support the need for biopsy.

Research is also ongoing as to the role of MRI in evaluating a mastectomy site after reconstruction with autogenous tissue. In one study of 23 patients who underwent mastectomy with autogenous tissue reconstruction, the MRI was able to clearly delineate the tissue that was transferred to the site from that which was native to the site.[35] While further study of this area is warranted, the preliminary data suggest that MRI can provide a helpful tool in the evaluation of the reconstructed breast.

As indicated previously, it is important to consider any woman who has already developed breast cancer as someone who is at greater than average risk of developing cancer in the contralateral breast. Furthermore, the greatest risk of contralateral disease exists in a population that is quite young at the time of initial diagnosis. Young age at diagnosis increases the likelihood that any subsequent cancer might be hidden in extremely dense breast tissue.

Because of this, more intensive screening of the contralateral breast with MRI may be considered in many of these patients.

4. Magnetic Resonance Imaging Guided Needle Localization: Technical Considerations for the Surgeon

Use of breast MRI in the scenarios discussed leads to detection of lesions that cannot be identified by mammography, sonography, or physical examination. For MRI-detected lesions warranting tissue diagnosis, biopsy must be guided by MRI, either with MRI-guided needle biopsy or MRI-guided needle localization (Figures 18.1 through 18.4). Recognizing the increasing role of breast MRI in the practice of the surgeon, there are several key technical points that should be made about surgical excision after MRI-guided needle localization.

Unlike most needle localization procedures, in which the most direct path to the lesion is taken when the localization wire is placed, the localization wires placed under MRI guidance often traverse a significant amount of the breast tissue. This occurs because the simplest way to perform the MRI-guided localization is to have the patient prone at the time of the localization procedure, thus rendering the medial breast relatively inaccessible. If the localizing wire was placed from a lateral approach for a medial lesion, the surgeon must bear in mind that the incision to be made should be over the end of the wire, not the

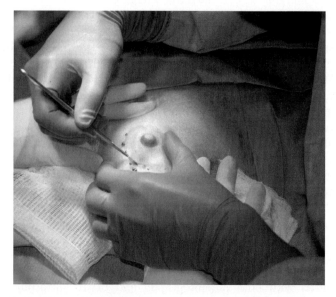

Figure 18.1. Intraoperative photograph of a women having surgical excision after MRI-guided needle localization. The wire, not seen on this image, was placed from a lateral approach. A periareolar incision is made to gain access to the lesion.

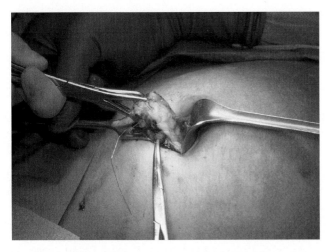

FIGURE 18.2. Intraoperative photograph showing removal of the tissue specimen after MRI-guided needle localization.

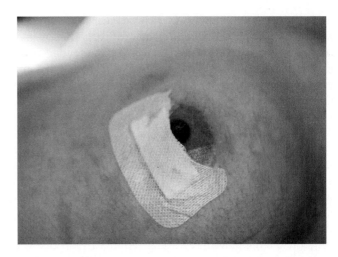

FIGURE 18.4. Intraoperative photograph of the breast after completion of MRI-guided localization and surgical excision. Sterile strips have been placed and a sterile dressing has been applied.

entrance point. If this is not taken into consideration, the surgeon could easily need to tunnel through a large area of breast tissue, increasing the risk of both infection and bleeding.

While the surgeon does not want to remove a large portion of tissue en route to the wire, it is important to consider performing a slightly more generous excision of the area in question than might be performed with either mammographic or sonographic localization. This is important due to the inability to visualize the lesion in question once the tissue is removed. Unlike mammographically or

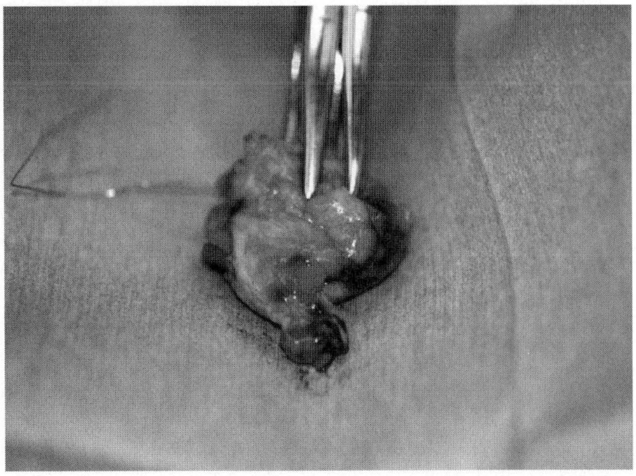

FIGURE 18.3. Intraoperative photograph of the specimen obtained after MRI-guided needle localization and surgical excision. The wire has been excised with the specimen. Specimen radiography (not shown) can confirm retrieval of the intact wire, but will not demonstrate the MRI-detected lesion, which was mammographically occult.

sonographically guided localization, in which specimen radiography or sonography, respectively, can confirm lesion retrieval, confirmation of removal of an MRI-detected lesion only comes with pathologic analysis. The surgeon is more likely to obtain the tissue in question with a wider excision.

When performing excision after MRI-guided needle localization, surgeons must also consider some of the unique properties of the localization wire. In contrast to the wire commonly used for mammographic and sonographic localization procedures, the titanium wire necessitated by its nonferrous (and thus nonmagnetic) nature is not as strong. This has several implications. First, if there is significant torque placed on the wire during the procedure, it can actually break. Second, the tip on the hook-end of the wire has more of a tendency either to break or to be cut during these procedures. Thus, it is extremely important to evaluate the wire after removal from the patient to determine that it is intact. One final property of the wire that is of importance is its heat-conductive properties. These titanium wires appear to have less resistance to heat conduction than the standard wire (G. Simkovich, PhD, personal communication) and, because of this, can transmit burns to the patient if electrocautery is used near them. For this reason, it is more appropriate to use a scalpel or sharp dissection scissor rather than cautery to remove the tissue in question.

5. Conclusions

Breast MRI can detect cancers that cannot be found by mammography or physical examination. However, breast MRI can have false-positive results. At our institution, among women who had high-risk screening breast MRI, a biopsy was recommended in 17%; cancer was found by MRI in 4%.[15] Among women with cancer who had contralateral breast MRI, a biopsy was recommended based on MRI findings in 32%; contralateral cancer was found by MRI in 5%.[20] Among women with cancer who had ipsilateral breast MRI, a biopsy was recommended based on MRI findings in 51%; additional sites of ipsilateral cancer were found by MRI in 27%.[21]

A surgeon who orders breast MRI should be aware of these data, and, perhaps even more importantly, should be aware of the outcomes from breast MRI at his or her own institution. The patient should understand the likelihood that breast MRI may lead to other tests, such as biopsy. In this manner, an informed decision can be made by the surgeon and the patient regarding whether to proceed with breast MRI. A surgeon who orders breast MRI should also be prepared to perform biopsy of nonpalpable, MRI-detected lesions that cannot be visualized by mammography or sonography.

As more is learned about MRI of the breast, more applications for its use in the management of the breast patient become apparent. For the surgeon who is intimately involved in all aspects of the care of such patients, understanding these potential applications and the technical issues involved with MRI-guided breast biopsies is becoming increasingly important. It is likely that breast MRI will have even greater impact as the technology disseminates, particularly methods for performing localization and biopsy under MRI guidance.

References

1. Day N, Warren R. Mammographic screening and mammographic patterns. *Breast Cancer Res*. 2000;2:247–251.
2. van Veen WA, Knotterus JA. Screening mammography. *Lancet* 2002;391:1701.
3. Tabar L, Bitak B, Tony HH, et al. Beyond randomized controlled trials: organized mammographic screening substantially reduces breast cancer mortality. *Cancer* 2001;91:1724–1731.
4. Ernster V, Barclay J, Kerlikowske K, et al. Incidence of and treatment for ductal carcinoma in situ. *JAMA*. 1996;275:913–918.
5. Kerlikowske K, Grady D, Rubin SM, et al. Efficacy of screening mammography: a meta-analysis. *JAMA*. 1995;273:149–154.
6. Carney PA, Migliortetti DL, Yankaskas BC, et al. Individual and combined effects of age, breast density, and hormone replacement therapy use on the accuracy of screening mammography. *Ann Intern Med*. 2003;138:168–175.
7. Easton DF, Bishop DT, Ford D, Crockford GP, and the Breast Linkage Consortium. Genetic linkage analysis in familial breast and ovarian cancer: results from 214 families. *Am J Hum Genet*. 1993;52:678–701.
8. Orel SG, Schnall MD. MR imaging of the breast for the detection, diagnosis, and staging of breast cancer. *Radiology* 2001;220:13–30.
9. Stoutjesdijk MJ, Boetes C, Jager GJ, et al. Magnetic resonance imaging and mammography in women with a hereditary risk of breast cancer. *J Natl Cancer Inst*. 2001;93:1095–1102.
10. Kuhl CK, Schmutzler RK, Leutner CC, et al. Breast MR imaging screening in 192 women proved or suspected to be carriers of a breast cancer susceptibility gene: preliminary results. *Radiology* 2000;215:267–279.
11. Warner E, Plewes DB, Shumak RS, et al. Comparison of breast magnetic resonance imaging, mammography, and ultrasound for surveillance of women at high risk for hereditary breast cancer. *J Clin Oncol*. 2001;19:3524–3351.
12. Page DL, Dupont WD, Rogers LW, Rados MS. Atypical hyperplastic lesions of the female breast: a long-term follow-up study. *Cancer* 1985;55:2698–2708.
13. Frykberg ER. Lobular carcinoma in situ of the breast. *Breast J*. 1999;5:296–302.
14. Bhatia S, Robison LL, Oberlin O, et al. Breast cancer and other second neoplasms after childhood Hodgkin's disease. *N Engl J Med*. 1996;334:745–751.
15. Morris EA, Liberman L, Ballon DJ, et al. MRI of occult breast carcinoma in a high-risk population. *AJR Am J Roentgenol*. 2003;181:619–626.
16. Kolb TM, Lichy J, Newhouse JH. Comparison of the performance of screening mammography, physical examination, and breast US and evaluation of the factors that influence them: an analysis of 27,825 patient examinations. *Radiology* 2002;225:165–175.
17. Fischer U, Kopka L, Grabbe E. Breast carcinoma: effect of preoperative contrast-enhanced MR imaging on the therapeutic approach. *Radiology* 1999;213:881–888.
18. Slanetz PJ, Edmister WB, Yeh ED, et al. Occult contralateral breast carcinoma incidentally detected by breast magnetic resonance imaging. *Breast J*. 2002;8:145–148.
19. Lee SG, Orel SG, Woo IJ, et al. MR imaging screening of the contralateral breast in patients with newly diagnosed breast cancer: preliminary results. *Radiology* 2003;226:773–778.
20. Liberman L, Morris EA, Kim CM, et al. MR imaging findings in the contralateral breast in women with recently diagnosed breast cancer. *AJR Am J Roentgenol*. 2003;180:333–841.
21. Liberman L, Morris EA, Dershaw DD, et al. MR imaging of the ipsilateral breast in women with percutaneously proven breast cancer. *AJR Am J Roentgenol*. 2003;180:901–910.
22. Davis PL, Staiger MJ, Harris KB, et al. Breast cancer measurements with magnetic resonance imaging, ultrasonography, and mammography. *Breast Cancer Res Treat*.1996;37:1–9.
23. Mumtaz H, Hall-Craggs MA, Davidson T, et al. Staging of symptomatic primary breast cancer with MR imaging. *AJR Am J Roentgenol*. 1997;169:417–424.
24. Krecke KN, Gisvold JJ. Invasive lobular carcinoma of the breast: mammographic findings and extent of disease at diagnosis in 184 patients. *AJR Am J Roentgenol*. 1993;161:957–960.
25. Weinstein SP, Orel SG, Heller R, et al. MR imaging of the breast in patients with invasive lobular carcinoma. *AJR Am J Roentgenol*. 2001;176:399–406.
26. Quan ML, Sclafani L, Heerdt A, et al. Magnetic resonance imaging detects unsuspected disease in patients with invasive lobular cancer. *Ann Surg Oncol*. 2003;10:1048–1053.

27. Baron PL, Moore MP, Kinne DW, et al. Occult breast cancer presenting with axillary metastases. *Arch Surg.* 1990;61: 431–434.

28. Jackson B, Scott-Conner C, Moulder J. Axillary metastasis from occult breast carcinoma: diagnosis and management. *Am Surg.* 1995;1995:61–431.

29. Orel SG, Weinstein SP, Schnall MD, et al. Breast MR imaging in patients with axillary node metastases and unknown primary malignancy. *Radiology* 1999;212:543–549.

30. Olson JA Jr, Morris EA, Van Zee KJ, et al. Magnetic resonance imaging facilitates breast conservation for occult breast cancer. *Ann Surg Oncol.* 2000;7:411–415.

31. Dewar JA, Arriagada R, Benhamous S, et al. Local relapse and contralateral tumor rates in patients with breast cancer treated with conservative surgery and radiotherapy. *Cancer* 1995;76:2260–2265.

32. Bernstein JL, Thomopson WD, Risch N, Holford TR. The genetic epidemiology of second primary breast cancer. *Am J Epidemiol.* 1992;136:937–948.

33. Padhani AR, Yarnold JR, Regan J, Husband JE. Magnetic resonance imaging of induration in the irradiated breast. *Radiother Oncol.* 2002;64:157–162.

34. Dao TH, Rahmouni A, Campana F, et al. Tumor recurrence versus fibrosis in the irradiated breast: differentiation with dynamic gadolinium-enhanced MR imaging. *Radiology* 1993;187:751–755.

35. Rieber A, Schramm K, Helms G, et al. Breast-conserving surgery and autogeneous tissue reconstruction in patients with breast cancer: efficacy of MRI of the breast in the detection of recurrent disease. *Eur Radiol.* 2003;13:780–787.

19
Magnetic Resonance Imaging Guided Needle Localization

Laura Liberman

Magnetic resonance imaging (MRI) can detect breast cancer that is mammographically and clinically occult. Although MRI has high (94%–100%) reported sensitivity in breast cancer detection, the reported specificity is lower (37%–97%).[1] Specificity can potentially be improved by careful analysis of lesion morphology and kinetics. However, definitive diagnosis of MRI-detected lesions that are suspicious or highly suggestive of malignancy requires biopsy. A breast MRI program should have capability for tissue sampling of lesions detected by breast MRI.

Magnetic resonance imaging guided localization presents numerous challenges.[2] Magnetic resonance imaging is usually performed with the patient prone, a position that enables ready access to the lateral but not the medial breast. In closed magnet systems, the patient must be removed from the magnet to gain access to the breast for localization. Lesion visibility often decreases with time after contrast injection as contrast washes out of the lesion and into the surrounding breast parenchyma. For MRI-guided surgical biopsy, confirmation of lesion retrieval is difficult because the lesion does not enhance ex vivo.

In spite of these challenges, several authors have reported success with MRI-guided needle localization for surgical biopsy[3–13] (Table 19.1). In published series of MRI-guided needle localization, the technical success rate was 98% to 100%; histologic analysis revealed cancer in 31% to 73% [of which up to half were ductal carcimoma in situ (DCIS)], and high-risk lesions such as atypical ductal hyperplasia (ADH) or lobular carcinoma in situ (LCIS) in up to 29% (Table 19.1). This chapter addresses equipment considerations for MRI-guided localization, discusses technique and results of MRI-guided needle localization for surgical biopsy using commercially available equipment at our institution, and makes suggestions for approaching specific challenging clinical situations.

1. Equipment Considerations

1.2. Closed Versus Open Magnets

Magnetic resonance imaging guided intervention requires imaging systems that allow visualization of small lesions with high spatial resolution to enable accurate needle placement, and that perform rapidly enough to allow dynamic as well as morphologic data and to minimize the procedure time. The 1.5 Tesla (T) closed magnets allow high signal-to-noise ratio and visualization of small lesions and have been validated for MRI-guided intervention.[14] Open magnets have potential advantages, including access to the breast from all angles and interactive real-time visualization of needle placement. However, closed magnets are more ubiquitous, have higher field strength and better field homogeneity, and are the systems for which most validation data exist for MRI-guided intervention. A system for MRI-guided biopsy must incorporate the possibility of performing biopsy in a closed system, requiring that the patient be removed from the bore of the magnet to gain access to the breast for the interventional procedure.

1.2. Free-Hand Versus Grid Compression

Magnetic resonance imaging guided interventions can be performed free-hand[9,15] or by using guidance methods, such as compression grid systems, that allow coordinates to be obtained.[12] The free-hand method has the advantage of allowing the needle to be angled, because it is not in a fixed orientation, but the potential disadvantage of a long examination time because repeat imaging is necessary to confirm needle placement. Open magnets that allow real-time imaging may be most amenable to the free-hand approach, as repositioning the needle and confirming needle location can be performed faster. For closed

TABLE 19.1. MRI-Guided Localization: Published Experience

Study/Year	N	Needle	Size (cm) (Mean Range)	No. Successful (%)	No. Cancer (%)	Invasive (%)	DCIS (%)	High Risk (%)	Time (min) (Mean Range)
Heywang-Kobrunner et al./1994[3]	11	NS	1.4 (0.6–1.5)	11 (100)	8 (73)	6 (55)	2 (18)	0 (0)	<1 h
Orel et al./1994[4]	11	18G	0.9 (0.3–2.0)	11 (100)	5 (45)	3 (27)	2 (18)	1 (9)	NS
Fischer et al./1995[5a]	15	NS	NS	15 (100)	5 (33)	5 (33)	0 (0)	0 (0)	NS
Fischer et al./1995[6a]	28	19.5G	NS	26 (93)	12 (43)	9 (32)	3 (11)	8 (29)	60 (40–90)[b]
Doler et al./1996[7a]	23	19.5G	NS	23 (100)	10 (43)	NS	NS	NS	NS
Kuhl et al./1997[8]	97	NS	NS	95 (98)	53 (55)	42 (43)	11 (11)	14 (14)	40 (30–60)
Daniel et al./1998[9]	19	20/21G	0.9[c] (0.3–6.0)	19 (100)	8 (42)	5 (26)	3 (16)	2 (11)	64 (up to 90)[d]
Fischer et al./1998[10a]	130	NS	NS	127 (98)	64 (49)	58 (45)	6 (5)	2 (2)[e]	NS (30–60)[f]
Orel et al./1999[11]	137	20G	1.2 (0.3–7.0)	134 (98)	57 (42)	40 (29)	17 (12)	NS	NS
Morris et al./2002[12]	101	18/20G	1.1[g] (0.2–8.0)	101 (100)	31 (31)	16 (16)	15 (15)	9 (9)	31[g] (15–59)
Taourel et al./2002[13]	264	NS	NS	259 (98)	95 (36)	76 (29)	19 (7)	6 (2)	NS

Abbreviations: N, number of lesions; NS, not stated. Percentages reflect proportion of all lesions (N). DCIS, ductal carcinoma in situ. High-risk lesions include atypical ductal hyperplasia (ADH), atypical lobular carcinoma (ALH), lobular carcinoma in situ (LCIS), and radial scar.

[a] There may be overlap between cases in Refs. 5–7 and 10, hence numbers should not be added together in meta-analysis.

[b] Reflects time average and range for all MR interventions (fine needle aspiration biopsy or localization).

[c] Approximate median: 10 (53%) of 19 lesions were smaller than 0.9 cm.

[d] Reflects total time that patient was in MR suite. Lower end of range not stated. Time from selection of skin entry site to deployment of hookwire was 60 min or less in all cases and averaged 17 min.

[e] Includes two radial scars. An additional 18 benign lesions classified as "dysplasia" are not included as high-risk lesions.

[f] Reflects time average and range for all MR interventions (fine needle aspiration, core biopsy, or localization).

[g] Median, not mean.

magnets, grid systems that allow more accurate initial needle placement may be preferable (Figure 19.1).

1.3. Prone Versus Supine Positioning

Breast MRI-guided intervention can be performed with the patient prone or supine. Although supine positioning has been used by some investigators,[7,16] prone positioning is usually preferable because breast coils may be used in the prone position; furthermore, the breast is pendant and away from the chest wall and needle direction is parallel to the chest wall. Some investigators have suggested that the prone oblique position facilitates access to the posterior tissues and axillary tail.[8]

1.4. Breast Immobilization

Breast immobilization is important in MRI-guided intervention for several reasons. Often the lesion becomes less evident during the procedure due to the transient nature of contrast enhancement; it is therefore essential to identify the lesion at the outset of the procedure and then to ensure that the lesion remains fixed in position. Furthermore, MRI-compatible needles are traditionally not as sharp as their non-MRI counterparts; breast immobilization is therefore necessary to help minimize lesion motion during needle placement. In addition to immobilizing the breast, mild compression may enable the entire breast to be imaged with fewer sagittal slices, shortening procedure time. It is important not to use excessive compression, which has been reported to interfere with lesion enhancement and visualization.[8,17]

Immobilization of the breast can be achieved by a thermoplastic mesh[18] or by immobilizing the breast between two compression plates[3] (Figure 19.1).[4,12] Compression plates, which allow access to the breast parallel to the direction of compression, are usually oriented in the mediolateral plane, although some noncommercially available

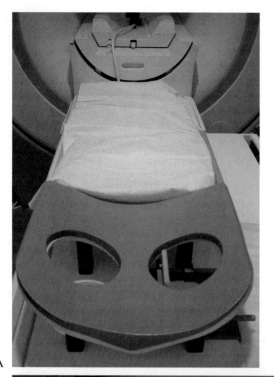

FIGURE 19.1. Equipment for MRI-guided needle localization. (A) Double breast coil (Open Breast Coil [Model OBC–63] MRI Devices, Waukesha, Wis.) in position in 1.5 T magnet (Signa, General Electric, Milwaukee, Wis.). For interventional MRI examinations, as for diagnostic studies, the patient lies prone with the breast, having biopsy breast in the dedicated breast coil, and enters the magnet feet first. (B) Breast MRI coil with compression grid (Biopsy Positioning Device Model MR-BI-160, MRI Devices) in place. (C) Close-up of compression grid for MRI-guided needle localization. This grid has crosshatches laterally and a flat plate medially. (D) Compression grid for MRI-guided localization with needle guide in place. The needle guide has multiple parallel holes that allow access for the localizing needle. (E) One of several commercially available MRI-compatible needle and wire combinations available for MRI-guided needle localization procedures (MR eye, Cook, Bloomington, Ind.). Useful features of this system include the 1-cm marks on the needle shaft, an adjustable plastic depth stop on the needle that can be set to the appropriate depth, and a reinforced portion (arrows) of the localizing wire.

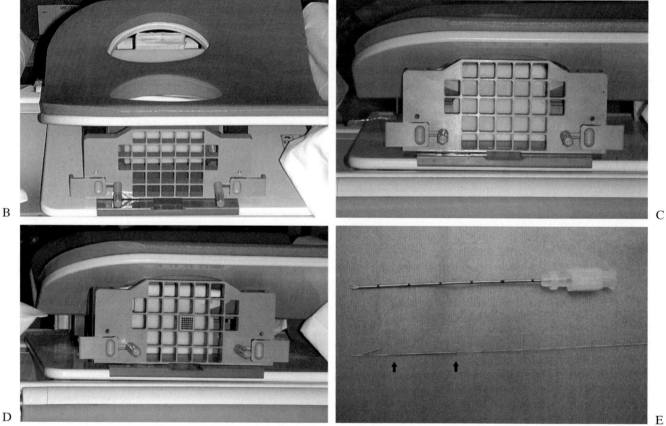

systems allow compression in the craniocaudal direction.[8] Compression plates have been manufactured with perforated holes,[4] flexible horizontal bands,[19] or fixed grid lines.[12] A breast biopsy coil is now available (Biopsy Breast Array Coil [model BBC] MRI Devices, Waukesha, Wis.) that has removable compression plates, enabling access to both the medial and lateral side of the breast with the patient in the prone position.

1.5. Fiducial Markers and Needle Guides

To accurately place a needle, the position of the lesion must be related to the overlying grid system. This can be accomplished by placing a fiducial marker on the grid system, usually close to the expected lesion location. The fiducial marker can be a vial filled with gadolinium-diaminotetra-ethyl penta-acetic acid (DTPA) or copper sulfate ($CuSO_4$) inserted into one of the grid holes or a vitamin E capsule taped to the grid and skin.[12] The fiducial marker is visualized as high signal on initial postcontrast images; needle insertion site can then be determined by measuring the lesion location relative to the fiducial marker. The depth of the lesion from the level of the grid and skin surface is calculated by multiplying the number of sagittal slices by the slice thickness.

To place the needle in the breast, an opening in the compression paddle is necessary. This can be accomplished in several ways. Grid systems may enable compression to be maintained while allowing a needle guide to be inserted into the desired hole to facilitate needle placement[12] [Figure 19.1(D)]. Alternatively, the compression paddle itself may have perforated holes.[4] Guidance for needle placement, by means of separate needle guide or holes in the compression plate, allows the needle to be straight and parallel to the chest wall. For free-hand localization procedures, the large opening in the compression paddle allows access but does not provide comparable breast immobilization.

1.6. Magnetic Resonance Imaging Compatible Needles

A variety of needles are now commercially available for MRI-guided needle localization [Figure 19.1(E)]. Conventional ferromagnetic needles cannot be used for MRI-guided localization procedures due to the high magnetic field. Nonferromagnetic materials such as stainless steel produce severe artifacts. Certain alloys and ceramic materials are ideal for use in MRI-guided interventions. Materials with increased nickel content such as iconel and other high nickel and low susceptibility alloys generate less artifact. Titanium wires and needles also have fewer artifacts but are difficult to manufacture and are less rigid than the alloys. Nonmetallic materials such as plastics and ceramics

may produce less artifact and are being investigated. Although artifact can be bothersome, artifact can be used to recognize the location of the wire or needle on MRI studies; the concept of *controlled artifact* should be considered in equipment design and selection of MRI intervention.

2. Breast Magnetic Resonance Imaging Technique and Interpretation at Memorial Sloan-Kettering Cancer Center

2.1. Breast Magnetic Resonance Imaging Technique

At our institution, diagnostic MRI examinations are performed with the patient prone in a 1.5T commercially available system (Signa, GE Medical Systems, Milwaukee, Wis.) using a dedicated surface breast coil. For most examinations to date, our imaging sequence has included a localizing sequence followed by a sagittal fat-suppressed T2-weighted sequence [4000/85 (repetition time msec/echo time msec)]. A T1-weighted three-dimensional, fat-suppressed fast spoiled gradient echo [17/2.4 (repetition time msec/echo time msec); flip angle, 35 degrees, bandwidth 31.25] sequence is then performed before and three times following a rapid bolus injection of 0.1 mmol/L gadopentetate dimeglumine (Magnevist®) per kilogram of body weight. Contrast material is administered as a rapid bolus injection through an indwelling intravenous catheter. Image acquisition starts immediately following contrast material injection and saline bolus. Images are obtained sagittally, for an acquisition time per volumetric acquisition approximately 2min each. Total imaging time for bilateral breast MRI with all sequences, including three postcontrast acquisitions, is approximately 35–40min.

Section thickness is 2–3mm without gap, using a matrix of 256×192 and field of view of 18–22cm. Frequency is in the anterior-posterior direction. Following the examination the precontrast images are subtracted from the first postcontrast images on a pixel-by-pixel basis. Maximum intensity projection (MIP) images are obtained in all examinations. Other MRI scanning protocols at our institution are discussed in Chapter 3.

2.2. Interpretation of Breast Magnetic Resonance Imaging Examinations

At our institution, breast MRI examinations are interpreted according to previously published criteria.[20] Studies are reviewed on soft copy using a picture archive and communication system (PACS; GE Medical Systems) that allows manual windowing and optimization of parameters. Magnetic resonance imaging examinations are interpreted in conjunction with other breast imaging studies, including mammograms and sonograms, when available. Mammographic parenchymal density is described on a scale of 1 to 4, where 1 is predominantly fatty, 2 is scattered fibroglandular densities, 3 is heterogeneously dense, and 4 is dense, as per the Breast Imaging Reporting and Data System (BI-RADS™).[21]

For MRI-detected lesions, level of suspicion is reported on a scale of 0 to 6 identical to the lesion assessment categories used in the BI-RADS lexicon.[21] Numerical categories are 0, needs additional imaging evaluation; 1, normal; 2, benign; 3, probably benign, recommend 6-month follow-up MRI; 4, suspicious; 5, highly suggestive of malignancy, or 6, proven cancer. Morphologic patterns that are referred for biopsy generally include spiculated or irregular margins, heterogeneous or rim enhancement or clumped enhancement in a ductal or segmental distribution.[20,22–26] Tiny foci of enhancement or stippled enhancement are morphologic features that do not generally prompt biopsy. Masses with smooth borders and homogeneous enhancement may be referred for biopsy, at the discretion of the radiologist interpreting the study. Classification is based primarily on lesion morphology, but kinetic features are visually assessed on the three postcontrast image acquisitions.[22] Quantitative kinetic curves are generated in specific cases at the request of the interpreting radiologist, such as for lesions with morphologic features considered to be *probably benign*.[27,28]

2.3. Correlative Sonography

For lesions interpreted as suspicious or highly suggestive of malignancy at MRI, correlative sonography is often performed to determine if the lesion is amenable to tissue sampling under sonographic guidance. If the lesion is not seen at sonography, MRI-guided localization is recommended. If the lesion is reliably identified by sonography or mammography, biopsy is usually performed under the guidance of those imaging modalities.

Some investigators have reported a sonographic correlate in up to 100% of MRI-detected lesions referred for biopsy.[29,30] However, in our experience, a sonographic correlate was found in only 23% of MRI-detected lesions referred for biopsy.[31] Although the frequency of cancer was higher among lesions that had sonographic correlates as compared with lesions that did not (43% vs. 14%, $P = 0.01$), absence of a sonographic correlate did not spare the need for biopsy of a suspicious MRI-detected lesion.[31] The lack of a sonographic correlate in a high proportion of MRI-detected lesions warranting biopsy emphasizes the importance of the capability to perform biopsy of lesions detected by MRI only.

3. Magnetic Resonance Imaging Guided Localization Technique

3.1. Positioning and Compression

At our institution, MRI-guided needle localization is performed as previously described[12] with the patient prone in a 1.5T magnet (Signa, GE Medical Systems) using a dedicated breast surface coil (Open Breast Coil [Model OBC–63] or Biopsy Breast Array Coil [Model BBC], MRI Devices, Waukesha, Wis.). The breast undergoing localization is placed in a dedicated biopsy compression device using a commercially available grid-localizing system or a slightly modified design of the commercially available model (Figure 19.2). In most cases, the medial aspect of the breast is first positioned flush against a compression plate. A lateral crosshatched grid is then firmly adjusted to immobilize the breast. A vitamin E capsule is used as a fiducial marker and is taped to the lateral grid over the expected lesion site, based on review of the diagnostic MRI examination (Figure 19.2C).

3.2. Imaging Before Needle Placement

An axial localizing T1-weighted MRI sequence is obtained, and the volume of interest selected to include the compression device and the vitamin E marker that is taped to the lateral grid (Figure 19.3A). Gadopentetate dimeglumine (Magnevist®), 0.1 mmol/L per kilogram of body weight, is then injected intravenously as a rapid bolus injection through an indwelling intravenous catheter. No precontrast image is obtained during the localization procedure, although such images were part of the initial diagnostic MRI examination.

Image acquisition starts immediately following contrast injection, using a three-dimensional, fat-suppressed fast spoiled gradient-recalled echo [17/2.4 (repetition time msec/echo time msec); flip angle, 35 degrees] sequence, with images obtained in the sagittal plane. Time of acquisition, usually less than 1 min, is variable, depending on the size of the breast and area covered. Section thickness of approximately 3 mm without gap, with a 256 × 192 matrix and a field of view of 18–22 cm, is used.

3.3. Determining Lesion Location

Images are reviewed at the workstation (Figure 19.3B). A cursor is placed over the lesion on the monitor, and its relationship to the skin surface and the vitamin E marker is determined by manually scrolling through sequential sagittal slices. The grid of the compression device is evident as low-signal intensity lines at the skin surface due to pressure indentation (Figure 19.3C); the plastic of the compression device is not visible on MRI. The vitamin E

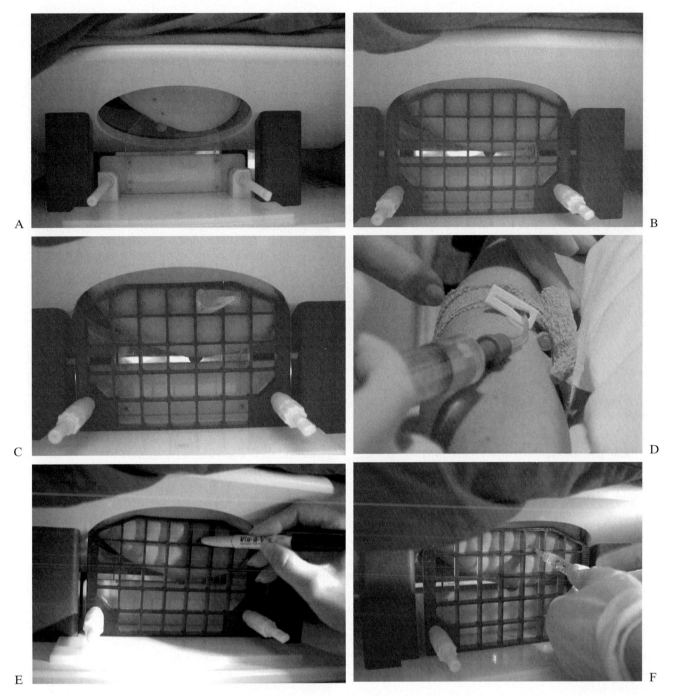

FIGURE 19.2. A 56-year-old woman with family history of breast cancer and prior biopsy showing atypia, who had abnormal breast MRI examination. (A) The patient is positioned prone with her breast in the dedicated breast coil. (B) The breast is positioned within the compression grid. This grid represents a slightly modified, earlier version of the grid shown in Figure 19.1. (C) A vitamin E capsule has been taped over the expected lesion site, based on review of MRI images. (D) After obtaining and reviewing axial localizing images to ensure that the breast and vitamin E marker are optimally included in the field of view, intravenous gadolinium is injected. (E) The expected lesion site is marked with a pen, based on review of MRI study after contrast injection on the day of the localization. (F) Local anesthesia is injected over lesion site.

(*Continued*)

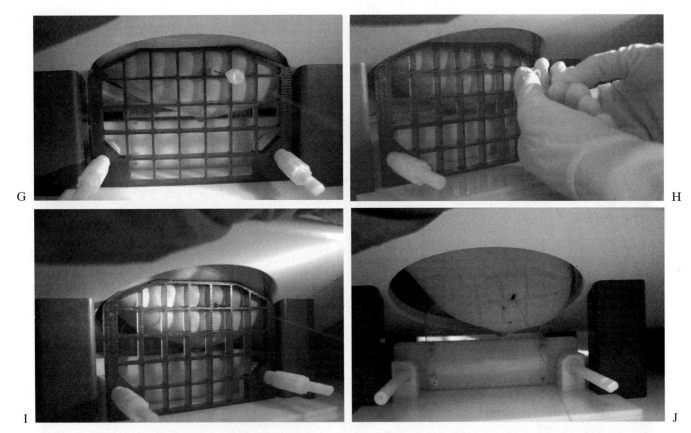

FIGURE 19.2. (*Continued*) (G) The localizing needle is placed, and its accurate position verified with repeat MRI. In this case, because the lesion was superficial, the radiologist elected to place the needle without using the needle guide. (H) If needle position is appropriate, the wire is deployed and the needle is removed. (I) The wire is left in place, and its accurate position confirmed with repeat MRI. (J) After appropriate wire position is docu-mented, the grid compression is removed, with the wire in place. Postlocalization two-view mammogram will be performed to demonstrate the location of the wire within the breast parenchyma and with respect to the nipple and chest wall. Labeled mammogram films are sent with the patient for use during surgery.

capsule is identified as an area of high signal intensity at the skin surface (Figure 19.3D). The skin entry site is determined based on visual assessment of the location of the lesion with respect to the grid lines, using the vitamin E capsule as a guide. The depth of the lesion from the skin surface is calculated as the difference between the depth of the skin surface and the depth of the sagittal slice containing the lesion.

After calculating the entrance site and lesion depth, the patient is withdrawn from the magnet. A mark is made on the skin overlying the lesion, and the skin is cleansed with alcohol and anesthetized with 1 to 2 mL 1% lidocaine HCl (Xylocaine®). A needle guide that is provided with the grid compression system can then be inserted into the grid hole overlying the anesthetized area. The needle guides are manufactured to have 18- or 20-gauge holes to accommodate various needle sizes. The needle guide is used to anchor and stabilize the needle and to enable insertion of the needle in a straight, perpendicular approach, without angulation. The MRI-compatible needle/hookwire (Leloc,

18 or 20 gauge, MRI Devices Daum Gmbtl; MRI Breast Lesion Marking System, 20 gauge, E-Z-EM Inc, Westbury, NY; or MReye, 20 gauge, Cook, Bloomington, Ind.) is then placed in one of the holes (through the needle guide, if used), closest to the marking on the skin.

The needle is inserted to the desired depth, approximately 5 to 10 mm deep to the lesion. If the needle guide is used, the radiologist must take into account the thickness of the needle guide attached to the grid, approximately 20 mm. For example, if the lesion is five slices deep to the skin, then the depth of insertion using the needle guide, in millimeters, is $(5 \times 3) + 20 + 10 = 45$ mm, where 5×3 indicates 5 slices each 3 mm thick, 20 is the thickness of the needle guide in the grid, and 10 mm is the desired depth of the tip of the wire beyond the lesion.

In some instances, the radiologist may choose to perform MRI-guided needle localization without the needle guide. The needle guide stabilizes the needle and increases the likelihood that it is straight, but deprives the radiologist of the opportunity to see exactly when the needle is piercing

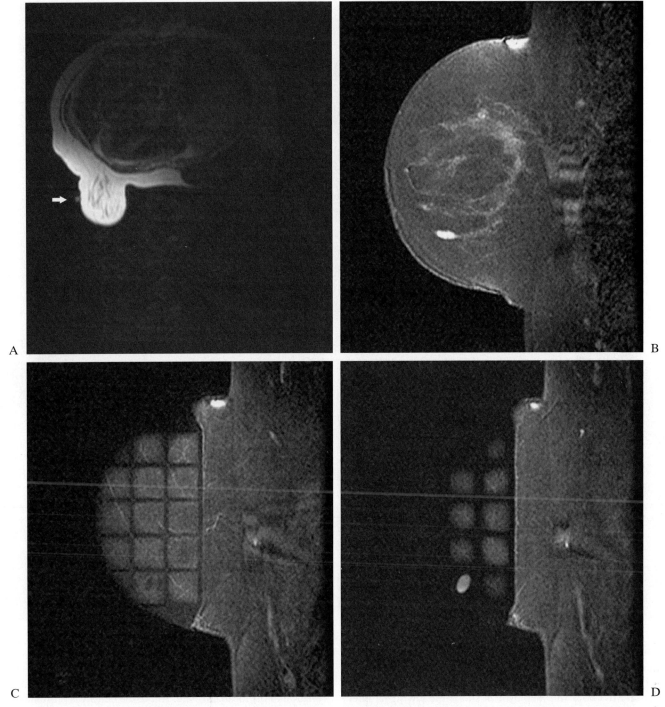

A

B

C

D

FIGURE 19.3. Representative images from left breast MRI-guided localization procedure in a 58-year-old woman who had a prior right mastectomy and reconstruction. (A) Axial localizing images show that the left breast is being gently compressed, as evidenced by slight flattening of the skin surface. The indentations of the grid lines are subtly seen at the lateral aspect of the breast, as is the vitamin E marker (arrow). (B) Sagittal MRI of the left breast after injection of intravenous gadolinium shows an enhancing mass in the inferior left breast. (C) Sagittal MRI of the left breast, more lateral image, shows the low signal intensity indentations of the grid lines on the skin. This slice is taken to represent the skin surface, and the depth of the lesion is calculated with respect to this level. For example, if the sagittal slice demonstrating the lesion is located 5 slices deep to this slice, then the depth of the lesion from the skin is 5 slices × 3 mm/slice = 15 mm. The desired location of the wire tip is 5 to 10 mm deep to the lesion. (D) Sagittal MRI of the left breast, even more lateral image, shows the high signal intensity vitamin E marker, which has been taped to the grid at the expected lesion site. The skin entry site is determined by scrolling back and forth on the workstation and relating the portion of the grid overlying the lesion to the portion of the grid containing the vitamin E marker.

(Continued)

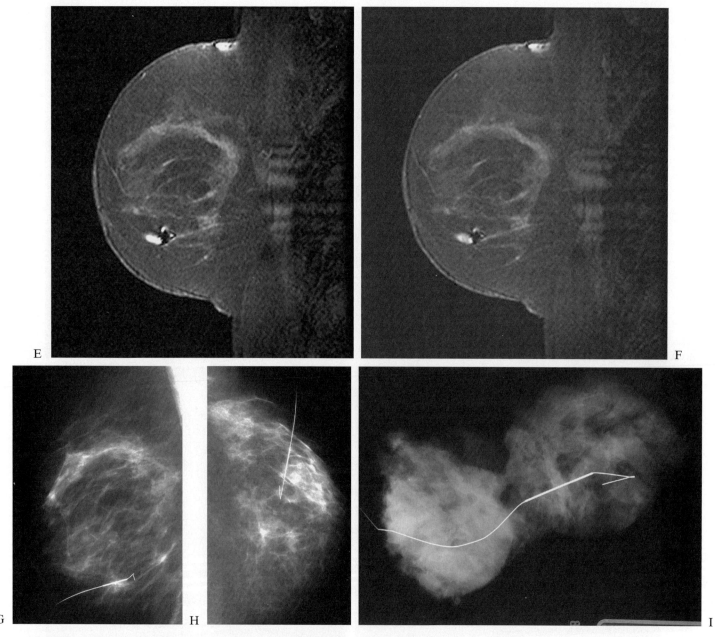

FIGURE 19.3. (*Continued*) (E) Sagittal MRI after needle place-ment shows the low signal intensity artifact from the needle immediately adjacent to the mass. The depth of the needle tip is determined by scrolling through sequential sagittal slices. (F) Sagittal MRI after wire deployment shows the low signal inten-sity artifact from the deployed wire at the posterior aspect of the lesion. (G) Mediolateral oblique view from two-view left mam-mogram obtained after localization shows the localizing wire in place. The reinforced portion is within a patchy area of parenchyma that was unaltered from multiple prior mammo-gram. (H) Craniocaudal view from two-view left mammogram again shows the deployed wire. (I) Specimen radiograph confirms retrieval of the localizing wire. Soft tissue density is present in the specimen, but no discrete mass is seen. Histologic analysis yielded infiltrating lobular carcinoma, for which the patient underwent subsequent mastectomy.

the skin rather than simply displacing it. It may be reasonable to forego the needle guide if the lesion is superficial and may be particularly helpful to forego the needle guide in specific scenarios, such as a lesion close to an implant. If the needle guide is not used, the radiologist simply inserts the needle to the desired depth, approximately 5 to 10mm deep to the calculated depth of the lesion.

3.4. Imaging After Needle Insertion

Sagittal T1-weighted images are then obtained to document the location of the needle. The needle is evident as a low signal intensity structure with adjacent susceptibility artifact [Figure 19.3(E)]. Visualization of the target lesion might be compromised by needle artifact on these images, especially if the lesion is small. Surrounding anatomic landmarks can be useful when verifying lesion depth. Also, the lesion may be less conspicuous due to washout of contrast material. However, identification of the target site is generally not a problem due to the ability to localize the lesion location relative to the vitamin E marker and the location of the tip relative to the desired depth, as well as analyzing surrounding landmarks. If the needle is too deep or too superficial, adjustments are made. When the needle tip is in good position, the wire is deployed by advancing the wire to the *mark*, indicating that the tip had emerged from the needle. The needle is then removed, leaving the wire in place, and a final series of T1-weighted images are obtained to document wire position [Figure 19.3(F)].

After localization, a two-view mammogram is obtained so that the surgeon can see the location of the wire with respect to the nipple, the chest wall, and the remainder of the breast tissue [Figure 19.3(G) and 19.3(H)]. These films are labeled, a labeled diagram is drawn, and the labeled films and diagram are sent to surgery with the patient. Specimen radiography can be performed to document retrieval of the localizing wire, but the lesions undergoing MRI-guided localization are generally not seen on the mammogram and are not identified on the specimen radiograph [Figure 19.3(I)].

4. Magnetic Resonance Imaging Guided Needle Localization: Memorial Sloan-Kettering Cancer Center Experience

4.1. Patient and Lesion Characteristics and Indications for Magnetic Resonance Imaging

In a study of 101 consecutive lesions in 69 women who had MRI-guided needle localization at Memorial Sloan-Kettering Cancer Center during a 17-month period,[12]

median age of women was 51 years (range, 28–79y). Magnetic resonance imaging guided localization was performed of a single lesion in 49 women and of two or more lesions in 20 women. Among 20 women with multiple (median, 2; range, 2–5) lesions, the lesions were unilateral in 17 and bilateral in 3; lesions were synchronous in 18 and metachronous in 2.[12]

The first 22 lesions had localization under an Institutional Review Board approved protocol that required a mammographic correlate for the MRI lesion; in these cases, the decision to biopsy had been made based on the findings at mammography. Among the subsequent 79 lesions, 1 had a mammographic correlate, 1 had both a mammographic and a sonographic correlate, and 1 had a sonographic correlate but no mammographic correlate; in these three women, MRI-guided localization was performed because of the existence of synchronous ipsilateral lesions identified only by MRI. Therefore, MRI guidance was necessary for localization in 76 (75%) of 101 lesions in the study. The indication for MRI that led to the detection of these 101 lesions was high-risk screening in 35 (35%), extent of disease assessment in a woman with known cancer in 35 (35%), and problem solving in 31 (31%).

4.2. Lesion Size and Location and Breast Density

In our study of 101 lesions that had MRI-guided needle localization for surgical biopsy, median lesion size was 1.1cm (range, 0.2–8.0cm). The lesion was located in the left breast in 53 (52%) and in the right breast in 48 (48%) lesions; 68 (67%) were lateral and 33 (33%) were medial. Breast parenchymal density was classified as ACR class 1 (fatty) in one (1%) lesion, class 2 (scattered fibroglandular densities) in 23 (23%) lesions, class 3 (heterogeneously dense) in 53 (52%) lesions, and class 4 (dense) in 24 (24%) lesions.

4.3. Histologic Findings

Histologic analysis of 101 lesions excised after MRI-guided needle localization revealed cancer in 31 (31%) lesions, high-risk lesions (LCIS or ADH) in 9 (9%), and benign findings in 61 (61%) (Table 19.1).[12] Cancer was found in 9 (38%) of 24 MRI lesions that had mammographic correlates and in 22 (29%) of 77 MRI lesions without mammographic correlates ($P = 0.57$).

Among 31 cancers, histologic findings were DCIS in 15 (48%) and invasive carcinoma in 16 (52%). Invasive caancers ranged in size from 0.1 to 2.0cm (median, 1.2cm). Histologic findings in 16 invasive cancers were invasive ductal carcinoma and DCIS in 8 (50%), invasive lobular cancer in 4 (25%), invasive ductal and lobular cancer and DCIS in 3, and invasive ductal carcinoma in 1 (6%).

4.4. Positive Predictive Value in Different Patient Subgroups

Cancer was found in 16 (46%) of 35 lesions referred for MRI-guided localization in women who had MRI for extent of disease assessment, 10 (32%) of 31 lesions referred for MRI-guided localization in women who had MRI for problem-solving, and 5 (14%) of 35 lesions referred for MRI-guided localizing in women who had MRI for high-risk screening.

The likelihood of cancer at MRI-guided localization was significantly higher if the indication for the diagnostic MRI examination was extent of disease assessment or problem-solving rather than high-risk screening (26/66 = 39% vs. 5/35 = 14%, $P < 0.02$). Of 16 cancers diagnosed at MRI-guided localization in women who had MRI for extent of disease assessment, the cancers diagnosed after MRI-guided localization were in the same breast as the index cancer in 12 (in the same quadrant in 10 and in a different quadrant in 2) and in the contralateral breast in 4.

4.5. Procedure Time, Accuracy, and Complications

The median time to perform MRI-guided needle localization was 31 min (range, 15–59 min). The median distance between the depth of the wire tip and the depth of the lesion was 1.0 cm (range, 0.0–3.4 cm). In 90 lesions in which the distance could be determined, the distance between the depth of the wire tip and the depth of the lesion was 1.0 cm or less in 48 (53%) lesions, 1.1 to 2.0 cm in 41 (46%) lesions, and more than 2.0 cm in 1 (1%) lesion.

Complications occurred in 3 (3%) of 101 lesions. In one woman who had MRI-guided needle localization of a solitary unilateral lesion, the wire tip broke off in the breast during deployment, requiring placement of a second wire; the tip, which was immediately adjacent to the lesion site, was successfully removed at surgery. In two other women, postoperative mammogram showed a retained wire fragment adjacent to the benign biopsy site. The reason for wire breakage is unknown, but our surgeons' impression is that some of the wires used for MRI-guided localization are weaker than those used for mammographically guided needle localization, with a propensity to break when approached by cautery. No other complications were encountered.

4.6. Follow Up

In all cases, surgical histology and imaging findings were considered concordant. Specimen radiography, performed in 13 lesions with mammographic correlates, confirmed lesion retrieval in all. Of the 101 lesion sites, 15 were not available for imaging follow up because the patient had ipsilateral mastectomy, due to ipsilateral cancer (n = 13) or prophylactically (n = 2). Postoperative MRI data are available in 33 (38%) of the remaining 86 lesion sites, including 19 (34%) of 55 lesions that yielded benign findings and 14 (45%) of 31 lesions that yielded carcinoma. The median time from surgery to the first follow-up MRI examination was 8 months (range, 1–24 mo).

Postoperative MRI of 33 lesion sites suggested complete excision of the MRI lesion in 29 (88%), partial lesion excision in 3 (9%), and a missed lesion in 1 (3%). In three lesions that yielded cancer at surgery, postoperative MRI confirmed partial excision of the lesion but suggested possible residual disease. These three lesions occurred in two women, both of whom had undergone MRI-guided needle localization of multiple synchronous lesions, yielding DCIS with close margins. Both women had subsequent re-excision, yielding DCIS in one and benign findings in one. In one woman with multiple synchronous lesions for which MRI-guided localization yielding multifocal invasive lobular cancer with positive margins, postoperative MRI suggested persistence of one of the lesions; subsequent MRI-guided needle localization and re-excision showed invasive lobular cancer in an intramammary lymph node.

Thirty-five lesion sites that had neither postoperative MRI nor subsequent mastectomy underwent postoperative mammograms at a median of 9 months (range, 4–20 mo) after biopsy, showing no suspicious findings. Eighteen lesion sites were not imaged postoperatively by mammography or MRI, but had stable clinical follow up.

4.7. Cancellations

During the time period in which these 101 lesions had MRI-guided localization, 5 additional lesions scheduled for MRI-guided needle localization were not visible on the day of the procedure and therefore were not localized. Therefore, among 106 lesions initially scheduled for MRI-guided needle localization, the procedure was canceled in five (5%).

These five lesions occurred in five women of median age 57 years (range, 31–71 y). All five of these women still had MRI-guided localization of other persistent suspicious lesions in the ipsilateral (n = 3) or contralateral (n = 2) breast. Three of these five women had follow-up MRI (median, 4 mo; range, 1–7 mo), which confirmed disappearance of the lesion. One woman had a follow-up mammogram 5 months after attempted localization, which showed no suspicious findings. One patient had prophylactic mastectomy of the ipsilateral breast 1 month after the date of MRI-guided localization; no evidence of cancer was identified.

5. Challenging Scenarios at Magnetic Resonance Imaging Guided Localization

5.1. Variation in Lesion Appearance and Canceled Cases

There may be variation in the appearance of the lesion between the diagnostic MRI examination and the images obtained on the day of the localization procedure, even if the diagnostic examination is performed in the same facility as the localization. This variation may be due to difference in positioning, compression, or phase of the menstrual cycle.[8,17,32] If the lesion is less conspicuous on the day of the localization procedure, delayed postcontrast imaging may be helpful; if the lesion is still not well seen, diminishing the compression, administration of additional intravenous contrast, and re-imaging may be of value. It may also be helpful to use adjacent landmarks, as often employed during mammographically guided needle localization of subtle lesions.

In a small proportion of cases, the lesion will not be evident on the initial postcontrast scan, on delayed images, or after diminishing compression and reinjection, in spite of a technically adequate study, as occurred 5% of lesions referred for MRI-guided needle localization in a study from our center.[12] If the lesion cannot be identified in spite of these maneuvers, the procedure is canceled. It is prudent to recommend short-term follow-up MRI in this scenario.

5.2. Decreasing Lesion Conspicuity During Localization

The lesion undergoing MRI-guided localization may become less conspicuous during the procedure. During the time it takes to perform the localization, contrast may washout from the lesion, and there may be progressive enhancement of the surrounding parenchyma. These factors both contribute to diminishing lesion visibility with time during MRI-guided localization or biopsy procedures. In order to deal with diminishing lesion conspicuity during localization or biopsy, the best approach is to make sure that the breast is thoroughly immobilized, to work quickly, to use adjacent landmarks, and to consider reinjecting a second dose of intravenous gadolinium if necessary.

5.3. Bilateral Localization

When bilateral localization is performed, one of two methods is employed. More often, following injection of contrast, both breasts are imaged and the lesions in each breast are localized simultaneously. Alternatively, each breast is imaged and localized separately, allowing for an adequate passage of time (approximately 20 min) following the initial contrast injection so that background

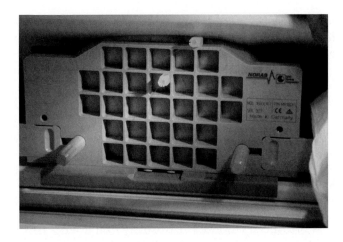

FIGURE 19.4. Photograph of needle localization procedure in a woman with two lesions, one of which was posterior to the localizing grid. Note placement of one of the two needles posterior to the grid, to localize this posterior lesion.

parenchymal enhancement does not obscure areas of suspicious enhancement in the second breast, when the patient is re-injected with contrast material for the second localization.

5.4. Posterior Lesions

Magnetic resonance imaging guided localization of posterior lesions can be difficult. In these cases, positioning of the patient by mammography technologists experienced in diagnostic mammography as well as stereotactic biopsy with the patient prone can be most valuable. In some cases, in spite of one's best efforts at positioning, the lesion may remain posterior and not included in the grid compression paddle. In such cases, the needle can be placed either posterior to the grid (Figure 19.4) or within the grid, as close to the lesion as possible; if the needle is placed within the grid, one can abandon the needle guide and (if safety allows) slightly angulate the needle toward the chest wall. If the wire is slightly anterior to the lesion, the radiologist should communicate this information to the surgeon; the surgeon can excise the wire and the tissue posterior to it (between the wire and the pectoral muscle).

5.5. Medial Lesions

Magnetic resonance imaging guided localization of medial lesions also poses technical challenges. Because of the geometry of some breast coils, if the patient lies prone with her breast in the breast coil, the needle can be placed from a lateral approach but not from a medial approach. For medial lesions, a lateral skin entry site is suboptimal because it requires that the needle and wire traverse a longer distance. When performing localization of medial lesions, we have found it helpful to position the patient in a prone oblique position rather than straight prone. For example, to localize a lesion in the medial left breast, the left breast can be placed in the right breast coil, making the medial aspect of the left breast accessible (Figure 19.5). This technique is most successful on women who are healthy and relatively thin; hip problems may make the oblique position less comfortable, and obesity may limit body access to the magnet in this position. To ensure that the images are properly acquired and annotated, the MRI technologist must be aware that the left breast is being imaged within the right breast coil.

A breast coil (Biopsy Breast Array Coil [Model BBC], MRI Devices) is now available that enables medial access with the patient in the prone position (Figure 19.6). This may facilitate MRI-guided interventional procedures for lesions that are in the medial aspect of the breast, although access to posteromedial tissue is somewhat limited.

5.6. Accordion Effect

During MRI-guided localization, the wire is deployed in a breast that is being compressed in a direction parallel to the direction of needle placement. This allows for an *accordion effect*: during compression, structures that were far apart are brought close together, and when compression is released, structures that were close together move further apart.[33] Any error in the depth direction (parallel to the axis of needle placement) can therefore be exaggerated when compression is released. Use of the minimal amount of compression necessary to achieve immobilization may minimize the likelihood of the accordion effect and may also prevent the impairment of contrast enhancement that has been described with excessive compression.[8,17]

5.7. Augmented Breasts

Like all interventions, MRI-guided interventions are challenging in augmented breasts. The informed consent conversation should include discussion of the possibility of implant rupture. When performing MRI-guided needle localization in an augmented breast, the following may be helpful. First, when positioning the patient, one can try to push the implant back, as if performing an Eklund view on the mammogram. Second, consider performing the localization without the needle guide. This enables the physician to know exactly when the needle is piercing the skin rather than displacing it. Third, it may be preferable to place the needle at the anterior aspect of the lesion, or even anterior to the lesion, depending on the proximity of the lesion to the implant. Fourth, axial reconstructions may help confirm that the needle is well positioned and away from the implant. Finally, if safe performance of wire localization does not seem feasible, consider alternatives to wire placement, such as injection of toluidine blue dye or marking the skin over the lesion using MRI guidance.

5.8. Confirming Lesion Retrieval

Confirmation of lesion retrieval remains an issue for MRI-guided localization. Imaging and histologic correlation plays an important role in this procedure, as in all breast biopsy procedures.[34] Use of an MRI-compatible, mammographically evident clip that can be placed after MRI-guided biopsy would be useful; specimen radiography could then document retrieval of the clip.[33,35] However, because the clip can be deployed distant from the lesion site, retrieval of the clip may support but does not confirm retrieval of the lesion.

Postoperative MRI, which can distinguish postoperative changes from residual tumor,[36,37] may be helpful. In a study from our institution, postoperative MRI suggested that the lesion was completely excised in 88%, partially excised in 9%, and missed in 3%.[12] The 3% miss rate is within the range of 0 to 18% miss rates for mammographically guided needle localization reported in a review of the literature by Jackman and colleagues.[38] The lesions that were partly excised or missed in our study all occurred in women who had MRI-guided localization of multiple synchronous ipsilateral lesions, yielding cancer extending to or close to the margins.[12] These findings are consistent with the results of Jackman and colleagues,[38] who reported that mammographically guided needle localization and surgical biopsy had a failure rate of 12% for patients with multiple ipsilateral lesions versus <2% for patients with single lesions ($P = 0.001$).

6. Advice and Caveats

For individuals embarking on performance of MRI-guided breast needle localization and biopsy procedures, we have several suggestions. It is helpful to begin with lesions that have mammographic correlates, so that lesion retrieval can be readily confirmed during the learning curve experience, and to collaborate with individuals expert in MRI physics. Magnetic resonance imaging technique should be standardized, so that the MRIs obtained during the diagnostic examination and the localization procedure can be readily compared. If possible, identify specific MRI technologists who will be involved in these procedures, and include the participation of mammography technologists experienced at breast localization and biopsy procedures. Postoperative MRI can be helpful to confirm lesion retrieval in women who have had MRI-guided localization; Frei and colleagues[37] have suggested that postoperative MRI may best be performed approximately 1 month after surgery, but

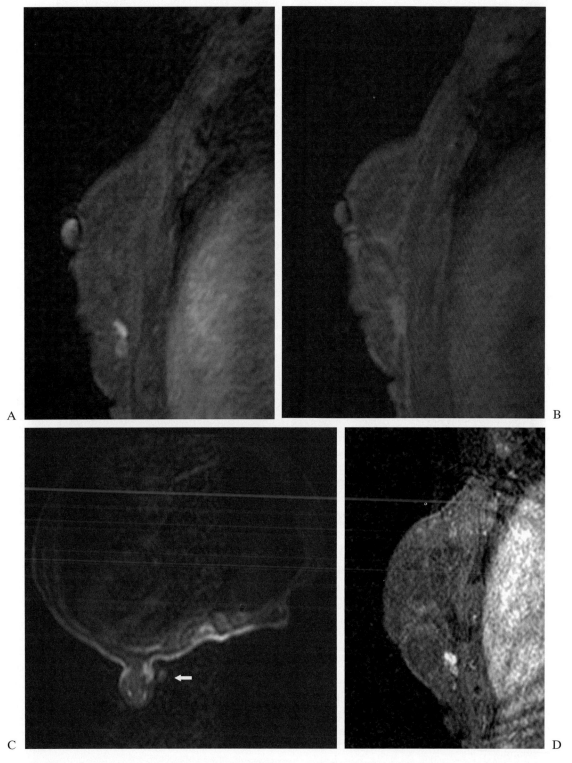

FIGURE 19.5. A 69-year-old woman with family history of breast cancer and prior excision of a radial scar. (A) Sagittal, T1-weighted image from high-risk screen MRI of the left breast immediately after contrast injection shows 1.3-cm irregular enhancing mass in the left lower inner quadrant, not seen by mammography or sonography. (B) Sagittal, T1-weighted, delayed image of the left breast after contrast injection shows washout of contrast from the lesion. Magnetic resonance imaging guided localization was recommended. (C) Magnetic resonance imaging guided needle localization of this medial lesion was performed with the patient in the prone oblique position, with her left breast in the right coil. The vitamin E marker (arrow) has been placed over the expected lesion site in the medial left breast. (D) Sagittal, contrast-enhanced, T1-weighted image obtained during MRI-guided needle localization shows the enhancing mass inferiorly.

(*Continued*)

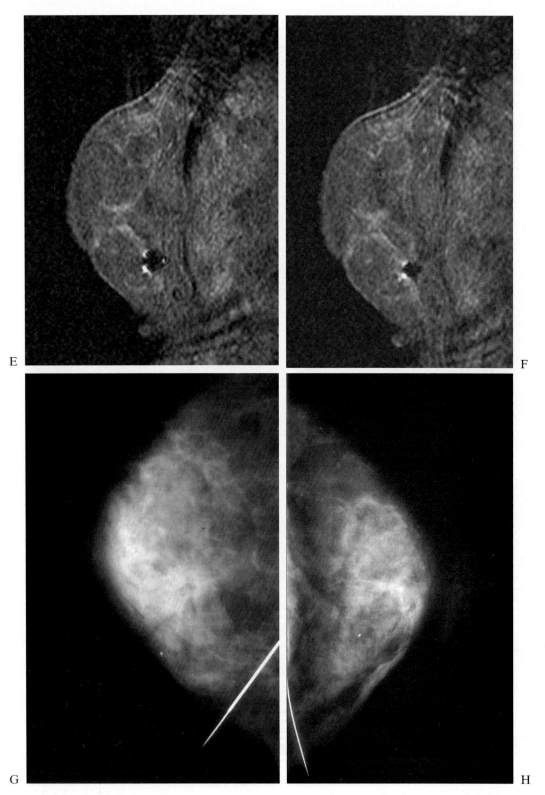

FIGURE 19.5. (*Continued*) (E) Sagittal, contrast-enhanced, T1-weighted image after needle placement shows the needle in the region of the mass. The mass is less evident, due to washout of contrast material, but the appropriate location can be discerned using adjacent parenchymal landmarks. (F) Sagittal, contrast-enhanced, T1-weighted MRI after wire deployment shows the wire in appropriate position. Again, the lesion is not seen due to washout of contrast, but the location can be determined by adjacent landmarks. (G) Collimated mediolateral oblique view of the left breast from two-view mammogram obtained after localization shows that the wire has deployed. The reinforced portion is partially imaged, but the tip could not be included due to the extreme posteromedial location, in spite of two attempts. (H) Craniocaudal view of the left breast from two-view mammogram obtained after localization again shows that the wire, placed from the medial aspect of the breast, has deployed. On this view, neither the reinforced portion nor the tip could be included on the mammogram due to the extreme posteromedial location, although the area was accessible to MRI-guided localization. Histologic analysis yielded infiltrating ductal carcinoma, tubular type, measuring 1.2 cm.

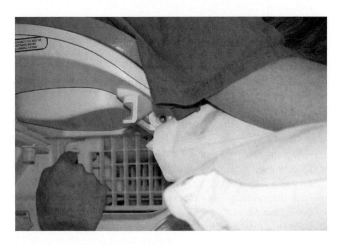

FIGURE 19.6. Example of a breast coil that allows access from either a medial or a lateral approach. In this photograph, the patient's right side is closer to the radiologist, and the right breast is resting on the white breast support. The left breast is in the grid, which has crosshatches on the lateral skin surface (not shown) and the medial skin surface (shown), enabling access to either surface for intervention.

our anecdotal experience suggests that an even shorter interval may be acceptable (e.g., 2 wks).

Magnetic resonance imaging can detect cancers that cannot be identified by other methods. However, no data as yet address the impact of MRI detection of breast cancer on survival, in the setting of screening, problem-solving, or assessment of extent of disease in women with known breast cancer. We report published experience from our institution and other centers, but breast MRI is still relatively early in its development, with persistent variation in technique and interpretation, and limited follow-up information. Furthermore, breast MRI is an expensive examination, and the cost-effectiveness of breast MRI and MRI-guided localization has yet to be determined.

7. Conclusions

Magnetic resonance imaging guided needle localization can be readily performed with commercially available equipment. Published reports indicate high technical success rate (93%–100%), high cancer yield (31%–73%), and high frequency of encountering high-risk lesions (up to 29%). At MSKCC, the positive predictive value of MRI-guided needle localization in our initial series of 101 lesions was 31%; among the cancers, approximately half were DCIS and half were invasive.[12] The median time to perform MRI-guided needle localization at our institution was 31 min.[12] We have now performed MRI-guided needle localization in over 1,000 lesions and are currently performing more than 300 of these procedures per year; with

the expanding clinical use of breast MRI, the use of breast MRI intervention continues to grow.

The ability to perform localizations is a necessary part of a breast MRI program. Ideal characteristics of the MRI localizing needle/wire combinations include sharpness, *scoring* (i.e., 1-cm marks on the needle shaft that can be used to adjust needle position), a visible mark on the wire that can be set to a specified position for deployment, a reinforced portion that the surgeon can identify intraoperatively, strength to resist breakage or cutting, and no problems with heating or deflection. Magnetic resonance imaging compatible biopsy systems should include compression devices to allow access to and immobilization of the entire breast, needle guides, and localizing markers. Excellent MRI-compatible equipment for needle localization is now available, with more equipment under development. This technology, and work evaluating its utility, is necessary to realize the potential of breast MRI in the detection and treatment of breast cancer.

References

1. Orel SG, Schnall MD, Newman RW, et al. MR imaging-guided localization and biopsy of breast lesions: initial experience. *Radiology* 1994;193:97–102.
2. Schnall MD. MR-guided breast biopsy. In: Lufkin RB, ed. *Interventional MRI.* St. Louis: Mosby; 2000:315–319.
3. Heywang-Kobrunner SH, Huynh AT, Viehweg P, et al. Prototype breast coil for MR-guided needle localization. *J Comput Assist Tomogr.* 1994;18:876–881.
4. Orel SG, Schnall MD, Newman RW, et al. MR imaging-guided localization and biopsy of breast lesions: initial experience. *Radiology* 1994;193:97–102.
5. Fischer U, Vosshenrich R, Bruhn H, et al. MR-guided localization of suspected breast lesions detected exclusively by postcontrast MRI. *J Comput Assist Tomogr.* 1995;19:63–66.
6. Fischer U, Vosshenrich R, Doler W, et al. MR imaging-guided breast intervention: experience with two systems. *Radiology* 1995;195:533–538.
7. Doler W, Fischer U, Metzger I, et al. Stereotaxic add-on device for MR-guided biopsy of breast lesions. *Radiology* 1996;200:863–864.
8. Kuhl CK, Elevelt A, Leutner CC, et al. Interventional breast MR imaging: clinical use of a stereotactic localization and biopsy device. *Radiology* 1997;204:667–675.
9. Daniel BL, Birdwell RL, Ikeda DM, et al. Breast lesion localization: a freehand, interactive MR imaging-guided technique. *Radiology* 1998;207:455–463.
10. Fischer U, Kopka L, Grabbe E. Magnetic resonance guided localization and biopsy of suspicious breast lesions. *Top Magn Reson Imaging.* 1998;9:44–59.
11. Orel SG, Schnall MD, Czerniecki B, et al. MRI-guided needle localization: indications and clinical efficacy [abstr]. *Radiology* 1999;213:454.
12. Morris EA, Liberman L, Dershaw DD, et al. Preoperative MR imaging-guided needle localization of breast lesions. *AJR Am J Roentgenol.* 2002;178:1211–1220.

13. Taourel PH, Sittek H, Boetes C, et al. MR-guided localization and surgery: results of a European multicenter study [abstr]. *Radiology* 2002;225:556.

14. Mumtaz H, Harms SE. Biopsy and intervention working group report. *J Magn Reson Imaging.* 1999;10:1010–1015.

15. Brenner RJ, Shellock FG, Rothman BJ, Giuliano A. Technical note: magnetic resonance imaging-guided pre-operative breast localization using "freehand technique." BrJ Radiol. 1995;68:1095–1098.

16. Fischer U, Vosshenrich R, Keating D, et al. MR-guided biopsy of suspect breast lesions with a simple stereotaxic add-on device for surface coils. *Radiology* 1994;192:272–273.

17. Kuhl CK, Leutner C, Mielcarek P, et al. Breast compression interferes with lesion enhancement in contrast-enhanced breast MR imaging. *Radiology* 1997;205:538.

18. Desouza NM, Coutts GA, Puni RK, Young IR. Magnetic resonance imaging guided breast biopsy using a frameless stereotactic technique. *Clin Radiol.* 1996;51:425–428.

19. Heywang-Kobrunner SH, Heinig A, Pickuth D, et al. Interventional MRI of the breast: lesion localisation and biopsy. *Eur Radiol.* 2000;10:36–45.

20. Liberman L, Morris EA, Lee MJY, et al. Breast lesions detected by MR imaging: features and positive predictive value. *AJR Am J Roentgenol.* 2002;179:171–178.

21. American College of Radiology (ACR). B1–RADS® Breast Imaging Reporting and Data System, Breast Imaging Atlas. Reston, VA.: American College of Radiology; 2003.

22. Kinkel K, Helbich TH, Esserman LJ, et al. Dynamic high-spatial-resolution MR imaging of suspicious breast lesions: diagnostic criteria and interobserver variability. *AJR Am J Roentgenol.* 2000;175:35–43.

23. Nunes LW, Schnall MD, Orel SG, et al. Breast MR imaging: interpretation model. *Radiology* 1997;202:833–841.

24. Nunes LW, Schnall MD, Siegelman ES, et al. Diagnostic performance characteristics of architectural features revealed by high spatial-resolution MR imaging of the breast. *AJR Am J Roentgenol.* 1997;169:409–415.

25. Nunes LW, Schnall MD, Orel SG, et al. Correlation of lesion appearance and histologic findings for the nodes of a breast MR imaging interpretation model. *Radiographics* 1999;19:79–92.

26. Nunes LW, Schnall MD, Orel SG. Update of breast MR imaging architectural interpretation model. *Radiology* 2001;219:484–494.

27. Kuhl CK, Mielcareck P, Klaschik S, et al. Dynamic breast MR imaging: are signal intensity time course data useful for differential diagnosis of enhancing lesions? *Radiology* 1999;211:101–110.

28. Morris EA. Illustrated breast MR lexicon. Semin Roentgenol. 2001;36:238–249.

29. Panizza P, De Gaspari A, Vanzulli A, et al. Accuracy of post-MR imaging second-look-sonography in previously undetected breast lesions [abstract]. *Radiology* 1997;205;489.

30. Dhamanaskar KP, Muradall D, Kulkarni SR, et al. MRI directed ultrasound: a cost effective method for diagnosis and intervention in breast imaging [abstract]. *Radiology* 2002;225:653.

31. LaTrenta LR, Menell JH, Morris EA, Abramson AF, Dershaw DD, Liberman L. Breast lesions detected with MR imaging: utility and histopathologic importance of identification with US. *Radiology* 2003;227:856–861.

32. Kuhl CK, Bieling HB, Gieseke J, et al. Healthy premenopausal breast parenchyma in dynamic contrast-enhanced MR imaging of the breast: normal contrast medium enhancement and cyclical-phase dependency. *Radiology* 1997;203:137–144.

33. Liberman L, Dershaw DD, Morris EA, et al. Clip placement after stereotactic vacuum-assisted breast biopsy. *Radiology* 1997;205:417–422.

34. Liberman L, Drotman MB, Morris EA, et al. Imaging-histologic discordance at percutaneous breast biopsy. *Cancer* 2000;89:2538–2546.

35. Harms SE. Technical report of the international working group on breast MRI. *J Magn Reson Imaging.* 1999;10:979–981.

36. Orel SG, Reynolds C, Schnall MD, et al. Breast carcinoma: MR imaging before re-excisional biopsy. *Radiology* 1997;205:429–436.

37. Frei KA, Kinkel K, Bonel HM, et al. MR imaging of the breast in patients with positive margins after lumpectomy: influence of the time interval between lumpectomy and MR imaging. *AJR Am J Roentgenol.* 2001;175:1577–1584.

38. Jackman RJ, Marzoni FA. Needle-localized breast biopsy: why do we fail? *Radiology* 1997;204:677–684.

20
Percutaneous Magnetic Resonance Imaging Guided Breast Biopsy

Laura Liberman

Breast cancers that cannot be detected by mammography or physical examination may be identified at magnetic resonance imaging (MRI).[1] In women at high risk of developing breast cancer, MRI detects a cancer occult to mammography and physical examination in 2% to 7%.[2] Among women with cancer in one breast, MRI detects additional sites of cancer in the ipsilateral breast in 6% to 34%[3] and detects an otherwise unsuspected contralateral cancer in 4% to 24%.[4] The sensitivity of MRI is high, reported as 94% to 100%, but it has lower specificity, ranging from 37% to 97%.[5] Biopsy of suspicious MRI-detected lesions is necessary for definitive diagnosis.

For MRI-detected lesions that can be seen on sonography, biopsy can be performed under sonographic guidance. However, *second-look* sonography fails to identify a sonographic correlate in up to 77% of MRI-detected lesions referred for biopsy.[6–8] Although cancer is more frequent among MRI-detected lesions that have a sonographic correlate rather than those that do not (43% vs. 14%, $P = 0.01$), absence of a sonographic correlate does not spare the need for biopsy.[8] The utility of breast MRI is therefore dependent on the availability of methods to perform biopsy of lesions detected by MRI only.

Percutaneous biopsy is being increasingly used for breast diagnosis. In prior studies of percutaneous biopsy using stereotactic or ultrasound guidance, percutaneous biopsy is less invasive, can be performed quickly, does not result in scarring or deformity, causes less anxiety for the patient, and can be performed at lower cost.[9] Magnetic resonance imaging guided percutaneous breast biopsy is a challenging endeavor for many reasons, including the requirement for equipment that will work in the MRI environment, need to remove the patient from the magnet to perform biopsy in closed systems, limited access to the medial and posterior breast, decreasing lesion conspicuity with time after contrast injection, necessity of precise targeting of small lesions, desirability of placing a localizing clip, and difficulties confirming lesion retrieval.[10] In spite of these challenges, several investigators have reported success with MRI-guided percutaneous biopsy.

This chapter discusses methods and results of MRI-guided percutaneous biopsy using a fine needle,[11–15] automated core needle,[15–20b] or vacuum-assisted biopsy probe,[21–26] and provides suggestions for MRI-guided percutaneous biopsy in specific challenging scenarios.

1. Fine Needle Aspiration Biopsy

Several investigators have reported results of fine needle aspiration biopsy under MRI guidance[11–15] (Table 20.1). In 1994, Fischer and colleagues[11] described a biopsy device with 57 puncture channels inserted into a surface coil designed primarily for eye and ear examinations. Fine needle aspiration biopsy, performed with a 19.5-gauge needle, yielded sufficient material in all cases, including four carcinomas, three fibroadenomas, and one intraductal hyperplasia, all of which were confirmed at subsequent surgical excision.

Although these preliminary results were encouraging, subsequent series of MRI-guided fine needle aspiration biopsy have had lower success rates. The most common problem has been insufficient samples, a problem also encountered at fine needle aspiration biopsy under stereotactic or ultrasound guidance.[27,28] In a study from the Radiologic Diagnostic Oncology Group V, Pisano and colleagues[27] reported that fine needle aspiration biopsy under stereotactic or ultrasound guidance had an insufficient sample rate of 34% (128 of 377). The insufficient sample rate was higher for fine needle aspiration under stereotactic (40%) than ultrasound guidance (9%), was higher for calcifications (46%) than masses (27%), and was higher if there was no on-site cytologist (31%) than if there was a cytologist present on site (15%). Insufficient samples are a major clinical limitation of image-guided fine-needle aspiration biopsy.

TABLE 20.1. MRI-guided Fine Needle Aspiration Breast Biopsy

Study/Year	No.	Needle Gauge	Size (cm) Mean (Range)	No. Successful (%)	No. Cancer (%)	Invasive (%)	DCIS (%)	High Risk (%)	Time (min) Mean (Range)
Fischer et al./ 1994[11a]	8	19.5	NS	8 (100)	4 (50)	NS	NS	NS	NS (30–60)
Fischer et al./ 1995[12a]	23	19.5	NS	20 (87)	7 (30)	NS	NS	NS	60 (40–90)[b]
Desouza et al./ 1996[13]	9	18	NS (0.2–1.7)	7 (78)	3 (33)	NS	NS	NS	90 (NS)[c]
Wald et al./ 1996[14]	18	22	1.8 (1.0–3.6)	11 (61)	2 (11)[d]	2 (11)	0 (0)	0 (0)	42 (30–80)
Fischer et al./ 1998[15a]	31	19.5	NS	28 (90)	7 (23)	NS	NS	NS	NS (30–60)[b]

Abbreviations: DCIS, ductal carcinoma in situ; N, number of lesions; NS, not stated. Percentages reflect proportion of all lesions (N).
[a] May be overlap between References 11, 12, and 15; numbers should not be added together in meta-analysis.
[b] Reflects time for MRI-guided interventions, including preoperative needle localization or needle biopsy.
[c] Reflects approximate time, including counseling, positioning, preparing patient, obtaining initial data set, performing biopsy, and postbiopsy care.
[d] A third infiltrating cancer was found at stereotactic core biopsy in lesion too posterior to undergo successful MRI-guided fine needle aspiration.

In subsequent investigations of MRI-guided fine needle aspiration biopsy, insufficient samples were encountered in 10% (3 of 31) lesions reported by Fischer and colleagues,[15] in 22% (2 of 9) lesions reported by Desouza and colleagues,[13] and in 17% (3 of 18) lesions reported by Wald and colleagues.[14] In the latter study, an additional 22% (4 of 18) lesions were inaccessible to the compression grid due to posterior location; hence the technical success rate in the study of Wald and colleagues[14] was 61% (11 of 18). These data indicate that fine needle aspiration biopsy under MRI guidance, like fine needle aspiration under stereotactic or sonographic guidance, has substantial limitations.

2. Automated Core Biopsy

Magnetic resonance imaging guided percutaneous biopsy has been performed with automated core needles[15–20b] (Table 20.2). Magnetic resonance imaging guided auto-

TABLE 20.2. MRI-guided Automated Core Breast Biopsy

Study/Year	No.	Needle Gauge	Size (cm) Mean (Range)	No. Successful (%)	No. Cancer (%)	Invasive (%)	DCIS (%)	High Risk (%)	Time (min) Mean (Range)
Orel et al./ 1995[16]	3	20	NS	1 (33)	1 (33)	1 (33)	0 (0)	NS	NS
Doler et al./ 1996[17]	2	14	NS	2 (100)	1 (50)	1 (50)	0 (0)	0 (0)	NS
Kuhl et al./ 1997[18]	5	16	NS	4 (80)[b]	4 (80)	4 (80)	0 (0)	0 (0)	40 (30–60)[a]
Fischer et al./ 1998[15]	4	NS	NS	4 (100)	1 (25)	1 (25)	0 (0)	0 (0)	NS (30–60)[a]
Kuhl et al./ 2001[19]	78	14	1.5 (0.6–3.0)	77 (99)	28 (36)[c]	23 (29)	5 (6)	2 (3)	60 (45–100)
Schneider et al./ 2002[20]	21	14	NS (0.5–1.7)	20 (95)	8 (38)	8 (38)	0 (0)	1 (5)	45 (40–65)
Chen et al./ 2004[20b]	35	14	1.5 (0.3–7.0)	34 (97)	8 (23)	7 (20)	1 (3)	5 (14)[d]	NS[e]

Abbreviations: DCIS, ductal carcinoma in situ; N, number of lesions; NS, not stated. Percentages reflect proportion of all lesions (N).
[a] Reflects time for MRI-guided interventions, including preoperative needle localization or needle biopsy.
[b] Fifth lesion, which gave insufficient material at core biopsy, yielded infiltrating ductal carcinoma at subsequent MRI-guided localization and surgical biopsy.
[c] The diagnosis of cancer was made by core biopsy in 27 (96%) of 28 cancers; in one infiltrating breast cancer, crushed specimen precluded histologic evaluation.
[d] Two lesions yielding atypical ductal hyperplasia at core biopsy yielded invasive ductal carcinoma at surgery.
[e] The time to perform the procedure is not stated in this study, but in a prior technical report of the method,[20a] the authors indicate an average procedure time from initial targeting sequence to final postbiopsy sequence of 47 min with standard deviation of 16 min.

mated core biopsy was reported by Orel and colleagues[16] using a 20-gauge needle in three lesions in 1995, by Doler and colleagues[17] using a 14-gauge needle in two lesions in 1996, by Kuhl and colleagues[18] using a 16-gauge needle in five lesions in 1997, by Fischer and colleagues[15] (needle gauge not specified) in four lesions in 1998 and by Chen and colleagues[20b] using a 14-gauge needle in 35 lessions in 2004 (Table 20.2). The largest series of MRI-guided core biopsy was reported by Kuhl and colleagues,[19] who used a 14-gauge automated needle in 78 lesions in 2001 (Table 20.2).

2.1. Technique

In the study by Kuhl and colleagues,[19] 78 lesions underwent MRI-guided 14-gauge automated core biopsy with patients semiprone in a 1.5 T magnet with the breast compressed between two plates featuring an MRI-visible fiducial system. The compression plates were perforated with 2-mm holes every 2.5 mm. A regular flexible circular surface coil was placed around the breast for imaging. Tissue was acquired with a variety of MRI-compatible, single-use, semiautomatic, 14-gauge automated core biopsy guns with a long throw and a 20-mm biopsy notch (Daum Medical Systems, Schwerin, Germany; Guerbet, Wurzberg, Germany; Somatex, Berlin, Germany).

The breast was gently compressed to achieve stabilization and immobilization. Intravenous sedation was given with 3 to 5 mg of midazolam (Dormicum®) or 5 to 10 mg of diazepam (Valium®) just before the contrast-enhanced series. Contrast-enhanced dynamic breast MRI was performed using 0.1 mmol/kg gadolinium-diaminotetra-ethyl penta-acetic acid (Gd-DTPA) (Schering, Berlin, Germany) injected intravenously. Parameters were equivalent to those used during diagnostic imaging (repetition time msec/echo time msec, 280/4.6; flip angle, 90 degrees). The field of view was 220 mm with an 80% rectangular field of view, yielding a 4-min acquisition time. In addition, T2-weighted turbo spin echo (SE) imaging (3000/120) was performed with the same parameters (acquisition time, 90 s). When the target lesion was identified on the post-contrast subtraction images, an attempt was made to identify the same lesion on the corresponding T2-weighted turbo SE images.

Coordinates of the lesion with respect to the fiducial system were obtained, and the needle trajectory was determined. Superficial and deep anesthesia were given with 10 to 15 mL of lidocaine (Xylocaine®) or bupivacaine (Carbostesin®). A skin nick was made with a scalpel, and the coaxial needle was placed and its position verified with the T2-weighted turbo SE sequence. Five to 11 core biopsy specimens were obtained, rotating the biopsy notch in a clockwise direction. If the position of the needle relative to the target lesion could not be determined, a second contrast-enhanced series [T1-weighted turbo SE imaging

before and after contrast injection (350/10); acquisition time, 90 s] was obtained with the needle in place; alternatively, contrast-enhanced T1-weighted turbo SE images with spectral-selective fat suppression were used (acquisition time, 2 min and 15 s).

2.2. Results

In the study by Kuhl and colleagues,[19] MRI-guided automated core biopsy was technically successful in 98% (77 of 78) lesions. The one technical failure occurred in a lesion considered "probably malignant" based on imaging findings, in which core biopsy yielded a crushed specimen for which no histologic evaluation was possible; subsequent surgical excision yielded invasive ductal cancer. In another lesion yielding radial scar at MRI-guided 14-gauge automated core biopsy, surgery revealed radial scar surrounded by invasive breast cancer. In 59 lesions with validation either by subsequent excision (n = 42), radiologic-pathologic correlation (n = 7), or follow-up MRI after at least 24 months (n = 10), the diagnostic accuracy of MRI-guided core biopsy was 98% (58 of 59): sensitivity was 96% (27 of 28), specificity 100% (31 of 31), positive predictive value 100% (27 of 27), and negative predictive value 98% (31 of 32). In a subsequent series of 21 lesions that had 14-gauge automated core biopsy in a vertically open 0.5 T magnet reported by Schneider and colleagues,[20] the technical success rate was 95% (20 of 21); in one medial lesion, the procedure was aborted due to pain.

Although these studies indicate that MRI-guided 14-gauge automated core biopsy can have high diagnostic yield, this method has potential limitations. A high proportion of lesions detected by breast MRI contain ductal carcinoma in situ (DCIS) or atypical ductal hyperplasia (ADH); a 14-gauge automated needle often underestimates the pathology of these complex lesions.[9] In addition, MRI-guided biopsy has the problem of the *vanishing target*—during the biopsy procedure, the lesion often becomes less conspicuous, due to washout of contrast material from the lesion and progressive enhancement of the surrounding breast parenchyma; for such lesions, it would be helpful to be able to acquire a larger volume of tissue than is possible with the 14-gauge automated needle. Finally, 14-gauge automated needles do not readily provide a mechanism for placement of an MRI-compatible localizing clip, which may be helpful for the small lesions that undergo MRI-guided biopsy.

3. Vacuum-Assisted Biopsy

Magnetic resonance imaging guided vacuum-assisted biopsy, pioneered by Dr. Sylvia Heywang-Kobrunner, has advantages compared with other biopsy methods for diagnosis of MRI-detected lesions[21–25] (Table 20.3). Vacuum-

TABLE 20.3. MRI-guided Vacuum-Assisted Breast Biopsy

Study/Year	No.	Needle Gauge	Size (cm) Mean (Range)	No. Successful (%)	No. Cancer (%)	Invasive (%)	DCIS (%)	High Risk (%)	Time (min) Mean (Range)
Heywang-Kobrunner et al./ 1999 [21a]	55	11	0.8 (NS)[b]	54 (98)	14 (25)	9 (16)	5 (9)	0 (0)	Slightly >1 h
Viehweg et al./ 2002 [23a]	280	11	NS	277 (99)	72 (26)	27 (10)	45 (16)	6 (2)	Slightly >1 h
Perlet et al./2002 [24a]	341[c]	11	NS	334 (98)[d]	84 (25)	37 (11)	47 (14)	17 (5)	70 (NS)[e]
Perlet et al./2002 [25a]	NS	11	NS	517 (NS)	196 (38)	134 (14)	62 (12)	16 (3)	NS
Liberman et al./ 2003 [26]	28	9	1.0 (0.4–6.0)	27 (96)	6 (22%)	5 (18)	1 (4)[f]	1 (4)	35 (24–48)[g]

Abbreviations: DCIS, ductal carcinoma in situ; N, number of lesions; NS, not stated. Percentages reflect proportion of all lesions (N).

[a] Reference 23 updates experience at University of Halle in Germany and includes cases in Reference 21. References 25 and 24 are multi-institutional collaborations which include University of Halle; Reference 25 includes cases in Reference 24 but degree of overlap with References 21 and 23 is uncertain. Numbers should not be added together in meta-analysis.

[b] Forty-one (75%) lesions measured 1 cm or less and 15 (27%) lesions measured 5 mm or less.

[c] Among 413 lesions initially referred for vacuum-assisted biopsy, 72 (17%) could not be performed.

[d] Seven unsuccessful vacuum-assisted biopsies were evident on the basis of postbiopsy MRI, imaging-histologic discordance, or both; all had prompt rebiopsy. The 334 lesions in which biopsy was successfully performed represent 93% of 361 lesions that could be seen on the day of the scheduled biopsy procedure.

[e] Time approximately 70 min for 1 lesion and 90 min for two lesions.

[f] In addition, in one lesion yielding LCIS and ADH at vacuum-assisted biopsy, surgery yielded DCIS. In another lesion that underwent biopsy in a woman with Paget's disease, the MRI target was excised at vacuum-assisted biopsy, yielding fibroadenoma; however, microscopic DCIS, occult at MRI, was found at the anterior margin of surgical resection.

[g] Median time was 35 (range, 24–48) min for biopsy of one lesion and 65 (range, 62–86) min for biopsy of two lesions.

assisted biopsy is a highly accurate procedure that is faster, less invasive, and less expensive than surgery and causes no deformity.[9,29] Vacuum-assisted biopsy has a higher technical success rate than fine needle aspiration biopsy, with fewer inadequate specimens. Compared with automated core biopsy, vacuum-assisted biopsy retrieves a larger volume of tissue, which can help compensate for decreasing lesion conspicuity during the MRI-guided biopsy procedure, and provides better characterization of complex lesions containing ADH and DCIS.[9] Vacuum-assisted biopsy also enables placement of a localizing clip that can be used for subsequent needle localization under mammographic guidance.[30]

Limited equipment is available for performing MRI-guided vacuum-assisted biopsy. The largest published experience is from Europe, using a biopsy system that is not yet commercially available in the United States. Other systems are commercially available, including the 9-gauge vacuum-assisted biopsy system used at our institution.

3.1. Vacuum-Assisted Biopsy in Europe

3.1.1. European Technique

The biopsy system used by Heywang-Kobrunner and colleagues[21] in 1999 consisted of three parts: a compression mechanism, a ring coil, and an aiming device. The compression device contained a medial and lateral compression plate consisting of plastic ribs that can be spread apart by a spacer. A marker tube, a small plastic vial filled with Gd-DTPA solution, was attached to the outside of the compression plate (parallel to the z axis of the magnet) and imaged as a dot on all transverse images; it served as reference for all measurements and allowed setting of the angle, height, and depth of needle insertion. The flexible ring coil could be inserted between the ribs of the compression plates so as not to interfere the access to the lesion. The aiming device, equipped with a long arm that allowed both medial and lateral access, was attached to the table outside the magnet and allowed insertion of the needle into the compressed breast at the calculated entry point, chosen angle, and depth. The aiming device was used to support the tissue acquisition device, which was the 11-gauge Mammotome (Biopsys/Ethicon Endo-Surgery, Cincinnati, Ohio).

The technique for MRI-guided vacuum-assisted biopsy with the Mammotome was described by Heywang-Kobrunner and colleagues[21] as follows. Intravenous sedation was provided with up to 5 mg of midazolamhydrochlorid. The patient was positioned prone on the biopsy table with her breast compressed moderately. The patient was moved into the magnet, and MRI examination was performed before and after intravenous injection of 0.1 mmol Gd-DTPA/kg using a high-resolution fast low angle shot (FLASH) three dimensional (3D) sequence [repetition time/echo time/flip angle (TR/TE/FA) = 14/7 ms/25 degrees, slice thickness 2 mm, FOV 200, matrix 256×256]. Based on these images, needle access (slice position, height, depth, and angle of needle insertion) were planned on a transverse slice through the lesion with respect to the marker tube.

An oblique line, representing the path of needle insertion, was chosen with the desired angulation by using specific software. The oblique line was then shifted parallel until it crossed the lesion. Point A was defined as the point where a vertical line through the marker tube intersects the oblique line through the lesion. Point B was defined as a point on the oblique line, 18 mm beyond (deep to) the center of the lesion; this point was chosen so that the tip of the vacuum-assisted device would be 18 mm deep to the center of the lesion, placing the center of the collecting chamber of the biopsy device at the center of the lesion. The vertical distance H between the outside margin of the marker tube and the oblique line (point A) was measured, indicating the height of needle insertion. The depth of needle insertion was measured as the relative shift between point A and B on the oblique line.

The patient was removed from the magnet and the aiming device aligned with the transverse slice that contained the lesion. A *substitute needle* (a nonmagnetic needle of the same length as the vacuum-assisted device) was mounted on the aiming device. The angle and height of insertion were set as previously calculated. Subcutaneous injection of 2 mL of 1% lidocaine was given for local anesthesia. The substitute needle was then advanced to the appropriate depth and detached from the needle holder. The needle holder was withdrawn, and the patient was placed back into the magnet. Magnetic resonance imaging examination was performed using a spin echo (SE) sequence (TR = 196 ms, TE = 15 ms, 3-mm slice thickness, 10% gap) to confirm appropriate location of the substitute needle.

If the substitute needle was in good position, the patient was moved out of the magnet, the substitute needle was removed, the vacuum-assisted device was mounted onto the aiming device, and the vacuum-assisted biopsy device was placed into the breast to the same position as the previous substitute needle. Additional local anesthesia was given by interstitial injection of 10 to 15 mL of a solution of 10 mL of lidocaine and 0.5 mL of vasopressin dissolved in 9.5 mL of saline. Vacuum-assisted biopsy was then performed, obtaining two to three full rotations around the clock at 1.5-h increments (eight specimens per rotation, therefore, 16 to 24 specimens). The vacuum-assisted biopsy device was then withdrawn and the patient moved back into the magnet for another set of MRIs before and after intravenous injection of 0.1 mmol Gd-DTPA/kg. This set of images was used to determine if the lesion was sampled or removed. If lesion sampling or removal were confirmed, the patient was turned supine and her breast compressed manually for 15 min.

3.1.2. Results from Europe

Several studies have reported the experience with MRI-guided Mammotome biopsy in Halle, Germany, alone and in collaboration with multiple institutions.[21–25] In 1999, Heywang-Kobrunner and colleagues[21] reported that MRI-guided vacuum-assisted biopsy was successful in 54 of 55 (98%) cases and yielded cancer in 14 of 54 (26%); the one failure was caused by incorrect use of the vacuum-assisted biopsy gun. Among 54 successful procedures, MRI examination performed immediately after biopsy suggested that removal of the MRI target was complete in 31 (57%), partial in 18 (33%), and difficult to assess due to bleeding in 5 (10%). All lesions in which the MRI target was removed measured 1 cm or less. Complete removal of the MRI target occurred in six lesions that yielded cancer at vacuum-assisted biopsy; among these, subsequent surgery revealed residual cancer in two (33%).

In an update of the multi-institutional experience, Perlet and colleagues[24] described 413 lesions referred for MRI-guided biopsy. In 72 (17%) of 413 lesions, MRI-guided biopsy could not be performed for the following reasons: lesion was no longer seen (n = 52, 13%), due to hormonal influences in 43, incorrect interpretation of original MRI study in 3, diffuse enhancement without focal abnormality in 3, and excessive compression in 3; biopsy not possible due to problems with the procedure (n = 14, 3%), including 3 patients who did not fit in the magnet with respect to the height of the biopsy coil, 1 patient with thin breasts, and 10 patients with problems of access related to design of the biopsy device; and other problems (n = 6, 1%), including 2 patients who refused biopsy, 2 in whom motion artifact limited interpretation of prebiopsy MRI study, and 2 patients in whom biopsy was not performed due to breakdown of the MRI unit.

Of 341 lesions that had MRI-guided vacuum-assisted biopsy, the procedure was unsuccessful in 7 (2%). Reasons for failure included patient motion (n = 2), operator failure (n = 1), breakdown of the MR unit (n = 1), biopsy performed but the lesion was still evident on postbiopsy MR images (n = 1), and strong bleeding that required termination of the procedure before obtaining sufficient tissue (n = 1) or led to hematoma that interfered with histologic assessment of biopsy specimens (n = 1). All seven failures were recognized on the basis of persistence of the lesion on postbiopsy MRI and/or imaging-histologic discordance. Of the 361 (413 – 52) lesions that were visible on the day of the scheduled biopsy procedure, biopsy was successfully performed in 334 (93%).

Among 334 lesions that yielded histologies for evaluation at MRI-guided Mammotome biopsy, histologic findings were carcinoma in 84 (25%), ADH in 17 (5%), of which 3 (18%) yielded DCIS at subsequent surgery, and benign in 223 (70%). In 19 (23%) of 84 lesions yielding cancer at vacuum-assisted biopsy, surgery showed no residual cancer; all of these lesions were smaller than 1 cm. In all other lesions yielding cancer at surgery, surgical histology confirmed vacuum-assisted biopsy findings. All benign diagnoses were confirmed by imaging-histologic correlation and by follow-up MRI at 12 to 36 months after biopsy. Among lesions yielding benign, concordant histology at MRI-guided biopsy, there were no missed cancers.

Complications were encountered in 16 of 341 (4.7%) lesions and included severe bleeding in 5 (1.5%) of 341 lesions, requiring a compression bandage in 2, suture in 1, and surgical drainage in 2; hematoma larger than 3 cm in 6 (1.8%) of 341 lesions, of which 1 developed a subsequent infection and 5 required no specific treatment; and vasovagal reaction in 5 (1.5%) of 341 lesions. The biopsy procedure lasted approximately 70 min for one lesion and 90 min for two lesions.

3.2. Vacuum-Assisted Biopsy at Memorial Sloan-Kettering Cancer Center

At our institution, MRI-guided vacuum-assisted biopsy is performed with a commercially available 9-gauge vacuum-assisted device (Automated Tissue Excision and Collection [ATEC] Breast Biopsy System, Suros Surgical Systems, Indianapolis, Ind). This method enables retrieval of a larger volume of tissue, with each specimen weighing 200 mg as compared with approximately 100 mg per specimen for 11-gauge Mamotome vacuum-assisted biopsy or 17 mg per specimen for 14-gauge automated needles.[9] The larger volume of tissue is useful for ensuring retrieval of vanishing targets and for characterizing the complex histologies (e.g., ADH and DCIS) often encountered in MRI-detected lesions. Furthermore, unlike the European device, which requires that each specimen be removed from the biopsy device before obtaining the next specimen, the system we use stores multiple specimens in a collecting area; this hastens the process by allowing the biopsy to proceed uninterrupted, with specimens retrieved after tissue acquisition is complete.

Magnetic resonance imaging guided vacuum-assisted biopsy can be performed quickly. During our learning curve experience, the average time to perform MR-guided vacuum-assisted biopsy of a single lesion was 35 min. This is faster than all other previous reports of MRI-guided percutaneous biopsy (Tables 20.1 through 20.3). We hypothesize that the ability to perform the biopsy quickly may contribute to higher accuracy. Because lesion conspicuity generally diminishes with time after contrast injection, sampling is dependent on identification of the lesion immediately after injection and immobilizing the lesion so that it remains in the same position. The faster the biopsy can be accomplished, the less likely that the lesion will move. A faster biopsy is more comfortable for the patient and enables increased throughput in the magnet.

3.2.1. Technique

The method currently used at our institution for MRI-guided vacuum-assisted biopsy is similar to that previously described.[26] The steps necessary to perform biopsy are illustrated in Figure 20.1, and images obtained during the biopsy procedure are shown in Figure 20.2.

3.2.1.1. Prebiopsy Preparation

Although MRI-guided biopsy is fast and well tolerated, the procedure can cause patient anxiety, particularly in the high-risk population undergoing breast MRI. At our institution, patients are pretreated as needed with oral benzodiazepines such as diazepam (Valium®), 5 mg orally × 1 to 2 doses, or lorazepam (Ativan), 0.5 mg orally × 1 to 2 doses on the morning of the procedure, as per discussion with the referring clinician.

Magnetic resonance imaging guided vacuum-assisted biopsy is not performed in patients on anticoagulants such as warfarin (Coumadin®). It is important to carefully consult with the referring clinician before scheduling the biopsy in these women. If percutaneous biopsy is considered the best diagnostic approach and if it is clinically acceptable to temporarily discontinue anticoagulation, Coumadin® may be stopped approximately 4 days before the procedure and the INR (international normalization ratio) checked the day before the biopsy; Coumadin® can be restarted after the biopsy is complete. If it is desirable to continue anticoagulation as long as possible, then on discontinuing the Coumadin®, the patient may start dalteparin (Fragmin®), a low-molecular-weight heparin, at a dose of 100 units per kilogram, injected subcutaneously twice a day, with the last dose given 24 h before biopsy. After the biopsy, the patient restarts both Fragmin® and Coumadin®, and then discontinues the Fragmin® when the INR approaches therapeutic level (approximately 2).

Routine prophylactic antibiotics are not indicated for MRI-guided biopsy. We prefer that patients avoid aspirin for 1 week and nonsteroidal anti-inflammatory agents for 48 h before the procedure, but they may take acetaminophen.

3.2.1.2. Targeting Images

The patient is positioned prone in the 1.5 T magnet (Signa, GE Medical Systems. Milwaukee, Wis.) using a dedicated surface breast coil (Open Breast Coil [Model OBC-63] or Biopsy Breast Array Coil [Model BBC], MRI Devices, Waukesha, Wis.). The breast undergoing biopsy is placed

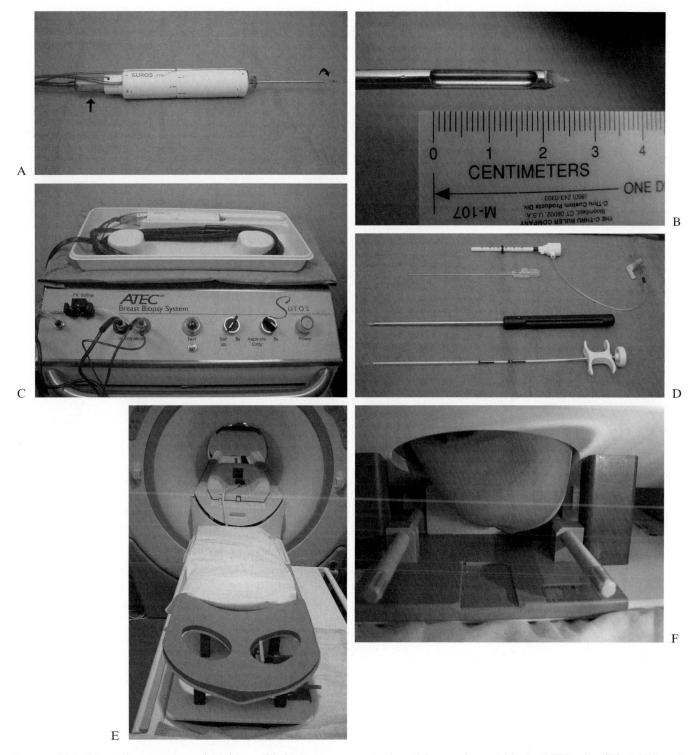

FIGURE 20.1. Magnetic resonance imaging guided vacuum-assisted biopsy: equipment and technique. (A) MRI-guided vacuum-assisted biopsy handpiece. Note the sampling notch (*mouth*) of the biopsy device (curved arrow). Specimens obtained during biopsy are stored in a specimen collecting cup (straight arrow), to be retrieved after tissue acquisition is complete. (B) Close-up view of mouth of biopsy needle. (C) Control module for MRI-guided vacuum-assisted biopsy. The biopsy handpiece is connected by tubing to the control module, and can be brought into the MRI suite for performing biopsy; the remainder of the control module remains outside the MRI suite. (D) Additional equipment for MRI-guided vacuum-assisted biopsy includes (from top to bottom) the white introducer, which is *scored* with marks every 5 mm to assist in setting the black depth stop, the plastic obturator, which serves as a placeholder for MRI; the sharp stylet, which creates the tract; and the clip introducer. (E) The double breast coil used for breast MRI-guided interventions. (F) The patient is positioned prone with her breast in the dedicated breast coil.

(Continued)

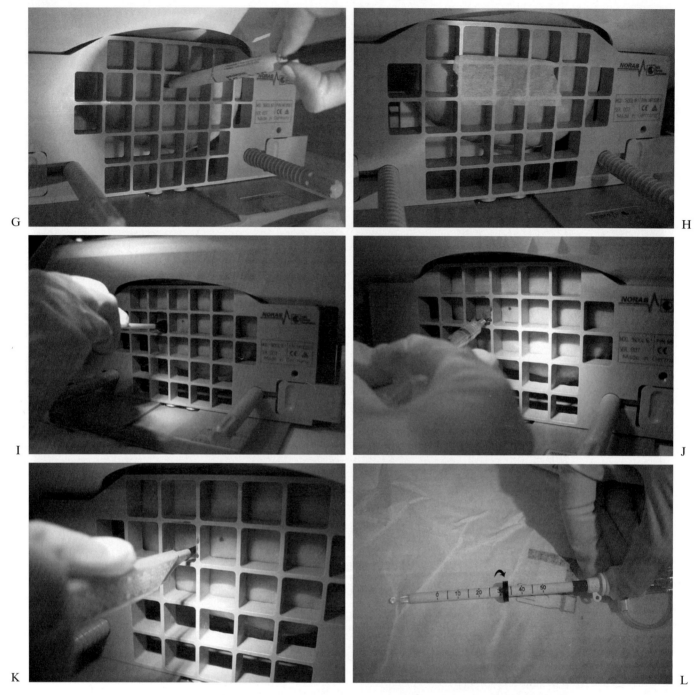

FIGURE 20.1. (*Continued*) (G) The breast is placed in the biopsy compression device. A mark is made on the skin over the expected lesion site, based on review of prior diagnostic MRI. (H) A vitamin E capsule is taped over the expected lesion site, to serve as a landmark for determining lesion location; MRI is then performed. (I) After the lesion is identified on MRI and its loca- tion determined, the skin overlying the lesion site is cleansed with iodine soap. (J) Local anesthesia is given, superficial (shown) and deep (not shown). (K) A skin nick is made with a scalpel. (L) The depth stop (arrow) of the introducer is set to the calculated depth of the lesion, based on review of the MRI study.

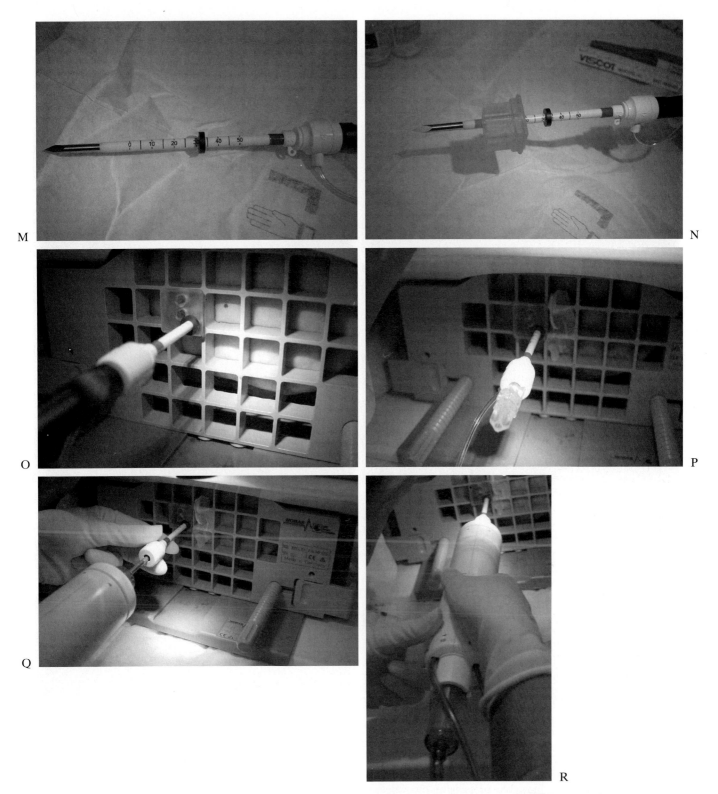

FIGURE 20.1. (*Continued*) (M) The stylet is placed inside the introducer. (N) The stylet and introducer are placed in the needle guide before attaching the needle guide to the grid. This enables the radiologist to ensure that the tip of the needle enters the scalpel incision. (O) The stylet is placed in the breast to create the tract. (P) The stylet is removed from the breast, leaving the introducer within, and replaced with the obturator to enable MRI confirmation of lesion location. When the introducer is positioned so that the depth stop is at the needle guide, the tip of the obturator indicates where the mouth of the biopsy device will be centered (ideally at the center of the lesion). (Q) The biopsy device is inserted into the introducer, after MRI confirmation of position and removal of the obturator. (R) With the biopsy device in place, tissue is acquired by stepping on a foot pedal. The specimens collect in the cup at the back of the device. The radiologist can rotate the device to acquire tissue from any direction. After tissue acquisition, the radiologist removes the biopsy device from the introducer, replaces it with the obturator, and performs MRI to determine if the lesion has been sampled.

(*Continued*)

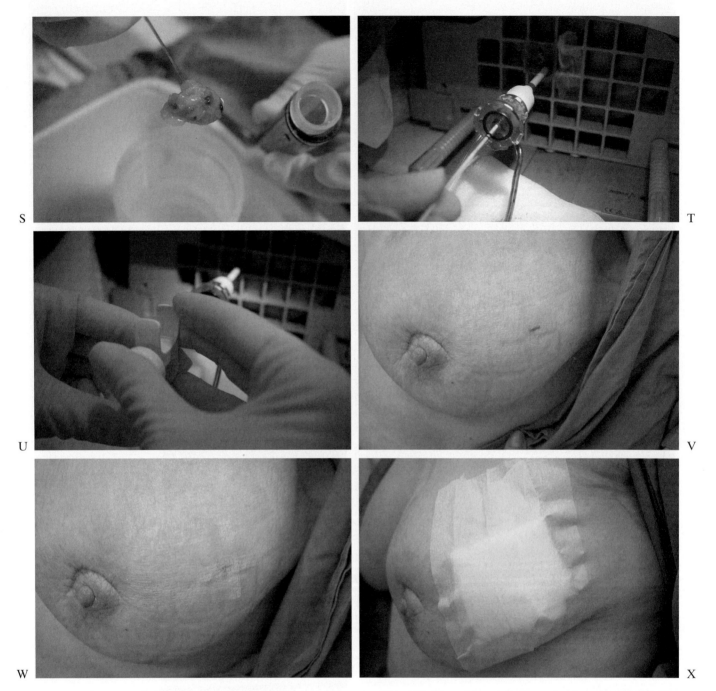

FIGURE 20.1. (*Continued*) (S) After tissue acquisition is complete, the technologists collect the specimens and place them in formalin. (T) If MRI confirms lesion sampling, the front end of the biopsy handpiece is placed back into the introducer, and the clip is inserted. (U) The clip is deployed by pressing on the squeeze handle. (V) The skin nick immediately after MRI-guided vacuum-assisted biopsy is much smaller than the periareolar scar the patient has from prior surgical biopsy. (W) The nick is covered by sterile strips. (X) The sterile strips are then covered with a sterile gauze bandage (shown) or other pressure dressing.

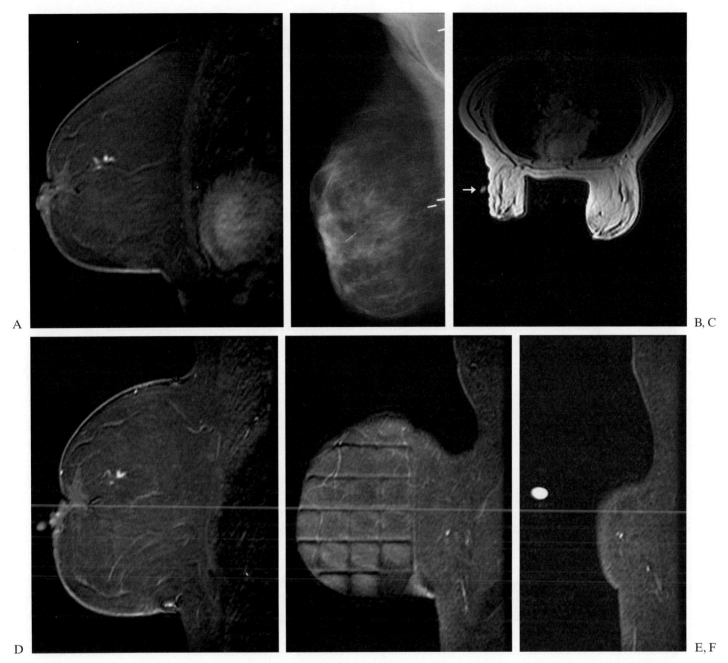

FIGURE 20.2. A 51-year-old woman status post prior left lumpectomy and irradiation, with suspicious lesion in the left breast on high-risk screening MRI. This woman's MRI-guided vacuum-assisted biopsy procedure is illustrated in Figure 20.1. (A) Sagittal, T1-weighted MRI obtained as high-risk screening examination shows clumped ductal enhancement in the 12:00 axis, suspicious for carcinoma. (B) Mediolateral oblique mammogram of the left breast shows postsurgical changes. The suspicious area identified on MRI is not seen at mammography. Note the small fragment of prior localizing wire in the retroareolar region. (C) Axial localizing MRI during MRI-guided vacuum-assisted biopsy shows vitamin E marker (arrow), which has been taped over the expected location of the lesion. The volume imaged should be selected to include this. (D) Sagittal, T1-weighted MRI after injection of intravenous gadolinium shows the area of clumped ductal enhancement, corresponding to the lesion referred for biopsy. (E) Sagittal, T1-weighted MRI shows low signal intensity lines due to pressure of the grid at the skin surface. By paging back and forth on sagittal images at the workstation, the lesion depth relative to the skin surface is determined. (F) Sagittal, T1-weighted MRI shows the vitamin E marker. By paging back and forth on sagittal images at the workstation, using the vitamin E marker as a reference point, the location of the skin entry site is determined.

(*Continued*)

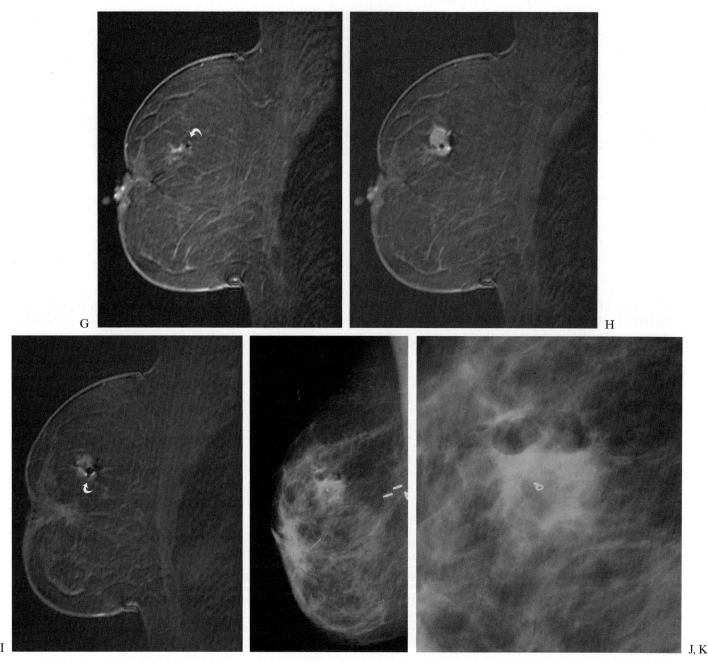

FIGURE 20.2. (*Continued*) (G) Sagittal, T1-weighted, MRI performed after placement of the obturator shows low signal at the posterior aspect of the lesion (arrow), indicating the location of the obturator tip. (H) Sagittal, T1-weighted MRI immediately after completion of tissue acquisition shows air and hematoma at the biopsy site. The obturator is evident as round low signal in the center of the hematoma. Note the air-fluid level is vertical; the patient is lying prone, so the air rises to the dependent (posterior) position. The lesion is no longer evident. (I) Sagittal, T1-weighted MRI after placement of the localizing clip shows low signal artifact at the deep (medial) aspect of the biopsy site (arrow), representing the clip. (J) Postbiopsy mediolateral oblique view mammogram shows the localizing clip has deployed at the biopsy site. The clip is in the expected location based on review of diagnostic MRI examination. (K) Collimated photograph of the biopsy site on the postbiopsy mammogram shows air and small hematoma, with the localizing clip in place. Histologic analysis yielded DCIS.

in a dedicated biopsy compression device using a commercially available grid-localizing system (Model BBC or Biopsy Positioning Device Model MR-BI-160, MRI Devices) or a slightly modified design of the commercially available model.

An axial localizing sequence is obtained, and the volume of interest selected to include the compression device and a vitamin E marker placed over the expected lesion site. Gadopentetate dimeglumine, 0.1mmol/L per kilogram of body weight, is injected intravenously as a rapid bolus injection through an indwelling intravenous catheter. Acquisition of sagittal images starts immediately following contrast injection using a T1-weighted 3D, fat-suppressed fast spoiled gradient echo [17/2.4 (repetition time msec/echo time msec); flip angle, 35 degrees, bandwidth 31.25] sequence is then performed. Section thickness is 3mm without gap, using a matrix of 256×192 and field of view of 18 to 22cm. Frequency is in the anterior-posterior direction. Time of acquisition, usually less than 2min, varies with breast size and area covered. The patient is then withdrawn from the magnet with her breast remaining in compression.

3.2.1.3. Determining Lesion Location and Desired Depth of Probe Insertion

After reviewing images at the console, a cursor is placed over the lesion on the monitor. The horizontal (x) and vertical (y) coordinates of the lesion are determined on the basis of the spatial relationship between the lesion, vitamin E marker, and grid lines. The depth (z) coordinate of the lesion is determined on the basis of the relationship between the lesion and the skin surface.

The skin surface is at the slice where the indentations from the grid are evident as low signal intensity lines. The depth of the lesion from the skin surface in millimeters (z) is calculated by determining the number of sagittal slices between the skin and the lesion and multiplying by 3 (to account for the 3-mm slice thickness).

3.2.1.4. Preparing the Probe

The introducer is the device through which the stylet (to create the tract), the obturator (for imaging confirmation of location), and the biopsy device (for tissue acquisition and placement of a localizing marker) are inserted into the breast. The *depth stop* on the introducer is set to the lesion depth. The introducer is *scored* in such a way to account for the thickness of the needle guide in the grid. Therefore, if the depth of the target is 30mm from the skin, the depth stop should be set to 30. The stylet is then placed inside the introducer as far as it will go. This is the initial device that will later be placed in the patient.

3.2.1.5. Placing the Device and Imaging to Confirm Location

A mark is made on the skin overlying the lesion, and the skin is cleansed with alcohol and anesthetized with 5mL of 1% lidocaine HCl 10mg/mL (Xylocaine®) and approximately 10mL 1% lidocaine 10mg/mL with epinephrine 1:100,000 (Xylocaine®) (Figure 20.1).

The appropriate hole of the needle guide is selected. The stylet and introducer are then placed through the needle guide in the appropriate orientation with the tip just protruding from the far side of the needle guide, and the tip of the stylet is placed in the skin at the site of the scalpel incision before attaching the needle guide to the grid. This helps to ensure that the biopsy device enters through the incision site, even when the needle guide obscures the incision site. A twisting motion is helpful when advancing the stylet. The stylet is advanced to the depth stop.

The stylet is removed, and the obturator is placed inside the white plastic introducer, to assist in MRI confirmation of location. The tray with the stylet is removed from the room before MRI. Magnetic resonance imaging examination is then performed to document location of the obturator, with the ideal location of the tip being at the site of the lesion. The scoring on the introducer is such that when the depth stop is advanced to the needle guide, the tip of the obturator is where the center of the collecting area of the biopsy device will be, which should ideally be at the center of the lesion.

3.2.1.6. Performing the Biopsy, Postexamination Images, and Collecting the Specimens

If positioning is appropriate, the obturator is removed and the biopsy device inserted. The control module is outside the MRI scanner; only the foot pedal and biopsy device come into the room with the magnet. The direction of tissue acquisition is chosen based on location of the introducer with respect to the lesion. Because each specimen weighs approximately 200mg, in general, we obtain 6 to 12 specimens. Tissue is acquired by stepping on the foot pedal. An audible beep is heard each time a specimen is acquired. The radiologist performing the biopsy controls the direction of tissue acquisition, by turning the arrow on the biopsy probe in the desired direction.

After tissue acquisition is complete, the biopsy device is removed, the obturator is reinserted, and postexamination MRI is performed to assess the completeness of tissue acquisition. While the postexamination images are being acquired, the technologist retrieves the samples from the collecting chamber and places them in formalin.

3.2.1.7. Placing the Clip

The clip (MammoMark Biopsy Site Marker, Artemis Medical, Hayward, Calif.) is a titanium clip attached to a resorbable collagen pledget. To prepare to place the clip, the blue tubing is peeled off from the biopsy handpiece, and the front end of the probe (with the *mouth*) is separated from the handpiece portion. The front end of the probe is then placed back into the introducer. The clip introducer is then placed inside the probe. Resistance is felt when it encounters the end of the mouth, indicating that it has reached the appropriate depth. The clip is deployed by pushing down on the handle. The clip introducer is then turned 180 degrees and removed, the biopsy handpiece is removed and inspected to make sure that the clip deployed, and the introducer is removed. *Postclip* sagittal MRI examination is performed to assess clip deployment. Subsequently, a two-view mammogram is obtained to determine the location of the clip with respect to the remainder of the breast parenchyma.

3.2.1.8. Postbiopsy Care of the Breast

After biopsy, compression with ice is held approximately 20 min to achieve hemostasis. The biopsy site is cleansed with alcohol and dried with sterile gauze. Sterile strips are placed over the biopsy site, and the patient is instructed to leave them on until they fall off; she may shower in the morning, but is asked not to take a bath or completely immerse the breast in water for a few days. She is also advised to refrain from heavy upper body exercises for a few days. A gauze bandage or pressure dressing is then placed over the sterile strips for 12 to 24h. The patient is also given the contact information for the radiologist and told when she will be contacted with the results.

3.3. Results

We performed a validation study of MRI-guided vacuum-assisted biopsy at Memorial Sloan-Kettering Cancer Center in 20 women with MRI-detected lesions who were scheduled for MRI-guided localization and surgical exci-

sion.[26] In this protocol approved by our Institutional Review Board, we performed MRI-guided vacuum-assisted biopsy with the Suros device, and then placed an MRI-compatible hookwire for subsequent immediate surgical excision. Results of the MRI-guided vacuum-assisted biopsy and surgical excision were reviewed and correlated.

In our validation study, vacuum-assisted biopsy was successfully performed in 19 (95%) of 20 women; in 1 woman, the biopsy device could not be introduced, and the vacuum-assisted biopsy was aborted. Of 27 MRI-detected lesions that had biopsy, median size was 1.0 cm (range, 0.4–6.4 cm). Histologic analysis showed cancer in 8 of 27 (30%) lesions and in 6 of 19 (32%) women; among these eight cancers, five were infiltrating and three were DCIS. In these 27 lesions, histology was benign at vacuum-assisted biopsy and at surgery in 19 (70%), cancer at vacuum-assisted biopsy in 6 (22%) (Figure 20.3), ADH at vacuum-assisted biopsy and DCIS at surgery in 1 (4%), and benign at vacuum-assisted biopsy with surgery showing microscopic DCIS that was occult at MRI in 1 (4%).

The median time to perform vacuum-assisted biopsy of a single lesion was 35 min (mean, 35; range, 24–48 min). The localizing clip, attempted in 26 lesions, was successfully placed in 25 of 26 (96%) and was retrieved on specimen radiography in 22 of 23 (96%). One complication occurred, a hematoma that resolved with compression. These preliminary results suggest that this method of MRI-guided vacuum-assisted biopsy is a fast, safe, and accurate alternative to surgical excision for the diagnosis of MRI-detected lesions.[26] Based on this validation study, we now offer MRI-guided vacuum-assisted biopsy as an alternative to surgical excision for MRI-detected lesions that are suspicious or highly suggestive of malignancy.

FIGURE 20.3. A 51-year-old woman status post prior right lumpectomy and irradiation. (A) Mediolateral oblique view of the right breast from screening mammogram shows moderately dense tissue with no suspicious findings. Coarse calcifications consistent with fat necrosis are present superiorly, at the lumpectomy site. (B) Sagittal, T1-weighted, contrast-enhanced image of the right breast from high-risk screening MRI examination shows two irregularly shaped, irregularly marginated heterogeneously enhancing masses in ductal orientation in the lower outer quadrant. These were not identified by mammography or sonography. The patient agreed to participate in our validation study of MRI-guided vacuum-assisted biopsy. (C) Sagittal, T1-weighted, contrast-enhanced image obtained during MRI-guided vacuum-assisted biopsy shows the two obturators evident as low signal intensity artifact (arrows) immediately adjacent to the enhancing lesions. Bright signal above the upper obturator may represent a small hematoma. (D) Sagittal, T1-weighted MRI after vacuum-assisted biopsy shows air and fluid at the site of the anterior lesion. Mild postbiopsy hematoma is evident at the site of the posterior lesion. The posterior clip and localization wire have been placed, and are evident as low-signal artifact posteriorly. (E) Sagittal, T1-weighted MRI after placement of the anterior clip and localization wire shows that the wires and clips have been placed, evident as low-signal artifact at the biopsy sites. Some of the air and hematoma previously present at the biopsy site has already been resorbed. (F) Collimated photograph of mediolateral oblique mammographic view of the right breast after biopsy and needle localization shows the localizing wires localizing the two clips. Histologic analysis of vacuum-assisted biopsy material yielded invasive ductal carcinoma and DCIS from the posterior lesion, and small foci of invasive carcinoma from the anterior lesion. Surgical excision, performed on the same day, showed invasive ductal carcinoma, 1.1 cm, and DCIS. The patient underwent subsequent mastectomy.

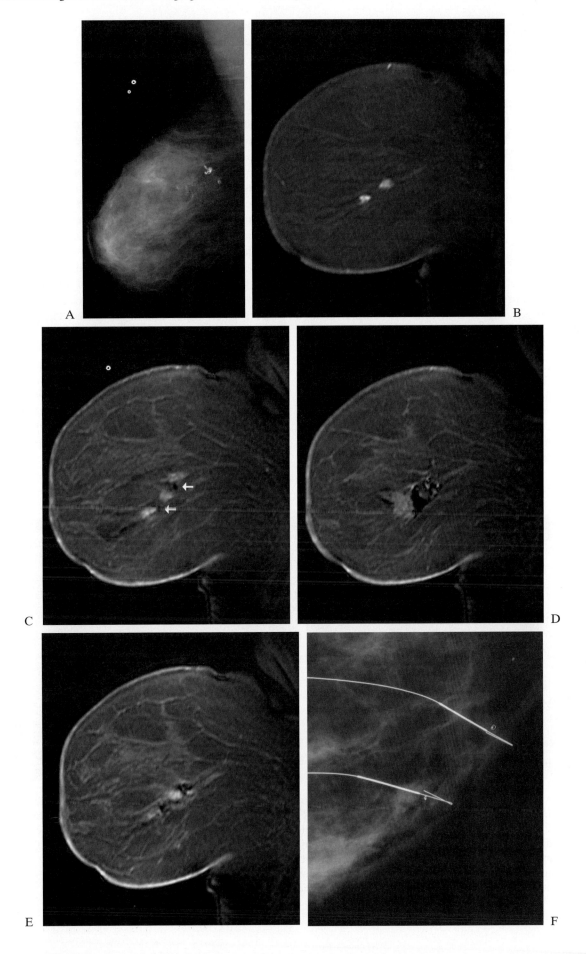

4. Challenging Scenarios at Magnetic Resonance Imaging Guided Vacuum-Assisted Biopsy

Many of the challenges posed by MRI-guided vacuum-assisted biopsy are similar to those posed by stereotactic biopsy with patients prone in a dedicated table. Some of the techniques described for stereotactic biopsy may be useful to overcome these challenges. Furthermore, it is helpful (if possible) to have technologists with expertise in stereotactic biopsy assisting with these procedures.

4.1. Posterior Lesions

The vacuum-assisted biopsy device is particularly helpful in performing biopsy of posterior lesions. Some posterior lesions cannot be captured within the biopsy grid, a problem that can also be encountered when performing stereotactic biopsy with the patient in the prone position.[31] If a lesion is close but posterior to the grid, the probe can be positioned adjacent to the lesion, and suction can be used to acquire tissue in the posterior direction to obtain diagnostic material (Figure 20.4). Automated core biopsy requires that the needle traverse a lesion to sample it. The ability to position the vacuum-assisted biopsy device adjacent to the lesion and still acquire tissue from the lesion is

another advantage of vacuum-assisted biopsy over automated core biopsy.

4.2. Thin Breasts

Thin breasts pose challenges for MRI-guided vacuum-assisted biopsy, as they do for stereotactic biopsy. The entire thickness of the tip and collecting area (mouth) of the probe must be within the breast to perform the biopsy. Maneuvers that assist in biopsy of thin breasts include raising a generous wheal of anesthetic and extrinsic circumferential pressure on the breast.[32] Use of the minimal amount of compression necessary may also be helpful, to maximize breast thickness as well as to avoid interfering with lesion enhancement.

Although no data yet address this issue, biopsy of thin breasts may be facilitated by use of a coil (Biopsy Breast Array Coil [Model BBC], MRI Devices) that has two parallel grids on either side of the breast. The grid on the side opposite to the skin entry site of the needle could function as a *reverse compression paddle*, such has been described for stereotactic breast biopsy; when the probe is placed deep into the breast, it displaces the skin and subcutaneous tissues into the overlying aperture on the side opposite the skin entry site without piercing the skin on the far side.[31] Alternatively, a reverse compression paddle could potentially be home built and taped to the far plate to accomplish the same goal.

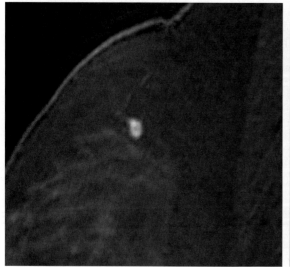
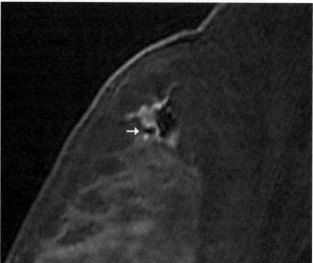

A   B

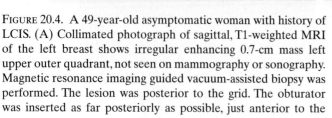

FIGURE 20.4. A 49-year-old asymptomatic woman with history of LCIS. (A) Collimated photograph of sagittal, T1-weighted MRI of the left breast shows irregular enhancing 0.7-cm mass left upper outer quadrant, not seen on mammography or sonography. Magnetic resonance imaging guided vacuum-assisted biopsy was performed. The lesion was posterior to the grid. The obturator was inserted as far posteriorly as possible, just anterior to the lesion. (B) Collimated photograph of sagittal T1-weighted MRI obtained after tissue acquisition shows a small hematoma with a vertical air-fluid level, and the clip (arrow) at the biopsy site. The lesion is no longer evident. Histologic analysis of material obtained at MRI-guided vacuum-assisted biopsy showed invasive lobular carcinoma. No residual carcinoma was found at surgery.

4.3. Medial Lesions

Although lateral lesions are more readily accessible for MRI-guided interventional procedures performed with the patient prone and with the breast to undergo biopsy in a dedicated breast coil, several approaches may facilitate access to medial lesions. Lesions that are only slightly medial to the plane of the nipple may undergo biopsy from a lateral approach. Lesions that are far medial in the breast underwent biopsy by placing the patient in the prone oblique position, with the breast of interest in the contralateral coil, as has been described for MRI-guided needle localization and surgical biopsy[33] and is discussed in the previous chapter (see Chapter 19). Finally, use of a breast coil that allows removal of the compression paddles on one side provides access to the medial aspect of the contralateral breast (see Figure 19–6).

4.4. Augmented Breasts

Augmented breasts pose challenges for MRI-guided percutaneous biopsy procedures, as they do for percutaneous biopsy under ultrasound or stereotactic guidance.[32] When performing a biopsy in a woman with an implant, several techniques are useful. First, one can attempt to push the implant back, similar to an Eklund view for mammography. Second, the biopsy handpiece can be placed at or slightly posterior to the lesion (if this can be accomplished safely), and then tissue can be acquired in the anterior direction (away from the implant).

4.5. Lesion That May Not Have Been Sampled

Careful review of the images from MRI study performed immediately after tissue acquisition is helpful to determine whether the lesion has been sampled. If these images suggest that the lesion has not been sampled, then repositioning and additional tissue acquisition may be appropriate. If the obturator is superficial to the lesion, the obturator is removed (leaving the introducer in place), the stylet advanced, and then the obturator replaced. If the obturator is deep to the lesion, the obturator and introducer are simply pulled back. Repeat MRI can then be performed to document appropriate positioning before repeat tissue acquisition. In lesions that exhibit rapid washout of contrast material where review of the images after biopsy leaves doubt as to whether the lesion was sampled, injecting a second dose of intravenous contrast before MRI may be helpful.

4.6. Clip Placement and Visualization

Some of the challenges posed by clip placement after MRI-guided vacuum-assisted biopsy are similar to those encountered during clip placement under stereotactic guidance and include failure to deploy and malposition due to the accordion effect.[30] In our validation study of MRI-guided vacuum-assisted biopsy,[26] the initial attempt at clip placement was successful in 20 of 26 (77%) lesions, and a second attempt was successful in 5 of 26 (19%) lesions; in 1 (4%) lesion, clip placement failed in spite of two attempts. It is our anecdotal impression that placing the clip in an anterior direction (ie., toward the floor) increases the likelihood of successful deployment. Careful inspection of the biopsy handpiece after its removal is essential; in all instances of unsuccessful clip deployment, the collagen pledget was visible in the mouth of the biopsy handpiece after its removal, and therefore failure of clip deployment was immediately apparent to the radiologist performing the biopsy. An immediate postbiopsy two-view mammogram is also necessary, to confirm clip deployment and to assess clip location.

Among the clips that deployed in our validation study,[26] the median maximal distance of the clip to the biopsy site (as judged by the position of the localizing wire) was 0.6 cm (range, 0.1–4.1 cm). The distance from the clip to the localizing wire was 1 cm or less in 19 of 25 (76%) lesions, 1.1 cm in 3 (12%) lesions, and 3 cm or greater in 3 (12%) lesions; the latter 3 lesions were all deep (i.e., medial) to the biopsy sites. Use of the least compression required may help to minimize the accordion effect. If the clip is distant from the biopsy site, use of MRI or mammographic landmarks (if the biopsy cavity is well seen on the immediate postbiopsy mammogram) may be necessary for subsequent localization.

One issue regarding clip placement that is unique to MRI-guided biopsy relates to the visibility of the clip on MRI. In our validation study,[26] the clip was evident as a low-signal focus measuring a median of 0.6 cm. In 4 (17%) of 24 lesions in which MRI was performed after clip deployment, the radiologist noted that the clip was difficult to distinguish from low-signal foci representing air; comparing images before and after clip placement is helpful in making this distinction. Further work, including exploration of different clip materials or different pulse sequences, may be helpful in improving clip conspicuity after placement.

5. Conclusion

Magnetic resonance imaging guided percutaneous biopsy can be accomplished with a variety of equipment, including fine needles, automated core needles, and vacuum-assisted biopsy probes. Fine needle aspiration biopsy under MRI guidance suffers from problems of insufficient specimens, as encountered in fine needle aspiration under stereotactic or ultrasound guidance. Magnetic resonance imaging guided automated core biopsy can have high diagnostic yield, but has potential problems of targeting small lesions that decrease in conspicuity during the biopsy procedure, histologic underestimation of lesions containing ADH and DCIS, and limited ability to place a localizing clip.

Vacuum-assisted devices may be advantageous for MRI-guided percutaneous breast biopsy, because vacuum-assisted biopsy can be performed quickly, removes a large volume of tissue, provides more accurate characterization of lesions containing ADH and DCIS, and enables placement of a localizing clip. Magnetic resonance imaging guided vacuum-assisted biopsy is a fast, safe, and accurate alternative to surgical excision for the diagnosis of MRI-detected lesions. Further work is necessary, including optimization of equipment and techniques for performing biopsy and placement of a localizing marker, evaluation of larger numbers of women, studies of cost effectiveness, and long-term follow up, so that we can offer women the benefits of MRI in breast cancer detection while minimizing surgical procedures for lesions that are benign.

References

1. Morris EA. Review of breast MRI: indications and limitations. Semin Roentgenol. 2001;36:226–237.
2. Morris EA, Liberman L, Ballon DJ, et al. MRI of occult breast carcinoma in a high-risk population. *AJR Am J Roentgenol.* 2003;181:619–626.
3. Liberman L, Morris EA, Dershaw DD, et al. MR imaging of the ipsilateral breast in women with percutaneously proven breast cancer. *AJR Am J Roentgenol.* 2003;180:901–910.
4. Liberman L, Morris EA, Kim CM, et al. MR imaging findings in the contralateral breast in women with recently diagnosed breast cancer. *AJR Am J Roentgenol.* 2003;180:333–341.
5. Orel SG, Schnall MD, Newman RW, et al. MR imaging-guided localization and biopsy of breast lesions: initial experience. *Radiology* 1994;193:97–102.
6. Panizza P, De Gaspari A, Vanzulli A, et al. Accuracy of post-MR imaging second-look-sonography in previously undetected breast lesions [abstract]. *Radiology* 1997;205:489.
7. Dhamanaskar KP, Muradall D, Kulkarni SR, et al. MRI directed ultrasound: a cost effective method for diagnosis and intervention in breast imaging [abstract]. *Radiology* 2002;225:653.
8. LaTrenta LR, Menell JH, Morris EA, et al. Breast lesions detected with MR imaging: utility and histopathologic importance of identification with US. *Radiology* 2003;227:856–861.
9. Liberman L. Percutaneous image-guided core breast biopsy. *Radiol Clin North Am.* 2002;40;483–500.
10. Schnall MD. MR-guided breast biopsy. In: Lufkin RB, ed. *Interventional MRI.* St. Louis: Mosby; 2000:315–319.
11. Fischer U, Vosshenrich R, Keating D, et al. MR-guided biopsy of suspect breast lesions with a simple stereotaxic

12. Fischer U, Vosshenrich R, Doler W, et al. MR imaging-guided breast intervention: experience with two systems. *Radiology* 1995;195:533–538.
13. Desouza NM, Coutts GA, Puni RK, Young IR. Magnetic resonance imaging guided breast biopsy using a frameless stereotactic technique. *Clin Radiol.* 1996;51:425–428.
14. Wald DS, Weinreb JC, Newstead G, et al. MR-guided fine needle aspiration of breast lesions: initial experience. *J Comput Assist Tomogr.* 1996;20:1–8.
15. Fischer U, Kopka L, Grabbe E. Magnetic resonance guided localization and biopsy of suspicious breast lesions. *Top Magn Reson Imaging.* 1998;9:44–59.
16. Orel SG, Schnall MD, Powell CM, et al. Staging of suspected breast cancer: effect of MR imaging and MR-guided biopsy. *Radiology* 1995;196:115–122.
17. Doler W, Fischer U, Metzger I, et al. Stereotaxic add-on device for MR-guided biopsy of breast lesions. *Radiology* 1996;200:863–864.
18. Kuhl CK, Elevelt A, Leutner CC, et al. Interventional breast MR imaging: clinical use of a stereotactic localization and biopsy device. *Radiology* 1997;204:667–675.
19. Kuhl CK, Morakkabati N, Leutner CC, et al. MR imaging-guided large-core (14-gauge) needle biopsy of small lesions visible at breast MR imaging alone. *Radiology* 2001;220:31–39.
20. Schneider JP, Schulz T, Horn LC, et al. MR-guided percutaneous core biopsy of small breast lesions: first experience with a vertically open 0.5T scanner. *J Magn Reson Imaging.* 2002;15:374–385.
20a. Lehman CD, Eby PR, Chen X, Dee KE, Thursten B, McCloskey J. MR imaging-guided breast biopsy using a coaxial technique with a 14-gauge stainless steel core biopsy needle and a titanium sheath. *AJR Am J Roentgenol.* 2003;181:183–185.
20b. Chen X, Lehman CD, Dee KE. MRI-guided breast biopsy: clinical experience with 140 gauge stainless steel core biopsy needle. *AJR Am J Roentgenol.* 2004;182:1075–1080.
21. Heywang-Kobrunner SH, Heinig A, Schaumloeffel-Schulze U, et al. MR-guided percutaneous excisional and incisional biopsy of breast lesions. *Eur Radiol.* 1999;9:1656–1665.
22. Prat X, Sittek H, Baath L, et al. European quadricentric evaluation of a breast MR biopsy and localization device: technical improvements based on phase-I evaluation. *Eur Radiol.* 2002;12:1720–1727.
23. Viehweg P, Heinig A, Amaya B, et al. MR-guided interventional breast procedures considering vacuum biopsy in particular. *Eur J Radiol.* 2002;42:32–39.
24. Perlet C, Heinig A, Prat X, et al. Multicenter study for the evaluation of a dedicated biopsy device for MR-guided vacuum biopsy of the breast. *Eur Radiol.* 2002;12:1463–1470.
25. Perlet CH, Prat X, Casselman JW, et al. European multicenter study on MR-guided vacuum biopsy of the breast: clinical results. *Radiology* 2002;225:556.
26. Liberman L, Morris EA, Dershaw DD, et al. Fast MRI-guided vacuum-assisted breast biopsy: initial experience. *AJR Am J Roentgenol.* 2003;181:1283–1293.

27. Pisano ED, Fajardo LL, Tsimikas J, et al. Rate of insufficient samples for fine-needle aspiration for nonpalpable breast lesions in a multicenter clinical trial: The Radiologic Diagnostic Oncology Group 5 study. *Cancer* 1998;82:678–688.

28. Pisano ED, Fajardo LL, Caudry DJ, et al. Fine-needle aspiration biopsy of nonpalpable breast lesions in a multicenter clinical trial: Results from the Radiologic Diagnostic Oncology Group V. *Radiology* 2001;219:785–792.

29. Pfarl G, Helbich TH, Riedl CC, et al. Stereotactic 11-gauge vacuum-assisted breast biopsy: a validation study. *AJR Am J Roentgenol.* 2002;179:1503–1507.

30. Liberman L, Dershaw DD, Morris EA, et al. Clip placement after stereotactic vacuum-assisted breast biopsy. *Radiology* 1997;205:417–422.

31. Philpotts LE, Tocino I, Lee CH. Canceled stereotactic 11-gauge vacuum-assisted suction biopsy of the breast. *AJR Am J Roentgenol.* 2001;176 (Suppl):45.

32. Jackman RJ, Lamm RL. Stereotactic histologic biopsy in breasts with implants. *Radiology* 2002;222:157–164.

33. Morris EA, Liberman L, Dershaw DD, et al. Preoperative MR imaging-guided needle localization of breast lesions. *AJR Am J Roentgenol.* 2002;178:1211–1220.

21
Image-Guided Ablation of Breast Cancer

Laura Liberman and Nanette Bracero

Progress in fighting breast cancer has been marked by development of effective, less invasive diagnostic and treatment techniques. In the past, the Halsted radical mastectomy[1] was the standard of care for the surgical management of invasive breast cancer. Breast conservation surgery created a revolution in breast cancer treatment, offering effective treatment while enabling breast preservation.[2] Other revolutions in breast cancer diagnosis and therapy have included percutaneous image-guided breast biopsy (for diagnosis)[3] and sentinel lymphadenectomy (for treatment).[4]

Image-guided tumor ablation is defined as the application under imaging guidance of chemical or thermal therapies to a specific focal tumor (or tumors) in an attempt to achieve eradication or substantial tumor destruction.[5] For image-guided ablation of breast cancer, most work to date has involved thermal methods that use heat or cold to kill tumor cells.[6] Methods of heating the tumor include laser ablation, radiofrequency ablation, and high-intensity focused ultrasound. Cooling the tumor can be accomplished through cryoablation. This chapter reviews research relating to percutaneous image-guided breast cancer ablation, and discusses the potential role of breast magnetic resonance imaging (MRI) in planning, targeting, monitoring, controlling, and follow up after image-guided ablative treatment.

1. Terminology

The Working Group on Image-Guided Tumor Ablation has proposed standardized language for reporting image-guided ablation procedures and outcomes.[5] The *index tumor* is the initially identified tumor before ablation. For thermal therapies, energy is said to be *applied*. The term *applicator* should be used to describe all devices used to apply the energy for thermal ablation: for example, laser applicators are *fibers*, radiofrequency applicators are *elec-*

trodes, and the applicators that freeze tissue during cryablation are *cryoprobes*.

According to the proposed standardized terminology, imaging serves five functions for image-guided ablation procedures: (1) planning, that is, assessment of tumor size, shape, and location within the organ and relative to blood vessels as well as other structures at risk during the ablation procedure; (2) targeting, that is, placement of the applicator or focusing the energy into the tumor (ideally with a method that can clearly delineate the tumor from surrounding tissue and that can provide real-time imaging and multiplanar capabilities); (3) monitoring, that is, viewing therapy effects during a procedure; (4) controlling, that is, tools and techniques used during the procedure to control the treatment; and (5) assessing treatment response.[5]

Standard terminology has also been proposed for describing pathologic and imaging findings after tumor ablation. The zone of cell death at pathologic examination should be called the *zone of coagulation* or *coagulation necrosis*. Most thermal treatments induce a central *white zone* of coagulation, usually thought to represent coagulated tissue, surrounded by a variable *red zone* of hyperemia. The Working Group on Tumor Ablation suggests that both measurements be reported. The term *ablation zone* refers to the radiologic region or zone of induced treatment effect (i.e., the area of gross destruction seen at imaging). The term *lesion* should be avoided because of potential confusion: *lesion* has been used to refer to the ablation zone and the underlying tumor to be ablated. The Working Group proposed the term *ablative margin* to refer to the 0.5- to 1.0-cm wide region beyond the border of the tumor that should ideally be ablated.[5]

Specific terms have also been proposed to describe outcomes. An ablation is *technically successful* if a tumor is treated according to the protocol and covered completely. The term *technical effectiveness* refers to a prospectively defined time point at which *complete ablation* of macroscopic tumor as seen at imaging follow up or another specified endpoint was achieved. *Debulking* refers to a procedure performed with the sole intent of decreasing the tumor burden. *Local tumor progression* refers to the development of foci of untreated disease in tumors that were previously considered to be completely ablated. The Working Group on Image-Guided Tumor Ablation also made recommendations regarding the classification of complications, pain, postablation syndrome, and follow-up imaging after treatment.[5]

2. Methods of Thermal Destruction

Thermal injury with heat or cold can result in cell death. Heating tumors with laser, radiofrequency, or focused ultrasound can result in coagulative necrosis. Alternatively, cryotherapeutic cooling techniques can kill cells by two mechanisms, depending on the cooling rate: extracellular ice, increased osmolarity of the extracellular fluid that is not frozen, and osmotic damage to cells (at low cooling rates) or in intracellular ice (at high cooling rates).[7,8]

The relationship between temperature and cell death has been studied by numerous investigators. Sapareto and Dewey[9] used mathematical modeling to calculate the thermal dose necessary in cancer therapy. Borrelli and colleagues[10] described the time-temperature relationship for killing of baby hamster kidney (BHK) cells. Rui and colleagues[11] described the relationship between thermal variables and the degree of freezing in human breast cancer cells and normal cells. These basic investigations are necessary to design clinical protocols for image-guided ablation.

Image-guided breast cancer ablation requires an imaging modality that has high sensitivity in breast cancer detection, that can delineate the cancer from the surrounding tissue, that enables monitoring and controlling of therapy effects during procedures, and that enables follow up of patients after treatment. Magnetic resonance imaging is advantageous for these purposes.[12] Magnetic resonance imaging may provide more accurate assessment of extent of disease than mammography or sonography, and hence is useful for treatment planning. The delineation of tumor from surrounding tissue provided by MRI is useful for targeting. Furthermore, MRI enables generation of temperature-sensitive maps that can be used to monitor heating or cooling during therapy. These MRI temperature maps can be made using T1-weighted images (due to the temperature sensitivity of the spin-lattice relaxation time, T1, which obeys a linear relationship over a small range of temperatures) or diffusion imaging.[13] Magnetic resonance imaging may also be useful for assessment of response after image-guided ablative treatment.

2.1. Laser Ablation

Laser ablation is the term used to describe all types of ablation with light energy. *Interstitial* or *direct* laser ablation is laser ablation applied via fibers directly inserted into the tissue. Laser ablation of solid tumors is accomplished by insertion of a thin optical fiber, which can be placed through a needle, into the target lesion.[14] The fiber delivers laser light energy from its tip that results in heating and coagulative necrosis of tumor cells. The use of a precharred fiber may result in a more predictable extent of necrosis.[15] Semiconductor diode laser and Nd:Yag pulse lasers have been used for laser ablation.[12] Laser *burns* measuring up to 1 cm can be generated by application of 2 to 2.5 W for approximately 500 s; use of multiple fibers or special *pull-back* methods can yield burns as large as 4 cm.[12]

Mumtaz and colleagues[15] described 20 women with symptomatic breast cancer who had laser ablation with a single fiber prior to surgical excision. Laser ablation was performed under ultrasound guidance through an 18-gauge needle, using low power (2 W/500 s). Treatment was monitored with ultrasound, which showed an irregular hyperechoic zone that correlated poorly with the histologic extent of laser-induced necrosis. Gadolinium-enhanced T1-weighted three-dimensional fast low-angle shot (FLASH) MRI was performed before and at a median of 48 h after laser treatment, before surgical resection (i.e., MRI was used for treatment planning and for follow up after treatment). Median diameter of enhancing masses on MRI prior to treatment was 21 mm.

Although early (4-hour) follow-up MRI failed to identify any laser effect, later (24–96) follow-up MRI scans showed a zone of nonenhancement within the residual enhancing tumor, which correlated with laser-induced necrosis found at surgery. The median diameter of the laser-induced necrosis on the gadolinium-enhanced images was 10 mm at MRI and at histologic analysis. Correlation coefficients between MRI and histologic findings were 0.80 for the laser-burn diameter and 0.86 for residual tumor. The area of laser-induced necrosis was completely within the tumor margins in 13 (65%) patients, extended beyond the margin of the invasive tumor in 5 (25%), and missed the tumor in 2 (10%). The data of Mumtaz and colleagues[15] suggest that delayed gadolinium-enhanced MRI can define the extent of laser-induced necrosis and residual tumor after laser ablation.

Dowlatshahi and coworkers[16] have published their experience with laser ablation of small breast cancers over a 7-year period from 1994 to 2002. In their study, 54 women with breast cancer (50 invasive, 4 in situ) of median diameter 12 (5–23) mm were treated by a stereotactically guided 805-nm laser beam via a fiber in a 16-gauge needle delivered to the cancer (Figure 21.1). Surgery was performed 1 to 2 weeks later (Figure 21.2).

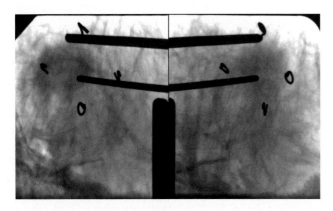

FIGURE 21.1. Stereotactic images demonstrating laser treatment of invasive ductal carcinoma in a 74-year-old woman. The lower needle is the laser probe, and the upper needle is the thermal probe. The metal markers serve as references. (Courtesy of Kambiz Dowlatshahi, MD, Professor of Surgery, Rush University, Chicago, IL.)

In this study, Dowlatshahi and coworkers[16] found no adverse effects. The average treatment time was 30 min. At pathology, the zone of laser-induced change was evident as a 2.5- to 3.5-cm hemorrhagic ring surrounding the necrotic tumor. The overall success rate for tumor ablation was 70%, which includes the learning curve, technical, and pro-

cedural changes over the study period. The authors state that under "steady conditions" in two groups of 14 patients, 93% and 100% of tumors showed complete necrosis, with clear histologic margins.

In the two studies of laser ablation discussed previously, MRI was not used for monitoring, or controlling the ablation procedure.[15,16] However, MRI may be useful for these aspects of image-guided laser ablation. Magnetic resonance imaging may identify acute laser-induced tissue changes that are poorly visualized with ultrasound[15] and not identified with stereotactic imaging.[16] Hall-Craggs[12] found that within 1 min of starting laser treatment, T1-weighted images obtained at high field strength show areas of low signal intensity around the fiber tip that persist during therapy, perhaps due to temperature changes and/or tissue coagulation. Temperature-sensitive MRI mapping during laser treatment may facilitate therapy, enabling identification of inadequate heating so that complete tumor ablation could be achieved in a higher proportion of patients.

2.2. Radiofrequency Ablation

Radiofrequency ablation refers to coagulation induction from all electromagnetic energy sources with frequencies less than 900 kHz, although most devices function in the 375 to 500 kHz range.[5] (Radiofrequency ablation is differ-

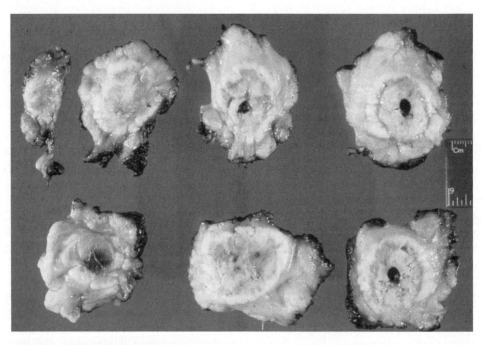

FIGURE 21.2. Gross serial sections of a 2.0-cm invasive ductal carcinoma in a 45-year-old woman who had stereotactic-guided laser treatment followed by lumpectomy 1 week later. The sections are 4 to 5 mm thick. The images on the far right best demonstrate the *bull's-eye* pattern in which the center represents the location of

the laser fiber, surrounded by the zone of coagulated tumor, a thin hyperemic zone, and adjacent fat necrosis. No residual tumor was found at surgery. (Courtesy of Kambiz Dowlatshahi, MD, Professor of Surgery, Rush University, Chicago, IL.)

ent from *microwave ablation*, a term used to describe electromagnetic methods that induce tumor destruction by using devices with frequencies greater than or equal to 900kHz.) Radiofrequency ablation requires insertion of a radiofrequency probe into the index tumor. Frictional heating occurs when the ions in tissue attempt to follow a rapidly changing alternating current flowing from an uninsulated electrode tip. This method has been used for ablation of tumors in the liver, prostate, bone, kidney, lung, and brain.[17]

The first clinical report of radiofrequency ablation in breast cancer was from Jeffrey and colleagues.[18] Five women with locally advanced (stage III) invasive breast cancer who were undergoing surgical resection of the tumor had radiofrequency ablation delivered intraoperatively, immediately prior to surgical excision. Under general anesthesia, a 15-gauge insulated multiple needle electrode was inserted into the index tumor under ultrasound guidance. Radiofrequency energy was applied according to a predetermined protocol for a period of up to 30min. Only a portion of the tumor was treated in order to assess the margin between ablated and nonablated tissue. Pathologic analysis included special cell viability staining with nicotinamide adenine dinucleotide (NADH)-diaphorase.

In these five women, the ablation zone extended around the radiofrequency electrode for 0.8 to 1.8cm. Hematoxylin-eosin staining showed complete cell death in two (40%) patients and a mixed pattern of necrotic and normal-appearing cells within the ablated tissue in three

(60%) women. Cell viability (NADH-diaphorase) stains showed complete cell death in four (80%) patients and a single focus of viable cells partially lining a cyst in one (20%) patient. The authors suggested that the technique warrants further study and may be most applicable for tumors smaller than 3cm in maximal diameter.

In pioneering studies performed at M.D. Anderson,[19,20] radiofrequency ablation was delivered through a 15-gauge needle electrode placed under real-time ultrasound guidance to 21 malignant lesions in 20 patients (Figure 21.3). A temperature of 95 °C was maintained for 15min at the tip of the prongs. Nicotinamide adenine dinucleotide-diaphorase staining was performed in addition to conventional pathologic analysis. Fornage and colleagues[20] reported complete ablation of the target lesion visualized on ultrasound in 21 of 21 (100%) lesions. In one patient who had received preoperative chemotherapy for a T2 invasive breast cancer, residual invasive and in situ carcinoma was found at surgery, although no residual lesion was identified by mammography or ultrasound after treatment. No adverse effects were identified.

Although these reports used ultrasound guidance for delivery of radiofrequency ablation, there are potential advantages of MRI rather than ultrasound to guide radiofrequency ablation. Ultrasound may underestimate the extent of tumor, particularly with respect to the in situ component; MRI may provide more accurate assessment of extent of disease and hence may be advantageous for treatment planning and targeting. With appropriate equipment, MRI could provide the potential ability to monitor

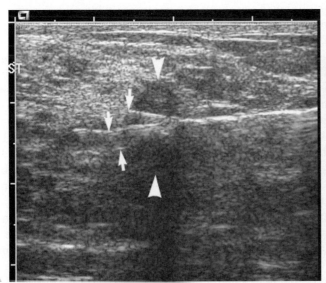
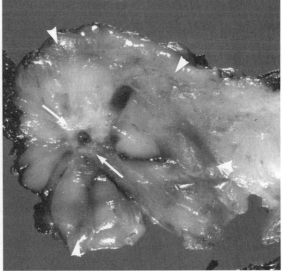

FIGURE 21.3. Ultrasound-guided radiofrequency (RF) ablation of a small breast cancer. (A) Longitudinal sonogram obtained immediately prior to RF ablation of a small breast cancer shows three of the RF ablation device's prongs (arrows) deployed in the center of the tumor (arrowheads). (B) Photograph of a post-RF ablation lumpectomy specimen shows a small carcinoma (arrows) in the center of the thermal lesion delineated by the hyperemic ring (arrowheads). (Courtesy of Bruno D. Fornage, MD, Professor of Radiology and Surgical Oncology, The University of Texas MD Anderson Cancer Center, Houston, TX.)

temperature changes during treatment, which were poorly assessed with ultrasound,[19,20] and could play a role in controlling the procedure as well as postablation follow up.

2.3. High-Intensity Focused Ultrasound

There are two methods of ultrasound ablation of tumors: (1) extracorporeal (transcutaneous) and (2) direct, with a needle-like applicator.[5] *High-intensity focused ultrasound* refers to the extracorporeal method, while *direct ultrasound ablation* refers to placing an applicator within the index tumor either percutaneously or via laparoscopic insertion.

High-intensity focused ultrasound has several advantages as a method for thermal destruction of breast tumors. Focused ultrasound can be accomplished noninvasively, without insertion of a probe. The ultrasound beams can be sharply focused and tailored to the desired volume; unlike laser and radiofrequency ablation, which rely on heat emanating from a point source, focused ultrasound enables targeting complex anatomic arrangement of tumors in three dimensions, and facilitates target ablation without damage to the surrounding or overlying tissues. The focus of the beam can be changed in real time, to accommodate movement during treatment. A potential disadvantage of focused ultrasound is longer treatment times.

Magnetic resonance imaging is useful in monitoring the changes that occur during focused ultrasound ablation. In a study of focused ultrasound lesions produced in dog's thigh muscle in vivo, Hynynen and colleagues[21] found that T2-weighted images demonstrated the lesions, and that the dimensions measured on MRI correlated with the postmortem measurements of tissue damage. In a subsequent study of sonications in rabbit thigh muscle, Hynynen and colleagues[22] used gradient-recalled acquisition in a steady state (GRASS) T1-weighted images, with contrast injected before or after the sonications. They found that MRI could be used to detect temperature elevations that did not cause tissue damage, and that contrast agent was useful in delineating the necrosed tissue volume. In another study, Cline and coworkers[13] showed that MRI temperature maps of muscle provided localization and dosimetry both in the focal region and in the near field.

In animal studies, McDannold and coworkers[23] showed a linear relationship between applied power and shifts in the proton resonant frequency. Fluctuations in the location of the focus about the target location were on the order of the resolution of the MRI examination. The temperature increase and lesion size varied significantly. Regions of tissue coagulation calculated from MRI data correlated well with posttherapy imaging. An ex vivo study of bovine kidney and liver by Graham and colleagues[24] used proton resonance frequency shift MRI thermometry during heating at 10-s intervals. Thermal coagulation occurred with heating at approximately 54 °C for 10s in both tissues

and could be predicted with approximately 625μm of spatial resolution.

Early work has been done using focused ultrasound in clinical patients with breast disease. Hynynen and colleagues[25] tested the feasibility of using MRI-guided focused ultrasound to treat 11 benign fibroadenomas of the breast. Target volumes were defined on T2-weighted images, and sequential sonications were delivered to treat the entire target. Temperature-sensitive phase-difference based MRI was performed to monitor localization of the focus and changes in temperature during therapy.

Magnetic resonance imaging monitoring of focused ultrasound treatment improved during the study period, with 82% (279/342) *hot spots* visible in the last seven treatments. Eight (73%) of the 11 lesions demonstrated complete or partial lack of contrast enhancement on posttreatment T1-weighted images. Three lesions did not show decrease in contrast enhancement, probably due to insufficient acoustic power and/or patient movement. One case of pectoralis muscle edema was identified 2 days after treatment; no other adverse effects were identified.

Preliminary work has also addressed the use of MRI-guided focused ultrasound to treat breast cancer (Figure 21.4). Gianfelice and colleagues[26] used MRI-guided focused ultrasound to treat 12 patients with invasive breast cancer prior to surgical resection. Anesthesia was provided with fentanyl citrate, 50μg per dose, one to four doses, and midazolam, 1mg per dose, two to four doses, intravenously as needed. Focused ultrasound ablation was performed with one of two systems, the Mark 1 system or the Mark 2 system (InSighte-TxSonics, Haifa, Israel).

To perform focused ultrasound ablation, the patient was placed prone on the treatment table and the breast was placed in the center of a ring-shaped MRI coil. Degassed water was placed between the breast and the ultrasound transducer to increase acoustic coupling; for the last five patients, the breast was placed in a gel-filled container. A series of T1-weighted spin echo images were obtained in the sagittal, transverse, and coronal planes, transferred to the focused ultrasound workstation, and used for the radiologist to manually draw an outline of the targeted lesion, including approximately 5mm of surrounding tissue. Determination of the treatment zone was made by the radiologist in conjunction with MRI and other imaging studies acquired prior to treatment.

The center of the lesion was sonicated with a noneffective dose (2–60W) of ultrasound energy to test the accuracy of lesion targeting. Then sonication was performed at therapeutic power levels (up to 400W) on multiple overlapping points until the target volume was ablated. Focused ultrasound treatments were verified by using MRI phase maps that showed temperature-dependent changes in resonant frequency. The number of sonications ranged from 12 to 52 and the total treatment duration was 35 to 133min; the total time required to perform MRI-guided

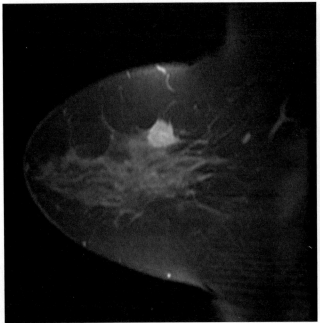
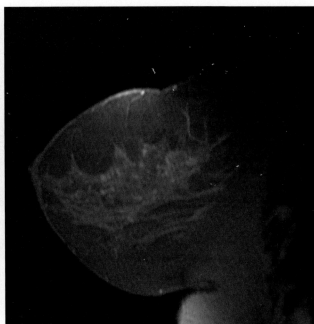

A

B

FIGURE 21.4. Focused ultrasound ablation of a cancer with residual disease at surgery. (A) Sagittal, T1-weighted, contrast-enhanced MRI in a 52-year-old woman with a nonpalpable, mammographically detected 1.6-cm mass. Ultrasound-guided core biopsy yielded infiltrating ductal carcinoma, moderately differentiated, with a minor component of DCIS, intermediate nuclear grade. Magnetic resonance imaging shows an irregular, heterogeneously enhancing mass, corresponding to the biopsy-proven cancer. The patient had focused ultrasound ablation of her tumor. (B) Sagittal, T1-weighted, contrast-enhanced MRI 6 days after focused ultrasound ablation (but before surgery) shows that the mass is no longer evident. At surgery, performed 1 day after this MRI, the surgeon indicated that grossly the treated tissue was clearly delineated from the surrounding tissue. Surgical histologic analysis showed showed a 1.4-cm invasive ductal carcinoma and no DCIS. Approximately 25% of the tumor appeared to be necrotic around the periphery, but the central portion of the tumor appeared viable. Numerous mitotic figures were present. Some adjacent normal tissue also appeared necrotic. Stromal edema and hemorrhage were also present. (Courtesy of Darrell N. Smith, MD, Assistant Professor of Radiology, Brigham and Women's Hospital, Boston, MA.)

focused ultrasound ablation and subsequent MRI was 2.0 to 2.5h.

Focused ultrasound ablation was well tolerated, with two minor skin burns in two (17%) patients and no other complications. The pain was graded by the patients as slight in four cases (33%) and moderate in eight (67%); three (25%) patients reported tenderness around the treatment zone. In three patients treated with the Mark 1 ultrasound system, a mean of 47% of the tumor within the target zone and a mean of 43% of the cancer tissue was necrosed. In nine patients treated with the Mark 2 ultrasound system, a mean of 95% of the tumor was within the target zone and a mean of 88% of the cancer was necrosed.

Residual viable cancer was present at surgery in 10 (83%) of the 12 patients. Residual cancer was found outside the targeted zone when targeting was poor (in two patients) or imperfect (in three patients), and residual tumor was found at the periphery of the tumor when targeting was accurate (in five patients). In two (17%) patients, no residual cancer was found (Figure 21.5). The authors concluded that thermal coagulation of small breast cancers by means of MRI-guided focused ultrasound ablation may be feasible, but that the data indicate the need to increase the total target area (e.g., by increasing the number of sonications).

2.4. Cryablation

Cryoablation or *cryotherapy* is the term used to describe all methods of destroying tissue by the application of low-temperature freezing.[5] Cryoablation requires insertion of a cryoprobe into the index tumor. The cryoprobe is cooled internally with a cryogen such as argon and insulated except at the tip. The uninsulated tip is inserted into the tumor; as heat is removed, the index tumor is frozen from the probe surface outward. The flow of freezing agent is stopped after the target volume has been frozen, and the tissue is allowed to thaw. After cryoablation, the frozen tissue is left is in situ, to be re-absorbed by the immune system over time.[11]

An advantage of cryoablation is that the cold itself provides some anesthesia. A disadvantage of cryoablation is

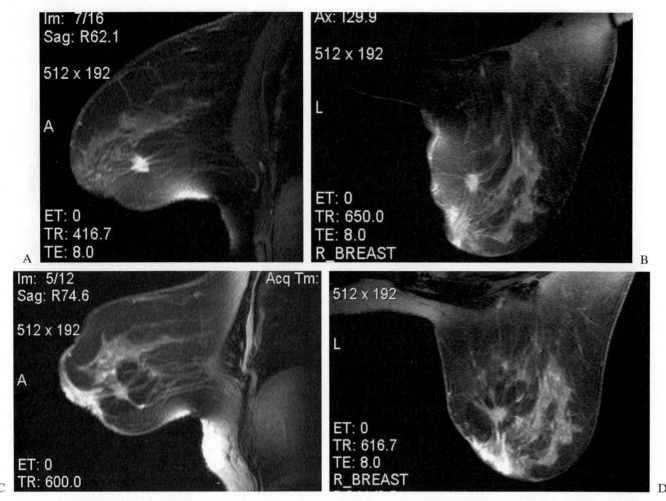

FIGURE 21.5. Focused ultrasound ablation of a cancer with no residual disease at surgery. (A) Sagittal T1-weighted image from contrast-enhanced MRI of 57-year-old woman who presented with suspicious mass on screening mammography shows an irregular, spiculated mass in the right lower inner quadrant. (B) Axial T1-weighted image from the same contrast-enhanced MRI shown in A shows the spiculated mass in the lower inner quadrant. Ultrasound-guided core biopsy yielded infiltrating ductal carcinoma. (C) Sagittal T1-weighted image from contrast-enhanced MRI performed 7 days after focused ultrasound ablation shows the spiculated mass, which demonstrates diminished enhancement by visual analysis as well as kinetic curves (not shown). (D) Axial T1-weighted image from the same postablation contrast-enhanced MRI shown in C demonstrates the spiculated mass with decreased enhancement as compared with the pre-ablation examination. The patient had subsequent lumpectomy 10 days after ablation. Surgical histologic analysis demonstrated total ablation of the neoplastic lesion with ablation of perilesional fat. (Courtesy of David Gianfelice, MD, Section Chief of Abdominal Imaging and Associate Professor of Radiology, Centre Hospitalier Universite, Montreal, Canada.)

that cell killing may be less effective, particularly if an insufficient number of freeze/thaw cycles are used. In a study of mice transplanted with mammary tumors,[27] the best results from cryoablation were obtained when using at least five freeze-thaw cycles at −180 °C. In a study of breast cancer cells and normal cells, a double freeze-thaw cycle significantly increased the extent of cell damage.[11]

Cryoablation has been used clinically in patients with breast disease. Rand and colleagues[27] used intraoperative cryoablation in conjunction with lumpectomy in a 77-year-old woman with a breast cancer measuring 2 cm at maximal diameter. The iceball was monitored with intraoperative real-time ultrasound guidance, which demonstrated the echogenic front edge of the iceball. Subsequent surgical excision showed complete necrosis of the tumor; only cell debris was detected at histologic analysis.

Cryoablation has been used to ablate benign fibroadenomas (Figure 21.6). Kaufman and colleagues[28] used a table-top cryoablation system with a 2.4-mm cryoprobe to

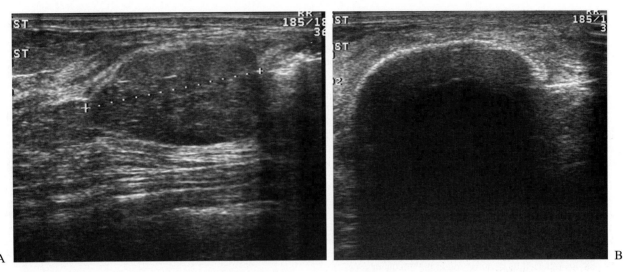

FIGURE 21.6. Cryoablation of a fibroadenoma. (A) Sonogram of the breast shows a large fibroadenoma. (B) Longitudinal sonogram obtained during cryoablation. The iceball and its associated acoustic shadow encompass the fibroadenoma. (Courtesy of Bruno D. Fornage, MD, Professor of Radiology and Surgical Oncology, The University of Texas MD Anderson Cancer Center, Houston, TX.)

treat 50 women with 57 core biopsy-proven fibroadenomas (mean diameter, 21 mm; range, 7–42 mm). Local anesthetic was used, and the cryoprobe was inserted under ultrasound guidance. Sterile saline was injected as needed between the lesion and the skin to protect the skin from cold injury. Treatment duration ranged from 6 to 30 min. The iceball engulfed the target lesion in each case. Local swelling and ecchymosis were transient postprocedural effects. Lesions showed progressive shrinkage and disappearance over 3 to 12 months. No skin injury was noted and cosmesis was excellent. No surgical follow up is available to quantify extent of histologic ablation in this study.

Pfleiderer and colleagues[29] evaluated the use of cryoablation under ultrasound guidance to treat 16 breast cancers in 15 women. The mean diameter of these lesions was 21 ± 8 mm. A 3-mm cryoprobe was placed in the tumor under ultrasound guidance, and two freeze-thaw cycles with durations of 7 to 10 min and 5 min, respectively, were performed. The size of the iceballs was monitored sonographically every minute, with the mean iceball diameter 28 ± 3 mm after the second freezing cycle. The patients had surgery within 5 days.

Among these 16 cancers, 3 (19%) had no residual tumor found after cryoablation; an additional 2 (13%) lesions had no residual invasive cancer but did have residual ductal carcinoma in situ (DCIS). All five of the tumors without residual invasive cancer at surgery measured less than 16 mm on the pretreatment imaging studies. In 11 (69%) tumors, all of which measured 23 mm or larger in maximal diameter on pretreatment imaging studies, cryoablation resulted in incomplete necrosis. These data suggest that cryoablation may obliterate the invasive component of a small tumor. Problems, however, were encountered with larger lesions or lesions with a significant in situ component.

Although the studies described used ultrasound to guide cryoablation, there may be advantages to the use of MRI for this purpose.[30,31] Ultrasound can identify the superficial edge of the iceball as an echogenic structure, but cannot image the posterior aspect of the iceball or the tissues deep to the iceball. Magnetic resonance imaging, on the other hand, could image both superficial and deep to the target lesion. Furthermore, MRI would be more sensitive in the identification of the in situ component of the tumor, which may enable more successful ablation.

3. Image-Guided Ablation of Breast Cancer: Problems

There are several potential problems with the use of image-guided ablation of breast cancer. Image-guided ablation would likely only be applicable to small breast cancers, tumors that have an excellent prognosis with current treatment methods. Any alternative to surgery would have to meet this high standard to be clinically acceptable. Most image-guided ablation methods require substantial anesthesia; hence, one of the main advantages of sparing surgery (avoiding anesthesia) is lost. Image-guided ablation techniques may require long procedure times (up to 2 h or more). Tumors close to the skin or chest wall may not be amenable to some methods of thermal

TABLE 21.1. Selected Studies of Percutaneous Image-guided Ablation of Breast Cancer

Investigator/Year	Method	No. Treated	No. Completely Ablated (%)	No. Partially Ablated (%)	No. Missed (%)	No. Complications (%)	Time (min)
Mumtaz/1996[15]	Laser	20	0 (0)	18 (90)	2 (10)	2 (10)[a]	NS[a]
Dowlatshahi/2002[16]	Laser	54	38 (70)	16 (30)	0 (0)	0 (0)	25–30
Jeffrey/1999[18]	RFA	5	0 (0)	5 (100)	0 (0)	0 (0)	30
Fornage/2004[20]	RFA	21[b]	20 (95)	1 (5)	0 (0)	0 (0)	NS[b]
Gianfelice/2003[26]	FUS	12	2 (17)	10 (83)	0 (0)	2 (17)[c]	35–133
Pfleiderer/2002[29]	Cryo	16[d]	3 (19)	13 (81)[d]	0 (0)	1 (6)[d]	41–64

Abbreviations: Cryo, cryoablation; FUS, focused ultrasound; NS, not stated; RFA, radiofrequency ablation.

[a] Complications were pain in two patients at 300 and 350 s, requiring stopping treatment. Time range was not recorded, but the authors indicate that lesions were treated at low power, 2 W/500 s (1000 J).

[b] Twenty-one malignant lesions in 20 patients were treated. The time range was not stated, but the authors indicate placement of the needle-electrode took 5–10 min and that a temperature of 95°C was maintained for 15 min.

[c] These two complications were minor skin burns. Of the 12 patients treated, pain was judged as slight in 4 (33%) and moderate in 8 (67%); 3 (25%) patients reported tenderness around the treatment zone.

[d] Sixteen tumors were treated in 15 patients. Among the 13 tumors that were partially ablated, 2 had complete ablation of the invasive component but had residual DCIS. The one complication was a seroma requiring aspiration; three patients required additional analgesia after the procedure.

ablation, due to the potential for injury of these adjacent structures.

Current breast cancer treatment is dependent on thorough histologic evaluation of the tumor, including assessment of margins. This information would have to be reliably obtained from a combination of pretreatment imaging and percutaneous needle biopsy for image-guided ablation to be a reasonable therapeutic approach. Whether this can be accomplished is unresolved.

In most studies of image-guided ablation of breast cancer followed by resection, residual tumor has been reported in a substantial proportion of women (Table 21.1), particularly at the tumor periphery. This may reflect a tendency to undertreat in the early trials, but also may indicate a limitation of these methods. Techniques that rely on a point source of thermal injury (such as laser ablation, radiofrequency ablation, and cryoablation) may drop off at the periphery. To obtain the temperatures necessary to reliably ablate the periphery may require an intolerable temperature at the source, particularly for larger tumors or lesions that have complex arrangements in three dimensions.

Treatment of invasive breast cancers currently requires surgical assessment of the axilla; for small breast cancers, this is often accomplished with sentinel lymph node biopsy. Even if image-guided ablation of the tumor can be accomplished, invasive cancers currently still require surgical assessment of the axilla; hence, image-guided ablation would not obviate the need for surgery. Furthermore, the impact of image-guided ablation on patterns of lymphatic drainage from the tumor site has not been determined; whether these procedures would impact on subsequent sentinel lymph node mapping is unknown.

Most of the experimental protocols described have been designed so that image-guided ablation is followed by resection soon thereafter, with cell killing assessed using special cell viability stains. The long-term effect of image-guided ablation on breast cancers in vivo has not yet been assessed. In addition to further studies of women who undergo image-guided ablation and subsequent excision, studies comparing recurrence rates in women who have ablation versus women who have standardized treatments may be necessary to determine if results are comparable; because the recurrence rate is so low with standard treatment, these studies will require large numbers of women and long-term follow up. The impact of image-guided ablation on physical examination, cosmesis, and imaging findings at long-term follow up also needs to be assessed, as do issues of patient tolerance and cost effectiveness. Use of MRI in percutaneous ablation will require development and optimization of appropriate equipment and techniques.

4. Summary and Conclusions

Image-guided ablation of breast cancer may be possible. However, it is likely to be applicable only to small breast cancers, tumors that have excellent prognosis with current treatment methods; hence, in order to be a reasonable therapeutic option, image-guided ablation must meet a high standard. Early studies have suggested that image-guided ablation techniques can be performed in patients and can result in cell death. Further investigation is necessary to determine if these methods will be acceptable in the future treatment of women with breast cancer. Breast

MRI, by providing a sensitive method for treatment planning, targeting, monitoring, controlling, and follow up after image-guided ablation, will likely play a major role in these future studies.

Acknowledgments. The authors gratefully acknowledge Kambiz Dowlatshahi, MD, Bruno D. Fornage, MD, David Gianfelice, MD, and Darrell N. Smith, MD, for contributing images illustrating their pioneering work in percutaneous image-guided ablation of breast lesions.

References

1. Halsted W. The results of radical operations for the cure of carcinoma of the breast. *Ann Surg.* 1907;46:1–19.
2. Fisher B, Redmond C, Fisher ER, et al. Ten-year results of a randomized clinical trial comparing radical mastectomy and total mastectomy with or without radiation. *N Engl J Med.* 1985;312:674–681.
3. Liberman L. Percutaneous image-guided core breast biopsy: state of the art at the millennium. *AJR Am J Roentgenol.* 2000;174:1191–1199.
4. Krag DN, Weaver DL, Ashikaga T, et al. The sentinel node in breast cancer: a multicenter validation study. *N Engl J Med.* 1998;339:941–946.
5. Goldberg SN, Charboneau JW, Dodd GD, et al. Image-guided tumor ablation: proposal for standardization of terms and reporting criteria. *Radiology* 2003;228:335–345.
6. Harms SE. MR-guided minimally invasive procedures. In: Schnall MD, Orel SG, eds. *Breast MR Imaging.* Philadelphia: Saunders; 2001:381–392.
7. Mazur P. Kinetics of water loss from cells at subzero temperatures and the likelihood of intracellular freezing. *J Gen Physiol.* 1963;47:347–369.
8. Mazur P. Cryobiology: the freezing of biological systems. *Science* 1970;168:939–949.
9. Sapareto SA, Dewey WC. Thermal dose determination in cancer therapy. *Int J Radiat Oncol Biol Phys.* 1984;10: 787–800.
10. Borrelli MJ, Thompson LL, Cain CA, Dewey WC. Time-temperature analysis of cell killing of BHK cells heated at temperatures in the range of 43.5C to 57.0C. *Int J Radiat Oncol Biol Phys.* 1990;19:389–99.
11. Rui J, Tatsuni KN, Dahiya R, Rubinsky B. Effect of thermal variables on human breast cancer in cryosurgery. *Breast Cancer Res Treat.* 1999;53:185–192.
12. Hall-Craggs MA. Interventional MRI of the breast: minimally invasive therapy. *Eur Radiol.* 2000;10:59–62.
13. Cline HE, Hynynen K, Hardy CJ, et al. MR temperature mapping of focused ultrasound surgery. *Magn Reson Med.* 1994;31:628–636.
14. Bown SG. Phototherapy of tumours. *World J Surg.* 1983;7: 700–709.
15. Mumtaz H, Hall-Craggs MA, Wotherspoon A, et al. Laser therapy for breast cancer: MR imaging and histopathologic correlation. *Radiology* 1996;200:651–658.
16. Dowlatshahi K, Francescatti DS, Bloom KJ. Laser therapy for small breast cancers. *Am J Surg.* 2002;184:359–363.
17. Mirza AN, Fornage BD, Sneige N, et al. Radiofrequency ablation of solid tumors. *Cancer J.* 2001;7:95–102.
18. Jeffrey SS, Birdwell RL, Ikeda DM, et al. Radiofrequency ablation of breast cancer: first report of an emerging technology. *Arch Surg.* 1999;134:1064–1068.
19. Singletary SE, Fornage BD, Sneige N, et al. Radiofrequency ablation of early-stage invasive breast tumors: an overview. *Cancer J.* 2002;8:177–180.
20. Fornage BD, Sneige N, Ross MI, et al. Small (≤2cm) breast cancer treated with US-guided radiofrequency ablation: feasibility study. *Radiology* 2004;231:215–224.
21. Hynynen K, Darkazanli A, Unger E, Schenck JF. MRI-guided noninvasive ultrasound surgery. *Med Phys.* 1993;20:107–115.
22. Hynynen K, Darkazanli A, Damianou CA, et al. The usefulness of a contrast agent and gradient-recalled acquisition in a steady-state imaging sequence for magnetic resonance imaging-guided noninvasive ultrasound surgery. *Invest Radiol.* 1994;29:897–903.
23. McDannold N, Hynynen K, Wolf D, et al. MRI evaluation of thermal ablation of tumors with focused ultrasound. *J Magn Reson Imaging.* 1998;8:91–100.
24. Graham SJ, Chen L, Leitch M, et al. Quantifying tissue damage due to focused ultrasound heating observed by MRI. *Magn Reson Med.* 1999;41:321–328.
25. Hynynen K, Pomeroy O, Smith DN, et al. MR imaging-guided focused ultrasound surgery of fibroadenomas in the breast: a feasibility study. *Radiology* 2001;219:176–185.
26. Gianfelice D, Khiat A, Amara M, et al. MR imaging-guided focused US ablation of breast cancer: histopathologic assessment of effectiveness- initial experience. *Radiology* 2003;227: 849–855.
27. Rand RW, Rand RP, Eggerding F, et al. Cryolumpectomy for carcinoma of the breast. *Surg Gynecol Obstet.* 1987;165: 392–396.
28. Kaufman CS, Bachman B, Littrup PJ, et al. Office-based ultrasound-guided cryoablation of breast fibroadenomas. *Am J Surg.* 2002;184:394–400.
29. Pfleiderer SOR, Freesmayer MG, Marx C, et al. Cryotherapy of breast cancer under ultrasound guidance: initial results and limitations. *Eur Radiol.* 2002;12:3009–3014.
30. Tacke J, Speetzen R, Heschel I, et al. Imaging of interstitial cryotherapy: an in vitro comparison of ultrasound, computed tomography, and magnetic resonance imaging. *Cryobiology* 1999;38:250–259.
31. Daniel BL, Butts K, Block WF. Magnetic resonance imaging of frozen tissues: temperature-dependent MR signal characteristics and relevance for MR monitoring of cryosurgery. *Magn Reson Med.* 1999;41:627–630.

II
Atlas

22
Normal Breast

1. Breast Density

1.1. Fatty

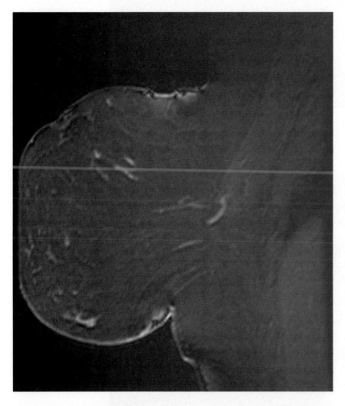

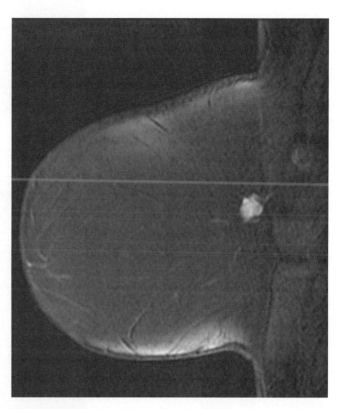

FIGURE 22.1. A 40-year-old woman with strong family history of breast cancer for screening magnetic resonance imaging (MRI) examination. The breast is almost entirely fat. Note normal vessels coursing through the pectoralis major muscle. These all subsequent images were performed after contrast administration using a sagittal fat suppressed T1 weighted image (MSKCC protocol) unless otherwise indicated.

FIGURE 22.2. A 41-year-old woman with almost entirely fatty breast presents with a mass on screening mammography. On ultrasound the mass was echogenic and very vascular. On MRI the mass is round and irregular and demonstrates homogeneous enhancement. At biopsy, an hemangioma was found.

1.2. Scattered Fibroglandular Densities

FIGURE 22.3. A 78-year-old woman with contralateral breast carcinoma. Magnetic resonance imaging demonstrates scattered fibroglandular densities with no suspicious findings. Note penetrating enhancing vessels in chest wall.

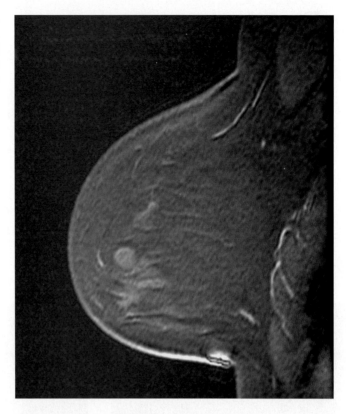

1.3. Heterogeneously Dense

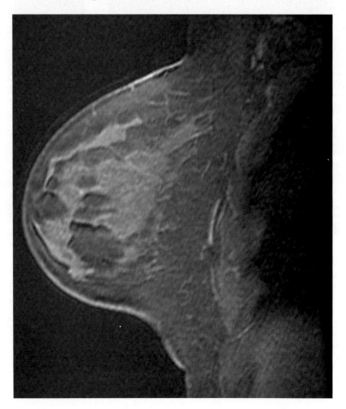

FIGURE 22.4. A 48-year-old status post lumpectomy and two re-excisions in the contralateral breast. Heterogeneously dense parenchyma is noted in this breast without significant enhancement. Note enhancing vessels penetrating the chest wall.

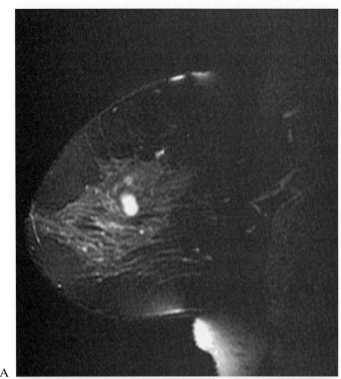

A

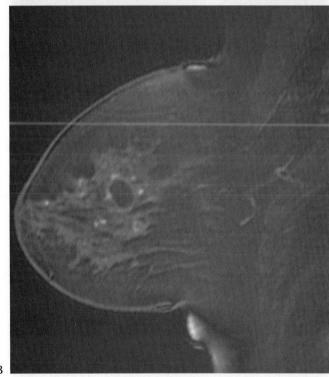

B

FIGURE 22.5. A 52-year-old woman status post lumpectomy in contralateral breast. (A) Heterogeneously dense breast shows a dominant cyst centrally on the T2-weighted image. (B) Postcontrast T1-weighted image demonstrates stippled enhancement, often seen with fibrocystic changes.

1.4. Dense

FIGURE 22.6. A 45-year-old woman with extremely complicated breasts and a prior history of breast cancer: Screening MRI examination. (A) Dense parenchyma with innumerable cysts are noted on the T2-weighted images. (B) Delayed postcontrast images taken 6 minutes after contrast administration demonstrate diffuse uptake in the breast parenchyma. Note that detection is compromised due to diffuse enhancement.

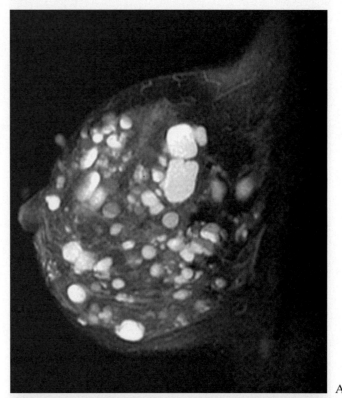

A

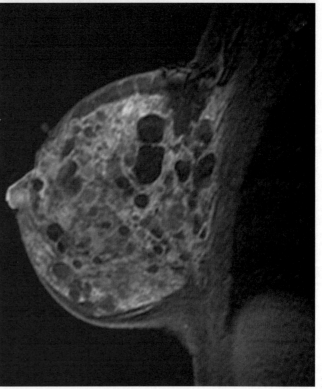

B

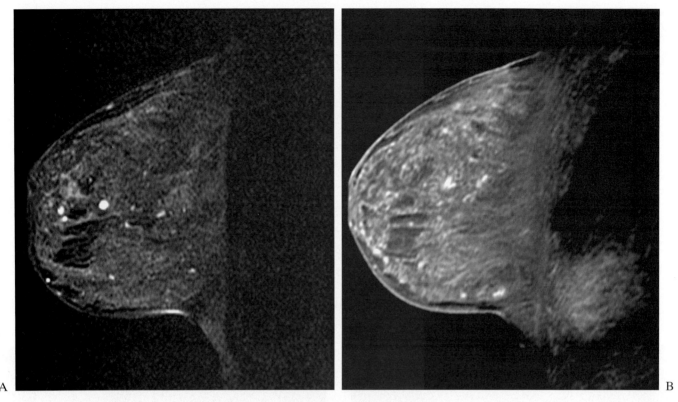

A   B

FIGURE 22.7. A 47-year-old woman with history of left breast biopsy yielding atypical duct hyperplasia. Breast is extremely dense. (A) T2-weighted images; a few high signal cysts are noted. (B) Post-contrast T1-weighted images; there is stippled enhancement.

2. Nipple

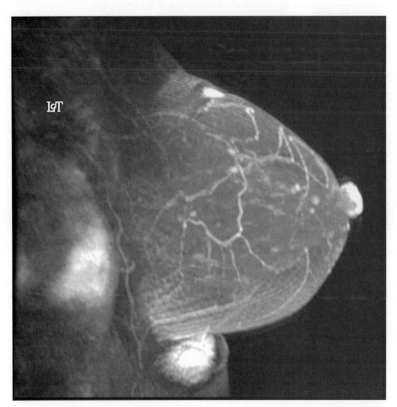

FIGURE 22.8. Maximum intensity projection of normal breast demonstrating minimal nipple enhancement.

23
Malignant Lesions

1. Distribution of Tumor

1.1. Unifocal Carcinoma

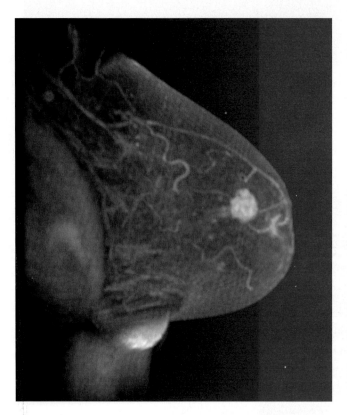

FIGURE 23.1. A 40-year-old woman presented with a palpable mass in the periareolar region. Ultrasound core biopsy yielded invasive ductal carcinoma, moderately differentiated and ductal carcinoma in situ (DCIS) solid type and intermediate nuclear grade. Maximum intensity projection (MIP) magnetic resonance imaging (MRI) examination demonstrated a unifocal mass corresponding to the carcinoma.

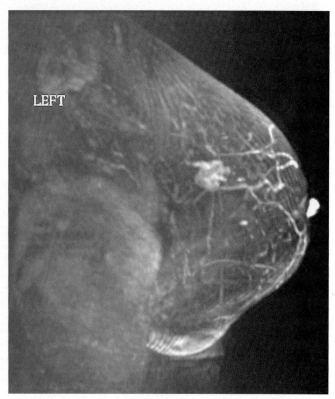

FIGURE 23.2. A 74-year-old woman with a dense mammogram presents with a palpable mass in the upper outer quadrant. Ultrasound core biopsy with subsequent surgical excision yielded invasive ductal carcinoma, not otherwise specified. Maximum intensity projection image demonstrates a unifocal carcinoma amenable to conservation.

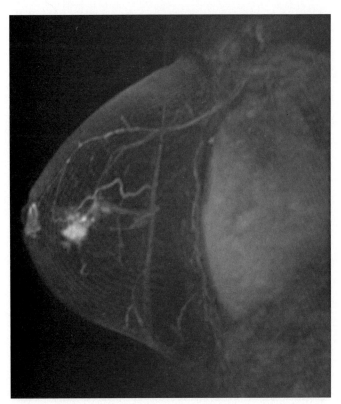

FIGURE 23.3. A 53-year-old woman with a strong family history developed an area of architectural distortion on mammography. Directed ultrasound of this region demonstrated a shadowing hypoechoic mass which was biopsied yielding DCIS, cribiform and papillary types, intermediate-to-high nuclear grade. Maximum intensity projection image demonstrates a unifocal irregular spiculated mass. The patient elected to undergo mastectomy, which demonstrated DCIS and no invasion.

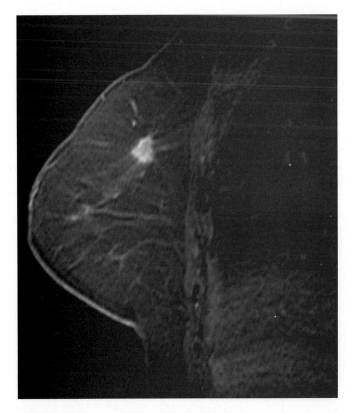

FIGURE 23.4. A 60-year-old woman with a spiculated mass noted on mammography in the upper breast. Fine needle aspiration yielded malignant cells. Magnetic resonance imaging confirmed the impression of unifocal carcinoma.

FIGURE 23.5. A 51-year-old woman status post stereotactic biopsy for calcifications yielded in situ and invasive carcinoma moderately to poorly differentiated with apocrine features. Calcifications were associated with the in situ carcinoma as well as benign breast tissue. Magnetic resonance imaging demonstrates a solitary spiculated mass compatible with the known carcinoma without additional findings.

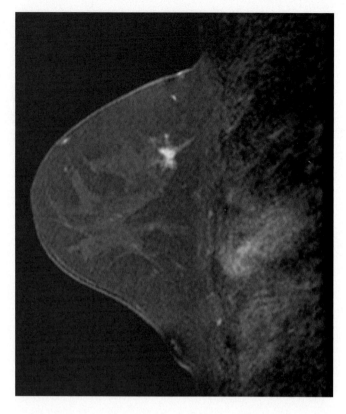

FIGURE 23.6. A 33-year-old woman who presented with a palpable mass. Ultrasound core biopsy demonstrated invasive ductal carcinoma, poorly differentiated with focal lobular growth pattern. She was then treated with neoadjuvant chemotherapy. She presents following this treatment course. Magnetic resonance imaging demonstrates a residual suspicious mass in the medial breast but no additional findings. At lumpectomy, a 1.9-cm invasive ductal carcinoma with extensive intraductal component was identified. Margins were close. The patient refused additional surgery.

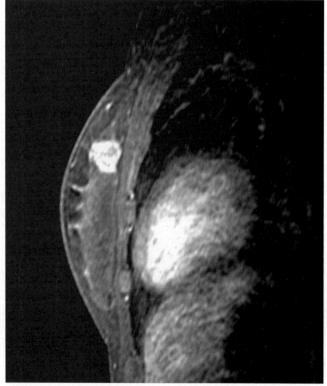

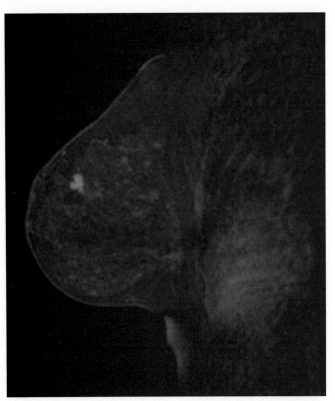

FIGURE 23.7. A 46-year-old woman with new calcifications in the upper breast. Stereotactic biopsy yielded invasive ductal carcinoma and DCIS, cribiform type with intermediate nuclear grade, apocrine cytology, and minimal necrosis arising in a background of atypical ductal hyperplasia. Magnetic resonance imaging demonstrated a unifocal finding.

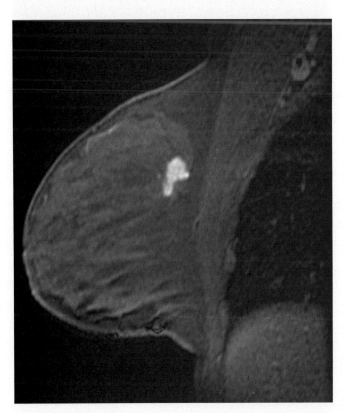

FIGURE 23.8. A 49-year-old woman with a palpable obscured mass on mammography. Pathology at percutaneous ultrasound guided core biopsy yielded invasive ductal carcinoma, histologic and nuclear grade II/III, confirmed at surgery. Magnetic resonance imaging demonstrates an irregular solitary mass.

FIGURE 23.9. A 58-year-old woman presents with palpable axillary lymph node. Aspiration yielded malignant cells compatible with breast primary. Mammogram was negative. (A) MRI demonstrated single dominant irregular mass in the inferior breast suspicious for breast primary. This was identified on directed ultrasound and biopsied yielding invasive ductal carcinoma, not otherwise specified, histologic and nuclear grade II/III. (B) Note contralateral breast screen by MRI detected DCIS, cribiform and micropapillary with intermediate nuclear grade.

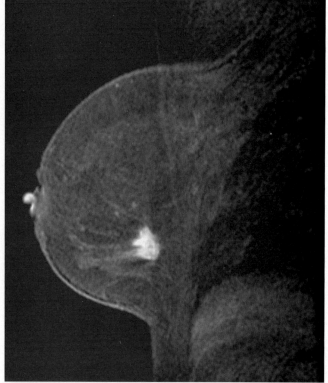

A

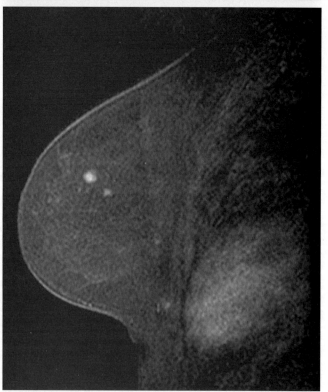

B

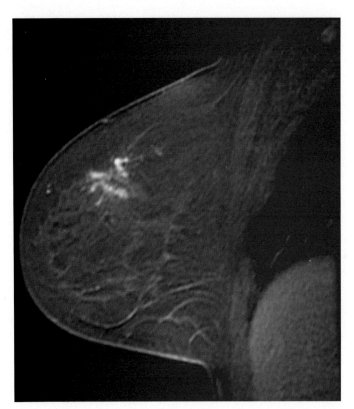

FIGURE 23.10. A 46-year-old woman status post breast conservation 4 years ago presents with a new spiculated mass on mammography. Magnetic resonance imaging demonstrates solitary mass that proved to represent recurrent invasive ductal carcinoma, histologic grade II/III and high nuclear grade III/III.

1.2. Multifocal Carcinoma

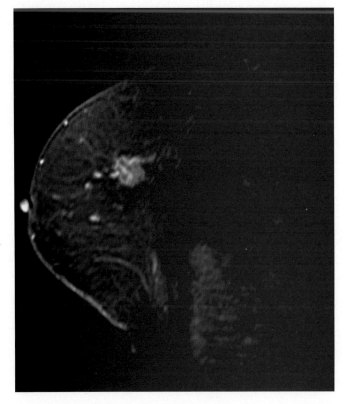

FIGURE 23.11. A 74-year-old woman with a palpable lump in the upper inner quadrant status post aspiration yielding malignancy. No mammographic correlate was present. Magnetic resonance imaging demonstrated a dominant mass with surrounding satellite nodules corresponding to invasive ductal carcinoma not otherwise specified and DCIS solid type of low nuclear grade.

FIGURE 23.12. A 65-year-old woman with palpable mass seen on mammography as a speculated mass. Percutaneous core biopsy yielded invasive lobular carcinoma and in situ carcinoma with ductal and lobular features. Maximum intensity projection demonstrates a dominant mass with satellite lesions. Based on the clinical examination, mastectomy was recommended and at surgery multiple nodules of invasive lobular carcinoma were found ranging in size from 0.3 to 1.8 cm.

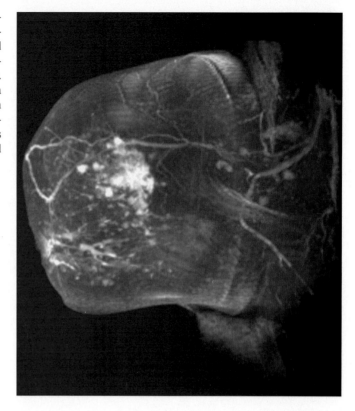

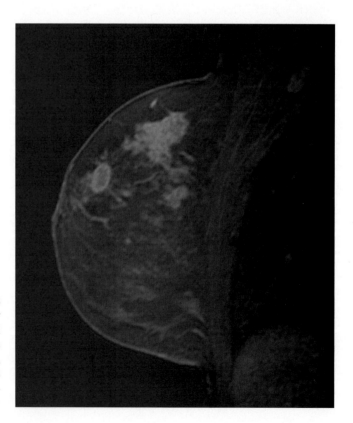

FIGURE 23.13. A 42-year-old woman presents with palpable breast masses in the upper outer quadrant. Core biopsy yielded invasive ductal carcinoma of both masses with an extensive intraductal component (EIC). At mastectomy, additional masses were identified and DCIS with high nuclear grade and moderate necrosis was found extensively.

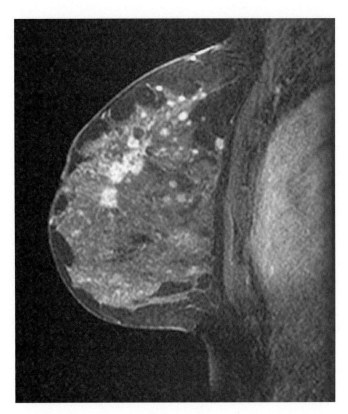

FIGURE 23.14. A 45-year-old woman with nipple retraction for several months had a mammogram that demonstrated a spiculated mass in the 12 o'clock axis. Due to breast density, MRI was performed which showed multiple irregular spiculated masses in the upper outer quadant. Bracketing of these masses was performed under magnetic resonance (MR) guidance to facilitate conservation. Pathology yielded multiple foci of invasive mammary carcinoma with mixed ductal and lobular features and positive margins. A mastectomy was subsequently performed with residual invasive mammary carcinoma found adjacent to the biopsy cavity.

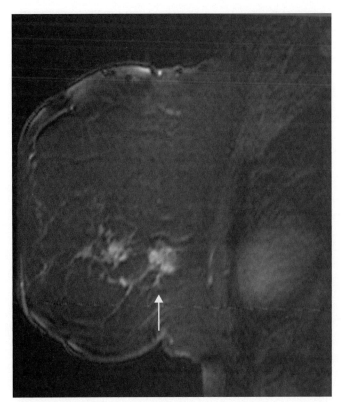

FIGURE 23.15. A 40-year-old woman with a palpable breast mass seen on mammography undergoes core biopsy yielding poorly differentiated invasive carcinoma and DCIS high nuclear grade with extensive necrosis. Magnetic resonance imaging performed for extent of disease assessment. In the posterior breast, the palpable irregular mass is seen (arrow) with anterior clumped enhancement suspicious for an intraductal component. Pathology at mastectomy yielded invasive carcinoma with an associated extensive intraductal component (EIC). The invasive and in situ tumor occupied a quadrant.

FIGURE 23.16. A 57-year-old woman with right bloody nipple discharge. Maximum intensity projection image demonstrates homogeneous segmental enhancement involving a ductal system. Pathology at excisional biopsy following MR localization (mammogram and ultrasound negative) demonstrate mulitfocal invasive carcinoma associated with EIC. Due to the disease extent the patient underwent mastectomy yielding abundant residual disease. Nodes were negative.

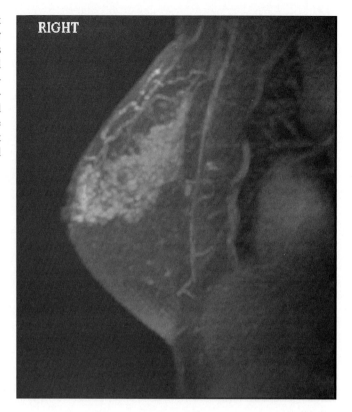

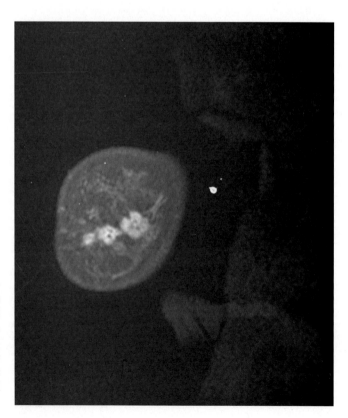

FIGURE 23.17. A 47-year-old woman presented with two palpable breast masses in the upper outer quadrant. Ultrasound identified three masses and all were biopsed. The two in the upper outer quadrant were poorly differentiated invasive ductal carcinoma and the third mass in the low axilla was a metastatic lymph node. A mastectomy was performed which confirmed multifocal disease.

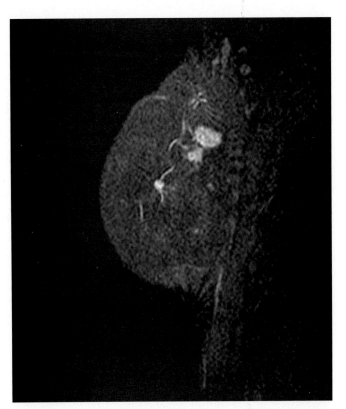

FIGURE 23.18. A 43-year-old woman who felt a right breast mass. Mammogram was negative but ultrasound identified three solid masses in the upper outer quadrant. All three were biopsied yielding moderately differentiated invasive ductal carcinoma, confirmed at surgery.

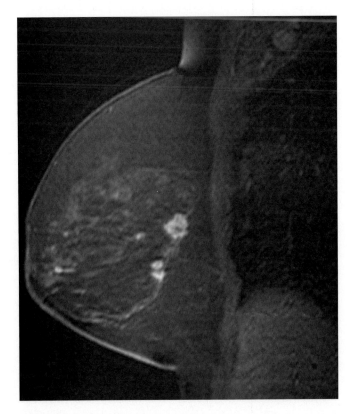

FIGURE 23.19. A 61-year-old woman with a new spiculated mass noted on mammography. Ultrasound was performed which showed two masses in the 8 and 9 o'clock positions. Both were biopsied yielding invasive mammary carcinoma, with predominantly lobular features. Magnetic resonance imaging demonstrates the two masses and no additional findings. The patient received breast conservation.

1.3. Multicentric Carcinoma

FIGURE 23.20. A 35-year-old woman status post excision of calcifications in the upper outer quadrant yielding invasive ductal carcinoma with close margins. Magnetic resonance imaging performed to assess disease extent. The postoperative seroma cavity is noted on the superior breast (arrow). In the interior breast clumped enhancement is identified representing DCIS and compatible with multicentric disease.

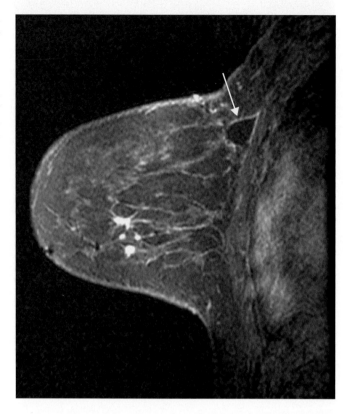

FIGURE 23.21. A 31-year-old woman with palpable left breast mass. Mammogram demonstrated multiple masses with associated pleomorphic calcifications in the upper outer quadrant. An ultrasound-guided core biopsy revealed invasive ductal carcinoma with apocrine features, histologic and nuclear grade III/III. The in situ component had associated calcifications. Magnetic resonance imaging examination demonstrated multiple masses that corresponded to the extent of calcifications noted on mammography. Mastectomy was performed.

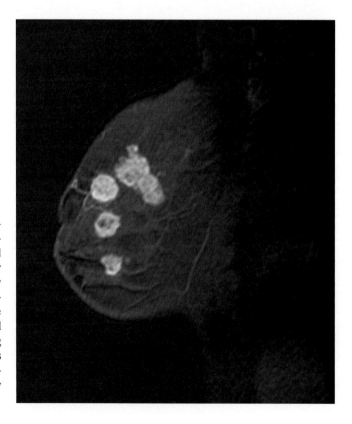

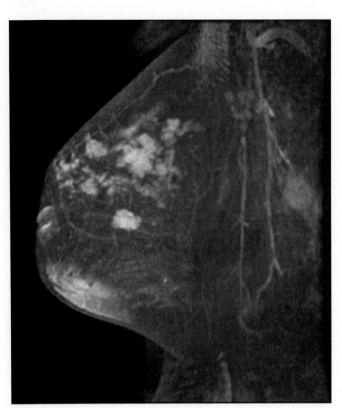

FIGURE 23.22. Maximum intensity projection image of multicentric disease. Invasive lobular carcinoma.

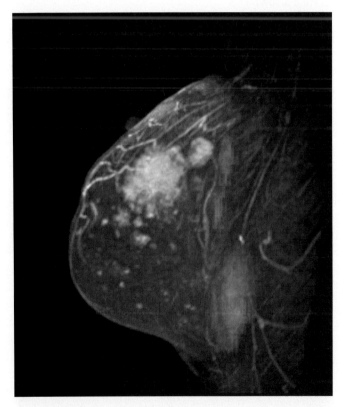

FIGURE 23.23. A 39-year-old woman with palpable masses in the upper outer quadrant. Ultrasound confirmed multiple contiguous masses. Two of these were biopsied in the 12 o'clock and 9 o'clock axes yielding poorly differentiated invasive ductal carcinoma and DCIS, intermediate grade with central necrosis. Maximum intensity projection confirms multicentric disease. A computed tomograph (CT) scan demonstrated multiple liver lesions that were biopsied yielding metastatic adenocarcinoma consistent with breast origin. She was started on systemic therapy.

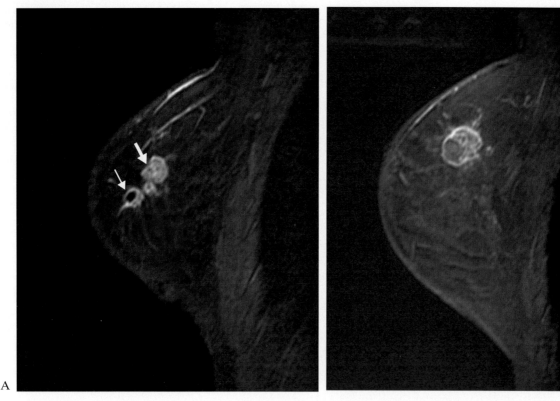

FIGURE 23.24. A 35-year-old woman status post bilateral reduction surgery had incidental invasive carcinoma noted on pathology. Magnetic resonance imaging performed to assess disease extent. In addition to the surgical changes from recent reduction surgery, a total of four masses (two shown) were found in the breast. (A) The lateral breast. Changes of reduction (thin arrow) can be seen next to the irregular carcinoma (thick arrow). (B) The central breast. Ultrasound confirmed the presence of solid lesions which were biopsied yielding invasive ductal carcinoma, histologic and nuclear grade III/III in multiple quadrants. The patient subsequently underwent mastectomy.

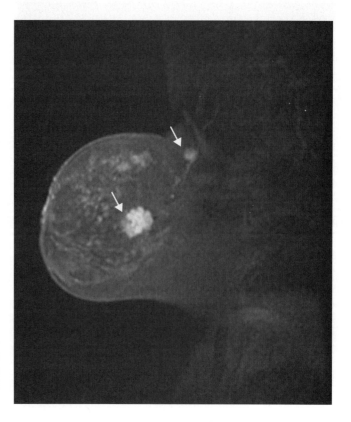

FIGURE 23.25. A 46-year-old woman with multicentric carcinoma, poorly differentiated. Two masses noted on MRI in the lateral breast were proven to represent poorly differentiated invasive ductal carcinoma (arrows).

1.4. Extensive Intraductal Carcinoma

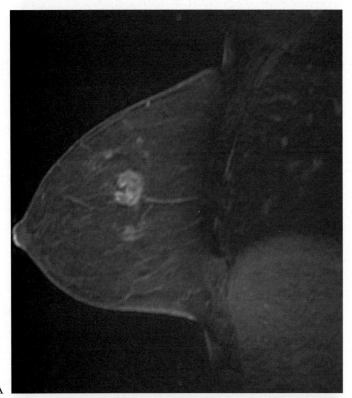

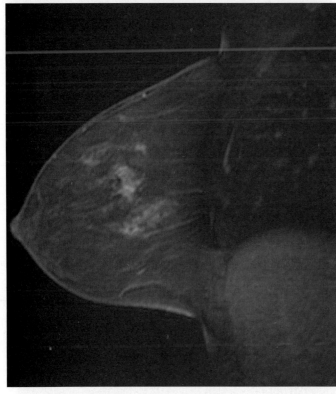

FIGURE 23.26. A 46-year-old woman underwent screening mammography that demonstrated a new 2-cm indistinct mass with associated pleomorphic calcifications. Ultrasound confirmed the presence of a solitary suspicious mass. Ultrasound core biopsy yielded DCIS, solid and comedo types, high nuclear grade, with lobular extension and foci of microinvasion. Magentic resonance imaging was performed for disease assessment. (A) A 1.6-cm rim enhancing mass was noted (B) with surrounding clumped enhancement. At pathology this represented invasive ductal carcinoma histologic and nuclear grade III/III in a background of DCIS, solid type with high nuclear grade and moderate necrosis. Ductal carcinoma in situ represented >25% of the tumor compatible with extensive intraductal component (EIC). Nodes were negative.

FIGURE 23.27. A 42-year-old woman with a spiculated mass noted on mammography. Ultrasound vacuum biopsy demonstrated invasive ductal carcinoma, poorly differentiated with focal lobular growth. Ductal carcinoma in situ, solid type of intermediate nuclear grade with minimal necrosis was also identified. Magnetic resonance imaging demonstrated a suspicious mass compatible with the known invasive component as well as extensive surrounding ductal clumped enhancement that was proved to represent EIC at surgery. The patient had five positive nodes at axillary dissection.

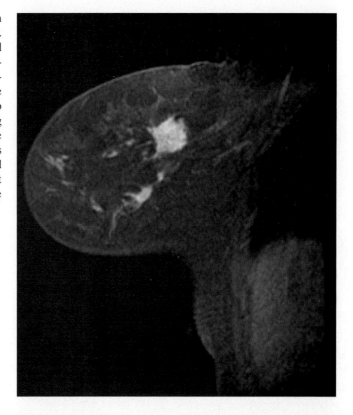

FIGURE 23.28. A 59-year-old woman status post excisional biopsy of two masses in the left breast yielding infiltrating ductal carcinoma and positive margins. Magnetic resonance imaging performed to assess extent of residual disease. Magnetic resonance imaging demonstrates a large postoperative seroma cavity and enhancement along the anterior margin compatible with residual disease. Note also the nodular enhancement of the skin suspicious for an early inflammatory component. Mastectomy demonstrated residual foci of infiltrating ductal carcinoma ranging in size up to 1.5 cm. Ductal carcinoma in situ was present constituting >25% of the tumor mass compatible with an extensive intraductal component. Tumor nodules were also noted involving the skin.

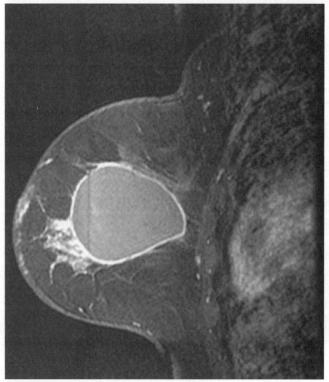

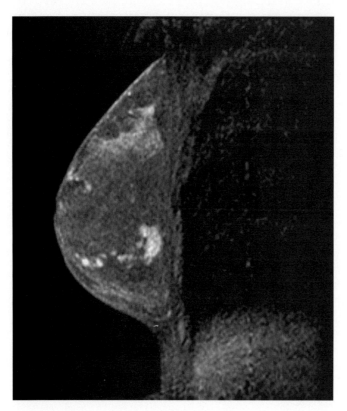

FIGURE 23.29. A 32-year-old with palpable breast nodularity. Mammogram demonstrates 5 cm of pleomorphic calcifications. Aspiration of the palpable area yielded malignant cells. Magnetic resonance imaging demonstrates an irregular mass in the posterior breast with associated irregular linear enhancement extending from the mass to the nipple. Several other masses were identified in the lower outer quadrant. Pathology at mastectomy yielded invasive ductal carcinoma not otherwise specified (NOS) histologic and nuclear grades III/III measuring 2 cm in greatest extent. Extensive intraductal component was present admixed with and away from the invasive component. In situ carcinoma was solid, cribiform typed with intermediate nuclear grade and extensive necrosis.

1.5. Locally Advanced Breast Carcinoma

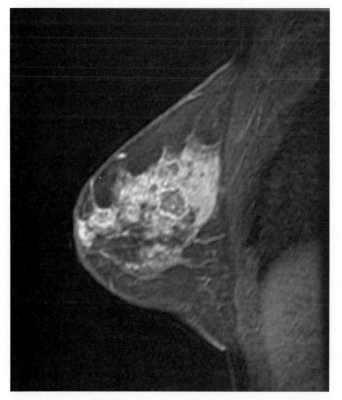

FIGURE 23.30. A 43-year-old woman with palpable abnormality. Outside fine needle aspiration positive for malignant cells. Mammogram demonstrates extensive calcifications in the upper outer quadrant and ultrasound demonstrates a suspicious lobulated mass. Ultrasound-guided biopsy demonstrated invasive moderately differentiated ductal carcinoma and intraductal carcinoma, solid type with minimal necrosis. Magnetic resonance imaging demonstrates extensive areas of abnormal enhancement suspicious for locally advanced breast carcinoma. The patient elected to have bilateral mastectomy. Extensive involvement by carcinoma was confirmed at surgery.

FIGURE 23.31. A 42-year-old woman presented with a negative mammogram and palpable retroareolar mass which was biopsied yielding invasive lobular carcinoma. The palpated mass was 3 cm and mastectomy was recommended. The patient seeks a second opinion. Magnetic resonance imaging confirms the presence of a large mass relative to breast size. Pathology at mastectomy demonstrated multiple foci of invasive lobular carcinoma involving the central breast and extending into all four quadrants.

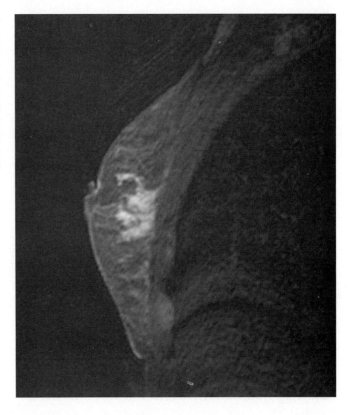

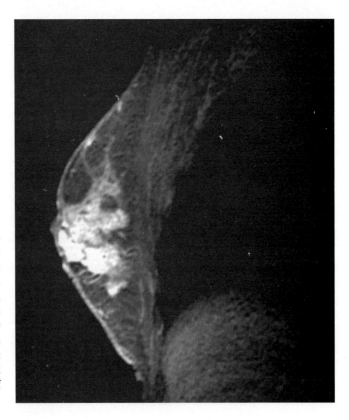

FIGURE 23.32. A 40-year-old with palpable breast mass. Mammography showed extensive pleomorphic calcifications compatible with locally advanced breast carcinoma. She underwent biopsy yielding poorly differentiated in situ and invasive mammary duct carcinoma and received preoperative chemotherapy with moderate response. Magnetic resonance imaging is performed following neoadjuvant therapy prior to mastectomy. A large central mass is identified occupying the majority of the breast, confirmed at surgery.

1.5.1. Complete Response to Chemotherapy

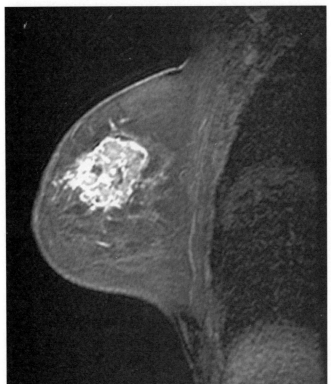

FIGURE 23.33. A 39-year-old woman who presents with (A) large palpable breast mass, core biopsy proven poorly differentiated invasive mammary carcinoma, ductal type. She also had palpable axillary nodes at presentation. She underwent preoperative chemotherapy with complete clinical response—no palpable breast mass or axillary nodes. (B) On MRI, minimal residual enhancement is identified. At mastectomy, no tumor was identified. Prominent fibroinflammatory changes and prominent foamy histiocytes were noted compatible with treatment effect. Nodes were negative.

A

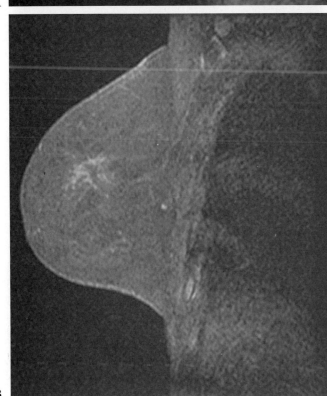

B

1.5.2. Partial Response to Chemotherapy

FIGURE 23.34. A 48-year-old woman with (A) palpable breast mass yielding invasive ductal carcinoma high grade with focal mucinous features and DCIS on ultrasound core biopsy. She refused mastectomy and elected to undergo preoperative chemotherapy. (B) The central irregular mass responded to the therapy though residual enhancement persists. Enlarged axillary lymph nodes are also less prominent. The patient ultimately refused breast surgery due to psychosocial reasons.

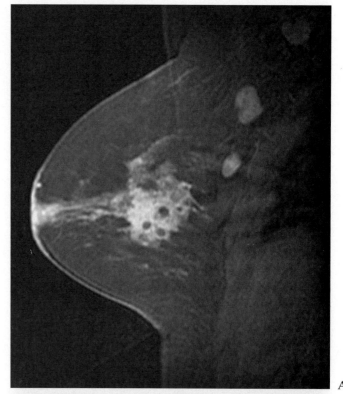

A

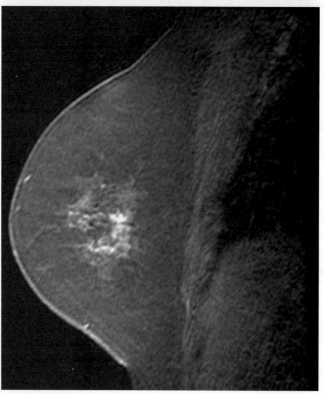

B

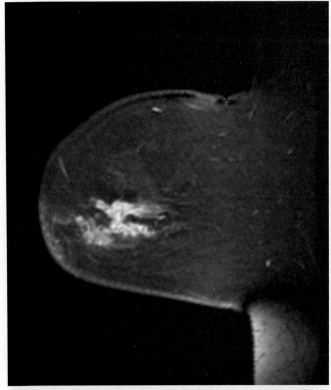

A

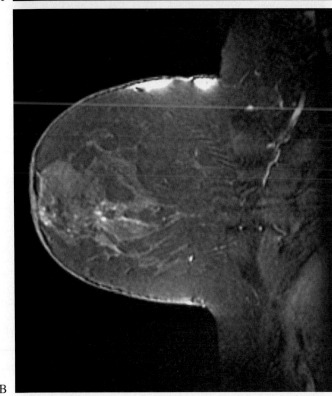

B

FIGURE 23.35. A 57-year-old with (A) clinical inflammatory breast carcinoma. Ultrasound core biopsy of a palpable mass yielded invasive ductal carcinoma, histologic and nuclear grade III/III with focal lobular pattern. She underwent preoperative chemotherapy with response clinically and by MRI. At mastectomy, invasive carcinoma is identified in the form of multiple tumor emboli in lymphatic vessels. Scattered microscopic foci of DCIS, cribiform and micropapillary types with high nuclear grade are present. (B) Post chemotherapy MRI demonstrates several tiny foci of enhacement in the region of the treated cancer.

1.5.3. No Response to Chemotherapy

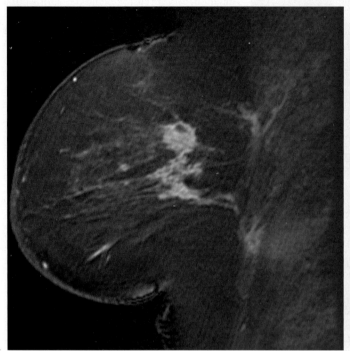
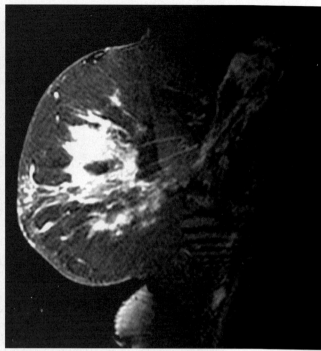

A
B

FIGURE 23.36. A 53-year-old woman presents with a large palpable mass in the upper outer quadrant that appears fixed to the chest wall. Pathology was invasive mammary carcinoma with vascular invasion. (A) MRI demonstrates a large infiltrating mass that extends into the pectoralis major muscle and chest wall. Due to chest wall involvement, neoadjuvent therapy was given with poor response. (B) Follow-up MRI scan shows enlargement and progression of the mass on adriamycin and cytoxan. The breast is retracted and involvement of the underlying muscles is still noted. The patient was switched to an alternative treatment with no effect and still progressed. A CT at this time demonstrated new liver and bone metastases.

2. Staging

2.1. Pectoralis Muscle Invasion

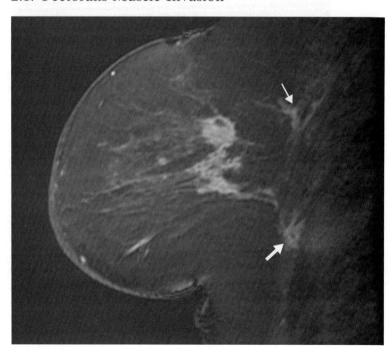

FIGURE 23.37. A 53-year-old with locally advanced breast carcinoma invading pectoralis major muscle (thin arrow) as well as chest wall (intercostal muscle) (thick arrow). Note that pectoralis muscle involvement does not change staging, however, chest wall involvement is stage IIIB.

2.2. Chest Wall Invasion

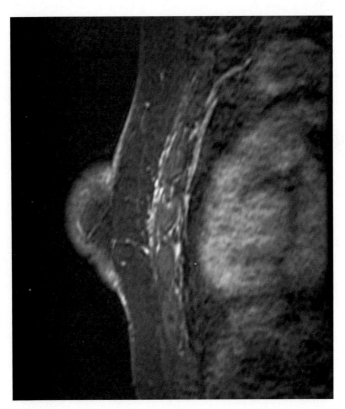

FIGURE 23.38. A 53-year-old woman with history of stage IIIB poorly differentiated invasive ductal carcinoma with perineural invasion. She underwent chemotherapy and radiation therapy following limited resection. She did well for 5 years until she presented with a skin nodule which was biopsied and demonstrated to represent recurrent mammary ductal carcinoma (stage IV disease). Bulky chest wall disease was also noted at this time. Magnetic resonance imaging was performed of the contralateral breast. Medially in the contralateral breast abnormal enhancement is identified along the chest wall musculature with extension into the intercostals muscles compatible with spread across the midline of known chest wall disease.

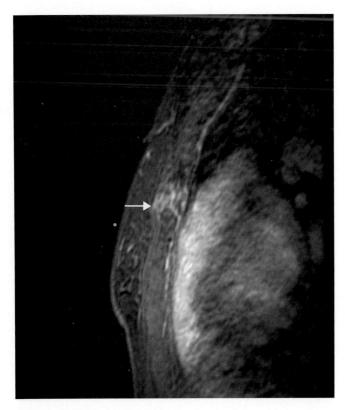

FIGURE 23.39. A 35-year-old woman presented with palpable mass noted to be invasive ductal carcinoma, high histologic grade, intermediate nuclear grade with associated DCIS, solid with intermediate nuclear grade. Excision was performed with negative margins. The patient presents 4 years later with a palpable mass medially in the treated breast. Pathology yielded invasive ductal carcinoma, moderately to poorly differentiated, focally invading skeletal muscle. Magnetic resonance imaging demonstrates a mass (arrow) that focally invades the chest wall involving intercostal muscles.

2.3. Nipple Invasion

FIGURE 23.40. A 60-year-old woman status post right lumpectomy 6 years ago presents with new nipple retraction. Magnetic resonance imaging demonstrates enhancing mass in right retroareolar region suspicious for recurrence. The recurrent tumor is causing nipple retraction.

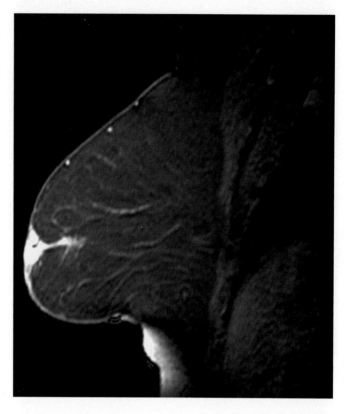

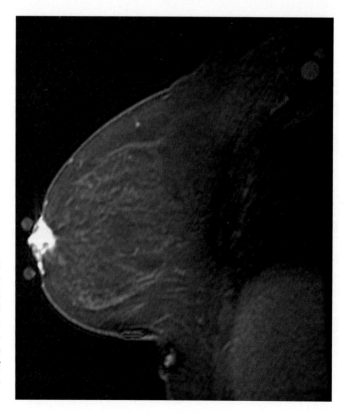

FIGURE 23.41. A 56-year-old woman had a left mastectomy 10 years ago presents with a palpable mass under the right nipple. Excisional biopsy yielded invasive carcinoma consistent with breast primary without in situ carcinoma. Subsequent mastectomy demonstrated invasive ductal carcinoma histologic and nuclear grade III/III with DCIS, cribiform type of intermediate nuclear grade and moderate necrosis.

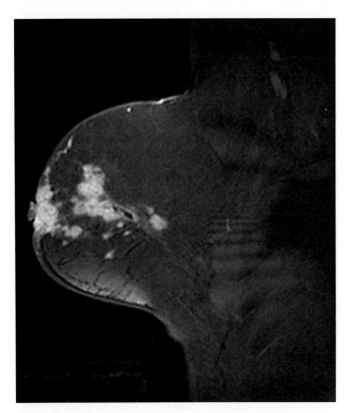

FIGURE 23.42. A 58-year-old woman with locally advanced breast carcinoma had MRI prior to chemotherapy. Note that the retroareolar mass invades the nipple and surrounding skin. Extensive involvement of the breast is also noted. On physical examination, she had thickened skin anteriorly with peau d'orange.

2.4. Nipple Discharge

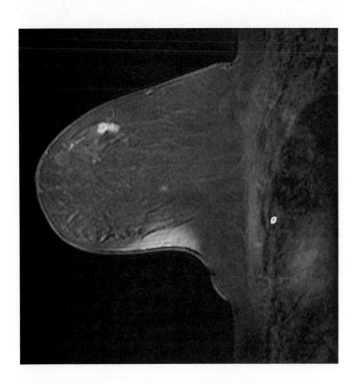

FIGURE 23.43. A 60-year-old woman post right lumpectomy 5 years ago for invasive ductal carcinoma with new left nipple discharge. Mammography was fatty with no suspicious findings. Magnetic resonance imaging showed an enhancing irregular mass with washout in the upper left breast. Patient underwent left breast major duct excision with preoperative ductogram and left segmental resection with preoperative MRI localization. Duct excision revealed intraductal papilloma and MRI localization revealed 5-mm invasive carcinoma. Sentinel lymph node biopsy was negative.

FIGURE 23.44. A 60-year-old woman with history of right lumpectomy 16 years ago presents with new left nipple bloody discharge. The mammogram was moderately dense with no suspicious findings. A ductogram demonstrated no suspicious filling defects however there were areas of narrowing and dilation that were mildly suspicious. MRI was performed that demonstrated a 1.3 cm mass in the upper outer quadrant that proved to represent invasive ductal carcinoma not otherwise specified with negative sentinel nodes. Duct excision in the region of the abnormal ductogram following preoperative ductogram demonstrated a sclerosed intraductal papilloma with focal atypia. The nipple discharge likely was on the basis of the papilloma and the invasive carcinoma was likely an incidental finding.

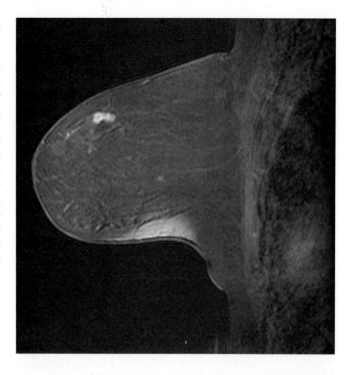

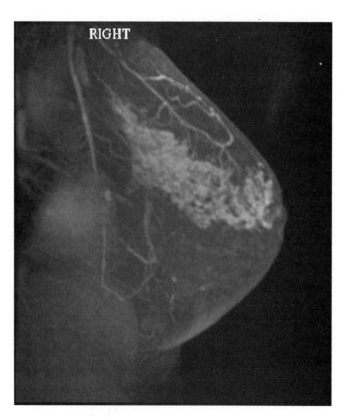

FIGURE 23.45. A 57-year-old with right bloody nipple discharge. No personal or family history of breast carcinoma. Mammography was heterogeneously dense with no abnormality. Maximum intensity projection image demonstrated a regional segmental area of heterogeneous enhancement yielding extensive DCIS with multifocal microinvasion. Right mastectomy performed with negative sentinel nodes.

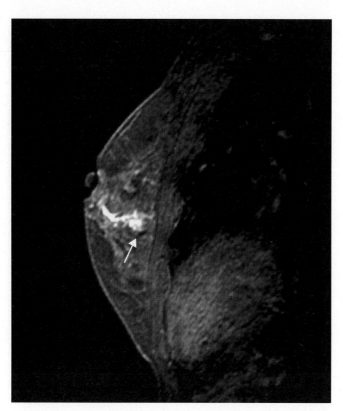

FIGURE 23.46. A 55-year-old with family history of breast cancer presents with spontaneous bloody left nipple discharge. Magnetic resonance imaging showed an irregular enhancing left breast mass that was seen on ultrasound (arrow). Localization and excision yielded papilloma with atypia. Note high signal in duct.

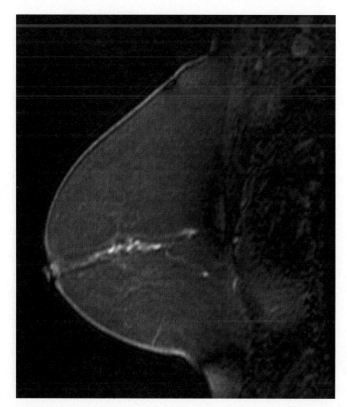

FIGURE 23.47. A 74-year-old woman with 3 months spontaneous serosanginous nipple discharge. Magnetic resonance imaging demonstrates a dilated central duct with proteinaceous debris that demonstrates enhancement. Directed ultrasound was negative as was mammography. Blind duct excision demonstrated low-to-intermediate nuclear grade DCIS.

FIGURE 23.48. A 57-year-old presents with bloody nipple discharge. Mammogram negative. Magnetic resonance imaging shows extensive ductal enhancement involving a segment. Pathology following MR localization bracketing demonstrated invasive ductal carcinoma NOS type and multifocal microinvasive carcinoma from 1 to 2 mm. Ductal carcinoma in situ also identified, papillary, cribiform, micropapillary with high nuclear grade and moderate necrosis. The DCIS was >25% of the tumor compatible with extensive intraductal component. Mastectomy was performed and sentinel node analysis was negative.

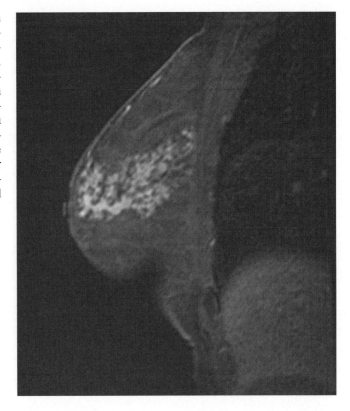

2.5. Skin Invasion, Inflammatory Carcinoma

2.5.1. Focal

FIGURE 23.49. A 65-year-old woman who noted a red mass in the medial breast 6 months ago. She thought that it was skin cancer and sought opinion from a dermatologist. A few months later she went for mammography that showed an irregular solid mass that infiltrated pectoralis muscle on ultrasound (not shown). Biopsy yielded invasive ductal carcinoma, moderately differentiated. She underwent preoperative chemotherapy. Breast MRI was performed which demonstrated a mass focally invading skin and no chest wall involvement. Following this, mastectomy was performed with 2-cm invasive ductal carcinoma NOS. The skin dermis was involved by direct extension. Skeletal muscle was negative for tumor.

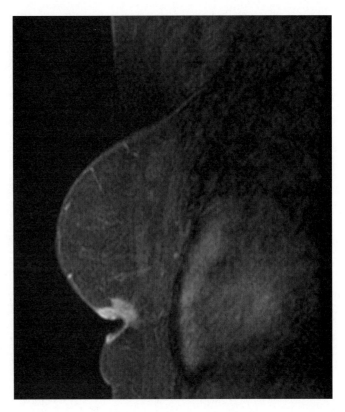

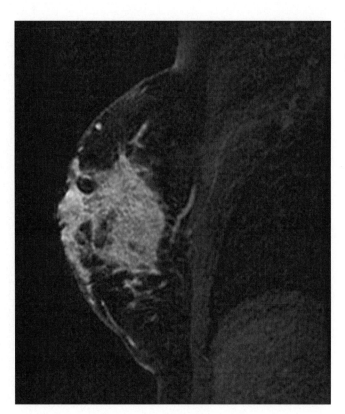

FIGURE 23.50. A 40-year-old with locally advanced breast cancer focally invading the skin surrounding the nipple. Pathology invasive ductal carcinoma.

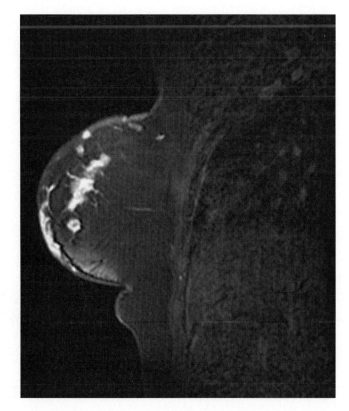

FIGURE 23.51. A 58-year-old woman with locally advanced breast cancer focally invading skin on MRI. Pathology yielded invasive ductal carcinoma 1.5 cm involving dermis with lymphatic permeation, histologic grade III, nuclear grade II. Ductal carcinoma in situ, solid type with moderate necrosis and moderate nuclear grade associated with the invasive tumor.

FIGURE 23.52. A 50-year-old woman palpated a mass that was poorly seen on both mammography and ultrasound. She underwent surgical excision that demonstrated poorly differentiated carcinoma with neuroendocrine features and marked necrosis. In situ carcinoma was not identified. Four centimeters of tumor was resected with wide positive margins. Physical examination after resection showed a 10-cm palpable mass. It was unclear how much represented residual disease or hematoma. Magnetic resonance imaging performed to evaluate residual disease. Extensive regional enhancement is present in the upper breast with focal skin invasion evidenced by thickening and abnormal enhancement. No hematoma was noted. Chemotherapy was ineffective for this patient and she died within the year due to metastatic neuroendocrine tumor arising from the left breast.

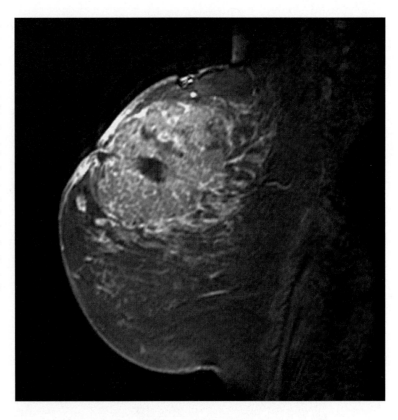

FIGURE 23.53. A 35-year-old woman presents with palpable mass. Breast biopsy yielded invasive mammary carcinoma poorly differentiated and focal DCIS with apocrine cytology. Skin punch biopsy was unremarkable, likely due to random sampling. Mastectomy yielded invasive ductal carcinoma, NOS type, histologic grade III/III, nuclear grade II/III measuring 15 cm in diameter. Associated DCIS, solid and cribiform types with high nuclear grade and minimal necrosis. The skin was involved by direct extension and tumor emboli were present in the deep dermal lymphatics. Tumor was present in all quadrants.

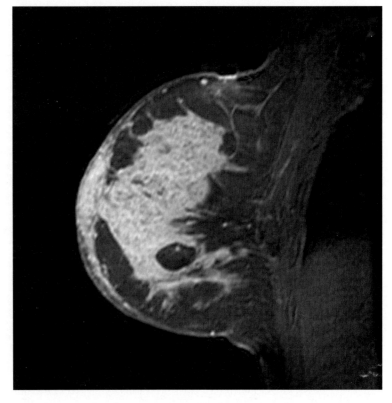

2.5.2. *Diffuse*

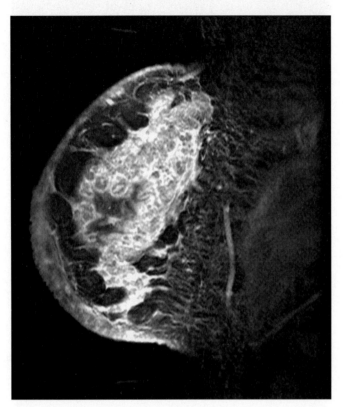

FIGURE 23.54. A 40-year-old woman who presented with a lump in her breast. Mammogram was negative. She sought surgical consultation and was found to have a red erythematous breast with palpable axillary adenopathy compatible with locally advanced breast carcinoma. Random core biopsy of the upper outer quadrant yielded in situ and invasive ductal carcinoma, moderately differentiated with focal lobular features. Focal lymphovascular invasion is identified. Magnetic resonance imaging demonstrates diffuse enhancement of the entire breast with associated diffuse skin thickening with associated enhancement. Findings are compatible with inflammatory carcinoma.

2.6. Paget's Disease

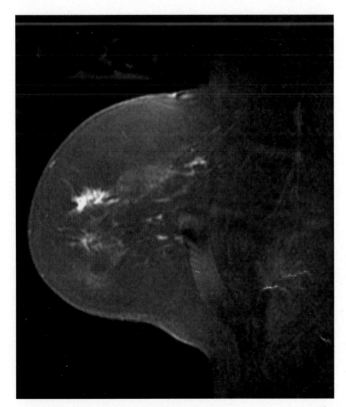

FIGURE 23.55. A 62-year-old woman presents with crustiness of the left nipple and biopsy proven Paget's disease. Tiny cluster of calcifications are noted in upper outer quadrant on mammography. Magnetic resonance imaging performed for extent of possible disease. In the upper outer quadrant a speculated mass is identified that measured 2.4 cm with associated multiple linear areas of enhancement suspected for extensive DCIS. Patient underwent left mastectomy yielding invasive ductal carcinoma and DCIS.

FIGURE 23.56. A 45-year-old woman with itching scaling and erythema of the left nipple. Biopsy showed extensive Paget's disease of the nipple. Mammography demonstrated a mildly dense parenchymal pattern with no suspicious findings. Magnetic resonance imaging showed extensive clumped linear enhancement extending over 9 cm in the breast that proved to represent intermediate-to-high nuclear grade DCIS without invasion. No calcifications were identified in the DCIS. Patient underwent mastectomy. Sentinel biopsy was negative.

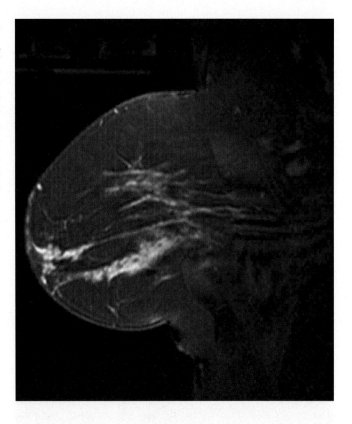

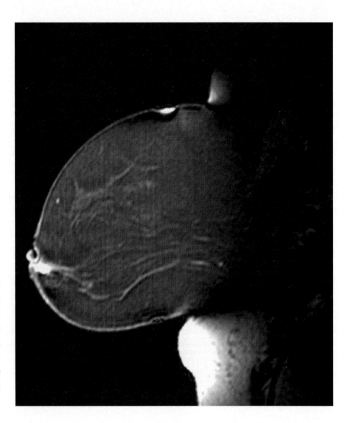

FIGURE 23.57. A 60-year-old woman status post left nipple bloody discharge. Punch biopsy of skin near nipple yielded invasive ductal carcinoma and DCIS—the nipple showed intraepidermal adenocarcinoma cells compatible with Paget's diease. Magnetic resonance imaging showed a 3-cm retroareolar left duct with enhancement that corresponded to residual DCIS.

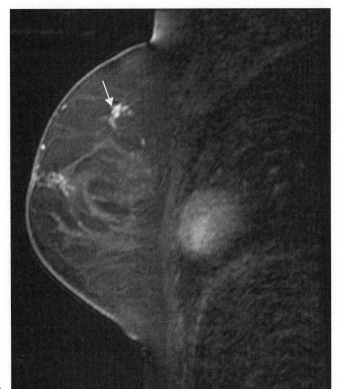

A

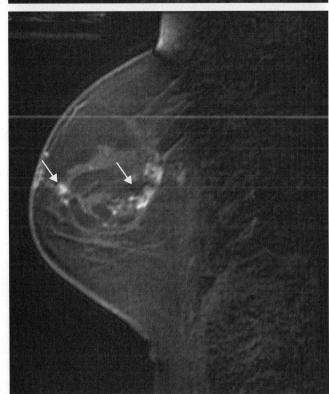

B

FIGURE 23.58. A 54-year-old patient who presented with left breast Paget's disease. Blind duct excision was performed yielding DCIS with positive margins. Sentinel lymph node was positive. Magnetic resonance imaging was performed to identify site of invasion and exclude residual disease. Mammography was initially negative and remained so. (A and B) MRI demonstrates multiple suspicious areas of enhancement throughout the breast (arrows). Directed ultrasound was attempted and core was performed of two areas with benign results, discordant with the MRI findings. Magnetic resonance imaging guided needle localization was performed in two separate quadrants yielding high-grade DCIS. A mastectomy was then performed. No area of invasion was identified at mastectomy. One positive lymph node was identified at completion axillary dissection.

2.7. Axillary Metastasis

FIGURE 23.59. A 53-year-old woman noted a mass in her breast 1 year ago. An aspiration reportedly was benign. Over the last 6 months she has noted the mass has grown larger and her nipple is inverted and has become red. Mammogram showed skin thickening and extensive pleomorphic calcifications. Core biopsy yielded poorly differentiated invasive ductal carcinoma. (A) MRI demonstrates a large central mass with skin thickening and enhancement compatible with inflammatory carcinoma. Irregular spiculated lymph nodes are noted compatible with metastatic disease with extranodal extension. (B) Follow-up MRI scan following chemotherapy demonstrates decrease in size of the mass as well as reduction in the axillary lymph nodes.

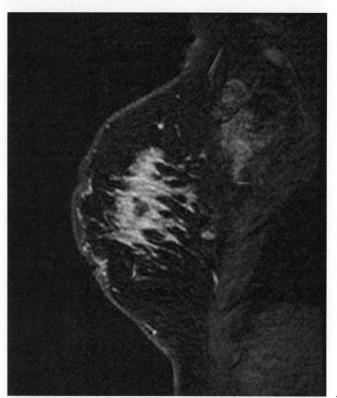

A

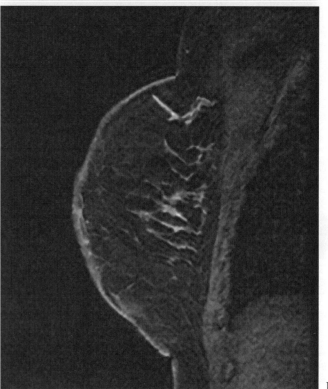

B

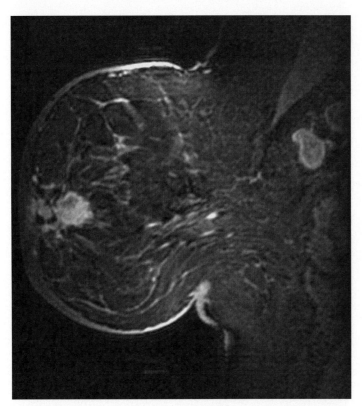

FIGURE 23.60. A 69-year-old woman noted new nipple retraction with a palpable mass. Mammography demonstrated a retroareolar mass (not shown). Magnetic resonance imaging (performed after several rounds of chemotherapy) confirms the presence of this finding as well as skin thickening and an irregular rim enhancing axillary lymph node that is suspicious for metastasis. Punch biopsy of the skin demonstrated poorly differentiated adenocarcinma involving dermal lymphatics consistent with breast primary. Mastectomy was performed, confirming the presence of a 2.5-cm carcinoma with skin involvement. Multiple metastatic nodes were present.

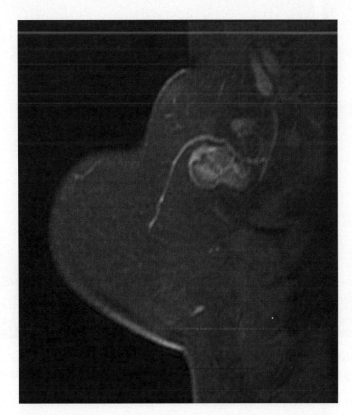

FIGURE 23.61. A 43-year-old woman status post lumpectomy for a 4-cm invasive ductal carcinoma of the left breast now has palpable right axillary adenopathy. Aspiration was positive for malignancy. Magnetic resonance imaging failed to identify any abnormality in the right breast that would be suspicious for occult malignancy. Irregular abnormal axillary lymph node is identified. Patient treated for stage IV disease.

FIGURE 23.62. A 60-year-old woman who underwent CT examination for cough and noted to have right breast mass. No recent mammogram. On mammography in the axillary tail a mass was identified which was thought to be a lymph node. Magnetic resonance imaging was performed to further evaluate. In the low axillary region, several masses are identified. The more posterior masses appear irregular round and exhibit rim enhancement and do not demonstrate fatty hilia. Because of their location (behind the pectoralis major muscle, thus, level I nodes) they are most likely metastatic nodes. The more anterior mass is irregular, demonstrates rim enhancement, and could represent an involved node or breast primary in the extreme axillary tail. Biopsy of this mass yielded poorly differentiated invasive ductal carcinoma with associated DCIS, solid type with high nuclear grade. Three of 19 nodes were positive for metastatic disease.

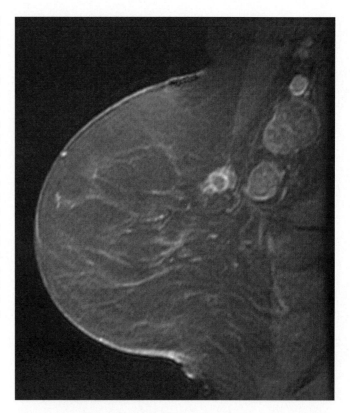

2.8. Axillary Metastasis with Unknown Primary

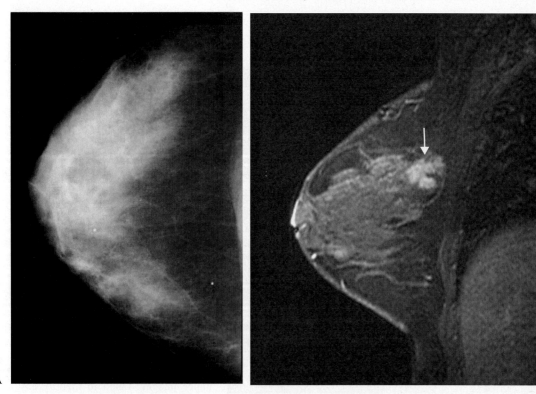

A

B

FIGURE 23.63. A 28-year-old woman presents with palpable right axillary lymph node. History of excision of a palpable right breast mass 1 year earlier yielding fibroadenoma. (A) Mammogram demonstrated extremely dense breasts with no suspicious findings. (B) MRI demonstrated a heterogeneously enhancing irregular mass (arrow) in the upper outer quadrant measuring 1.1 cm. Directed ultrasound confirmed the presence of the mass and ultrasound core biopsy was performed yielding infiltrating ductal carcinoma high grade. Patient was then treated in a single stage procedure with negative margins and negative axillary node dissection.

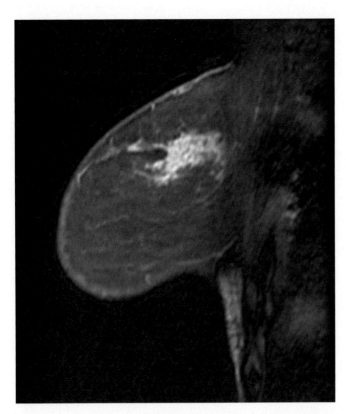

FIGURE 23.64. A 47-year-old with history of right breast DCIS and ovarian cancer presents with palpable left axillary adenopathy, biopsy positive for metastatic poorly differentiated adenocarcinoma with extracapsular extension. Mammogram is mildy dense with no suspicious findings. Magnetic resonance imaging demonstrates a large enhancing heterogeneous mass in the upper outer quadrant (shown) with smaller surrounding masses (not shown). All were visible on ultrasound and biopsied yielding high grade invasive ductal carcinoma in two areas compatible with multicentric disease. The patient underwent left mastectomy with multiple foci of invasive ductal carcinoma found throughout the breast and 15 positive lymph nodes.

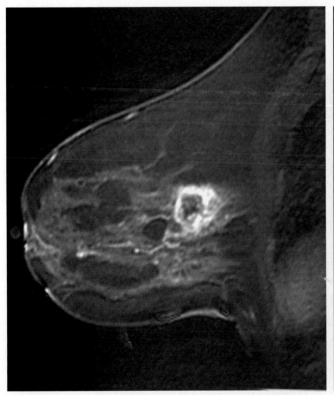

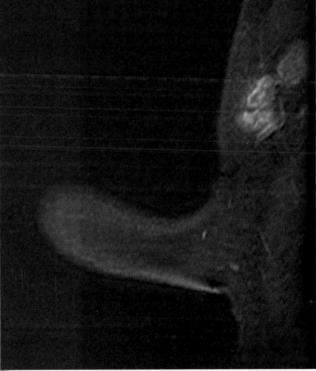

A   B

FIGURE 23.65. A 44-year-old woman with strong family history of breast cancer and prior benign right breast biopsy presents with palpable left axillary adenopathy. (A) MRI demonstrated findings compatible with multicentric disease (one mass shown) and (B) multiple abnormal axillary lymph nodes. Following confirmation of multicentric disease by ultrasound core biopsy, left mastectomy yielded demonstrated two separate foci of poorly differentiated ductal carcinoma in two separate quadrants with 16 positive nodes.

FIGURE 23.66. A 64-year-old presents with left axillary mass, fine needle aspiration positive for adenocarcinoma. Mammogram was heterogeneously dense and MRI demonstrated enlarged metastatic left axillary lymph node and clumped enhancement in the upper outer quadrant which proved to represent metastatic carcinoma in intramammary lymph nodes. As no other MR abnormality was identified, the patient was treated with whole breast radiation following complete axillary node dissection yielding two positive nodes. The patient has been free of disease for 3 years.

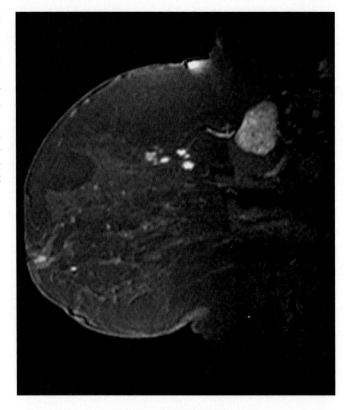

FIGURE 23.67. A 62-year-old with right axillary adenopathy. Aspiration yielded adenocarcinoma suspicious for breast primary. Mammogram mildly dense and negative. Magnetic resonance imaging demonstrated 7-mm mass corresponding to patient's occult carcinoma. Magnetic resonance imaging localization yielded invasive ductal carcinoma high grade with negative margins. The patient underwent radiation therapy.

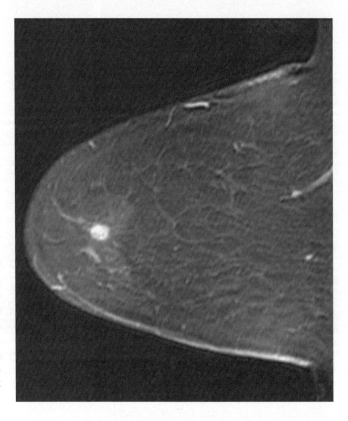

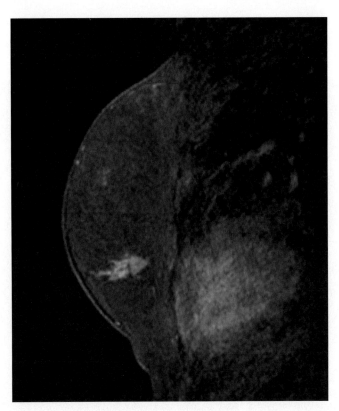

FIGURE 23.68. A 50-year-old woman with left axillary lymph node metastatic adeno carcinoma with focal extranodal extension. Mammogram was extremely dense with no suspicious findings. Magnetic resonance imaging demonstrates irregular mass in lower inner quadrant extending over 3 cm from skin to chest wall. Mastectomy yielded high-grade invasive ductal carcinoma.

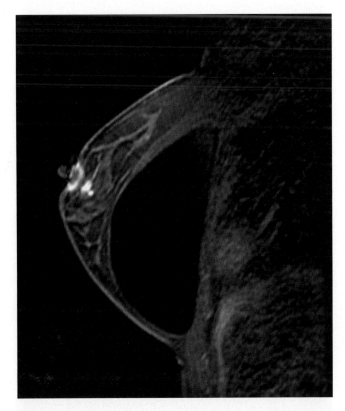

FIGURE 23.69. A 42-year-old woman with left axillary lymph node positive for adenocarcinoma. Bilateral subpectoral implants are present. The breasts are heterogeneously dense on mammography with no suspicious findings. Magnetic resonance imaging demonstrates 7-mm nodular enhancement in the retroareolar region yielding invasive ductal carcinoma and high grade DCIS and axillary dissection yielded three positive nodes. The area was localized under ultrasound guidance.

3. Metastasis

3.1. Parenchyma

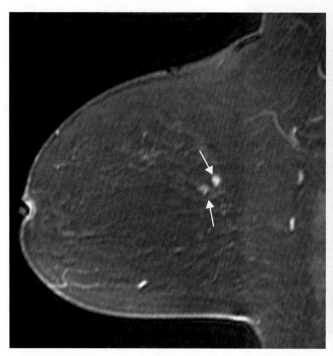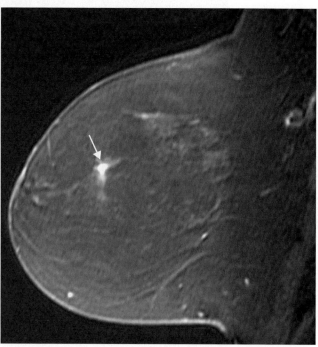

A   B

FIGURE 23.70. A 53-year-old woman with history of left ocular melanoma clinically without evidence of disease until screening mammogram demonstrated new bilateral nodules (A and B). She underwent multiple excisions yielding melanoma metastases to the breasts. There is no other evidence of disease. As lesions difficult to see by mammography, follow up by MRI performed. Magnetic resonance imaging demonstrated several ill-defined masse (arrows), biopsy proven melanoma metastases.

3.2. Skin

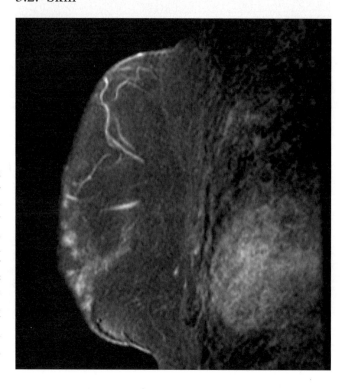

FIGURE 23.71. A 66-year-old woman who 8 years ago had breast-conserving therapy for 0.7-cm invasive ductal carcinoma with 37 negative nodes. She underwent radiation therapy and was placed on Tamoxifen® for 2 years, which was then discontinued due to vaginal bleeding. She now presents with multinodular skin recurrence in the medial breast. Magnetic resonance imaging demonstrates multiple nodular areas of enhancement within the skin, compatible with locally recurrent stage IV breast cancer. She was treated with mastectomy and hormonal therapy and is doing well 3 years later.

4. Invasive Carcinoma

4.1. Invasive Ductal

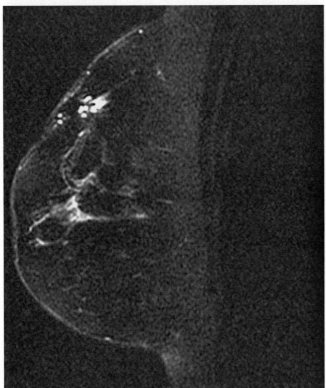

FIGURE 23.72. A 51-year-old woman status post lumpectomy and axillary node dissection of the left breast upper outer quadrant yielding mucinous carcinoma 8 years ago. Now has abnormal mammogram with increasing fullness at the lumpectomy site. Stereotactic biopsy of this finding demonstrated recurrent mucinous carcinoma. Magnetic resonance imaging performed to ensure the absence of other findings. Unifocal (A) high signal mass on T2 demonstrates (B) enhancement on the postcontrast T1-weighted images in the superior breast.

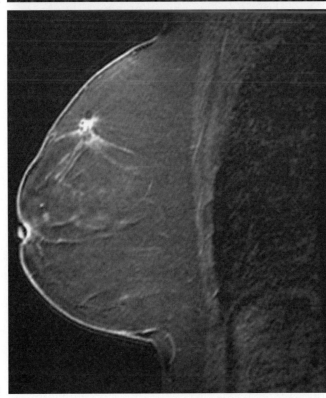

FIGURE 23.73. A 39-year-old woman presented with palpable masses in the upper outer
quadrant. Needle biopsy yielded invasive
ductal carcinoma poorly differentiated and
DCIS intermediate nuclear grade with central
necrosis. Due to extent of disease she underwent preoperative chemotherapy prior to
surgery.

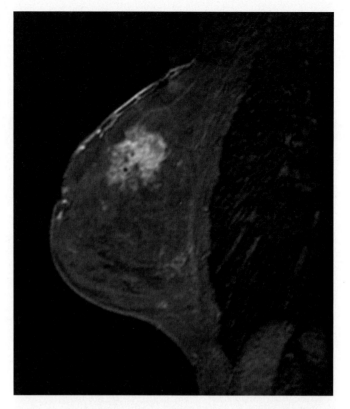

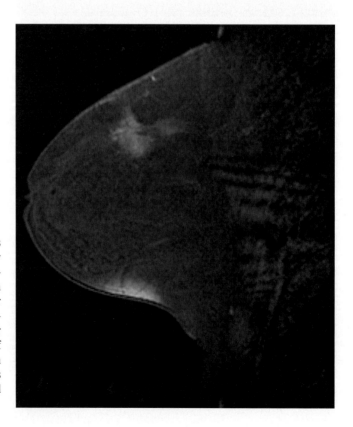

FIGURE 23.74. A 43-year-old woman status
post neoadjuvant chemotherapy for poorly
differentiated invasive ductal carcinoma. Magnetic resonance imaging demonstrated a
mildly enhancing mass in the upper outer
quadrant with plateau kinetics. She was conserved with surgical excision of the upper
outer quadrant. At pathology a single focus of
high-grade residual ductal carcinoma 3 mm in
size. Associated extensive reactive changes
were present. The MRI findings overestimated
the extent of residual disease.

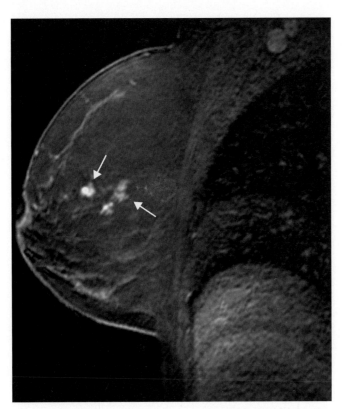

FIGURE 23.75. A 59-year-old woman presents with metastatic axillary adenopathy, unknown primary. Mammogram was negative. Magnetic resonance imaging examination demonstrates enhancement in the central breast (arrows) and nodular enhancement extending towards the nipple. Directed ultrasound following was negative. Magnetic resonance imaging guided needle localization yielded poorly differentiated invasive ductal carcinoma associated with lymphocytic infiltration and associated high-grade DCIS. Positive margins were found with subsequent re-excision. Patient then underwent completion mastectomy.

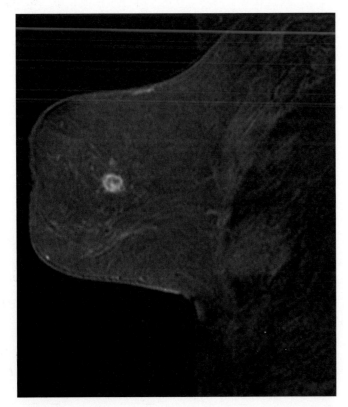

FIGURE 23.76. A 35-year-old woman with high risk underwent screening MRI examination yielding occult invasive ductal carcinoma. Nodes were negative. Note rim and central enhancement.

FIGURE 23.77. A 53-year-old woman had a new area of distortion in the 12 o'clock axis of her breast. Stereotactic biopsy yielded DCIS, cribiform and papillary types with intermediate-to-high nuclear grade. Magnetic resonance imaging performed which demonstrated a highly suspicious spiculated mass. At mastectomy (patient preference), an 1.8-cm mass-like area of DCIS involving sclerosing adenosis was found with no invasion. Other areas of DCIS were found in separate quadrants.

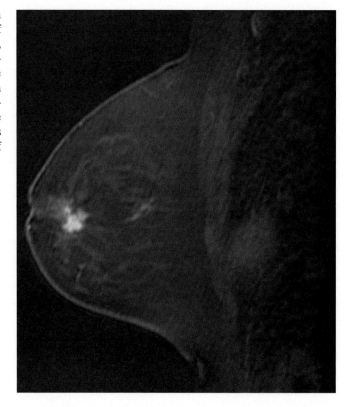

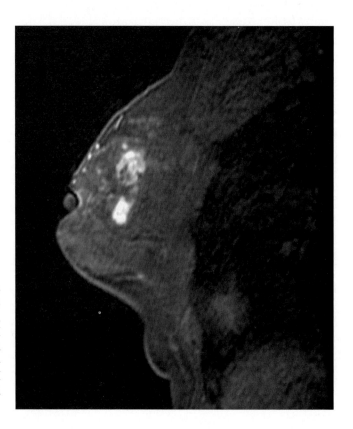

FIGURE 23.78. A 45-year-old woman presents status post excisional biopsy of a palpable lump that yielded invasive ductal carcinoma, histologic grade III/III, nuclear grade II/III with extensive intraductal component. In situ tumor is solid and cribiform types of intermediate nuclear grade and minimal necrosis. MRI demonstrates residual masses concordant with the pathological findings.

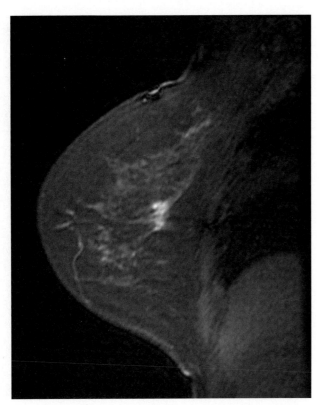

FIGURE 23.79. A 58-year-old woman had a mass identified in the breast on CT scan performed for pneumonia. Mammogram demonstrated calcifications that underwent stereotactic biopsy with clip placement. Pathology yielded DCIS solid, high nuclear grade with focal necrosis. MRI demonstrates an irregular mass adjacent to the biopsy site (not shown). At surgical excision, multiple foci of invasive mammary carcinoma were identified with mixed ductal and lobular features. Margins were negative.

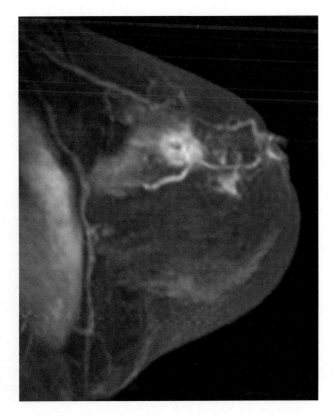

FIGURE 23.80. A 39-year-old with pregnancy-related carcinoma. One year after delivery and still breastfeeding she presented with palpable left axillary node, aspirated and positive for malignant cells. Maximum intensity projection of the left breast demonstrates two adjacent masses that proved to represent invasive ductal carcinoma, NOS, histologic grade III/III, nuclear grade II/III. Extensive intraductal component present with in situ component solid type, high nuclear grade, and minimal necrosis. The patient underwent mastectomy and chemotherapy.

FIGURE 23.81. A 36-year-old with palpable mass yielding invasive ductal carcinoma with focal lobular features, nuclear grade II/III, and vascular invasion.

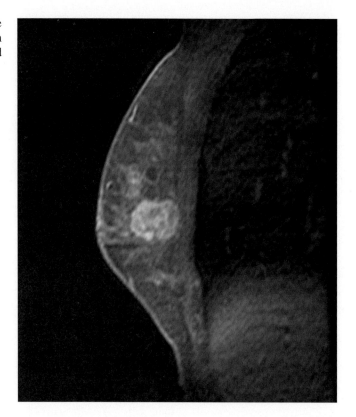

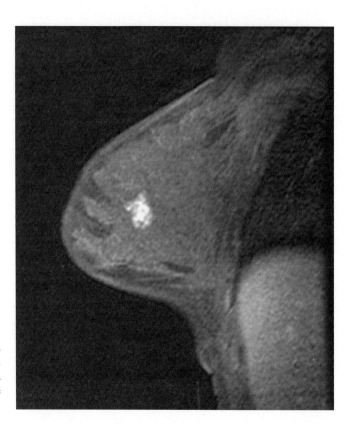

FIGURE 23.82. A 31-year-old presented with a palpable mass in an extremely dense breast. Pathology yielded invasive ductal carcinoma with focal lobular features, histologic grade III/III, nuclear grade II/III measuring 1.4 cm.

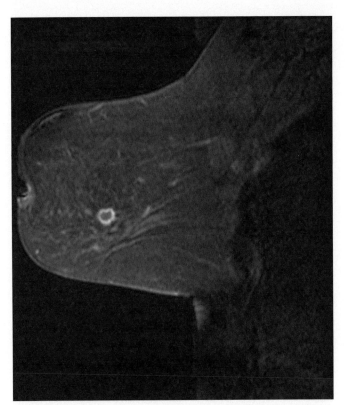

FIGURE 23.83. A 54-year-old woman with axillary metastasis of suspected breast primary. Conventional imaging negative. Magnetic resonance imaging demonstrates a unifocal rim-enhancing mass that was identified on directed ultrasound and biopsied yielding moderately differentiated invasive ductal carcinoma compatible with the patient's primary tumor.

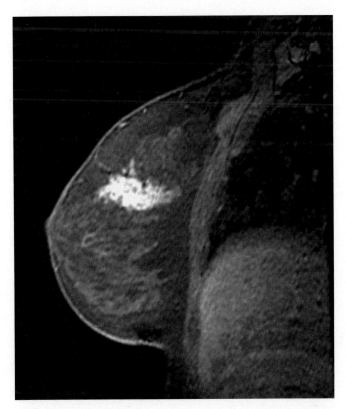

FIGURE 23.84. A 51-year-old woman presents with palpable mass. Mammogram was negative and ultrasound demonstrated subtle abnormality. Ultrasound-guided biopsy was performed which yielded invasive ductal carcinoma moderately to poorly differentiated with DCIS, cribiform type with intermediate nuclear grade and minimal necrosis. Due to the subtle imaging findings, MRI was performed which clearly demonstrated abnormality in the 12 o'clock axis. Pathology yielded invasive carcinoma and EIC.

FIGURE 23.85. A 38-year-old woman presents with palpable mass. Excisional biopsy yielded invasive ductal carcinoma, histologic grade III/III, and nuclear grade III/III with DCIS, solid and cribiform, high nuclear grade and necrosis. Note dominant rim enhancing mass with numerous surrounding nodules.

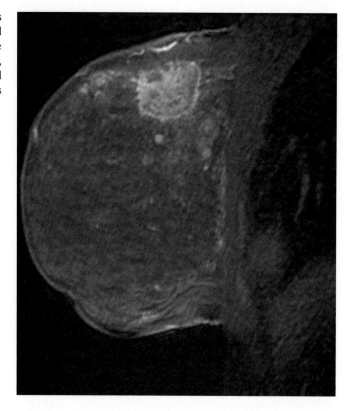

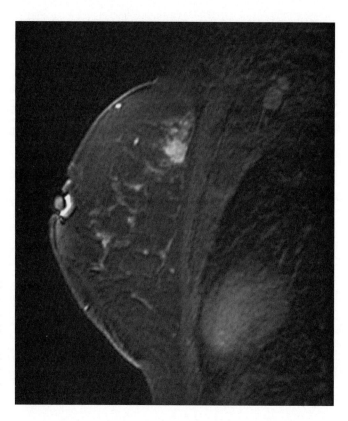

FIGURE 23.86. A 39-year-old with strong family history presents with subtle architectural distortion on mammography seen best on one view. Magnetic resonance imaging demonstrates the irregular mass in the superior breast that demonstrates washout kinetics. Ultrasound-guided core biopsy yielded invasive ductal carcinoma, moderately differentiated.

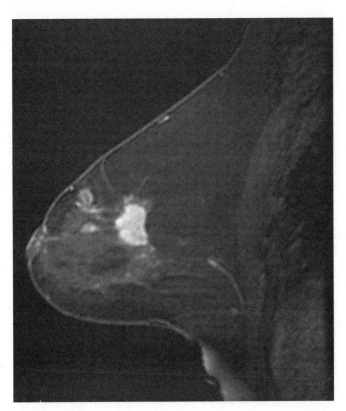

FIGURE 23.87. A 55-year-old woman with dense breasts and a spiculated mass noted on mammography. Core biopsy yielded invasive mammary carcinoma with mixed ductal and lobular features and low-grade DCIS. Surgical excision yielded invasive ductal carcinoma NOS with lobular features, histologic grade III/III, and nuclear grade II/III. Note that the carcinoma on MRI is lobulated and smoothly contoured.

4.2. Invasive Lobular

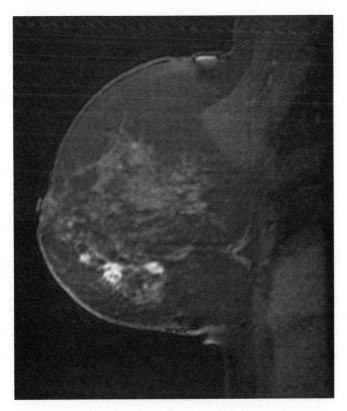

FIGURE 23.88. A 64-year-old woman demonstrates a spiculated mass in the lower breast on mammography. Ultrasound investigation disclosed two adjacent masses and both were biopsied yielding invasive lobular carcinoma. Magnetic resonance imaging confirmed the presence of these masses and did not detect additional disease. The patient was successfully treated with lumpectomy.

FIGURE 23.89. A 58-year-old woman status post mastectomy 3 years ago presents for screening MRI examination with negative mammography. A small oval homogeneously enhancing mass is noted in the lower breast with plateau kinetics. Ultrasound directed over this region was negative. Magnetic resonance localization and excisional biopsy yielded widespread multicentric invasive lobular carcinoma extending to the margins. Magnetic resonance imaging underestimated the extent of disease when compared to pathology.

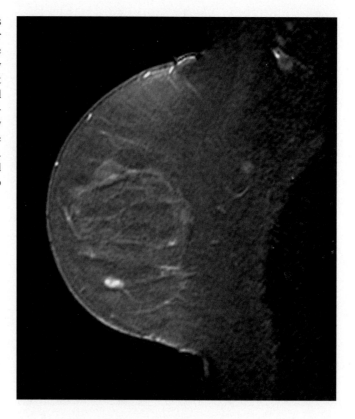

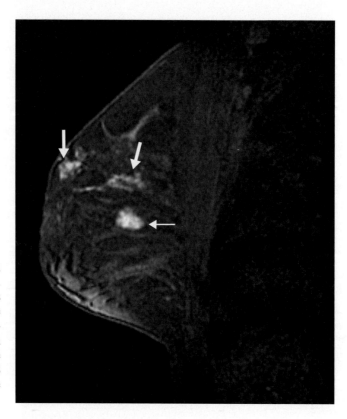

FIGURE 23.90. A 38-year-old woman with palpable right upper outer quadrant mass. On mammography a 2-cm spiculated mass was identified. Core biopsy yielded invasive lobular carcinoma. Magnetic resonance imaging identified multiple suspicious masses in several quadrants. At mastectomy invasive lobular carcinoma (thin arrow) and DCIS (thick arrows) were only identified in the upper outer quadrant.

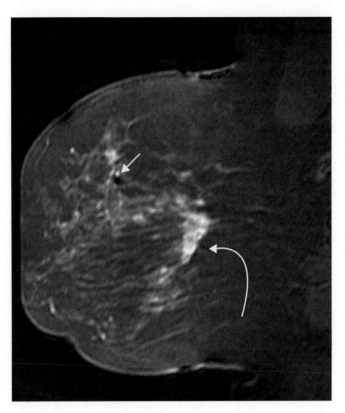

FIGURE 23.91. A 56-year-old with a subtle area of a symmetry on mammograph. Stereotactic core biopsy of the area with clip placement yielded invasive lobular carcinoma. Magnetic resonance imaging performed to evaluated disease extent. Clip artifact is noted in the superior breast (arrow). Away from the biopsy site is an irregular mass (curved arrow) that demonstrates washout kinetics. An attempt at conservation was made with bracketing of the area but margins were positive and the patient subsequently underwent mastectomy.

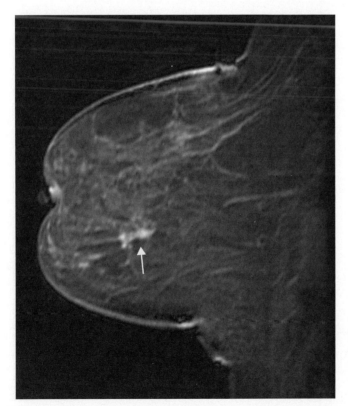

FIGURE 23.92. An 81-year-old woman with new spiculated mass on mammography. A corresponding 7-mm mass was identified on ultrasound. Biopsy yielded invasive lobular carcinoma. Magnetic resonance imaging confirms the mass (arrow) but does not detect additional disease. At mastectomy (patient preference) no other foci of carcinoma were found.

FIGURE 23.93. A 59-year-old woman with dimpling of the skin. A vague area of architectural distortion was identified on mammography. This was biopsied under stereotactic guidance yielding invasive lobular carcinoma. Magnetic resonance imaging demonstrates disease confined to the quadrant (arrows). Negative margins were obtained after two surgical excisions.

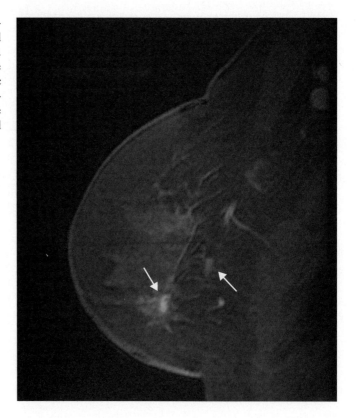

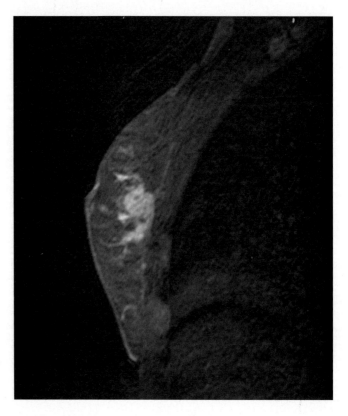

FIGURE 23.94. A 42-year-old woman with a palpable mass and negative mammogram. Ultrasound demonstrated a large mass that was biopsied yielding invasive lobular carcinoma. MRI confirmed the mass and demonstrated more extensive disease than ultrasound. At mastectomy, multiple foci of invasive lobular carcinoma were identified involving multiple quadrants.

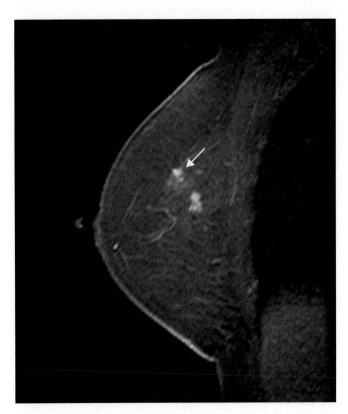

FIGURE 23.95. A 58-year-old woman with palpable mass and negative mammogram. Ultrasound demonstrates a mass that was biopsied yielding invasive lobular carcinoma. Magnetic resonance imaging confirms this finding and notes an additional mass (arrow) that proved to be a separable carcinoma. Both were removed at surgery. Nodes were negative.

5. Ductal Carcinoma In Situ

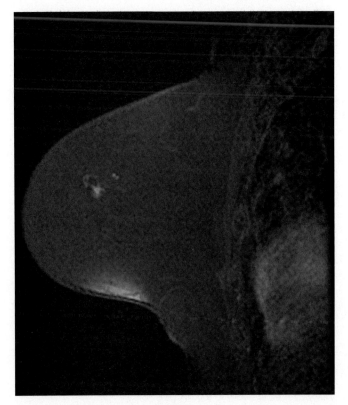

FIGURE 23.96. A 79-year-old woman with strong family history of breast cancer. Magnetic resonance imaging showed a spiculated mass that was biopsied yielding low grade DCIS.

FIGURE 23.97. A 43-year-old woman status post stereotactic biopsy for small cluster of calcifications yielding DCIS. Mother had breast cancer at 55 years. Magnetic resonance imaging demonstrates segmental clumped enhancement (arrows) representing micro-papillary DCIS with intermediate nuclear grade in the inferior breast adjacent to the site of biopsy.

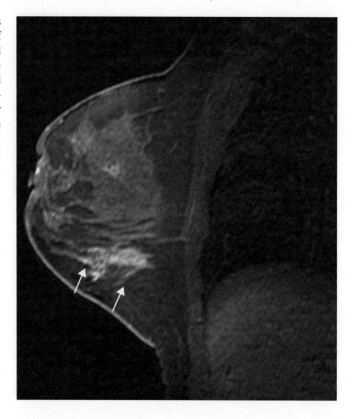

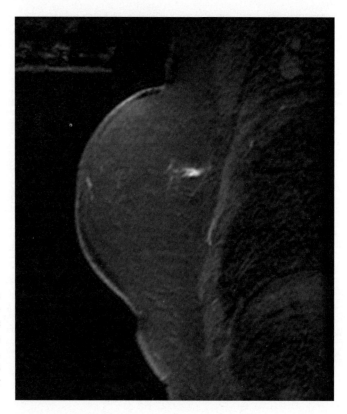

FIGURE 23.98. A 38-year-old woman with stage IV breast carcinoma considering reconstruction surgery of the left breast. Magnetic resonance imaging has performed to evaluate for any underlying findings prior to surgery. Linear enhancement in the superior breast is noted which proved to represent high nuclear grade DCIS.

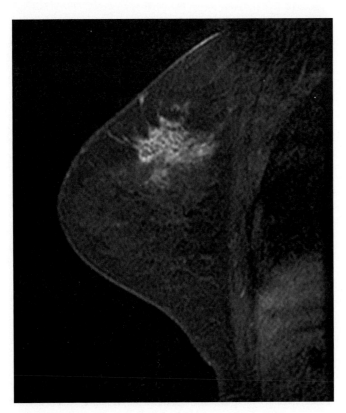

FIGURE 23.99. A 32-year-old woman with biopsy proven carcinoma undergoes MRI to assess for disease extent. A large spiculated mass in the right breast was identified (not shown) and in the left breast an irregular area of regional enhancement was noted (shown). Pathology yielded intraductal carcinoma papillary and cribiform with central necrosis, intermediate-to-high nuclear grade.

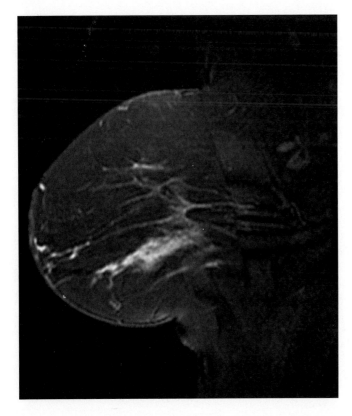

FIGURE 23.100. A 45-year-old with extensive Paget's disease of the left nipple and normal mammogram undergoes MRI examination which demonstrates irregular clumped linear enhancement extending over multiple quadrants suspicious for extensive underlying malignancy. Enhancement on this image is in a ductal orientation. Pathology at mastectomy demonstrated DCIS, solid cribiform and micropapillary types with high nuclear grade and minimal necrosis. No areas of microinvasion were identified.

FIGURE 23.101. A 52-year-old woman who developed a new cluster of calcifications on mammography. Stereotactic biopsy was performed yielding DCIS with mixed ductal and lobular features, solid and cribiform types, intermediate grade. Calcifications were associated with the DCIS. Magnetic resonance imaging was performed to assess extent of disease. Segmental branching enhancement was identified in the superior breast with involvement of one quadrant. Pathology showed at excision extensive DCIS with positive margins. A few foci of microinvasion were noted. The patient then underwent mastectomy and sentinel node sampling. Ductal carcinoma in situ was noted in two quadrants and nodes were negative.

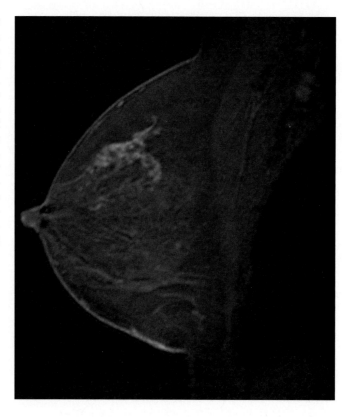

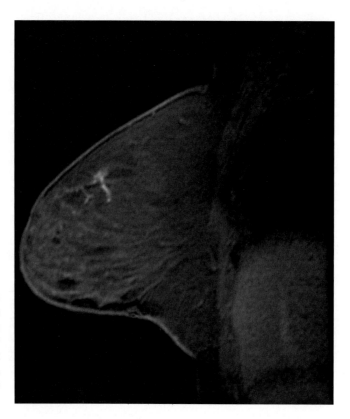

FIGURE 23.102. A 55-year-old woman with history of bilateral DCIS not treated with radiation therapy. Bilateral MRI examination performed which demonstrated a linear branching area of suspicious enhancement in the superior breast. Pathology showed DCIS, cribiform and solid types of intermediate grade.

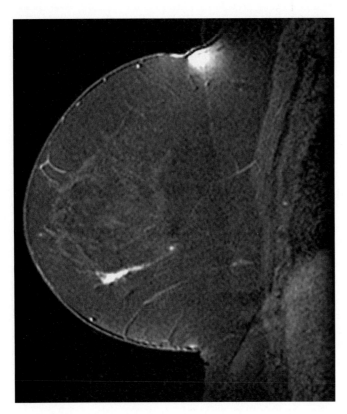

FIGURE 23.103. A 60-year-old woman with a history of mastectomy 11 years ago presents with hematoma of the remaining breast and no history of trauma. Mammography was negative aside from a mass that on ultrasound was thought to be a small hematoma. Magnetic resonance imaging demonstrates linear irregular enhancement along a ductal distribution away from the hematoma. Pathology of the linear enhancement was DCIS, cribiform and micropapillary, low nuclear grade with minimal necrosis. The hematoma had no associated malignancy.

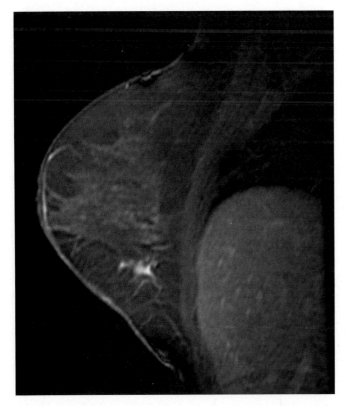

FIGURE 23.104. A 52-year-old woman with strong family history has multiple calcifications on mammography along the 6 o'clock axis of the right breast spanning 5 cm. A single area was biopsied under stereotactic guidance yielding DCIS, intermediate nuclear grade. Magnetic resonance imaging demonstrates segmental clumped enhancement that corresponds to the area of abnormality on mammography. At surgery microinvasive ductal carcinoma was identified. Subsequent sentinel nodal analysis was negative.

FIGURE 23.105. A 45-year-old woman with right breast bloody nipple discharge. A palpable mass in the right breast was aspirated yielding malignant cells. Mammogram was dense with no suspicious masses or calcifications. Ultrasound was performed over the palpable area and a corresponding solid mass was identified. Due to young patient age, breast density and clinical presentation, bilateral MRI was performed. MRI demonstrated an extensive regional area of clumped enhancement that extended from the chest wall to the subareolar region involving more than one quadrant that was suspicious for extensive multicentric carcinoma. Ultrasound guided core biopsy of the solid palpable mass yielded DCIS, solid type with intermediate nuclear grade. At mastectomy, extensive DCIS, intermediate to high nuclear grade with extensive necrosis was found in multiple quadrants. A sentinel node biopsy was negative.

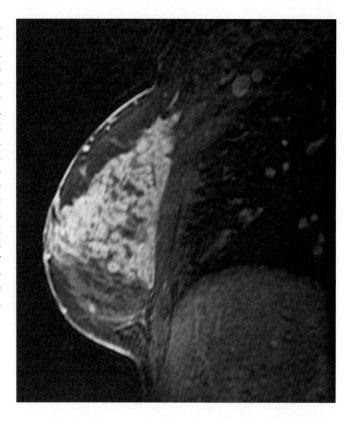

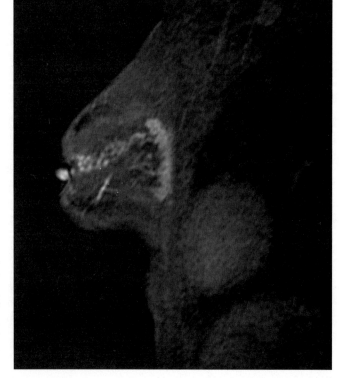

FIGURE 23.106. A 37-year-old woman with recent excisional biopsy yielding DCIS in the upper left breast. Margins were positive. Magnetic resonance imaging performed for residual disease and demonstrates triangular segmental enhancement compatible with residual disease and extensive involvement of the breast. Pathology yielded DCIS solid and cribiform with intermediate-to-high nuclear grade involving a quadrant. Mastectomy was performed and sentinel nodes were negative.

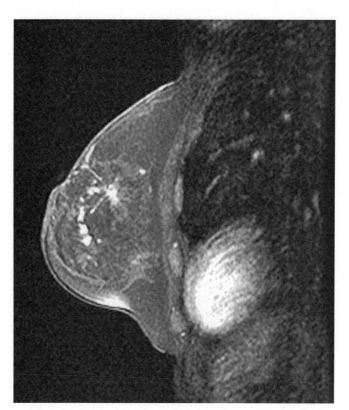

FIGURE 23.107. A 52-year-old woman with extensive DCIS and postoperative residual calcifications noted on postoperative mammogram. Assess for residual disease. Magnetic resonance imaging shows linear and clumped areas of enhancement near and away from the lumpectomy site. Pathology was DCIS, solid, cribiform and flat types of intermediate nuclear grade and moderate necrosis.

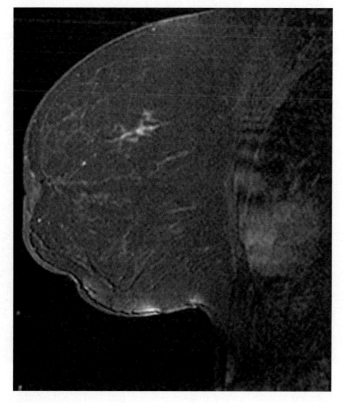

FIGURE 23.108. A 48-year-old woman presents with bloody nipple discharge. She had subsequent excision showing benign papillomatosis. She then developed a mass in the upper breast that was biopsied yielding intraductal papillary carcinoma with focal areas of invasion. Excision was performed with negative margins and axillary node dissection was negative for metastasis. She then developed bloody nipple discharge again and MRI was performed. Magnetic resonance imaging demonstrates linear branching enhancement in the upper breast that corresponded to multiple foci of intraductal carcinoma, papillary and cribiform arising in association with atypical ductal hyperplasia.

FIGURE 23.109. A 47-year-old woman with history of invasive lobular carcinoma presents for MRI screening. Mammogram is negative. Irregular mass noted in superior breast is confirmed on ultrasound and biopsied yielding apocrine DCIS with focal necrosis. At excision, microinvasive moderately differentiated ductal carcinoma with extensive DCIS was present. The patient went on to mastectomy.

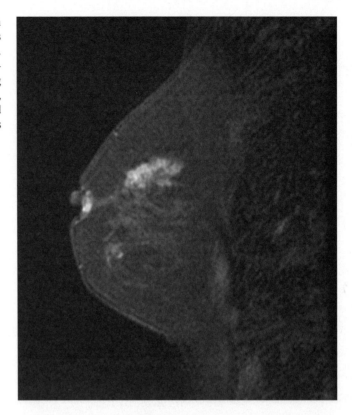

6. Other Tumors

6.1. Lymphoma

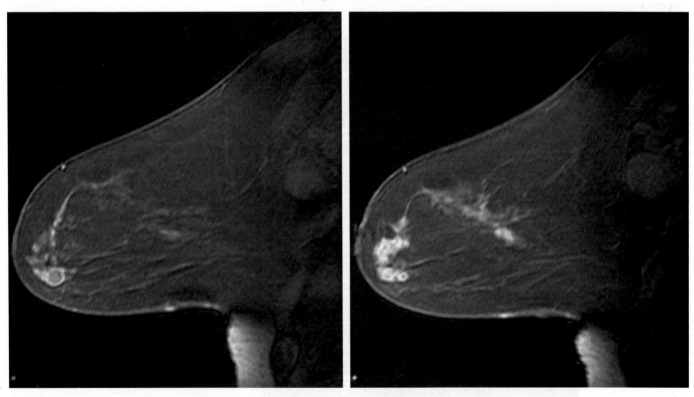

A

B

FIGURE 23.110. A 54-year-old woman with a history of non-Hodgkin's lymphoma presents with three new left breast masses and axillary adenopathy. She had no evidence of disease elsewhere in the body. Magnetic resonance imaging performed to evaluated extent of disease. (A and B) MRI demonstrated multiple masses. All but one had a sonographic correlate. Surgical excision of all areas yielded low-grade B-cell lymphoma involving breast tissue.

6.2. Phyllodes

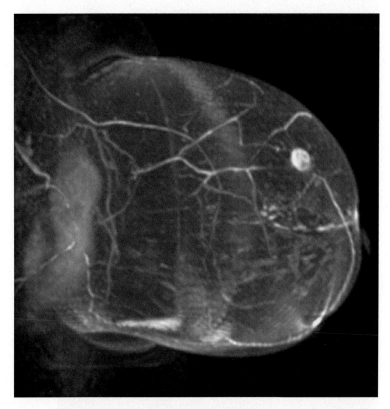

FIGURE 23.111. A 45-year-old woman with right mastectomy developed a new left breast mass on screening MRI examination (maximum intensity projection shown). It was verified on ultrasound and a core biopsy was performed yielding fibroepithelial tumor with increased stromal celularity. The differential diagnosis includes a cellular fibroadenoma and phyllodes tumor. Excision was performed yielding benign phyllodes tumor.

6.3. Angiosarcoma

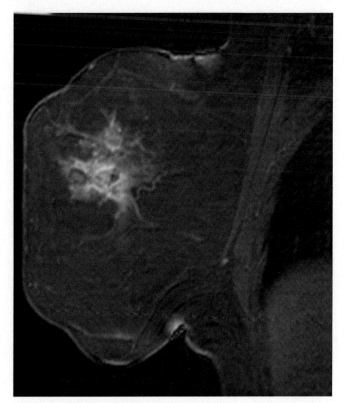

FIGURE 23.112. A 41-year-old woman noticed a palpable right breast mass 2 months ago. Biopsy yielded low-grade angiosarcoma. She was treated with mastectomy.

7. Recurrence

7.1. At the Lumpectomy Site

FIGURE 23.113. A 50-year-old woman treated with breast conserving therapy 1 year ago presents with palpable axillary recurrence following chemotherapy and radiation therapy. Magnetic resonance imaging performed to exclude recurrence in the breast. Initial carcinoma was 1.5-cm invasive ductal carcinoma, histologic and nuclear grade III/III. Negative margins were found on the second excision. Sentinel lymph node negative. She underwent total mastectomy with multiple foci of invasive ductal carcinoma identified ranging from 0.2 to 1.1 cm.

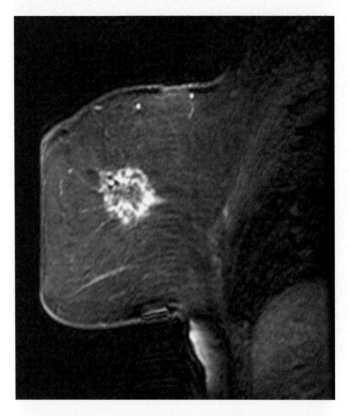

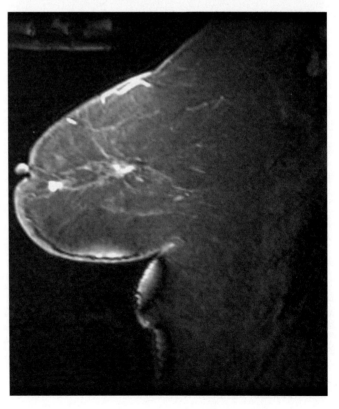

FIGURE 23.114. A 57-year-old woman status post quadrentectomy yielding in situ and invasive ductal carcinoma NOS type 2.7 cm. In situ was cribiform, papillary type with extension into lobules. Histologic and nuclear grades III/III. Margins negative. Treated with chemotherapy without radiation therapy. Magnetic resonance imaging performed demonstrates several ill-defined masses proven to represent recurrent invasive carcinoma.

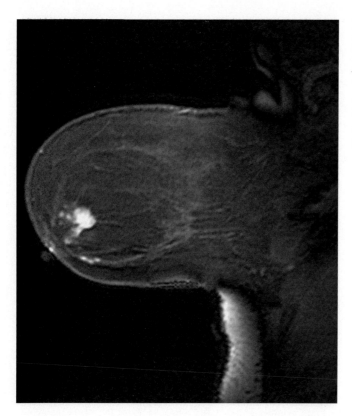

FIGURE 23.115. A 43-year-old woman status post conservation for invasive lobular carcinoma followed by chemotherapy and radiation therapy now presents with breast thickening. Magnetic resonance imaging demonstrates recurrent mass in the anterior breast proven to represent invasive mammary carcinoma with mixed ductal and lobular features.

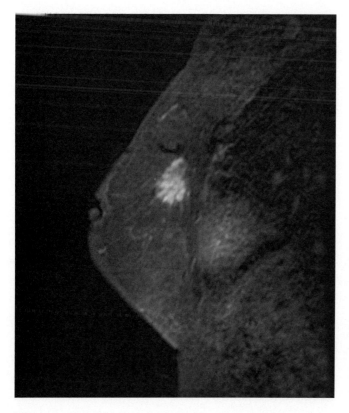

FIGURE 23.116. A 71-year-old diagnosed with stage II invasive ductal carcinoma breast cancer with 10/19 positive nodes. She received three cycles of chemotherapy and refused more. Full course of radiation therapy given. Presents now with peri-incisional fullness. At the lumpectomy site an irregular mass was identified and documented on ultrasound. Core biopsy yielded invasive ductal carcinoma treated with mastectomy and hormonal therapy.

FIGURE 23.117. A 42-year-old treated 5 years ago for invasive and in situ ductal carcinoma. Invasive component with histologic and nuclear grades III/III and in situ component cribiform, solid and comedo type with high nuclear grade and comprising >25% of the tumor compatible with EIC. Margins were negative following the second re-excision and lymph nodes were negative. Patient now presents with new calcifications on mammography. Stereotactic biopsy yielded recurrent DCIS, high nuclear grade, and extensive necrosis. Mastectomy performed. Maximum intensity projection shows linear branching enhancement in the superior breast compatible with recurrent DCIS.

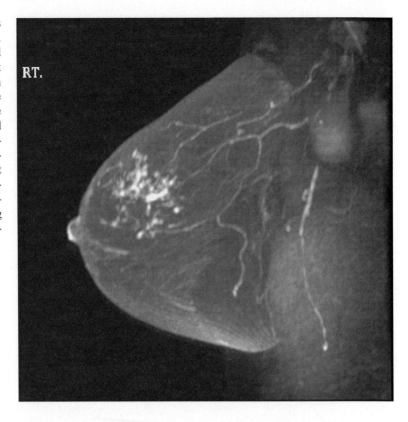

FIGURE 23.118. A 57-year-old woman with history of bilateral lumpectomies and bilateral augmentation. She has been treated with chemotherapy and radiation therapy to both breasts. She presents with palpable nodularity in the left upper outer quadrant. Mammography failed to note any suspicious findings but was limited due to the presence of the implants. Magnetic resonance imaging demonstrates two suspicious irregular masses that were biopsied under ultrasound guidance yielding invasive ductal carcinoma, moderately to poorly differentiated. Bilateral total mastectomies were performed.

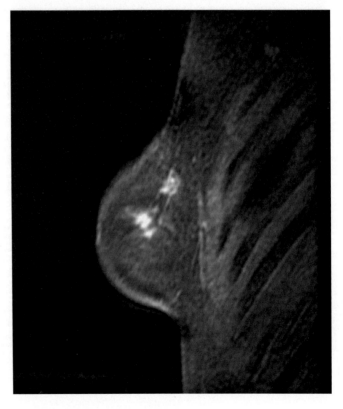

7.2. Elsewhere in Breast

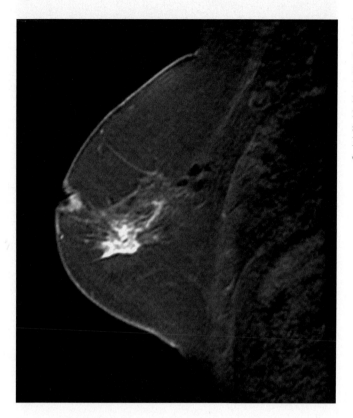

FIGURE 23.119. A 63-year-old woman with a history of DCIS 1 year ago treated with excision and no radiation presents with a new mass on mammography that was biopsied under ultrasound guidance yielding invasive mammary carcinoma with ductal and lobular features. Magnetic resonance imaging demonstrates an irregular mass anterior to the lumpectomy site compatible with recurrent carcinoma.

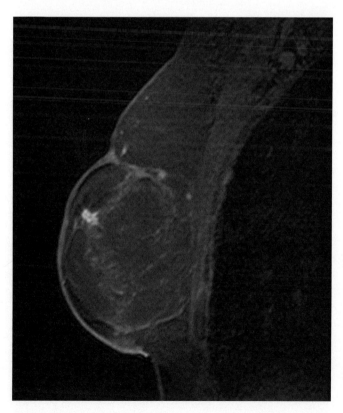

FIGURE 23.120. A 50-year-old initially presented with a mass 5 years ago in the breast in Central America. Biopsy yielded invasive ductal carcinoma. No initial mammogram was performed. Re-excision was reportedly negative though axillary nodal dissection yielded eight positive nodes. She underwent full courses of chemotherapy and radiation therapy and now presents for follow up. Magnetic resonance imaging demonstrates an irregular suspicious mass anterior and inferior to the lumpectomy site. Directed ultrasound over this region discloses a mass that was biopsied yielding invasive mammary carcinoma with mixed ductal and lobular features, poorly differentiated which was morphologically similar to the patient's prior mammary carcinoma. Patient subsequently underwent total mastectomy.

FIGURE 23.121. A 44-year-old woman underwent screening mammography that identified a nonpalpable mass that proved to represent multiple foci of invasive ductal carcinoma, poorly differentiated with lobular growth pattern. Re-excision demonstrated residual multiple foci of invasive carcinoma ranging in size from 0.3 to 0.9 cm. Final margins were negative. She underwent full course of chemotherapy and radiation therapy. She now presents 2 years later with new calcifications elsewhere in the breast. Stereotactic biopsy yielded invasive ductal carcinoma, histologic grade III, nuclear grade II. Ductal carcinoma in situ, solid and cribiform typed, intermediate nuclear grade extensive necrosis. Magnetic resonance imaging demonstrates multiple irregular masses throughout the breast. Pathology of the mastectomy specimen yielded recurrent invasive mammary carcinoma with ductal and lobular features that involved the entire breast. Ductal carcinoma in situ was of the same type and involved all quadrants. Note skin enhancement representing inflammatory component confirmed at surgery.

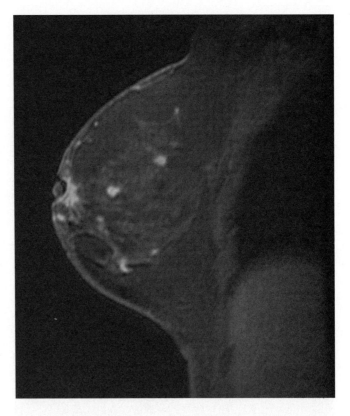

FIGURE 23.122. A 48-year-old woman status post stereotactic biopsy for calcifications showing DCIS, solid type with high nuclear grade and moderate necrosis. Calcifications were present in the DCIS and benign breast tissue. Re-excision was performed which yielded invasive ductal carcinoma NOS type, histologic and nuclear grade III/III measuring 0.4 cm and associated EIC, solid type with high nuclear grade and extensive necrosis. No involvement of the surgical margins was noted. Nodes were negative. The patient underwent radiation therapy. At that time she had a normal MRI examination. Six months later she underwent repeat MRI, which demonstrated abnormal clumped enhancement anterior to the lumpectomy site in the lower breast. Mammography and ultrasound were negative. Biopsy showed DCIS, high nuclear grade, and moderate necrosis. The patient then underwent completion mastectomy.

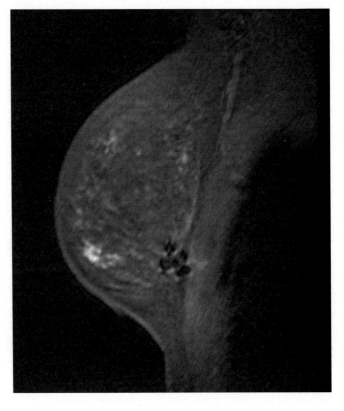

8. Residual

8.1. At the Excisional Biopsy Site

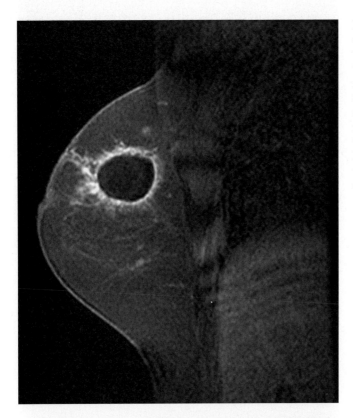

FIGURE 23.123. A 60-year-old woman with 2-cm infiltrating lobular carcinoma, classical type of the right breast status post excision with positive margins. Magnetic resonance imaging demonstrates a small amount of nodular enhancement anterior to the seroma cavity. Re-excision yielded infiltrating mammary carcinoma poorly differentiated with innumerable foci ranging up to 1.2 cm. Magnetic resonance imaging underestimated the extent of residual disease and the patient ended up having mastectomy.

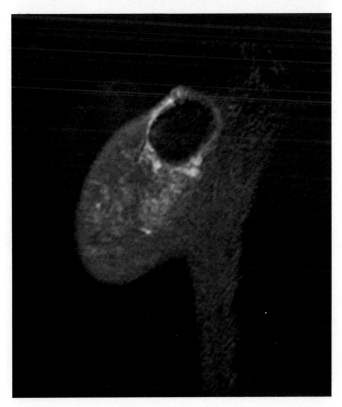

FIGURE 23.124. A 48-year-old with suspicious calcifications noted on routine mammogram of the left breast proven to represent well-differentiated infiltrating ductal carcinoma, pure tubular type with three separate foci measuring up to 2.4 cm. Posterior margin was positive. Magnetic resonance imaging performed demonstrated nodular enhancement along the inferior and posterior margins of the seroma cavity suspicious for residual disease. Re-excision demonstrated low-grade DCIS, micropapillary and cribiform types.

FIGURE 23.125. A 37-year-old presented with a palpable left breast mass. Mammography demonstrated heterogeneously dense breasts with no focal finding. Biopsy yielded 2.5-cm infiltrating ductal carcinoma with positive margins. No calcifications were noted in the carcinoma. Postoperative mammogram was unremarkable. Magnetic resonance imaging demonstrates anterior to the seroma cavity clumped patchy enhancement that showed residual high-grade DCIS, cribiform architecture, with extensive necrosis Margins were negative at re-excision.

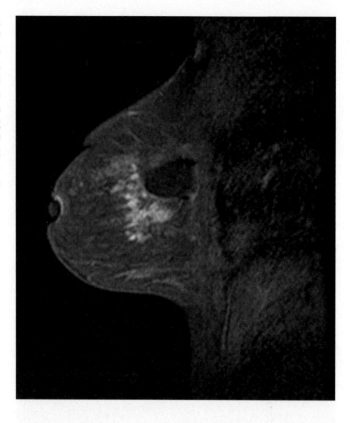

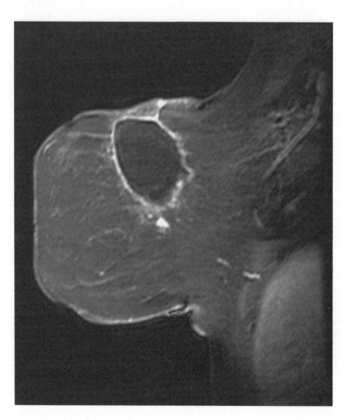

FIGURE 23.126. A 68-year-old with 1.5-cm moderately differentiated infiltrating ductal carcinoma in the right breast with several separate foci of invasive carcinoma measuring 0.2 and 0.5 cm. Associated DCIS cribiform, solid, papillary with low-to-intermediate nuclear grade was identified. A few foci of DCIS approached the inked margins. Magnetic resonance imaging was performed for residual disease and demonstrates a single small mass inferior to the surgical site. Re-excision showed a few foci of atypical ductal hyperplasia and LCIS but no residual carcinoma.

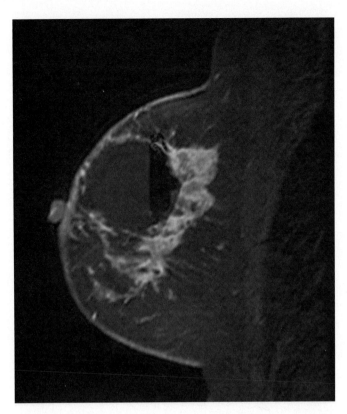

FIGURE 23.127. A 42-year-old who sought bilateral reduction surgery was noted to have a palpable nodule on examination. On ultrasound the palpable abnormality was solid. Excisional biopsy yielded invasive lobular carcinoma extending to cauterized margins. Magnetic resonance imaging performed to assess residual disease. The patient opted for bilateral mastectomy which demonstrated residual invasive lobular carcinoma measuring at least 7 cm and 4 of 16 positive axillary nodes.

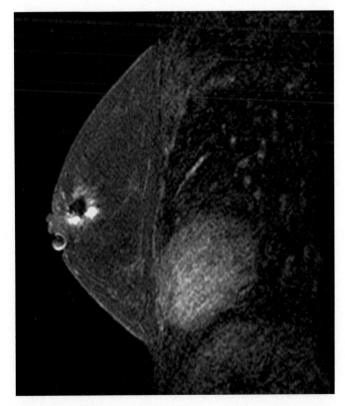

FIGURE 23.128. A 40-year-old presented with left breast mass yielding moderately differentiated invasive ductal carcinoma measuring 1.1 cm with associated DCIS and DCIS extending to an unspecified margin. The postoperative seroma was small and demonstrated thick enhancement. No residual was found at re-excision.

FIGURE 23.129. A 50-year-old with new calcifications on mammography status post stereotactic biopsy positive for DCIS. Excisional biopsy was performed yielding foci suspicious for microinvasive ductal carcinoma and extensive DCIS, solid, cribiform, and papillary types with high nuclear grade and moderate necrosis. Ductal carcinoma in situ extended to all margins. Magnetic resonance imaging following excision demonstrates extensive enhancement around the seroma caity confirmed at surgery. Patient ultimately underwent mastectomy.

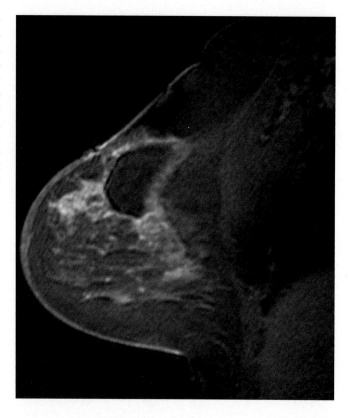

FIGURE 23.130. A 65-year-old woman with spiculated mass on mammography thought to represent radial scar. Excisional biopsy performed which demonstrated DCIS solid and cribiform types with low-to-intermediate nuclear grade and minimal necrosis portions of which involved the radial scar. A few foci of DCIS were close to the superior margin. Postoperative MRI demonstrates thick nodular enhancement around the seroma cavity. Reexcision showed florid ductal hyperplasia with focal atypia and fibrocystic changes and no residual carcinoma.

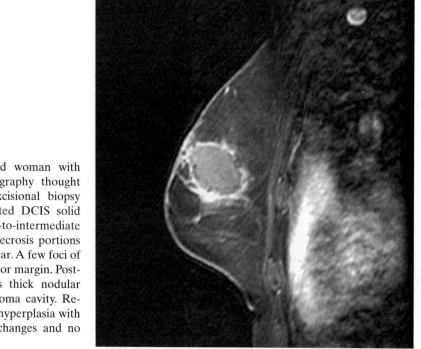

8.2. In the Same Quadrant

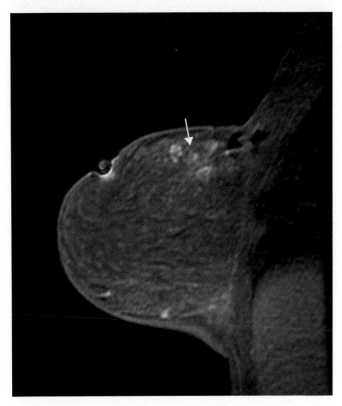

FIGURE 23.131. A 52-year-old woman who developed a 2-cm area of calcifications in the upper outer quadrant. At surgical excision following needle localization these were shown to be associated with atypical ductal hyperplasia. Because so few calcifications were identified on the specimen radiography, rebiopsy was planned. Prior to surgery, MRI was performed which showed suspicious clumped enhancement (arrow) in the upper outer quadrant extending to the nipple. This was shown to represent DCIS, cribiform type with low nuclear grade and no necrosis. Calcifications were associated with benign breast parenchyma.

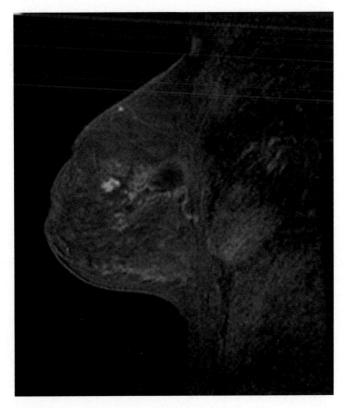

FIGURE 23.132. A 37-year-old presented with palpable breast mass. Mammogram demonstrated subtle asymmetry but ultrasound showed a suspicious 2.5-cm mass that was biopsied yielding invasive ductal carcinoma NOS, histologic and nuclear grades III/III and high-grade DCIS with extensive necrosis. Invasive carcinoma was within 0.5 cm of the superior margin and DCIS was 0.6 cm from the anterior and superior margins. Magnetic resonance imaging performed for assessment of residual disease. Nodular enhancement was seen surrounding the lumpectomy site in the same quadrant. These were not identified on ultrasound. Magnetic resonance needle localization demonstrated several foci of DCIS, high grade with extensive necrosis adjacent and away from the lumpectomy site. The patient then underwent completion mastectomy. Nodes were negative.

FIGURE 23.133. A 52-year-old woman who had a small cluster of pleomorphic calcifications in the upper outer quadrant. Subsequent excisional biopsy yielded invasive ductal carcinoma with poor differentiation and underlying lymphatic invasion. She then underwent wide excision with sentinel node biopsy with carcinoma close to the inked margins. Micrometastases were noted in three sentinel lymph nodes. Magnetic resonance imaging demonstrated areas of clumped enhancement posterior to the lumpectomy site. A second, wide re-excision was performed which found focal microinvasive ductal carcinoma and DCIS, solid type with high nuclear grade and moderate necrosis. Axillary node dissection was negative.

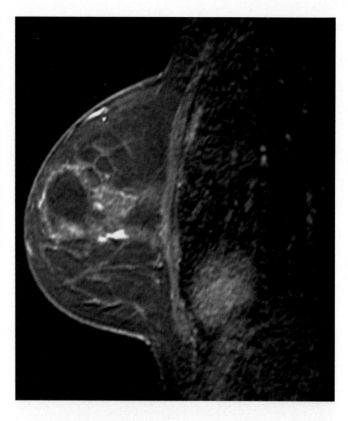

FIGURE 23.134. A 45-year-old woman with dense breasts and strong family history of breast carcinoma initially presented with a palpable abnormality and no corresponding mammographic or ultrasound abnormality. A wide excision had already been performed prior to the MRI yielding DCIS, micropapillay, papillary and cribiform types with intermediate nuclear grade and moderate necrosis. Magnetic resonance imaging demonstrates extensive residual segmental clumped enhancement posterior and anterior to the lumpectomy site extending from the chest wall to the subareolar region. After a further attempt at conservation with positive margins, a completion mastectomy was finally performed.

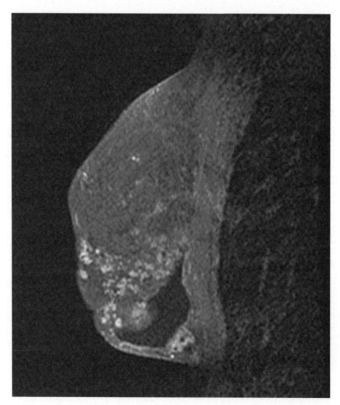

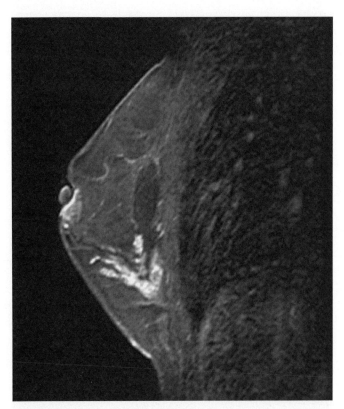

FIGURE 23.135. A 37-year-old BRCA1-positive patient with a palpable breast mass. Mammography demonstrated extensive pleomorphic calcifications in the lower outer quadrant. The posterior extent of the tumor could not be identified on mammography. On ultrasound there was an ill-defined mass that was inseparable from the chest wall and invasion was suspected. Magnetic resonance imaging was performed to stage the patient and assess the chest wall. Invasion of the chest wall muscles was confirmed on MRI (not shown) and enhancement anterior to the lumpectomy site was noted which involved an entire quadrant compatible with residual carcinoma. The patient underwent preoperative chemotherapy with excellent response. At mastectomy, two residual foci of invasive carcinoma were found, 2 mm each.

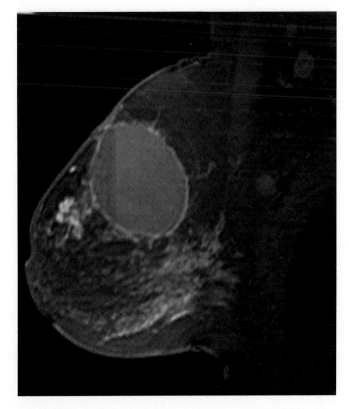

FIGURE 23.136. A 39-year-old with no family history but a history of LCIS and atypical ductal hyperplasia presented initially with a palpable mass that represented 5-cm invasive mammary carcinoma with mixed ductal and lobular features extending to the inked margin. Magnetic resonance imaging performed for residual disease assessment. Magnetic resonance imaging shows suspicious enhancing nodule anterior to the lumpectomy site, proved to represent residual invasive lobular carcinoma at mastectomy. Additional foci were identified at and away from the biopsy site (not shown).

8.3. In a Separate Quadrant

FIGURE 23.137. A 39-year-old with palpable left breast cancer and outside excisional biopsy and axillary node dissection yielding invasive ductal carcinoma, histologic and nuclear grade III/III, 2.7 cm with vascular invasion. She then received three cycles of chemotherapy and presented to our institution. On pathologic review, surgical margins could not be assessed. Magnetic resonance imaging performed to evaluate possible residual disease. In a quadrant separate from the lumpectomy site, multiple small enhancing masses were identified suspicious for multi-centric disease. Ultrasound was able to identify several of these which were biopsied yielding invasive ductal carcinoma, histologic and nuclear grade III/III. Mastectomy was performed.

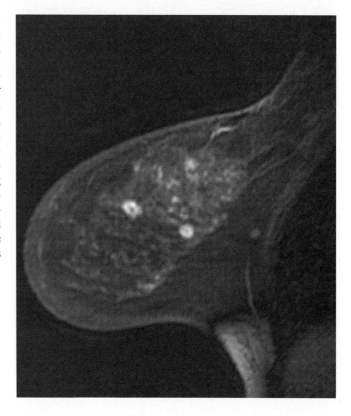

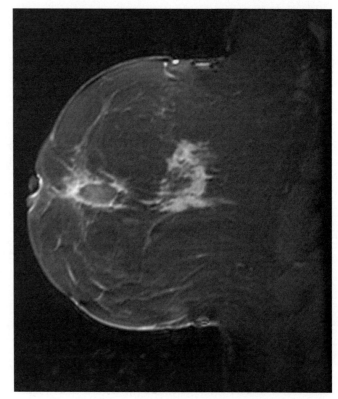

FIGURE 23.138. A 51-year-old woman with new 1.6-cm microlobulated obscured mass noted on mammography in the retroareolar region. Outside needle localization and surgical excision yielded DCIS, cribiform and micropapillary with intermediate nuclear grade and moderate necrosis. Margins were close. Magnetic resonance imaging performed for residual disease. Magnetic resonance imaging demonstrates the lumpectomy site in the anterior breast, however, separate from the lumpectomy site is a large mass posteriorly that yielded two foci of invasive ductal carcinoma, moderately differentiated ranging in size 0.8 to 2.5 cm. Ductal carcinoma in situ was also identified, solid, cribiform, and micropapillary types with intermediate nuclear grade and extensive necrosis.

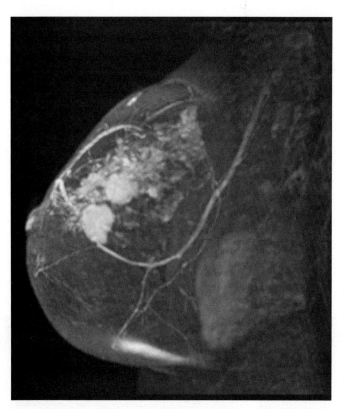

FIGURE 23.139. A 39-year-old woman presented with a palpable abnormality in the upper inner quadrant. On mammography two masses were identified with associated pleomorphic calcifications. The disease on mammography was confined to a single quadrant. MRI was performed to assess disease extent which confirmed the impression of two dominant masses with surrounding clumped enhancement. The enhancement involved more than one quadrant compatible with multicentric disease. The patient received mastectomy. Pathology yielded two sites of invasive ductal carcinoma and DCIS was identified in both upper quadrants. Axillary node dissection was negative.

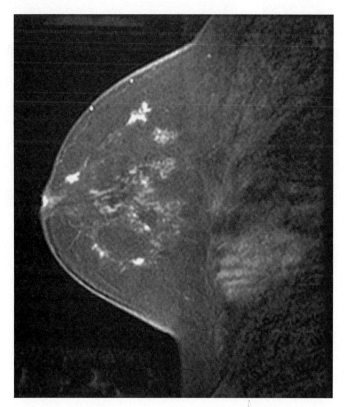

FIGURE 23.140. A 57-year-old woman underwent excisional biopsy yielding 4.5-cm invasive ductal carcinoma with apocrine features, histologic and nuclear grade III/III with associated DCIS, solid type with high nuclear grade and extensive necrosis. Magnetic resonance imaging was performed to assess residual disease. In multiple quadrants ill-defined masses were identified representing multifocal invasive ductal carcinoma.

24
High-Risk Lesions

1. Atypical Duct Hyperplasia

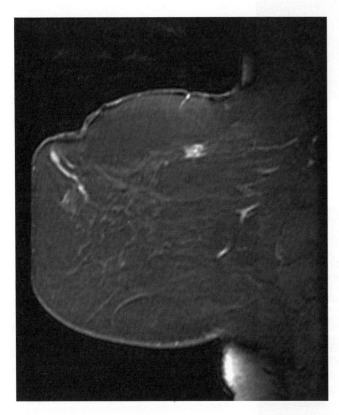

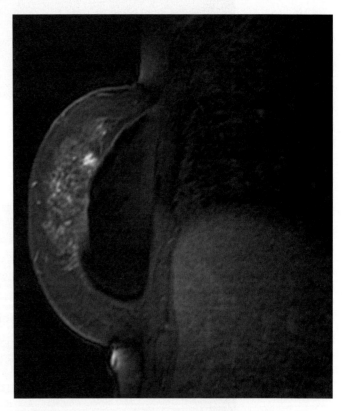

FIGURE 24.1. A 60-year-old (high-risk) woman undergoes screening contrast enhanced magnetic resonance imaging (MRI) that demonstrates clumped enhancement in the superior breast. No ultrasound correlate was identified. Subsequent magnetic resonance (MR) needle localization and surgical excision showed atypical ductal hyperplasia.

FIGURE 24.2. A 63-year-old woman with silicone implants had MRI for assessment of palpable nodularity. MRI demonstrates an irregular mass adjacent to the implant. This was localized under MRI guidance using a skin marker. Pathology yielded atypical ductal hyperplasia.

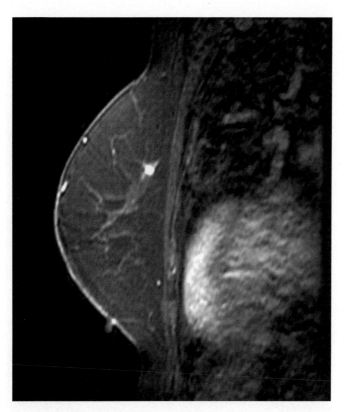

FIGURE 24.3. A 49-year-old woman with prior benign biopsies yielding atypical ductal hyperplasia and lobular carcinoma in situ undergoes screening. An irregular mass seen posteriorly in the breast was not identified on mammogram or ultrasound. MRI needle localization with surgical excision yielded markedly atpical ductal hyperplasia.

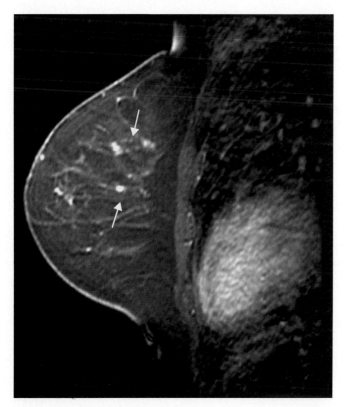

FIGURE 24.4. A 60-year-old woman status post right mastectomy underwent MRI evaluation of left breast. Clumped enhancement was noted centrally in the breast (arrows). MRI needle localization yielded atypical duct hyperplasia.

2. Atypical Lobular Hyperplasia

FIGURE 24.5. A 46-year-old woman with infiltrating lobular carcinoma of the left breast scheduled for left mastectomy. MRI performed to screen right breast. Focal clumped enhancement was identified in the superior breast proven to represent atypical lobular hyperplasia focally at the level of lobular carcinoma in situ (classical type).

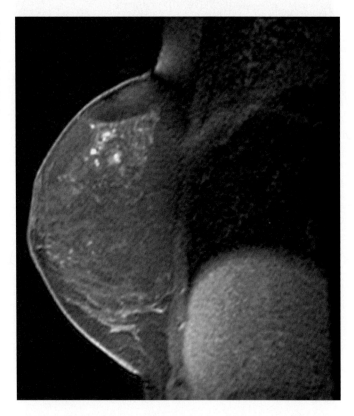

3. Lobular Carcinoma In Situ

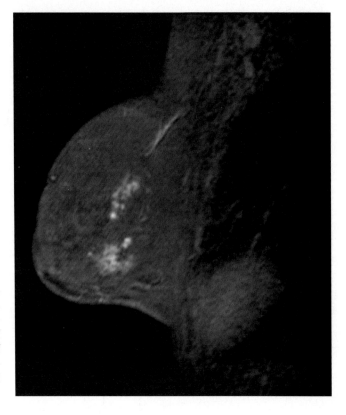

FIGURE 24.6. A 50-year-old woman presents with palpable mass right breast, biopsy proven infiltrating lobular carcinoma. Patient is scheduled for right mastectomy. MRI screening of the left breast demonstrates two areas of patchy enhancement for which needle localization was performed and pathology found lobular carcinoma in situ (LCIS).

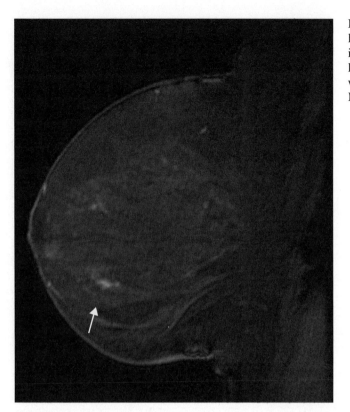

FIGURE 24.7. A 59-year-old woman with prior history of breast biopsy yielding LCIS. Screening MRI demonstrates suspicious clumped linear enhancement (arrow) for which biopsy was suggested. The area was localized under MR guidance yielding LCIS.

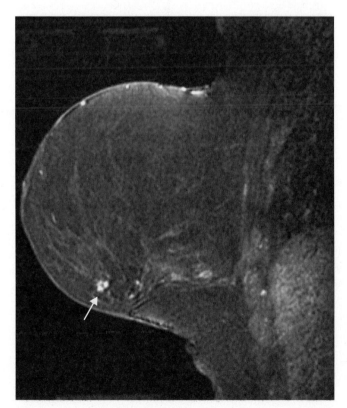

FIGURE 24.8. A 60-year-old woman with family history of breast carcinoma. Prior reduction mammoplasty and benign biopsy in the upper outer quadrant yielding benign results. In the lower right breast there is clumped enhancement (arrow) with plateau kinetics. Magnetic resonance localization yielded LCIS.

FIGURE 24.9. A 56-year-old status post bilateral breast biopsies yielding bilateral infiltrating ductal carcinoma (not shown). MRI performed for staging. Patchy areas of enhancement are noted superiorly (arrows) that yielded LCIS at surgery. The patient opted for bilateral mastectomy.

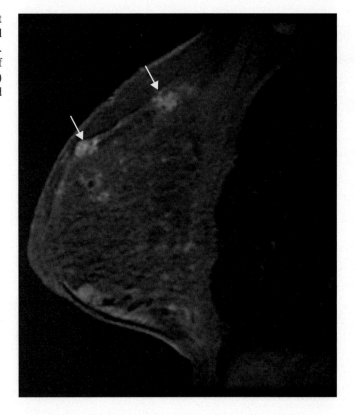

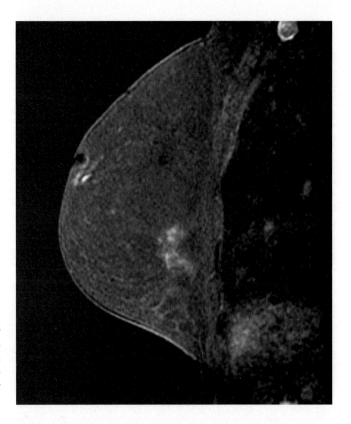

FIGURE 24.10. A 62-year-old woman status post left lumpectomy for ductal carcinoma in situ (DCIS). Screening MRI performed. Clumped nodular enhancement in the posterior breast was identified and subsequently localized yielding LCIS.

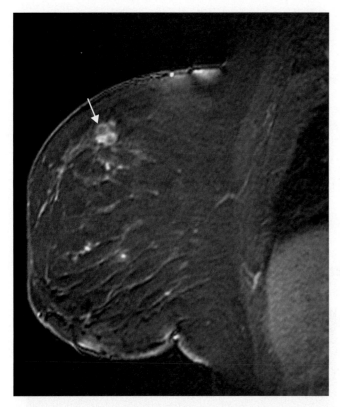

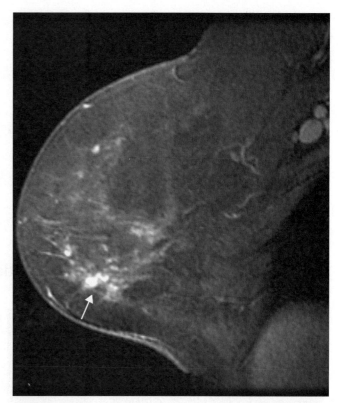

FIGURE 24.11. A 44-year-old woman with a strong family history of breast carcinoma. The patient developed clumped enhancement in the superior breast (arrow) when compared to prior screening MRI examinations. Pathology was LCIS and proliferative fibrocystic changes.

FIGURE 24.12. A 69-year-old woman with normal mammogram had MRI which showed two suspicious areas of clumped enhancement in the right breast. One of these (not shown) proved to represent DCIS at surgery. The other (shown in the interior breast (arrow)) proved to represent LCIS.

4. Radial Scar

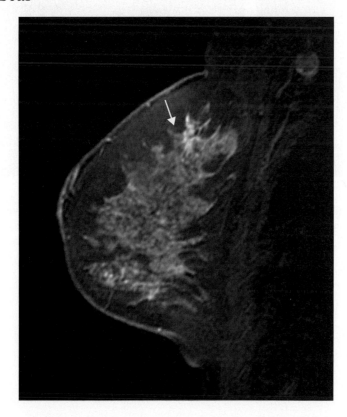

FIGURE 24.13. A 50-year-old woman with contralateral breast cancer undergoes contralateral screening MRI. At the time of contralateral mastectomy biopsy of the spiculated area (arrow) in the left breast was performed yielding radial scar.

25
Benign Lesions

1. Fibroadenoma

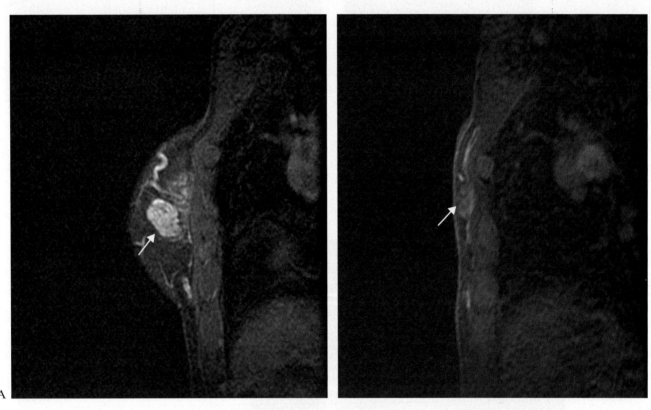

A   B

FIGURE 25.1. A 44-year-old woman status post biopsy for a sono-graphically evident mass yielding 1-cm benign phyllodes tumor and atypical lobular hyperplasia. (A and B) Contrast enhanced magnetic resonance imaging (MRI) demonstrated two additional masses medially (arrows). Both were removed at surgery and demonstrated to represent fibroadenomas.

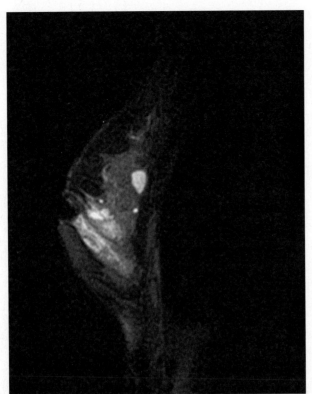

A

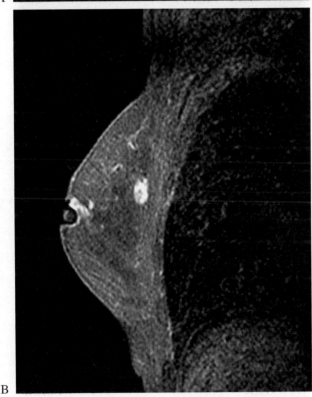

B

FIGURE 25.2. A 54-year-old woman at high risk for breast cancer undergoes screening MRI. (A) High signal mass noted on the T2-weighted image corresponds to (B) an oval, irregular enhancing irregular mass. Biopsy of the enhancing mass demonstrates myxomatous fibroadenoma.

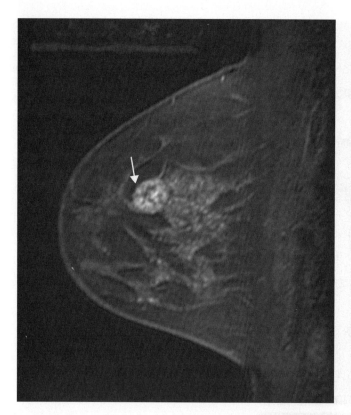

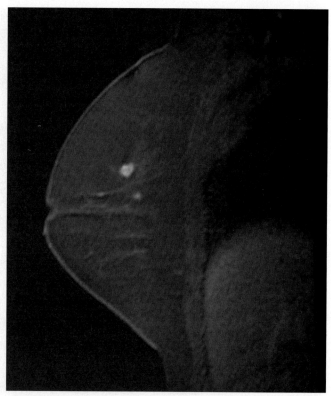

FIGURE 25.3. A 46-year-old woman presented with palpable right breast mass proved to be invasive ductal carcinoma. Left breast MRI demonstrated fibroadenoma (arrow) not detected on mammogram.

FIGURE 25.4. A 60-year-old woman preoperative for left mastectomy had screening MRI examination of the right breast demonstrating a circumscribed mass which was seen on targeted ultrasound following MRI and yielded fibroadenoma.

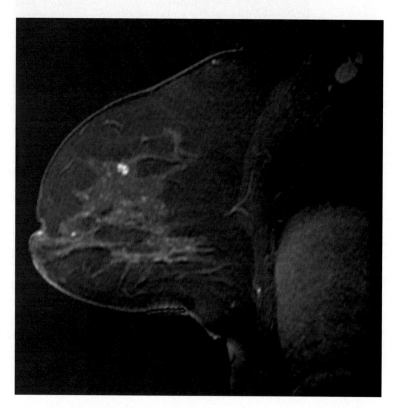

FIGURE 25.5. A 66-year-old with bilateral calcifications and right breast mass proved to represent invasive ductal carcinoma. Left breast MRI showed two small masses (one shown) which were not seen on ultrasound and localized under MRI guidance yielding fibroadenoma.

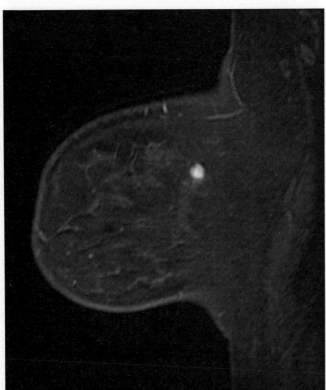

A

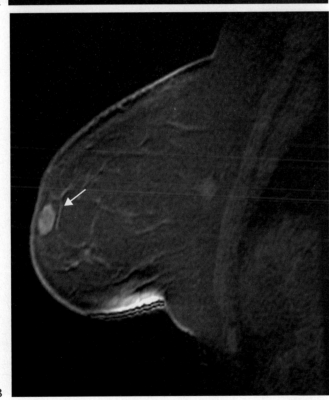

B

FIGURE 25.6. A 35-year-old woman with history of Hodgkin's disease and thyroid cancer undergoes screening MRI. (A) Post-contrast T1-weighted image demonstrates an irregular mass that proved to be a myxomatous fibroadenoma on ultrasound biopsy. (B) Nonenhancing well-circumscribed mass (arrow) that is intermediate signal on precontrast T1-weighted image that was proven to represent sclerotic fibroadenoma.

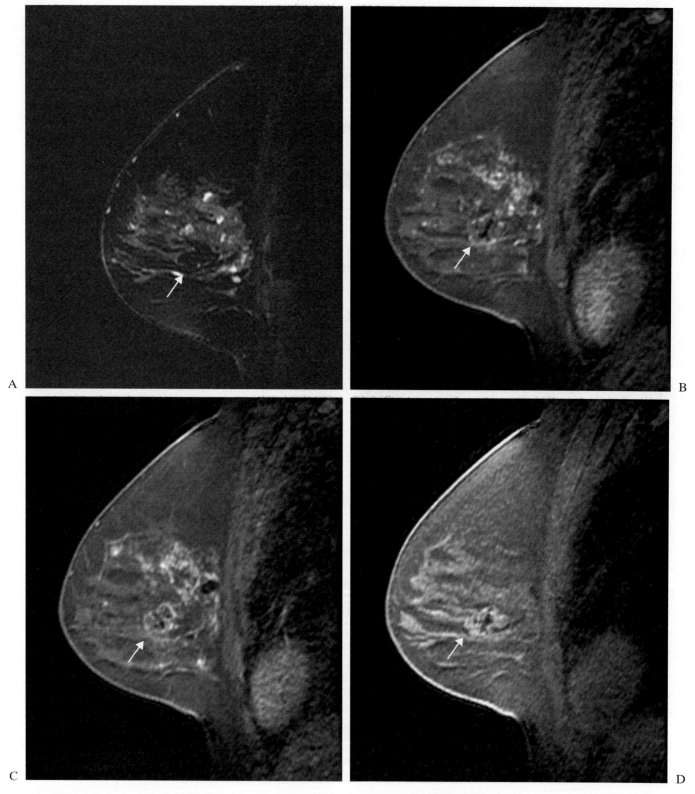

FIGURE 25.7. A 47-year-old woman with prior right lumpectomy for breast cancer. (A) In the lower breast a fibroadenoma was identified that corresponded to a mammographic finding that was stable for many years and characteristic for a benign calcified fibroadenoma. The mass is low signal on T2 (arrow). (B and C) Almost no enhancement is noted of the mass on the postcontrast images (arrows). (D) Precontrast image demonstrates central low signal that corresponded to the calcifications seen on the mammogram.

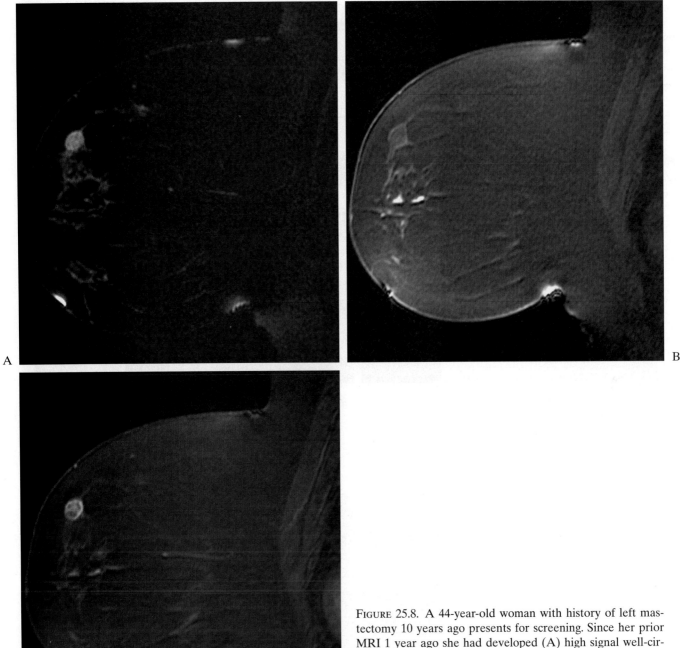

A

B

C

FIGURE 25.8. A 44-year-old woman with history of left mastectomy 10 years ago presents for screening. Since her prior MRI 1 year ago she had developed (A) high signal well-circumscribed mass on T2 that was evident on ultrasound and biopsied yielding fibroepithelial tumor. The mass was (B) isointense to breast parenchyma on the precontrast image and demonstrates (C) rim enhancement on the postcontrast image. Margins were smooth. Subsequent excision yielded cellular fibroadenoma, concordant with the MRI findings.

FIGURE 25.9. A 38-year-old woman 1 year following lumpectomy for invasive lobular carcinoma undergoes screening MRI. Mass identified that undergoes biopsy under ultrasound yielding fibroadenoma.

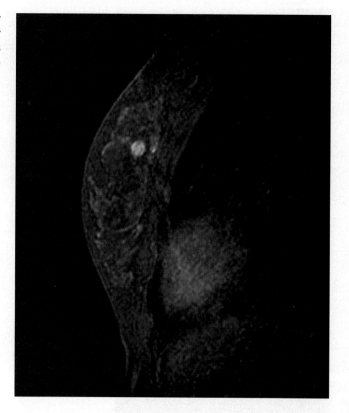

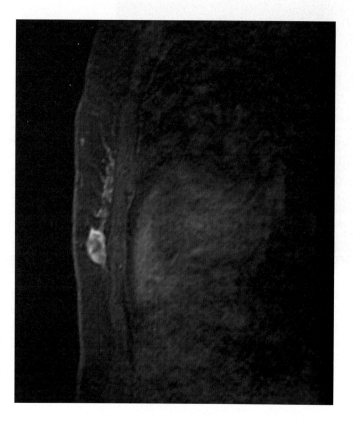

FIGURE 25.10. A 45-year-old woman with strong family history undergoes screening MRI. Several masses were identified (one shown) which underwent ultrasound guided biopsy yielding multiple fibroadenomas.

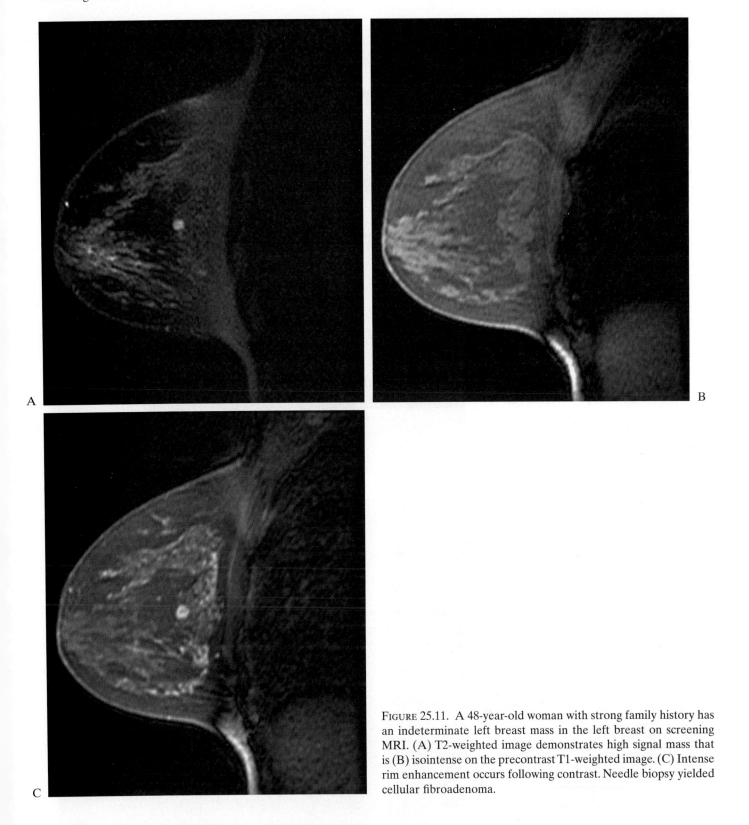

FIGURE 25.11. A 48-year-old woman with strong family history has an indeterminate left breast mass in the left breast on screening MRI. (A) T2-weighted image demonstrates high signal mass that is (B) isointense on the precontrast T1-weighted image. (C) Intense rim enhancement occurs following contrast. Needle biopsy yielded cellular fibroadenoma.

2. Cysts

2.1. Inflammatory

FIGURE 25.12. A 48-year-old woman status post left mastectomy and right reduction mammoplasty. Breast parenchyma is dense with cystic alteration. A small cyst in the posterior breast demonstrates rim enhancement (arrow).

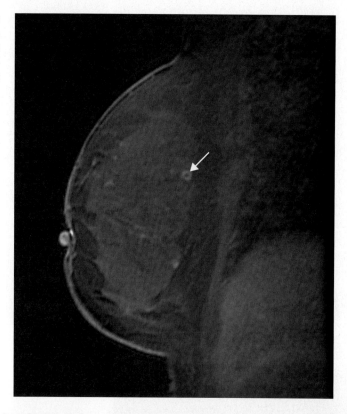

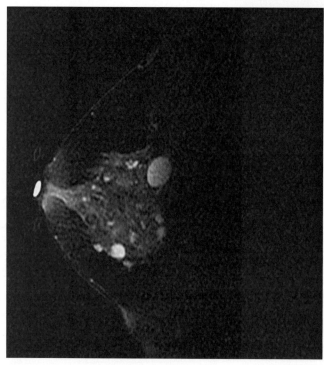

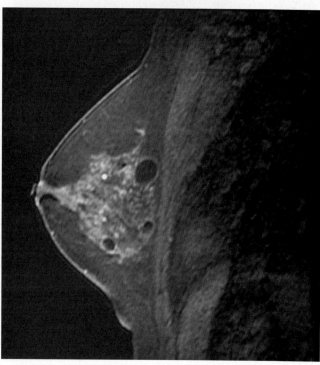

A

B

FIGURE 25.13. A 48-year-old woman with cervical carcinoma and a strong family history of breast cancer undergoes Screening bilateral MRI examination. The breast is extremely dense and cystic. (A) T2 weighted image documents multiple high signal cysts. (B) On the postcontrast images several of these enhance peripherally compatible with imflammatory cysts.

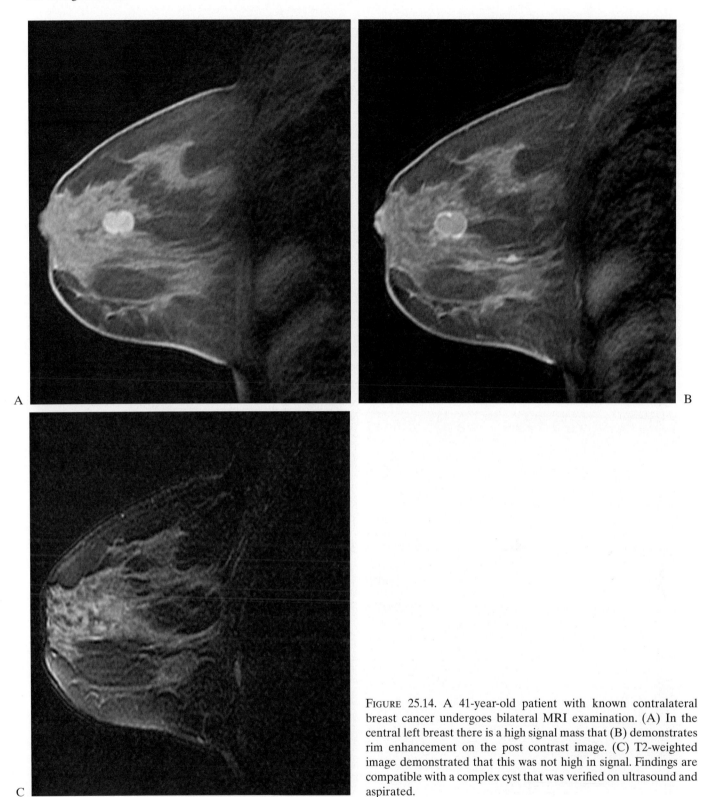

FIGURE 25.14. A 41-year-old patient with known contralateral breast cancer undergoes bilateral MRI examination. (A) In the central left breast there is a high signal mass that (B) demonstrates rim enhancement on the post contrast image. (C) T2-weighted image demonstrated that this was not high in signal. Findings are compatible with a complex cyst that was verified on ultrasound and aspirated.

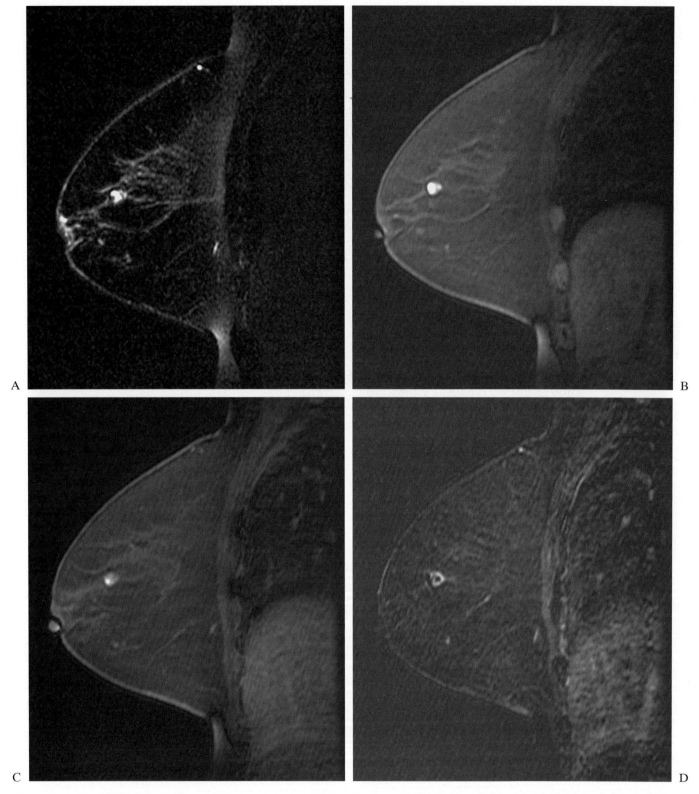

FIGURE 25.15. A 57-year-old patient with contralateral DCIS diagnosed on stereotactic biopsy performed for new calcifications. Magnetic resonance imaging performed for assessment of disease extent. (A) A high signal cyst is noted on T2-weighted image. (B) On the precontrast T1-weighted image this is high in signal. (C) Following contrast injection, rim enhancement is seen compatible with inflammatory changes. (D) Subtraction imaging confirms enhancement.

2.2. Fluid/Fluid Layer

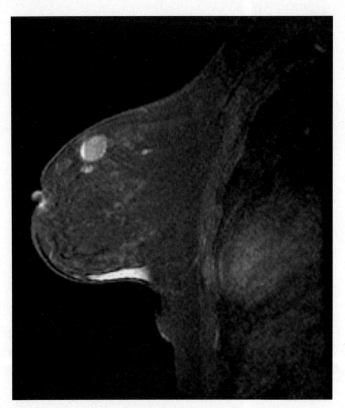

FIGURE 25.16. A 67-year-old woman with history of bilateral cysts on hormone replacement therapy now stopped for 3 months. Note fluid-fluid layer in dominant cyst superiorly in breast.

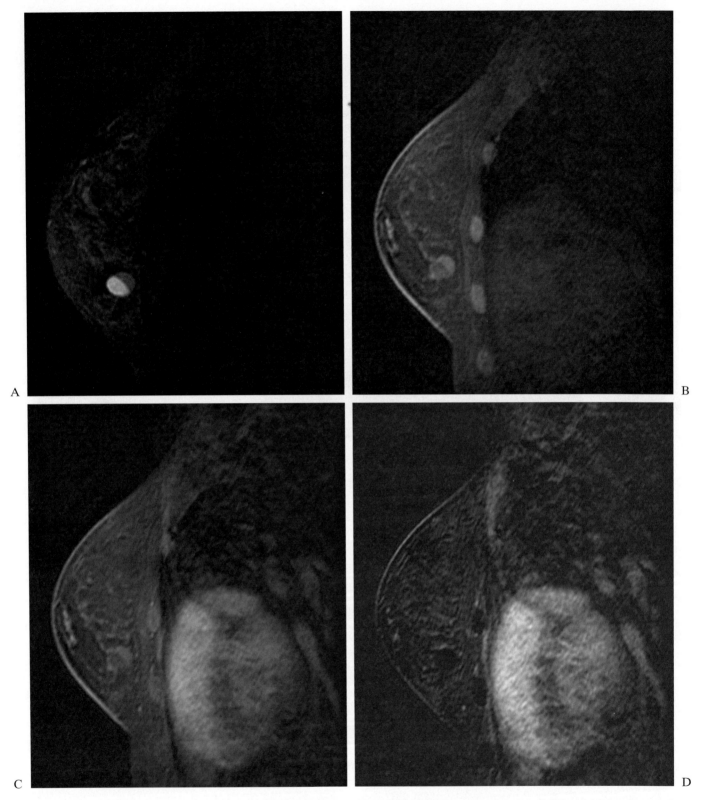

FIGURE 25.17. A 62-year-old woman with left breast DCIS status post re-excision with close margins. (A) T2 demonstrates a high signal mass with fluid fluid layer. (B) Pre- and (C) postcontrast T1-weighted images demonstrate slightly high signal mass that does not enhance as confirmed on the (D) subtraction image.

3. Lymph Nodes

3.1. Intramammary

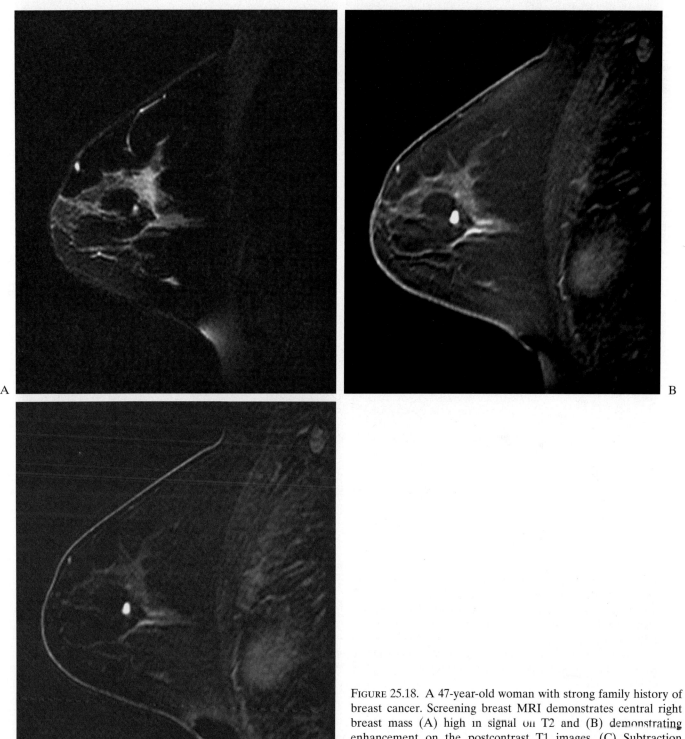

FIGURE 25.18. A 47-year-old woman with strong family history of breast cancer. Screening breast MRI demonstrates central right breast mass (A) high in signal on T2 and (B) demonstrating enhancement on the postcontrast T1 images. (C) Subtraction imaging confirms presence of enhancing mass. Ultrasound-guided fine needle aspiration was performed confirming impression of intramammary lymph node.

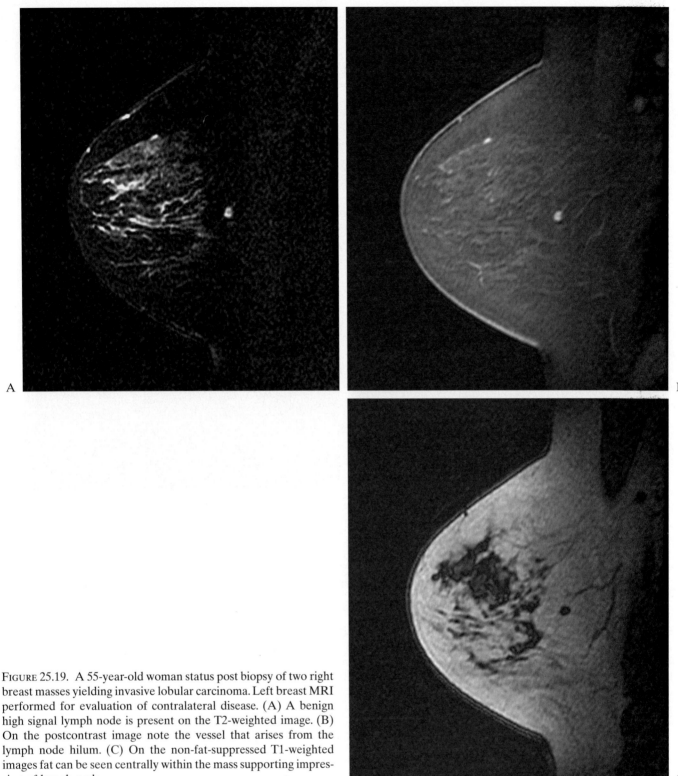

FIGURE 25.19. A 55-year-old woman status post biopsy of two right breast masses yielding invasive lobular carcinoma. Left breast MRI performed for evaluation of contralateral disease. (A) A benign high signal lymph node is present on the T2-weighted image. (B) On the postcontrast image note the vessel that arises from the lymph node hilum. (C) On the non-fat-suppressed T1-weighted images fat can be seen centrally within the mass supporting impression of lymph node.

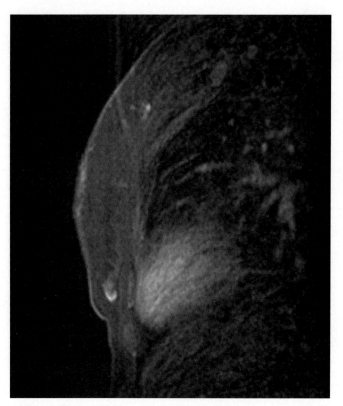

FIGURE 25.20. A 26-year-old woman with extremely dense breasts and palpable nodule in the left breast upper outer quadrant. In the posterior lower inner quadrant on postcontrast T1-weighted MRI a reniform mass is identified with radiating vessels compatible with lymph node.

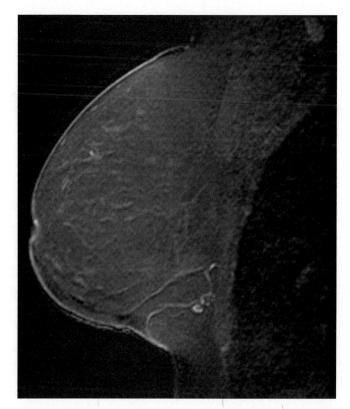

FIGURE 25.21. A 53-year-old woman status post right lumpectomy for poorly differentiated invasive mammary carcinoma with mixed ductal and lobular features. Magnetic resonance imaging demonstrates benign appearing lymph node in the posterior breast adjacent to the chest wall.

FIGURE 25.22. A 66-year-old woman with right breast carcinoma. Magnetic resonance imaging demonstrates reniform lobulated mass in the upper outer quadrant of the left breast that was high in signal on T2 and demonstrated washout kinetics compatible with a lymph node.

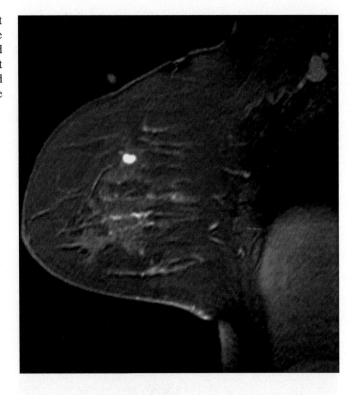

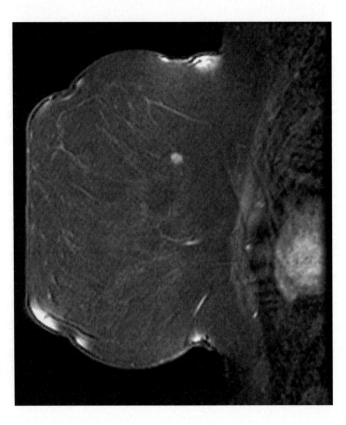

FIGURE 25.23. A 51-year-old woman with right breast carcinoma. Benign intramammary lymph node identified on MRI performed for staging.

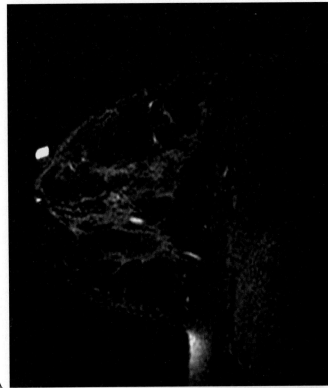

A

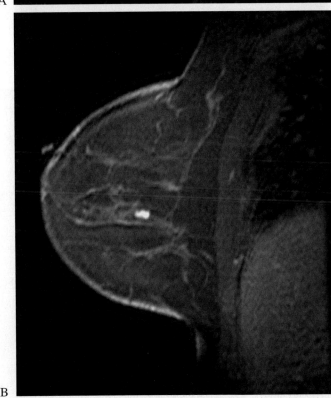

B

FIGURE 25.24. A 44-year-old woman with family history of breast cancer as well as multiple other cancers. Screening MRI protocol patient. Lymph node in an uncharacteristic location (central breast) and with uncharacteristic appearance. (A) MRI demonstrates lobulated oblong mass with high signal on T2 and (B) strong enhancement with washout characteristic of a lymph node. Subsequent mammogram 9 months following MRI showed development of 1.5-cm linear calcifications in a different quadrant of the breast that proved to represent DCIS at stereotactic biopsy.

3.2. Axillary

FIGURE 25.25. A 43-year-old woman status post left lumpectomy 2 years ago yielding invasive ductal carcinoma with axillary metastases. Patient now presents with palpable right axillary adenopathy. Fine needle aspiration yielded adenocarcinoma resembling the prior contralateral carcinoma. Magnetic resonance imaging documents presence of enlarged irregular heterogeneous node without fatty hilum compatible with metastatic involvement.

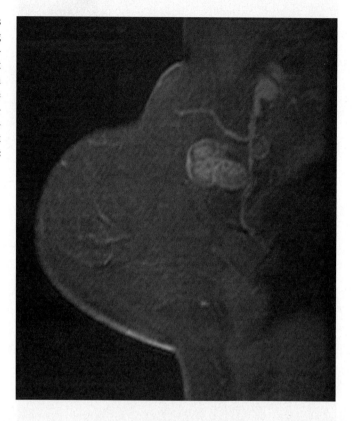

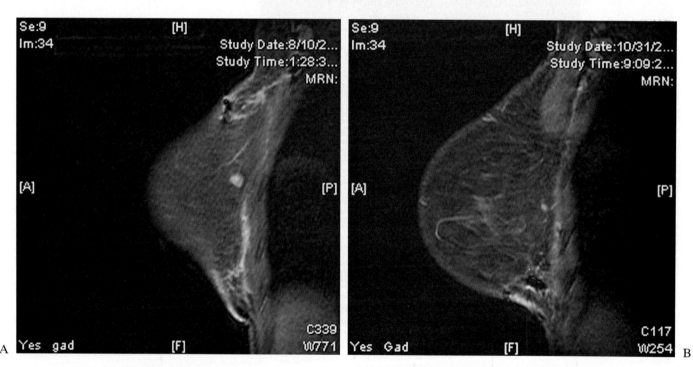

FIGURE 25.26. A 49-year-old woman who underwent biopsy for a palpable abnormality yielding invasive ductal carcinoma with positive margins. MRI performed to assess residual disease. No residual disease was noted. (A) Incidental note was made on the initial post operative MRI examination of a prominent lymph node, likely reactive from the recent surgery in the breast. (B) A follow up examination one year later demonstrates marked decrease in size of the lymph node compatible with reactive node.

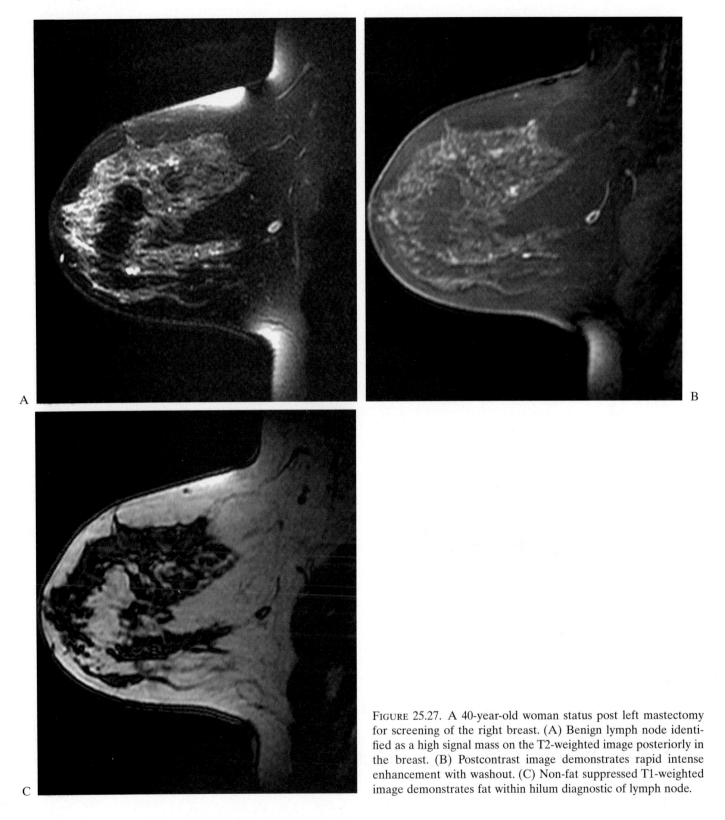

FIGURE 25.27. A 40-year-old woman status post left mastectomy for screening of the right breast. (A) Benign lymph node identified as a high signal mass on the T2-weighted image posteriorly in the breast. (B) Postcontrast image demonstrates rapid intense enhancement with washout. (C) Non-fat suppressed T1-weighted image demonstrates fat within hilum diagnostic of lymph node.

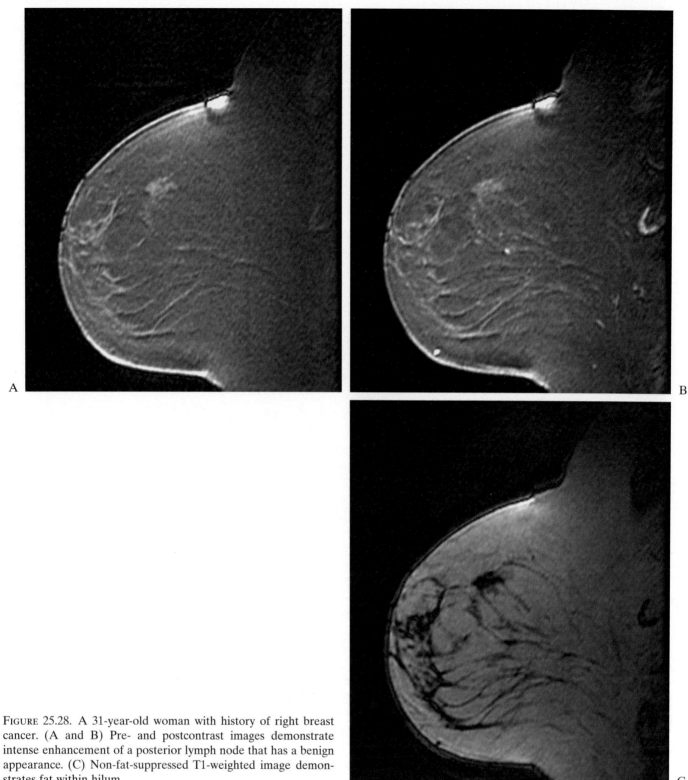

FIGURE 25.28. A 31-year-old woman with history of right breast cancer. (A and B) Pre- and postcontrast images demonstrate intense enhancement of a posterior lymph node that has a benign appearance. (C) Non-fat-suppressed T1-weighted image demonstrates fat within hilum.

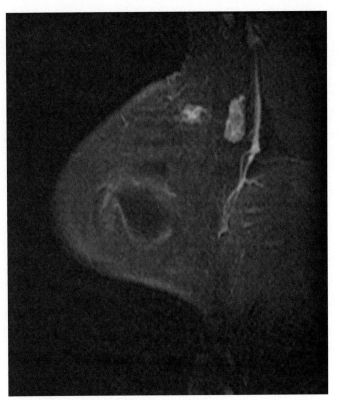

FIGURE 25.29. A 55-year-old woman with 20-year history of bilateral implants staus post removal with incidental invasive carcinoma found at time of removal. Subsequently patient underwent left mastectomy. Now presents with right axillary adenopathy. Axillary dissection yielded 24/25 positive nodes with extranodal extension. Magnetic resonance imaging demonstrates irregular lymph nodes suspicious for metastatic involvement.

3.3. Reactive

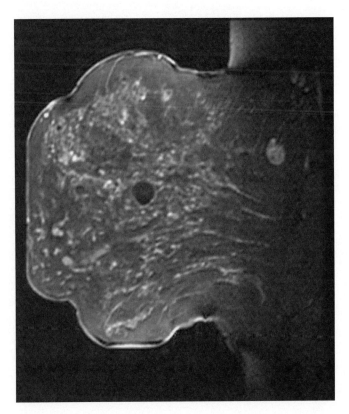

FIGURE 25.30. A 40-year-old with history of normal mammogram and normal physical examination presents with outside nuclear medicine scan suspicious for malignancy. Bilateral MRI demonstrated a mass in the right upper inner quadrant which was subsequently identified on ultrasound and biopsied yielding benign findings of fibroadenomatoid hyperplasia, fibrosis, cysts. Follow-up MRI examination demonstrates low axillary level I lymph node compatible with reactive node as follow up MRI demonstrated interval decrease in size. Breast parenchyma shows cystic changes with stippled enhancement.

FIGURE 25.31. A 58-year-old woman status
post left mastectomy 5 years ago now presents
with new right breast mass on mammography.
Ultrasound confirmed presence of mass and
biopsy yielded invasive ductal carcinoma histologic and nuclear grade III/III. Note that
location of carcinoma can be confused with
axillary adenopathy.

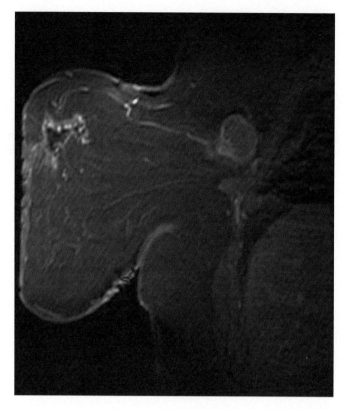

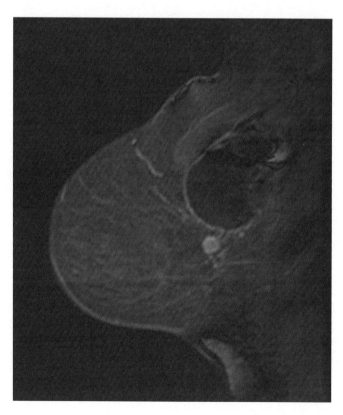

FIGURE 25.32. A 78-year-old woman status
post excision of poorly differentiated invasive
ductal carcinoma with close margins. Sentinel
lymph node biopsy also performed which was
negative. Enhancing mass identified next to
seroma cavity from sentinel node biopsy.
Ultrasound-guided biopsy demonstrated
benign lymphoid tissue with no evidence of
malignancy compatible with benign intramammary lymph node.

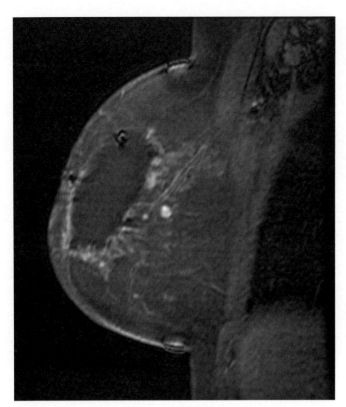

FIGURE 25.33. A 41-year-old woman status post excision of invasive lobular carcinoma. Magnetic resonance imaging performed to rule out residual disease. Magnetic resonance imaging demonstrates large postoperative seroma cavity with artifact from surgical clips. A 3-mm enhancing mass posterior to the seroma cavity was identified, which was confirmed on ultrasound. Subsequent biopsy yielded benign intramammary lymph node. Residual invasive lobular carcinoma (1.5mm) was found at re-excision.

4. Duct Ectasia

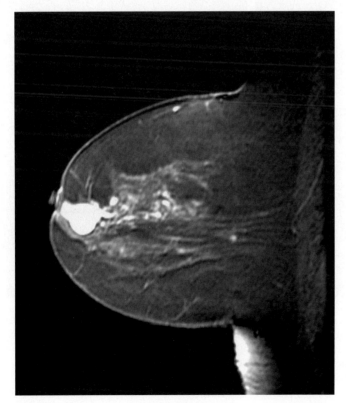

FIGURE 25.34. A 56-year-old woman with strong family history of breast cancer. Screening protocol study. Postcontrast fat-suppressed T1-weighted images show dilated retroareolar lactiferous sinus with high signal material likely representing proteinaeous or hemorrhagic debris.

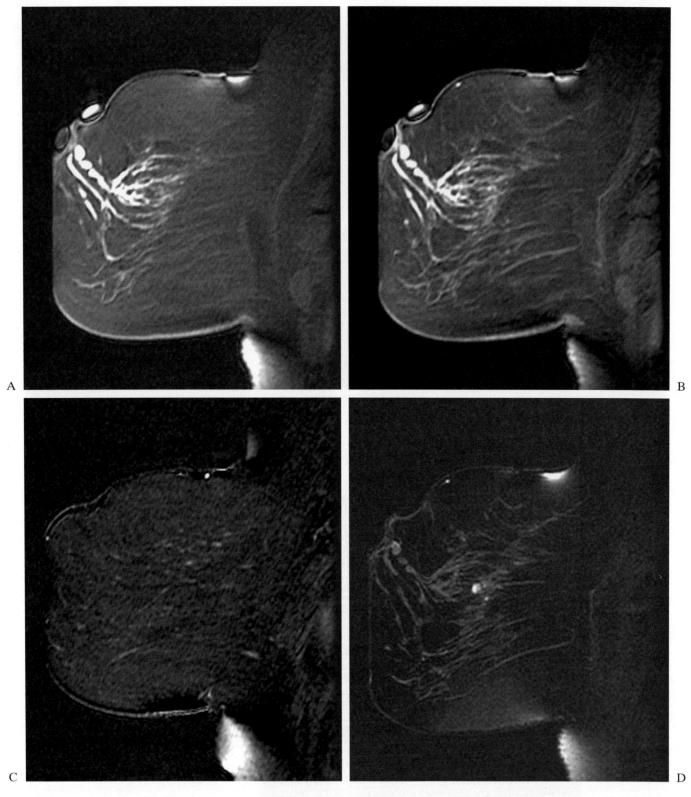

A

B

C

D

FIGURE 25.35. A 60-year-old high-risk patient with history of lobular carcinoma in situ (LCIS) and atypical duct hyperplasia. (A) High signal material is noted in dilated ducts that arborize in a segmental duct distribution on the precontrast image com-patible with duct ectasia. (B) Following contrast injection it appears that no enhancement occurs which is (C) confirmed on the subtraction views. (D) Corresponding T2-weighted image of duct ectasia.

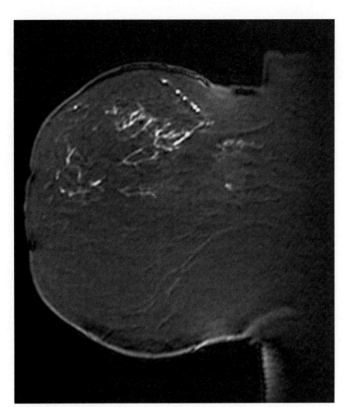

FIGURE 25.36. A 56-year-old woman with history of intraductal papillomatosis and atypia (precontract fat supressed T1-weighted images) demonstrates segmental dilation of a ductal system in the upper breast with high signal content.

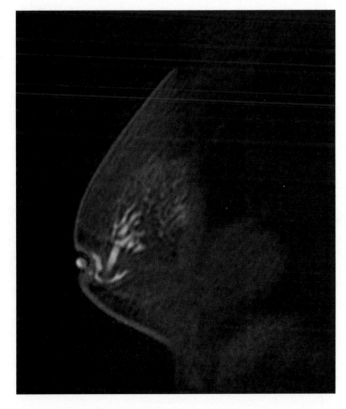

FIGURE 25.37. A 62-year-old woman with history of left breast DCIS. Retroareolar prominence of ducts is noted on screening MRI examination.

FIGURE 25.38. A 58-year-old woman with history of bilateral invasive ductal carcinoma. Maximum intensity projection demonstrates ductal dilation in the retroareolar region.

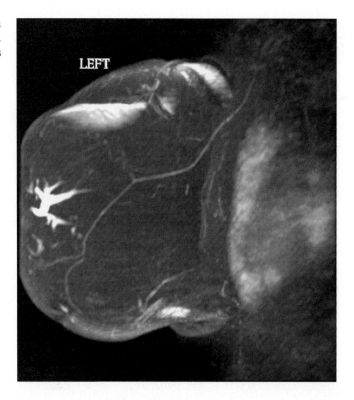

5. Papilloma

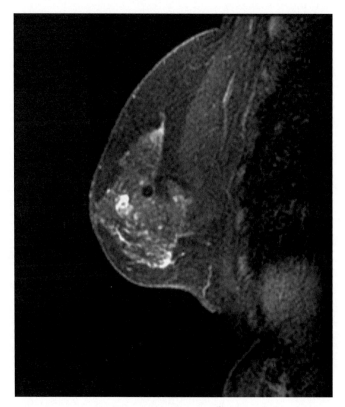

FIGURE 25.39. A 43-year-old woman status post left lumpectomy. Magnetic resonance imaging demonstrates irregular mass in the retroareolar region which was seen on ultrasound, biopsied percutaneouly yielding papilloma. Subsequent surgical excision demonstrated an 8-mm sclerosing intraductal papilloma.

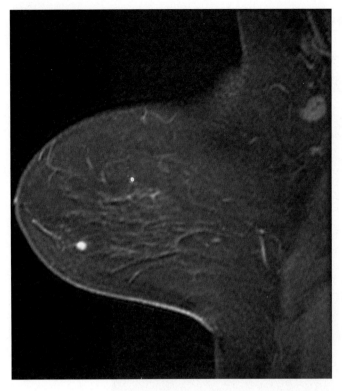

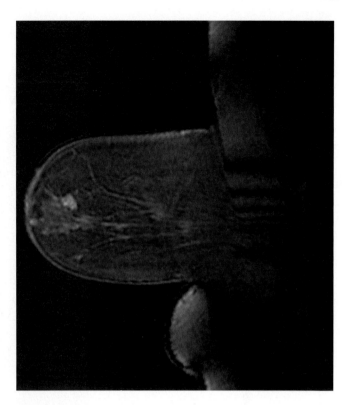

FIGURE 25.40. A 48-year-old woman status post left lumpectomy for invasive ductal carcinoma and DCIS 7 years ago. Magnetic resonance imaging demonstrates round homogeneously enhancing mass in the right breast that was identified on ultrasound and biopsied yielding papillary lesion with focal moderate ductal hyperplasia. Surgical excision was recommended due to the pathology and a 3-mm intraductal papilloma with biopsy site changes were found.

FIGURE 25.41. A 55-year-old woman with right breast carcinoma underwent staging MRI examination. Left breast demonstrated a suspicious mass that proved to represent intraductal sclerosing papillomatosis with florid duct hyperplasia.

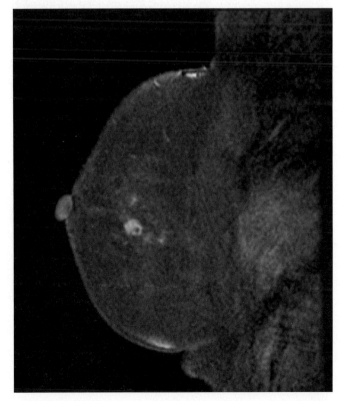

FIGURE 25.42. A 45-year-old woman presents with nipple discharge and negative mammogram. Magnetic resonance localization of the enhancing mass performed prior to duct excision. Mass corresponded to an intraductal papilloma.

6. Fibrocystic Changes

FIGURE 25.43. A 44-year-old high-risk patient with prior history of benign biopsy yielding atypical duct hyperplasia, radial scar, papilloma. Subsequent bilateral benign biopsies yielded benign findings including fibrocystic changes. (A) MRI demonstrates a dominant cyst on the T2-weighted image and (B) diffuse stippled enhancement throughout the remainder of the parenchyma.

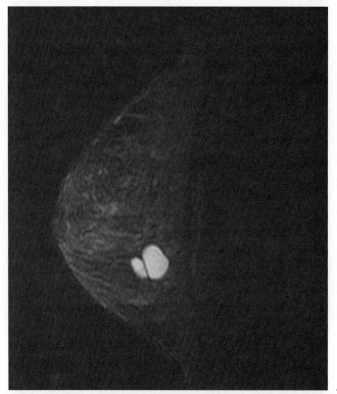

A

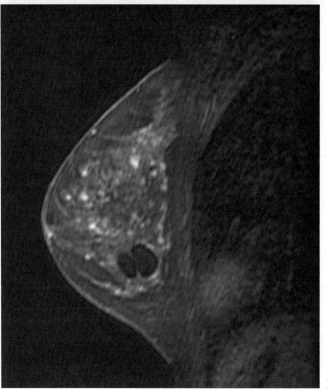

B

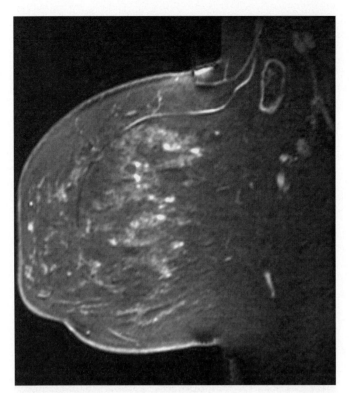

FIGURE 25.44. A 44-year-old woman with strong family history participating in screening study. Background stippled enhancement noted.

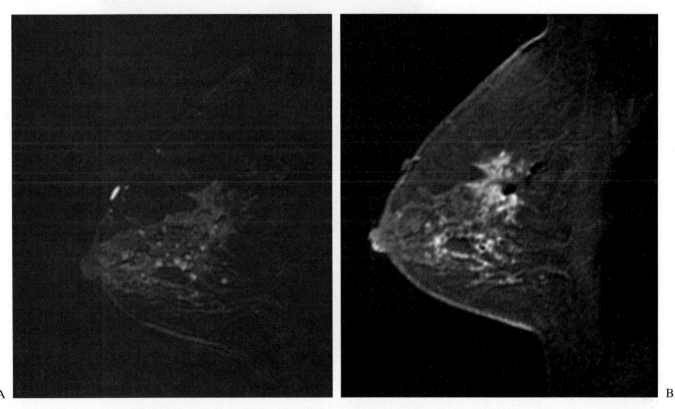

A   B

FIGURE 25.45. A 47-year-old woman with strong family history status post lumpectomy right breast and benign left breast biopsy (artifact from clip identified). (A) Multiple tiny high signal cysts are noted scattered throughout the breast parenchyma fat sup- pressed on T2 weighted imaging. (B) Patchy stippled enhance- ment on the post contrast fat suppressed T1 weighted image iden- tified compatible with fibrocystic changes.

FIGURE 25.46. A 52-year-old woman status post right breast excisional biopsy for invasive ductal carcinoma with positive margins. Magnetic resonance imaging performed for disease extent. (A) In the contralateral breast stippled enhancement is seen on the postcontrast fat-suppressed T1-weighted images. (B) Cysts are seen on the fat-suppressed T2-weighted images.

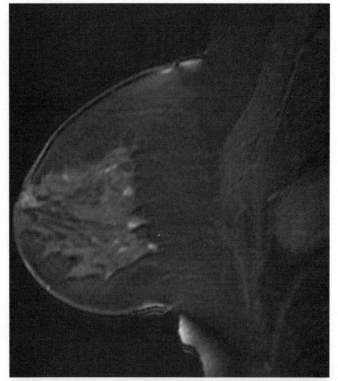

A

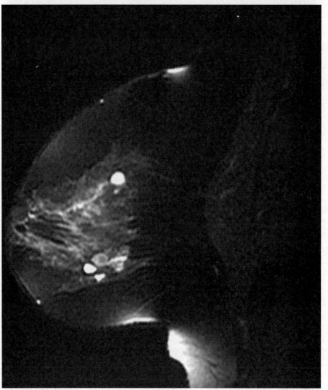

B

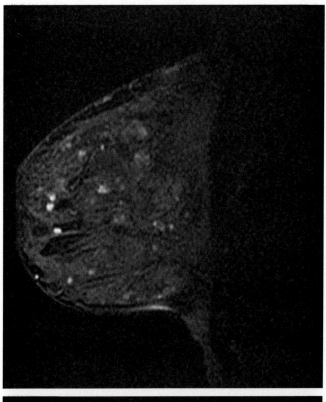

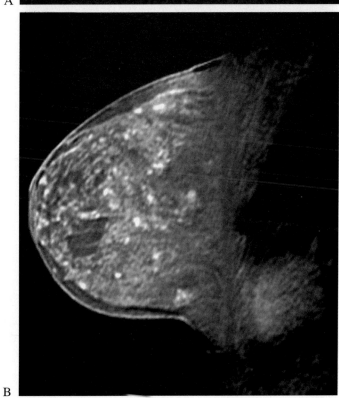

FIGURE 25.47. A 47-year-old status post multiple fine needle aspirations for bilateral cysts and excisional bipsy yielding ductal hyperplasia. Strong family history. (A) Breast are extremely dense with multiple cysts, seen on T2-weighted image. (B) Following contrast injection, stippled enhancement is seen.

A

B

FIGURE 25.48. A 40-year-old woman status post bilateral benign biopsies yielding focal LCIS on the left and fibroadenomas on the right. Presents for screening MRI. (A) Dense breasts demonstrate cysts on fat suppressed T2-weighted image. (B) Stippled enhancement noted on the post contrast fat suppressed image.

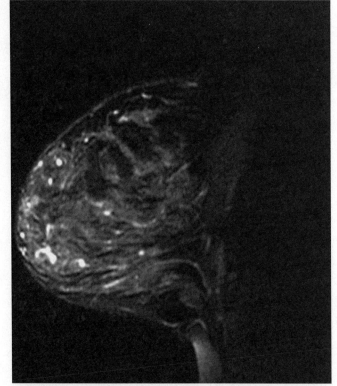

A

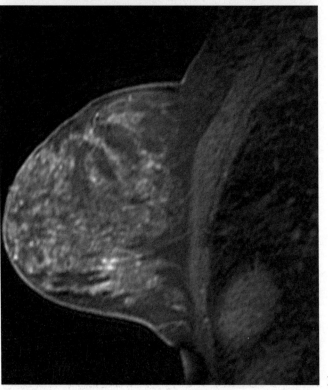

B

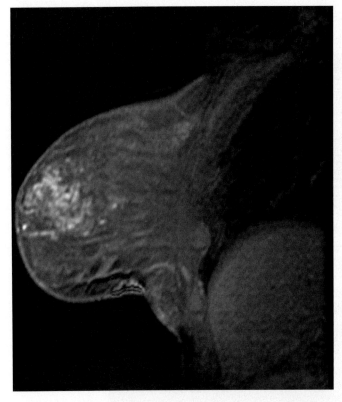

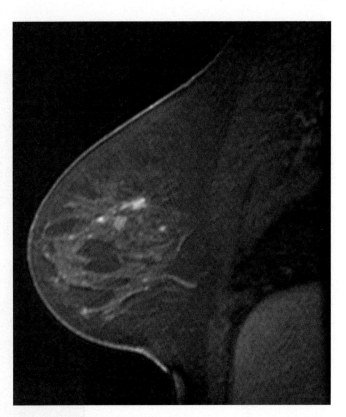

FIGURE 25.49. A 46-year-old woman with history of DCIS and LCIS in the left breast and palpable right breast lesion. Corresponding to the area of palpable abnormality is a regional area of stippled enhancement that was recommended for biopsy. Magnetic resonance vacuum biopsy yielded fibrocystic changes including ductal hyperplasia, sclerosing adenosis, fibrosis, apocrine metaplasia, and cysts.

FIGURE 25.50. A 46-year-old woman status post stereotactic biopsy of the left breast yielding DCIS. Contralateral right breast at MRI examination demonstrates clumped enhancement florid proliferative changes including sclerosing intraductal papillomas and microscopic radial scars.

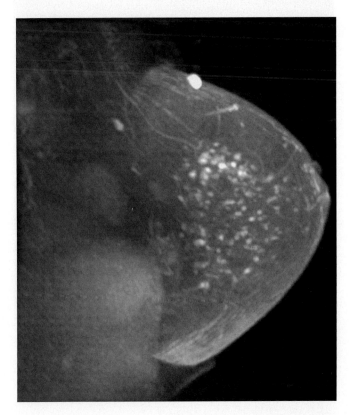

FIGURE 25.51. Maximum intensity projection (MIP) of benign stippled enhancement in a dense breast.

7. Abscess

FIGURE 25.52. A 55-year-old woman noticed lump in right breast upper outer quadrant. Mammography showed a 2.5-cm spiculated mass that was biopsied 2 months ago yielding invasive ductal carcinoma and DCIS. Patient presents with an inflamed breast and fluid collection that was aspirated yielding inflammation without malignancy. Magnetic resonance imaging performed to assess for residual or recurrent disease. (A) MRI demonstrates large septated mass with surrounding edema on T2-weighted image. (B) The abscess enhances peripherally on the postcontrast T1-weighted images but there is no evidence of gross residual or recurrent disease.

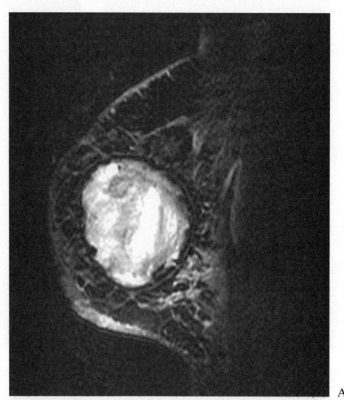

A

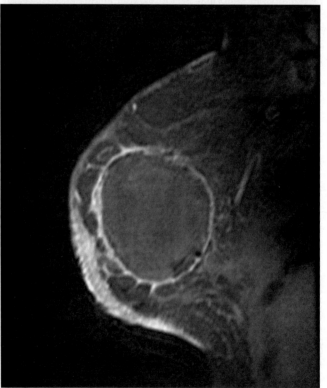

B

8. Duct Hyperplasia

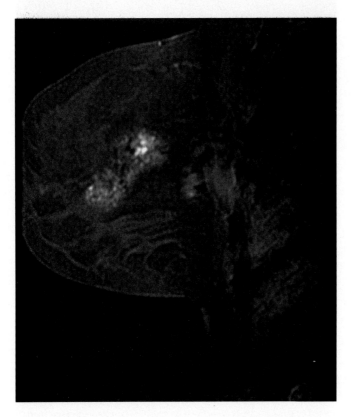

FIGURE 25.53. A 36-year-old woman with palpable lump in the upper outer quadrant of the left breast. Mammogram demonstrates dense breast tissue with no focal finding. Magnetic resonance imaging shows patchy enhancement that demonstrates plateau kinetics corresponding to the palpable abnormality. Biopsy yielded benign breast tissue with ductal hyperplasia without atypia.

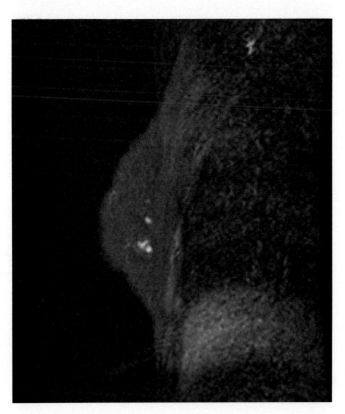

FIGURE 25.54. A 46-year-old woman with strong family history underwent screening MRI. Irregular enhancement in the lower inner quadrant was noted with plateau kinetics. At MR localization and biopsy this was proven to represent duct hyperplasia.

FIGURE 25.55. A 42-year-old woman with peri-incisional fullness following benign excisional biopsy. Magnetic resonance imaging was performed to evaluate excisional site. Elsewhere in the breast a small focus of enhancement was identified which underwent MR needle localization and surgical excision yielding ductal hyperplasia.

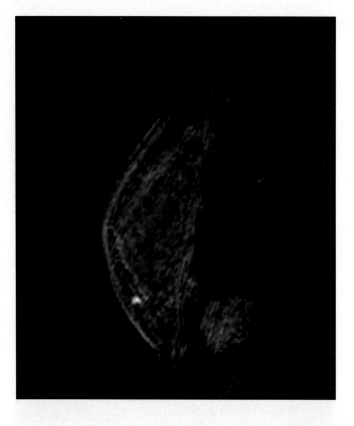

FIGURE 25.56. A 54-year-old woman status post aspiration of a 1-cm irregular mass in the 5 o'clock axis of the left breast yielding adenocarcinoma. The area was localized under ultrasound however surgical excision disclosed atypical ductal hyperplasia without evidence of needle tract. Magnetic resonance imaging performed to assess for residual suspicious mass. Magnetic resonance imaging showed suspicious enhancement in the superior breast away from the biopsy site (not shown). This was localized and demonstrated florid ductal hyperplasia without atypia.

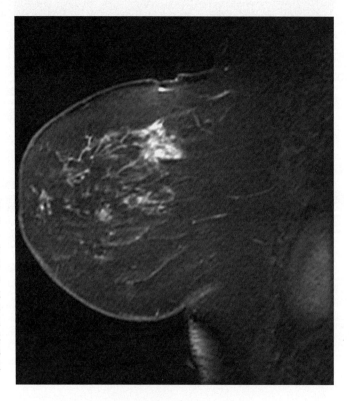

9. Sclerosing Adenosis

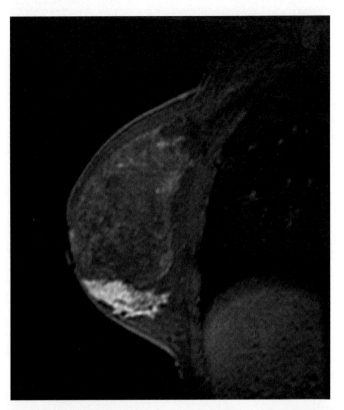

FIGURE 25.57. A 33-year-old woman with stage III ovarian dysgerminoma. Family history of breast cancer. Magnetic resonance imaging performed for screening demonstrates homogeneous regional enhancement in the lower breast. Magnetic resonance vacuum biopsy demonstrated florid sclerosing adenosis, radial sclerosing lesions, and stromal fibrosis. Surgical excision was recommended which confirmed the benign histology.

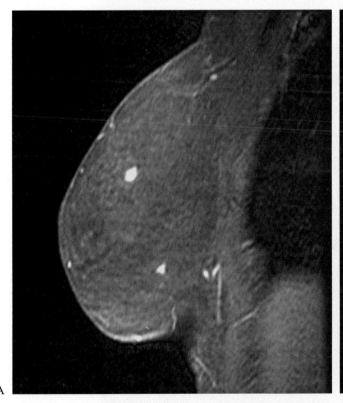

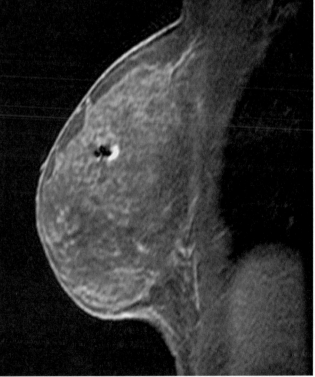

A   B

FIGURE 25.58. A 51-year-old high risk woman with history of atypical duct hyperplasia at benign biopsy underwent screening MRI. (A) An oval smooth homogeneously enhancing mass in the superior breast was identified exhibiting plateau kinetics. Biopsy was recommended. Ultrasound failed to demonstrate a correlate. As this examination was performed prior to MR biopsy capability, (B) MR needle localization was performed. Pathology yielded sclerosing adenosis and stromal fibrosis.

10. Adenomyoepithelioma

FIGURE 25.59. A 52-year-old woman with contralateral DCIS undergoes staging MRI examination that demonstrated enhancing 8-mm mass in the central breast (arrow) that underwent biopsy under ultrasound guidance yielding adenomyoepithelioma.

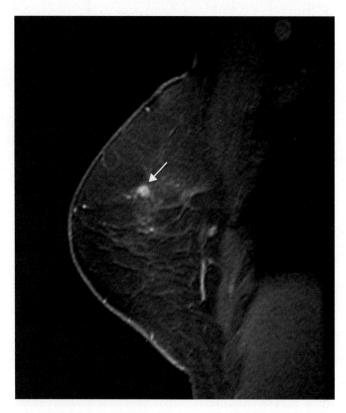

11. Fibrosis

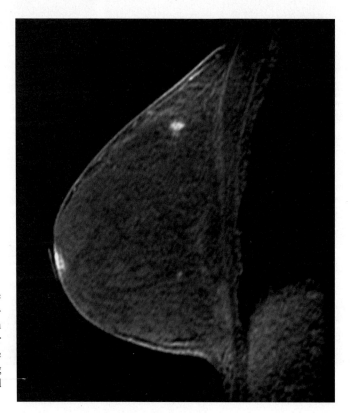

FIGURE 25.60. A 39-year-old gene-positive patient with extremely dense breasts undergoes screening MRI which demonstrates an irregular enhancing mass in the superior breast. Directed ultrasound found a correlate which was biopsied percutaneously yielding fibrosis. Excisional biopsy was recommended to ensure benign results confirming fibrosis.

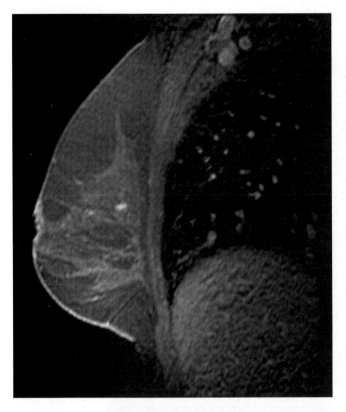

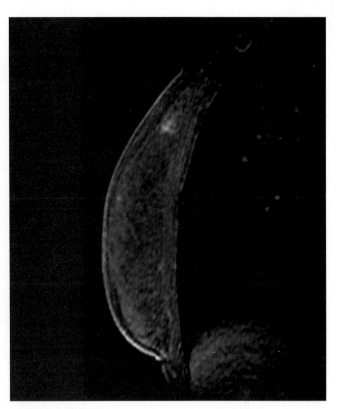

FIGURE 25.61. A 35-year-old woman status post mastectomy 3 years ago. Screening MRI demonstrates small irregular mass in the posterior breast with suspicious morphology but plateau kinetics. Biopsy yielded dense stromal fibrosis.

FIGURE 25.62. A 42-year-old woman with palpable abnormality in the 6 o'clock axis that underwent fine needle aspiration yielding findings suspicious for adenocarcinoma. Subsequent surgical excision showed benign findings at the aspiration site. Magnetic resonance imaging performed to exclude any suspicious findings. In the superior breast a small irregular enhancing mass was identified which proved to be fibrosis.

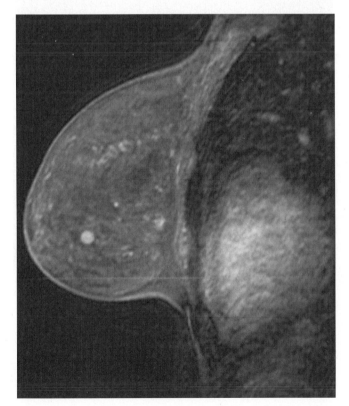

FIGURE 25.63. A 48-year-old woman presents with two palpable masses in the right breast that are proven to represent invasive ductal carcinoma. Magnetic resonance imaging performed for extent of disease. In the contralateral breast a homogeneously enhancing round smooth mass with plateau enhancement was identified. Due to the presence of contralateral disease this was considered suspicious and MRI-guided needle localization yielded fibrosis.

FIGURE 25.64. A 35-year-old woman status post mastectomy with (A) suspicious irregular mass identified on screening MRI of the contralateral breast. Due to continuous kinetics this was followed at 6 months without change in the findings. (B) At this time patient desired removal and fibrosis was found at surgery following MR needle localization.

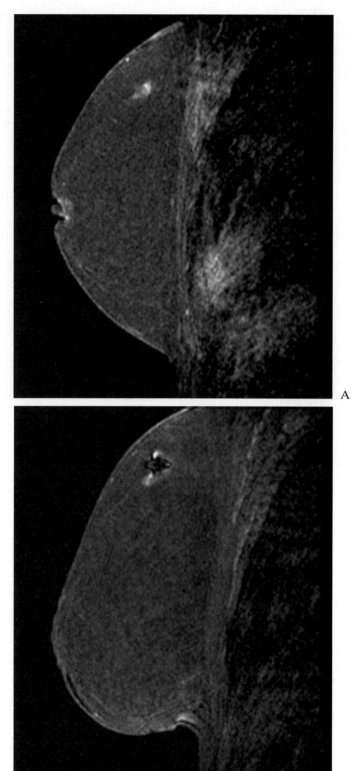

A

B

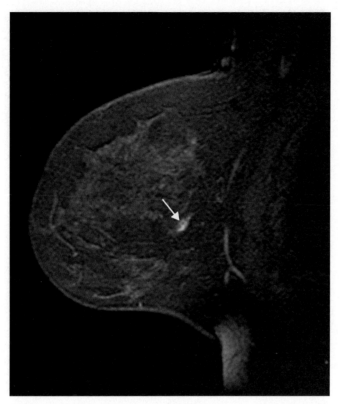

FIGURE 25.65. A 42-year-old woman status post right mastectomy with palpable thickening left breast. Mammogram and screening ultrasound were negative. History of prior benign biopsy in the lower outer quadrant yielding pseudoangiomatous stromal hyperplasia (PASH). Patient underwent surgical excision of the mass noted on MRI and the palpable thickening. The mass (arrow) yielded dense fibrosis and the palpable area yielded duct hyperplasia.

12. Pseudoangiomatous Stromal Hyperplasia

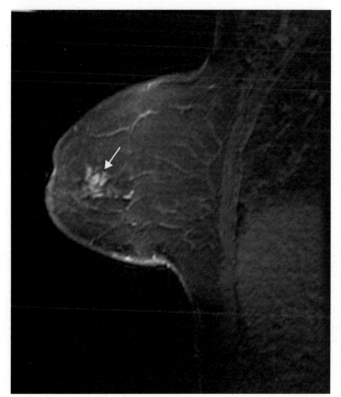

FIGURE 25.66. A 54-year-old woman with ovarian carcinoma and fibrocystic disease on hormonal replacement therapy, presents with abnormal screening MRI. Magnetic resonance imaging demonstrated progressive clumped enhancement (arrow) in the right breast and MRI needle localization was performed yielding PASH.

FIGURE 25.67. A 34-year-old woman with abnormal mammogram which demonstrates asymmetry. Breast MRI demonstrates a small enhancing mass in the posterior breast that proved to represent PASH.

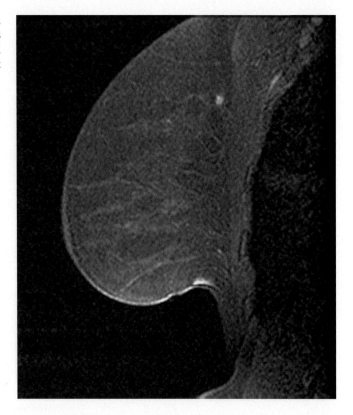

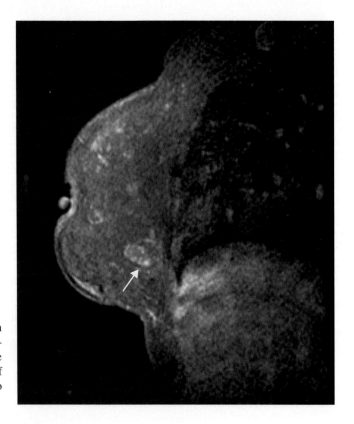

FIGURE 25.68. A 45-year-old woman with strong family history of breast cancer undergoes screening MRI examination. Breasts are extremely dense and there is a focal area of enhancement inferiorly (arrow) that proves to represent PASH.

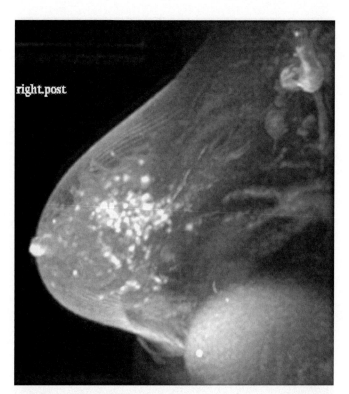

FIGURE 25.69. A 54-year-old woman status post contralateral mastectomy undergoes screening MRI which demonstrates regional clumped enhancement yielding PASH.

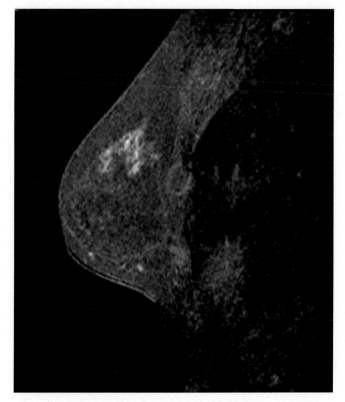

FIGURE 25.70. A 44-year-old woman status post right mastectomy for Paget's disease 13 years ago presents with new bloody nipple discharge. Magnetic resonance imaging shows a large area of enhancement in the upper breast that underwent excision yielding PASH and no carcinoma.

FIGURE 25.71. A 63-year-old woman with left breast density seen on one view. Magnetic resonance imaging confirmed the presence of a finding in the superior breast (arrow). Magnetic resonance localization and biopsy yielded PASH.

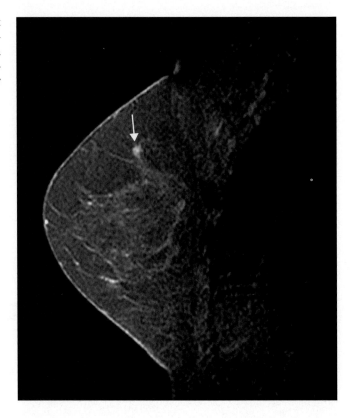

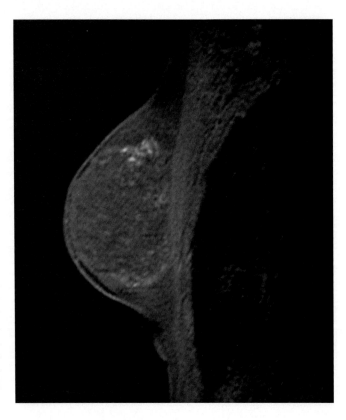

FIGURE 25.72. A 44-year-old woman with history of LCIS for high-risk screening. Magnetic resonance imaging demonstrates an irregular mass in the superior breast. Mammogram was dense without abnormality. No ultrasound correlate was identified. Magnetic resonance imaging guided needle localization demonstrated stromal fibrosis, PASH, adenosis, and apocrine metaplasia.

13. Skin Lesions

13.1. Sebaceous Cyst

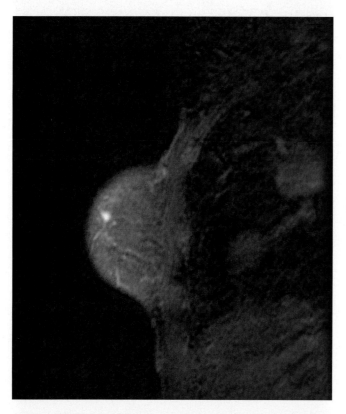

FIGURE 25.73. A 43-year-old woman had suspicious calcifications on baseline mammogram demonstrated to represent DCIS on stereotactic biopsy. The patient had conservation therapy and radiation therapy. Follow-up mammogram 1 year later showed new calcifications at the lumpectomy site demonstrated to represent recurrent DCIS. She was recommended for mastectomy and seeks a second opinion. No additional lesions were identified on MRI other than the recurrence at the lumpectomy site. Incidental enhancement of a cutaneous lesion demonstrated compatible with known sebaceous cyst.

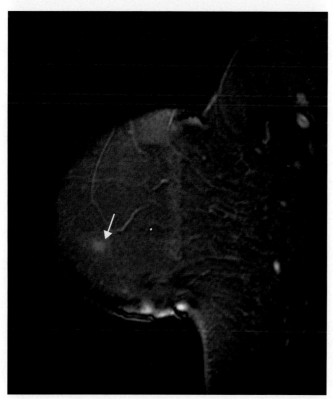

FIGURE 25.74. A 42-year-old woman with strong family history (sister diagnosed at age 27) status post bilateral reduction surgery. No suspicious areas of enhancement on MRI. Incidental sebaceous cyst noted (arrow).

13.2. Skin Thickening After Surgery

FIGURE 25.75. A 65-year-old woman status post excisional biopsy for a palpable mass yielding invasive lobular carcinoma. Post-biopsy changes are noted inferiorly in the breast. Incidental note is made of focal skin thickening (arrow) without enhancement compatible with postoperative changes.

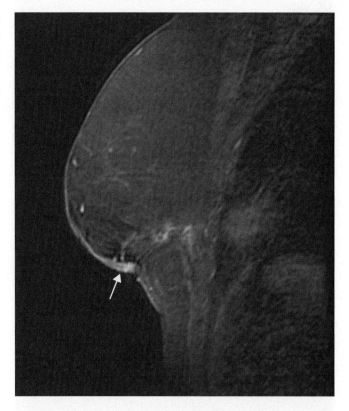

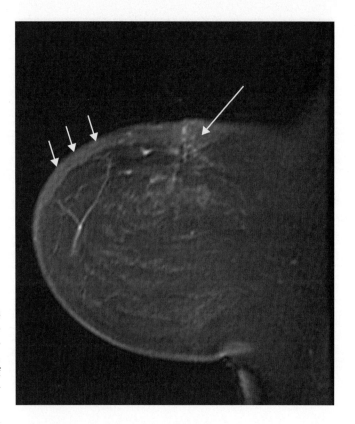

FIGURE 25.76. A 38-year-old woman status post lumpectomy for invasive lobular carcinoma 3 months ago with close margins. Undergoes MRI to assess for residual disease. Distortion is noted superiorly at the site of biopsy (long arrow). Note adjacent skin thickening (short arrows).

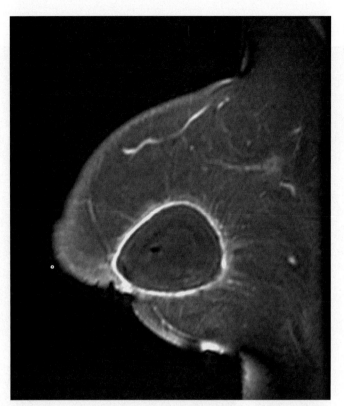

FIGURE 25.77. A 53-year-old woman status post lumpectomy for invasive lobular carcinoma with close margins. Magnetic resonance imaging performed for assessment of residual disease. Thin rim enhancement is noted around the seroma cavity. No bulky residual disease is noted. Note postoperative skin thickening.

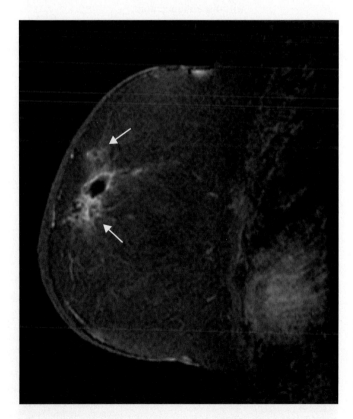

FIGURE 25.78. A 46-year-old woman status post excisional biopsy yielding intraductal papillary carcinoma. Magnetic resonance imaging demonstrates residual disease (arrows) surrounding the biopsy cavity. Skin thickening noted.

13.3. Skin Thickening After Radiation

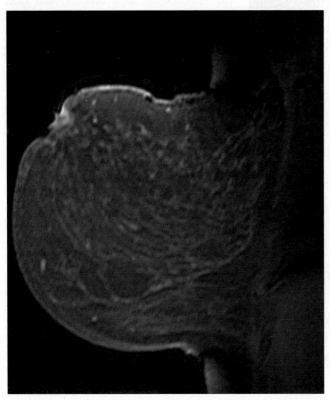

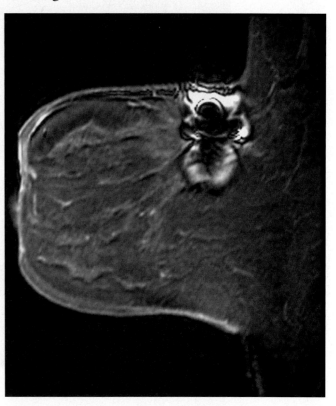

FIGURE 25.79. A 47-year-old woman with a history of locally advanced right breast cancer status post neoadjuvant chemotherapy with complete response. Superior retraction of the nipple is seen as well as skin thickening.

FIGURE 25.80. A 60-year-old woman status post left lumpectomy followed by radiation therapy with significant artifact from clips placed at lumpectomy. Note skin thickening in the anterior breast without enhancement.

14. Gynecomastia

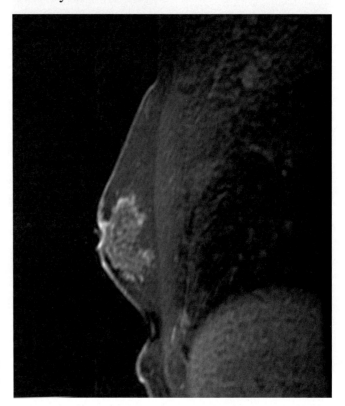

FIGURE 25.81. A 53-year-old man status post radical prostatectomy 4 years ago on hormone therapy with a rising PSA.

26
Findings Following Intervention

1. Excisional Biopsy

1.1. Immediate Sequelae Following Intervention

1.1.1. Clips

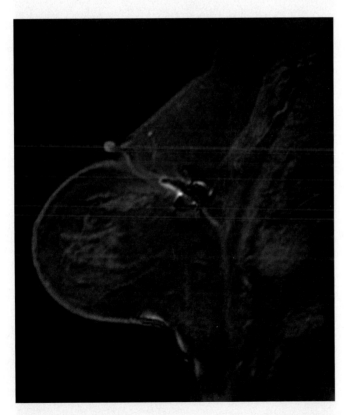

FIGURE 26.1. A 42-year-old woman status post lumpectomy 1 year ago for poorly differentiated breast carcinoma. Multiple clips are noted posteriorly at the lumpectomy site (marked with a cutaneous marker). Note scar extending to the skin.

FIGURE 26.2. A 45-year-old woman 1 year after lumpectomy for invasive ductal carcinoma well-to-moderately differentiated. Susceptibility artifact from titanium clips placed at the lumpectomy site is noted. Generally these are used to identify the lumpectomy site for boost radiation.

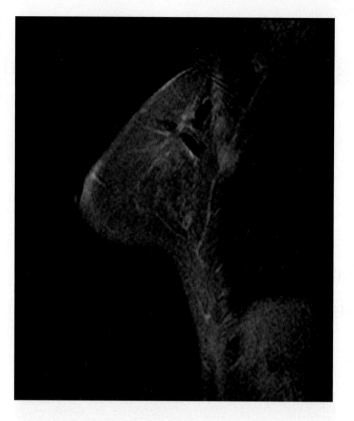

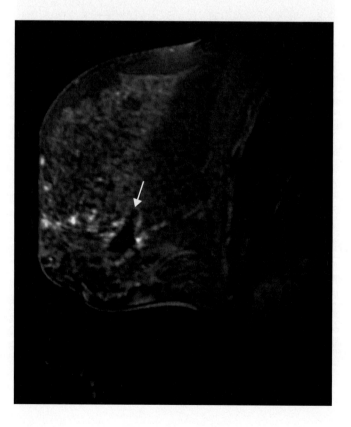

FIGURE 26.3. A 37-year-old woman with a palpable mass had a mammogram that demonstrated calcifications. These underwent stereotactic biopsy yielding ductal carcinoma in situ (DCIS) with microinvasion. Magnetic resonance imaging (MRI) performed following stereotactic biopsy. Note artifact from clip (arrow) and surrounding clumped enhancement in a ductal distribution that represented residual DCIS.

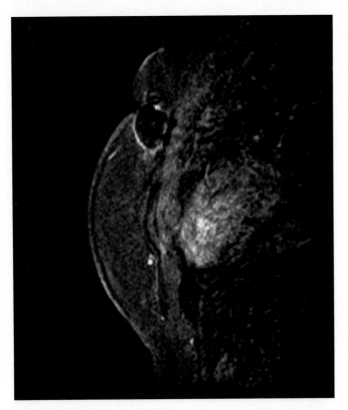

FIGURE 26.4. A 47-year-old woman underwent screening MRI that identified an occult carcinoma (not shown). Following excisional biopsy 2 weeks ago a seroma cavity is seen superiorly in the breast with associated susceptibility artifact from clips. Note thin rim enhancement that is an expected finding following recent surgery.

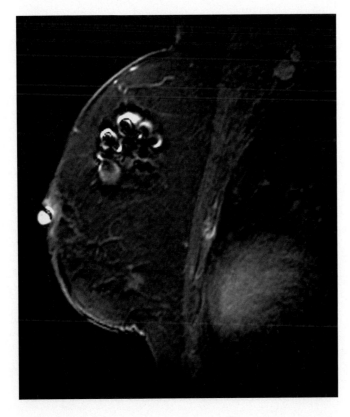

FIGURE 26.5. A 54-year-old woman 10 years following lumpectomy for moderately differentiated invasive ductal carcinoma. Abundant artifact from multiple clips is noted at the lumpectomy site limiting evaluation.

FIGURE 26.6. A 36-year-old woman status post lumpectomy for poorly differentiated invasive ductal carcinoma 1 year ago. Minimal enhancement is still noted at the surgical site with clips.

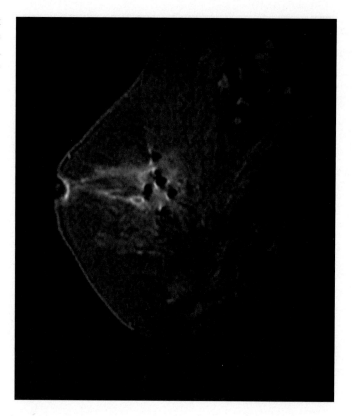

1.1.2. Hematoma and Seroma

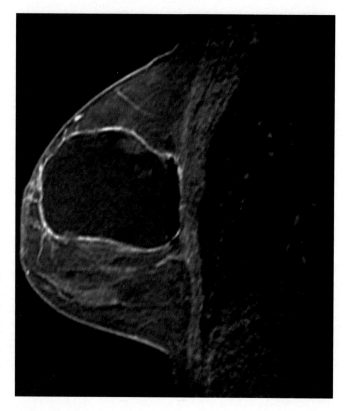

FIGURE 26.7. A 52-year-old woman following lumpectomy for invasive ductal carcinoma with close margins. Magnetic resonance imaging performed 3 weeks following initial surgery (performed elsewhere) to assess for residual disease. Note large postoperative seroma cavity with air-fluid level (patient is prone). Thin symmetric enhancement is noted surrounding the cavity.

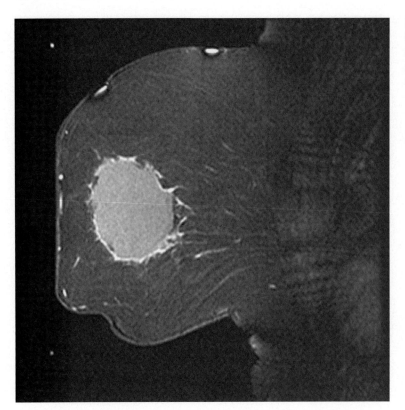

FIGURE 26.8. A 65-year-old woman 2 weeks following conservation for DCIS with positive margins. Magnetic resonance imaging demonstrates high signal postoperative collection with enhancement at the surgical margins.

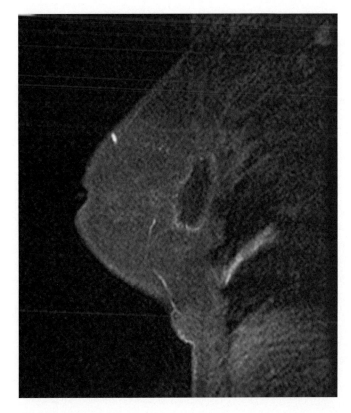

FIGURE 26.9. A 25-year-old woman 2 months following excision of calcifications yielding DCIS. Note the absence of enhancement surrounding the collection at the lumpectomy site.

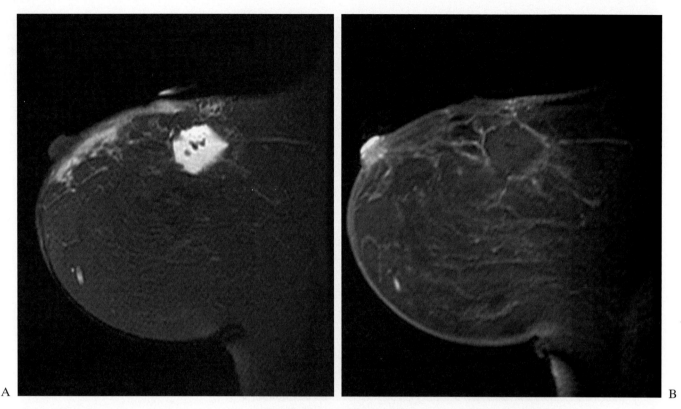

A   B

FIGURE 26.10. A 38-year-old woman status post lumpectomy 2 weeks ago for invasive lobular carcinoma with positive margins. (A) T2-weighted image demonstrates high signal postoperative collection compatible with seroma. Note high signal edema supe- riorly in the breast and adjacent skin thickening from the surgery. (B) No suspicious enhancement is noted on the postcontrast T1- weighted image. Note normal nipple enhancement.

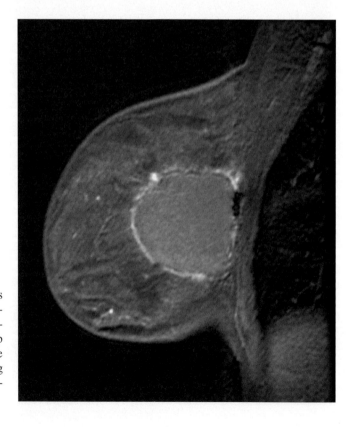

FIGURE 26.11. A 53-year-old woman status post surgery yielding invasive ductal carci- noma and LCIS. Margins were close. MRI per- formed 4 weeks following surgery. Note clip artifact along the posterior aspect of the seroma cavity. Nodular enhancement along the anterior surface was localized prior to re- excision and LCIS was found at pathology.

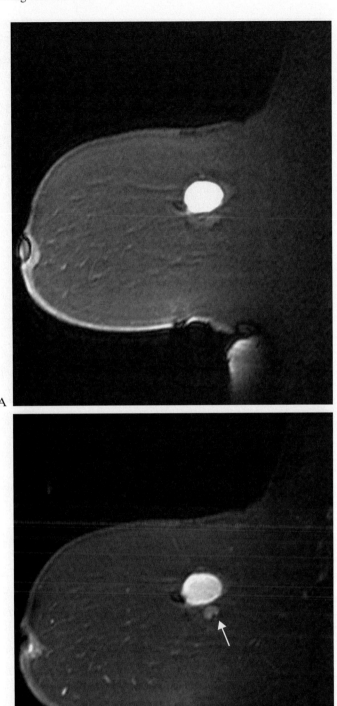

FIGURE 26.12. A 52-year-old woman 7 years following lumpectomy for DCIS. (A) Pre- and (B) postcontrast images demonstrate a chronic egg-shaped hematoma (confirmed on multiple prior mammograms) at the surgical site. Note adjacent enhancing lymph node (arrow).

FIGURE 26.13. A 47-year-old woman status
post lumpectomy for DCIS. (A) MRI performed 2 months following surgery demonstrates a postoperative seroma cavity. (B) MRI
performed 2 weeks later demonstrates interval
reduction of the seroma cavity without suspicious findings.

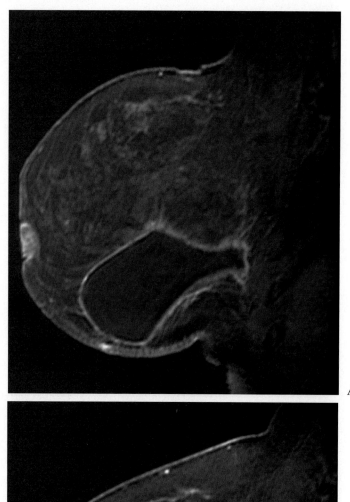

A

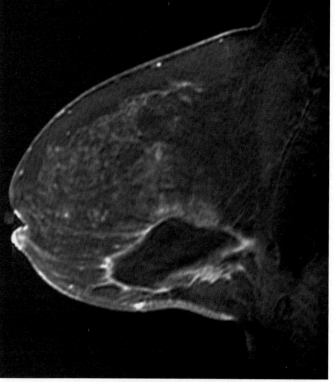

B

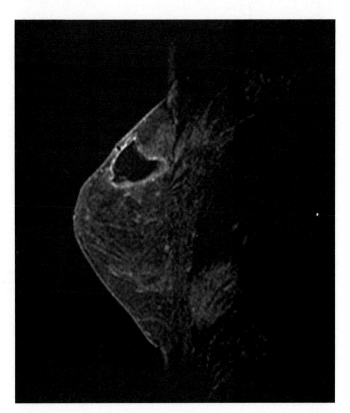

FIGURE 26.14. A 42-year-old with occult primary breast carcinoma metastatic to the axilla underwent excision of the primary in the upper breast with negative margins. Magnetic resonance imaging identifies a normal seroma cavity 3 weeks following excision.

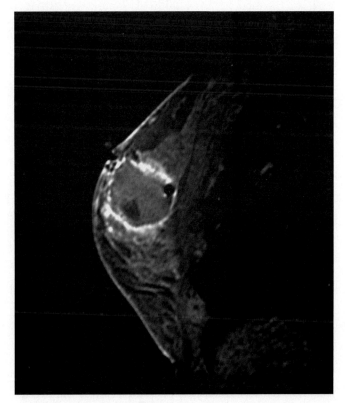

FIGURE 26.15. A 48-year-old woman with left breast invasive ductal carcinoma with close margins. MRI performed 2 weeks after surgery demonstrates postoperative collection with thick rim enhancement at the periphery. Re-excision demonstrated lobular carcinoma in situ (LCIS) but no residual malignancy.

FIGURE 26.16. A 68-year-old woman who was treated for breast cancer 6 years ago presents with new calcifications at the lumpectomy site. Excision demonstrated a few foci of intermediate grade DCIS. Patient refused mastectomy and MRI was performed to ensure the absence of any suspicious findings. Two weeks following surgical excision a large postoperative seroma cavity is noted with thin enhancement at the periphery of the cavity. No additional findings were noted.

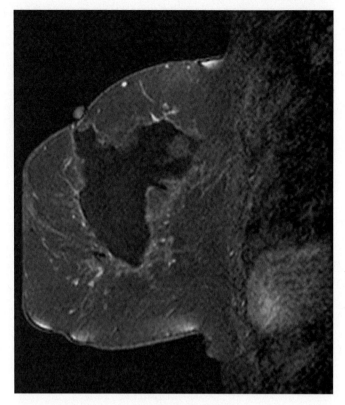

1.2. Delayed Sequelae

1.2.1. Fat Necrosis

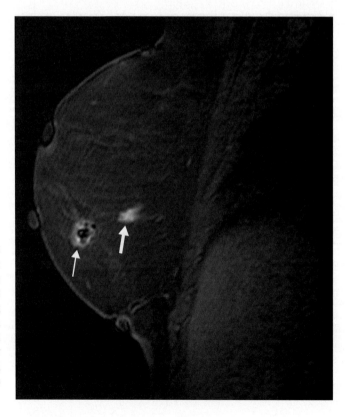

FIGURE 26.17. A 58-year-old woman with history of left mastectomy with reduction mammoplasty of the right breast. Note the reduction scar inferiorly is marked with a skin marker. In the lower breast a rim enhancing mass with central low signal is noted (thin arrow) and a more mass-like area (thick arrow) is noted posterior to this area. Biopsy of both yielded fat necrosis, hemorrhage, foreign body giant cell reaction, likely from the reduction surgery.

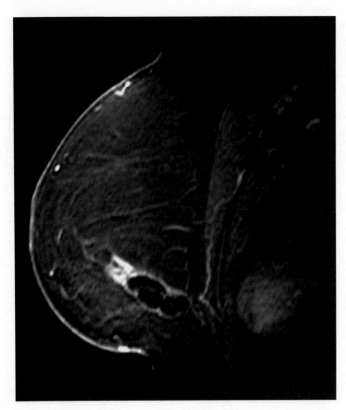

FIGURE 26.18. A 58-year-old woman status post bilateral reduction mammoplasty 5 years ago. Along the inferior surgical site, a rim-enhancing lobulated mass with central low signal is noted. Anterior to this region is a mass-like area of enhancement that demonstrated plateau kinetics. The low signal area was thought to be benign fat necrosis but biopsy of the mass was recommended. Pathology yielded fat necrosis, foreign giant cell reaction.

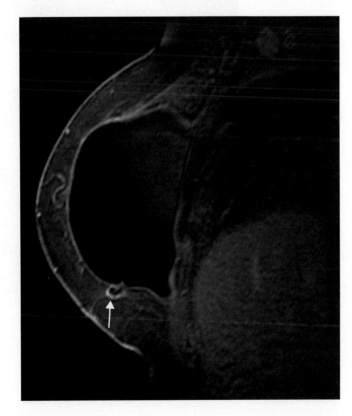

FIGURE 26.19. A 50-year-old woman status post lumpectomy inferiorly in the augmented breast. At the surgical site, rim enhancement of a low signal structure is noted compatible with fat necrosis (arrow).

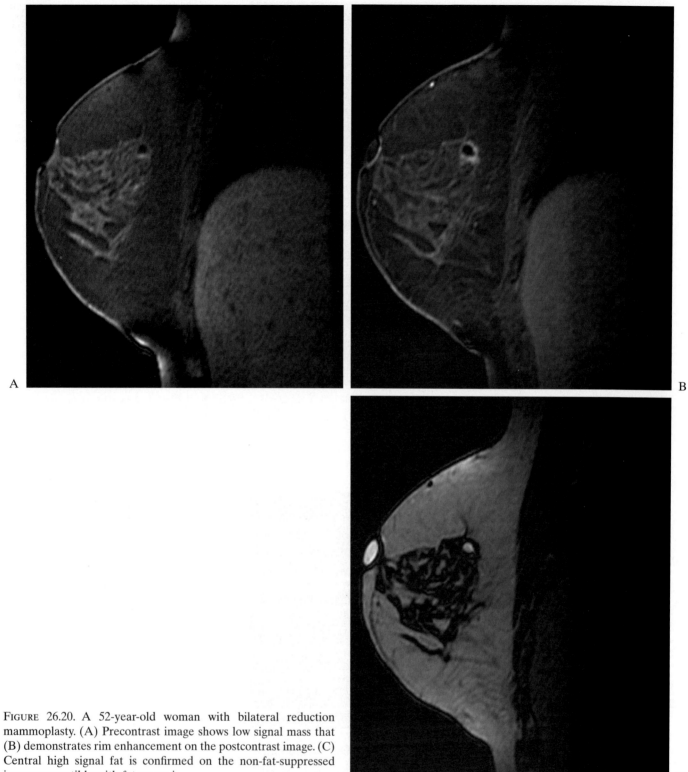

FIGURE 26.20. A 52-year-old woman with bilateral reduction mammoplasty. (A) Precontrast image shows low signal mass that (B) demonstrates rim enhancement on the postcontrast image. (C) Central high signal fat is confirmed on the non-fat-suppressed image compatible with fat necrosis.

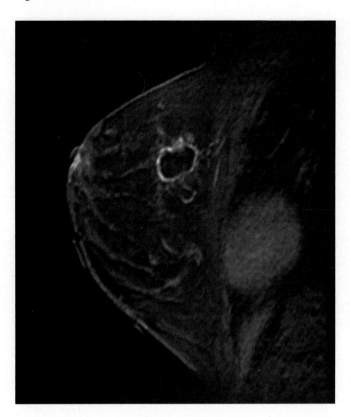

FIGURE 26.21. A 35-year-old woman status post bilateral reduction mammoplasty. Superiorly in the breast is a low signal mass with rim enhancement typical for fat necrosis. This was confirmed on the non-fat-suppressed image.

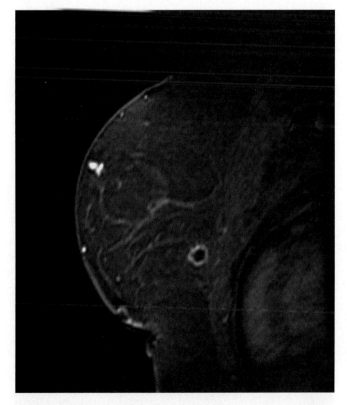

FIGURE 26.22. A 56-year-old woman status post bilateral reduction surgery and lumpectomy. Pathology was moderately differentiated in situ and invasive ductal carcinoma with close margins. Magnetic resonance imaging performed for residual disease assessment. Magnetic resonance imaging demonstrates a low signal intensity mass inferiorly in the breast with rim enhancement compatible with fat necrosis from prior reduction. Lumpectomy site (not shown) did not demonstrate residual disease.

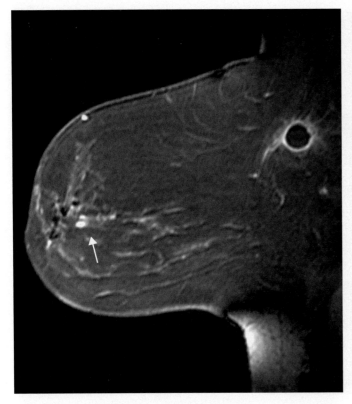

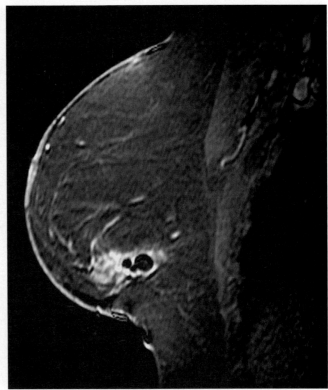

FIGURE 26.23. A 43-year-old woman with history of lumpectomy and sentinel node biopsy. In the axillary tail of the breast a rim-enhancing mass of low signal is seen marking the sentinel node biopsy site. Clips in the retroareolar region are present marking the lumpectomy site. Adjacent clumped enhancement (arrow) represents residual DCIS.

FIGURE 26.24. A 57-year-old woman following remote reduction breast surgery. Rim enhancing mass inferiorly corresponds to fat necrosis.

1.2.2. Nipple Inversion

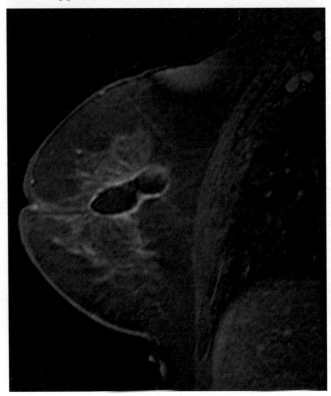

FIGURE 26.25. A 56-year-old woman with history of right breast cancer status post lumpectomy 2 years ago for invasive ductal carcinoma and DCIS. Recent re-excision at the lumpectomy site has been performed for suspicious palpable finding with benign results. Centrally in the breast there is a postoperative fluid collection with retraction of the nipple.

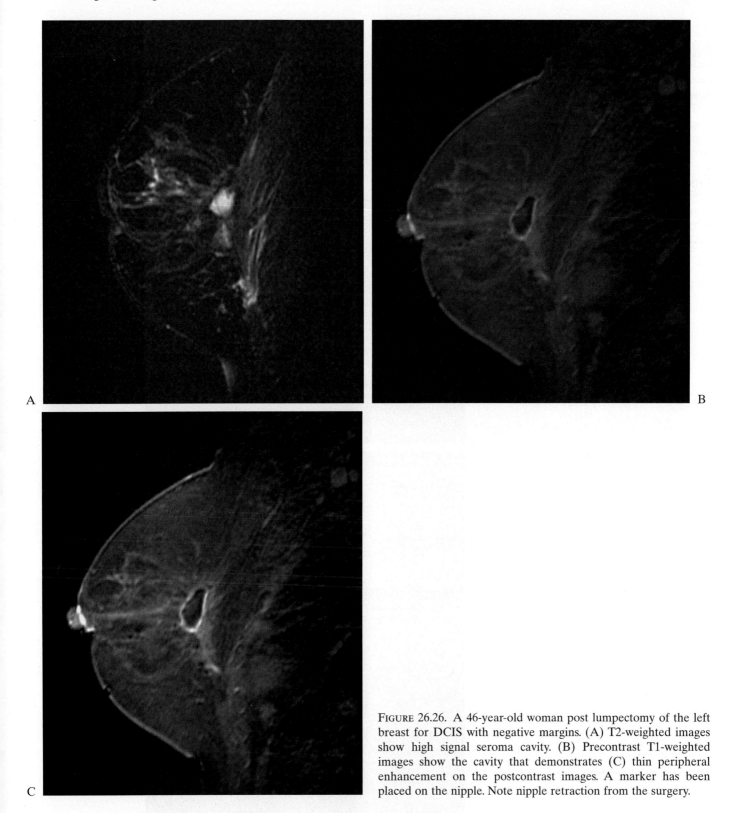

A

B

C

FIGURE 26.26. A 46-year-old woman post lumpectomy of the left breast for DCIS with negative margins. (A) T2-weighted images show high signal seroma cavity. (B) Precontrast T1-weighted images show the cavity that demonstrates (C) thin peripheral enhancement on the postcontrast images. A marker has been placed on the nipple. Note nipple retraction from the surgery.

1.2.3. Scar

FIGURE 26.27. A 55-year-old woman with bilateral silicone implants had breast MRI that demonstrated enhancement (not shown) not confirmed on mammography or ultrasound. Magnetic resonance localization and excisional biopsy demonstrated fat necrosis with no carcinoma. (A) Three months after surgery the scar resembles a spiculated mass. No seroma cavity was identified 3 months following surgery. (B) Follow-up MRI examination 6 months later demonstrates improvement of the postoperative changes with residual enhancement still noted.

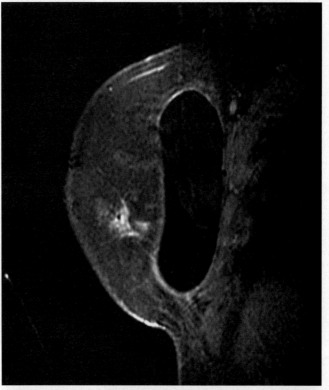

A

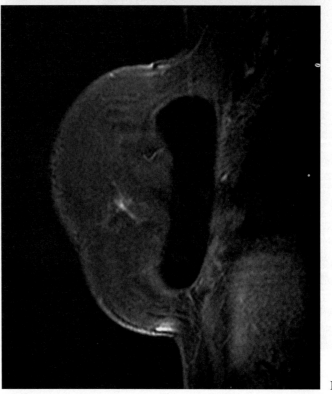

B

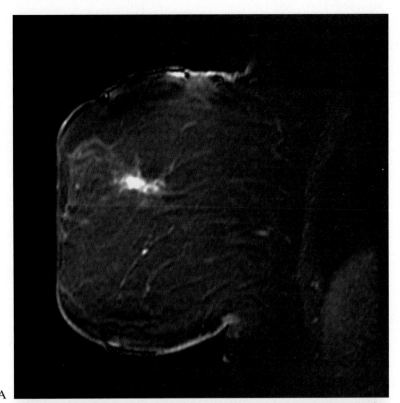

A

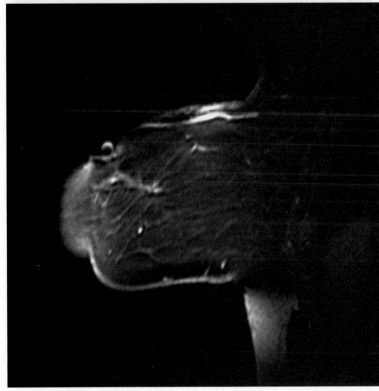

B

FIGURE 26.28. A 52-year-old woman with abnormal ultrasound for which surgical excision was performed yielding LCIS. (A) MRI performed 4 months following surgery demonstrates irregular enhancement at the biopsy site. (B) Follow-up MRI 6 months later demonstrates near complete resolution of the postbiopsy changes. Note poorer positioning of the breast on this examination.

FIGURE 26.29. A 31-year-old woman with right mastectomy. Patient underwent benign biopsy in the left retroareolar region yielding fibrosis and fibrocystic changes. (A) MRI was obtained two months following benign biopsy. (B) Eight months following benign biopsy, enhancement of the postoperative site has reduced markedly compatible with resolving postoperative changes.

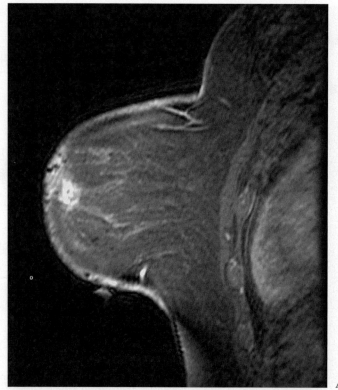

A

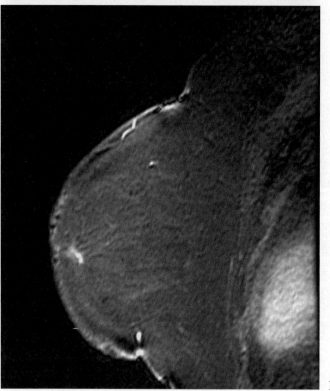

B

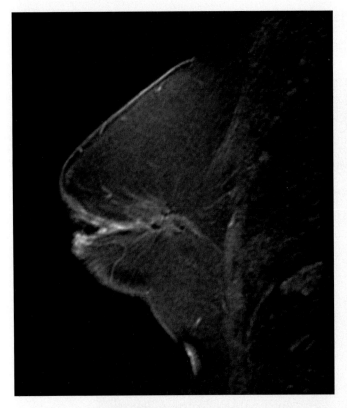

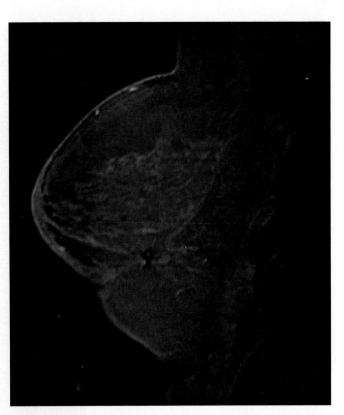

FIGURE 26.30. A 66-year-old woman with history of left breast lumpectomy for invasive ductal carcinoma 10 years ago. Magnetic resonance imaging demonstrates distortion, nipple retraction, and scarring in the central breast at the site of lumpectomy.

FIGURE 26.31. A 59-year-old woman with a history of invasive ductal carcinoma 3 years ago. Distortion extending to the skin is noted with associated focal skin retraction compatible with scarring.

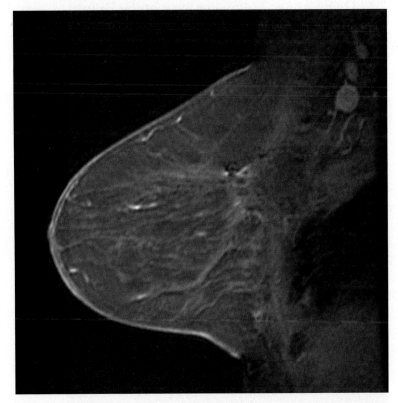

FIGURE 26.32. A 48-year-old woman had a new spiculated mass on mammography that was excised yielding invasive ductal carcinoma, moderately differentiated. At the lumpectomy site posteriorly, nonenhancing distortion is noted with a few clips.

2. Needle Biopsy

2.1. Clips Following Needle Biopsy

FIGURE 26.33. A 45-year-old woman following stereotactic biopsy for calcifications in the central right breast yielding DCIS. Clumped enhancement is noted anterior to the clip (arrow) in the central breast suspicious for residual DCIS, confirmed at surgery.

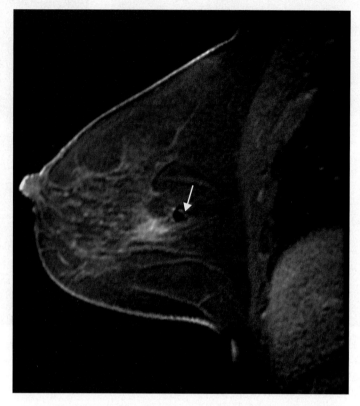

2.2. Hemorrhage Following Stereotatic Biopsy

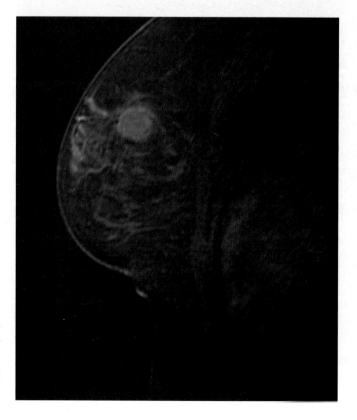

FIGURE 26.34. A 65-year-old woman with a history of right mastectomy now presents with abnormal mass on MRI. Magnetic resonance guided vacuum biopsy was performed. High signal postbiopsy hematoma is noted at the biopsy site.

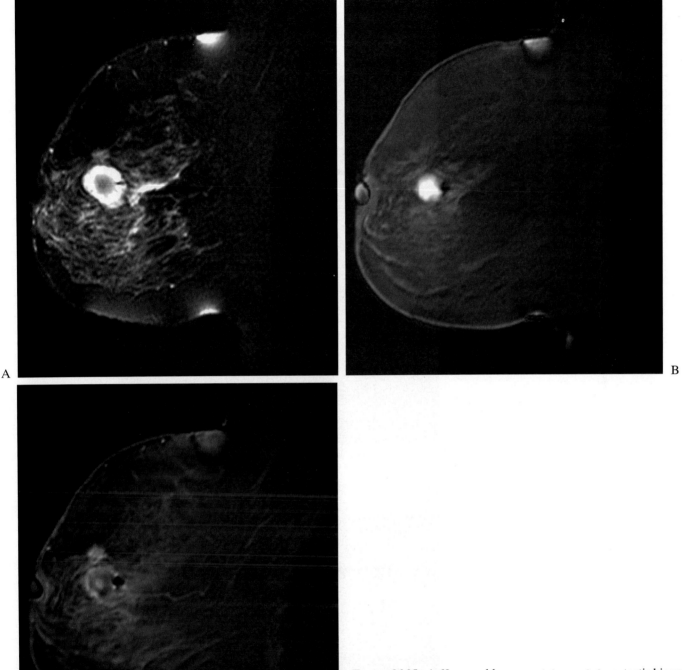

A

B

C

FIGURE 26.35. A 60-year-old woman status post stereotactic biopsy yielding invasive ductal carcinoma with lobular features. (A) T2-weighted image demonstrates peripheral high signal mass at biopsy site. (B) Precontrast T1-weighted image demonstrates high signal hematoma. (C) Postcontrast image demonstrates signal void from clip, hematoma, and residual spiculated mass superior to the hematoma.

3. Reconstructive Surgery

3.1. Mammoplasty

FIGURE 26.36. A 57-year-old woman with history of bilateral reduction mammoplasty. Note fat necrosis in the inferior breast.

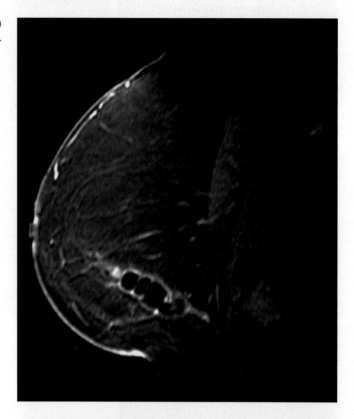

FIGURE 26.37. A 59-year-old woman with right mastectomy and left mastopexy 1 year ago. Curvilinear scar is noted in the anterior breast extending into the upper inner quadrant where postoperative enhancement is identified. This resolved on follow-up MRI examination.

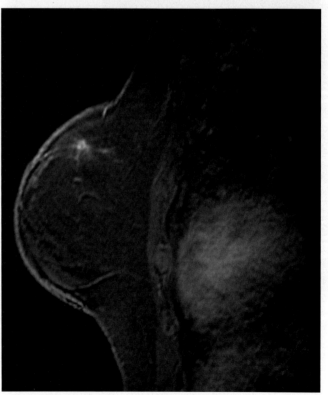

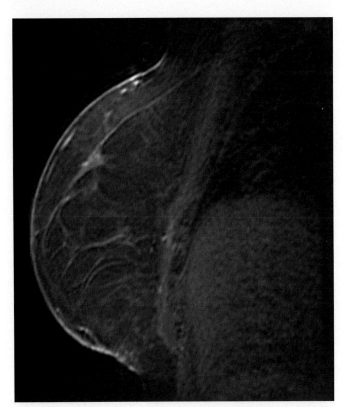

FIGURE 26.38. A 63-year-old woman with bilateral reduction surgery 6 years ago. Note curvilinear scar anteriorly in the upper breast.

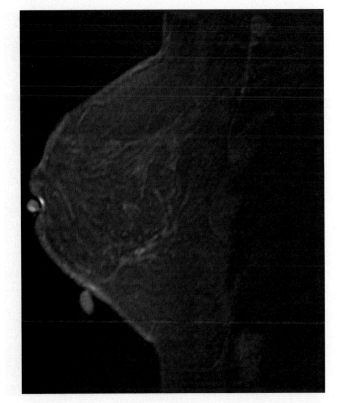

FIGURE 26.39. A 46-year-old woman status post bilateral reduction 6 months ago yielding LCIS of both breasts. Magnetic resonance imaging performed for high-risk screening. Skin marker was placed on reduction scar inferiorly. Note that it corresponds to a linear scar in the lower breast.

FIGURE 26.40. A 41-year-old woman with right mastectomy had left breast reduction 5 months ago. Enhancement along the scar is still identified.

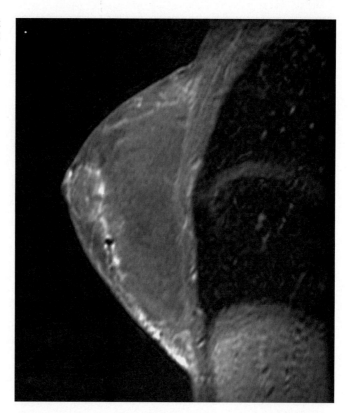

3.2. Transverse Rectus Abdominis Muscle Flap

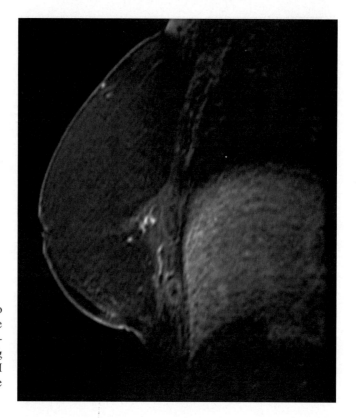

FIGURE 26.41. A 48-year-old woman who underwent right mastectomy and transverse rectus abdominis muscle (TRAM) reconstruction 7 years ago. Magnetic resonance imaging demonstrates normal appearance of TRAM flap with muscle and vascular pedicle in the lower inferior breast.

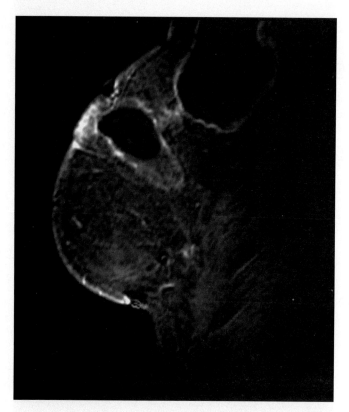

FIGURE 26.42. A 44-year-old woman with TRAM flap reconstruction following mastectomy. Note extensive fat necrosis (low signal masses with peripheral enhancement) in the upper outer TRAM, a site of possible devascularization. This patient presented with a hard palpable abnormality. Aspiration was negative. Magnetic resonance imaging was performed to assess for any suspicious underlying masses. None were identified.

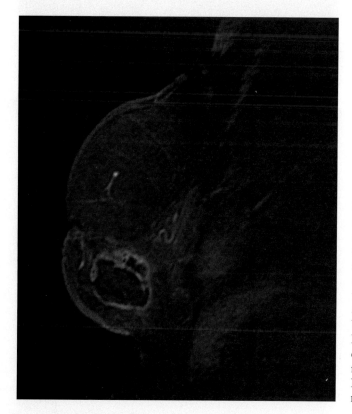

FIGURE 26.43. A 49-year-old woman who underwent TRAM reconstruction 5 months ago following mastectomy for stage III breast cancer. Erythema immediately occurred in the skin over the TRAM flap and a questionable axillary node was palpated. Punch biopsy of the skin was negative as was the axillary node aspirate. The patient then developed a palpable mass inferiorly over the lower TRAM site. Magnetic resonance imaging was ordered to exclude recurrence. Extensive fat necrosis is noted over the area of palpable abnormality. Patient went to surgery for skin changes. No malignancy was identified.

27
Pitfalls in Analysis of Carcinomas

1. Atypical Appearance of Carcinomas

1.1. Diffuse Carcinoma

FIGURE 27.1. A 43-year-old woman with palpable thickness in the upper outer quadrant. Mammogram demonstrates extensive pleomorphic calcifications in the upper outer quadrant and a lobulated 3-cm mass on ultrasound. Contrast enhanced magnetic resonance imaging (MRI) demonstrated extensive involvement of the breast with multiple contiguous masses coalescing in the upper outer quadrant. Core biopsy was performed yielding moderately differentiated invasive ductal carcinoma and ductal carcinoma in situ (DCIS) solid type with minimal necrosis and high nuclear grade. Mastectomy was performed yielding multiple foci of invasive carcinoma ranging in size from 0.8 to 2.2 cm. Extensive intraductal component was present. More than two quadrants were involved with tumor. Note that diffuse enhancement may be mistaken for benign parenchymal enhancement. Kinetics (not shown), clinical history and correlation with other imaging modalities aid in arriving at the correct diagnosis.

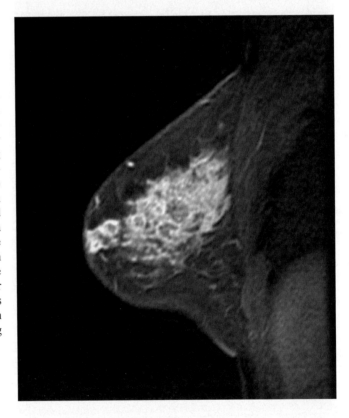

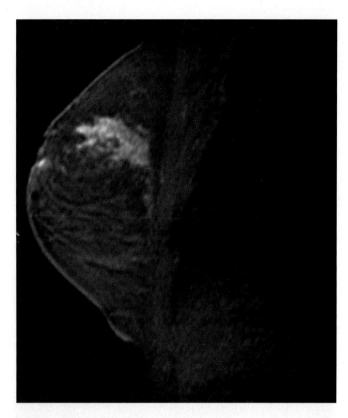

FIGURE 27.2. A 39-year-old woman with palpable mass corresponded to architectural distortion on mammography. Ultrasound demonstrated two adjacent masses in the area of abnormality measuring 1.1 amd 2.3 cm. Magnetic resonance imaging performed to assess extent of disease. Confluent intense enhancement is identified in the superior breast. Excisional biopsy demonstrated multifocal invasive mammary carcinoma with mixed ductal and lobular features, histologic grade III/III and nuclear grade II/III with widely positive margins. Completion mastectomy demonstrated tumor in three out of four quadrants.

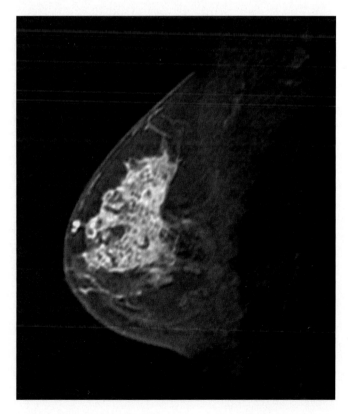

FIGURE 27.3. A 53-year-old woman with a palpable breast mass. Mammography was negative and ultrasound suspected the presence of multiple masses. Core biopsy of one of these demonstrated invasive carcinoma with ductal and lobular features. Palpable axillary adenopathy was aspirated and shown to be metastatic. Magnetic resonance imaging was performed to evaluate disease extent. Regional heterogeneous enhancement is present in the upper breast compatible with locally advanced breast carcinoma. Patient then underwent preoperative chemotherapy with clinical response. At mastectomy 4 cm of residual carcinoma was identified with a background of fibroinflammatory changes. Nodes were negative following chemotherapy.

1.2. High Signal Carcinoma on T2

FIGURE 27.4. A 60-year-old woman underwent chest computed tomography (CT) for shortness of breath where a mass was noted in the breast. Mammogram demonstrated an irregular mass confirmed on ultrasound. Referred for MRI for extent of disease assessment. Solitary spiculated mass identified on MRI that is high in signal on T2 (shown). Pathology yielded invasive ductal carcinoma poorly differentiated histologic grade II/III and nuclear grade III/III and DCIS solid type with high nuclear grade.

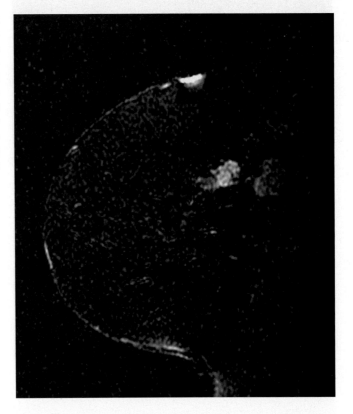

1.3. Obscured

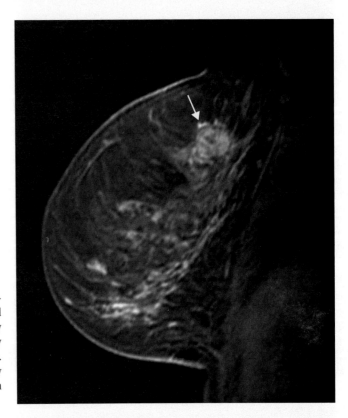

FIGURE 27.5. A 62-year-old woman with interval development of a noncalcified lobulated obscured mass. Ultrasound-guided biopsy yielded invasive ductal carcinoma, moderately differentiated with mucinous component. MRI demonstrates irregular heterogeneously enhancing mass (arrow) difficult to distinguish from background enhancement.

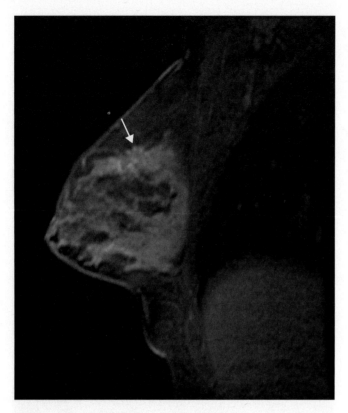

FIGURE 27.6. A 28-year-old woman recently postpartum and breastfeeding presented with palpable mass. Mammography demonstrated a spiculated mass with questionable extension into the pectoralis muscle and possible skin on outside evaluation. Magnetic resonance imaging performed demonstrates diffuse enhancement of the dense parenchyma (compatible with postpartum status) with obscuration of the irregular mass in the superior breast (arrow). No skin or chest wall involvement was seen. The patient underwent mastectomy that demonstrated 2-cm invasive ductal carcinoma histologic grade III/III, nuclear grade III/III.

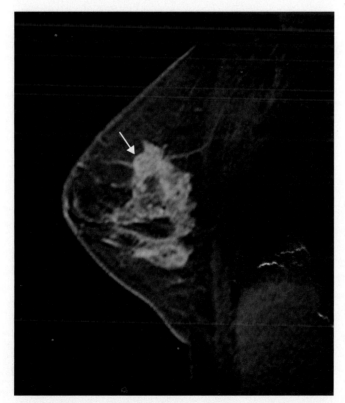

FIGURE 27.7. A 38-year-old woman presents with palpable mass with negative mammography. Ultrasound demonstrated an irregular mass that was biopsied yielding moderately differentiated invasive ductal carcinoma with multiple foci of lymphovascular emboli. Magnetic resonance imaging demonstrates an obscured mass in the superior breast (arrow) that enhances similarly to what may be interpreted as background parenchyma. Spiculation can be appreciated. Right breast excision yielded multiple foci of invasive ductal carcinoma ranging in size from 1.2 to 1.8 cm. The surrounding enhancement was likely in retrospect adjacent tumor.

FIGURE 27.8. A 33-year-old woman with palpable breast mass. Mammogram demonstrates an irregular obscured mass with adjacent calcifications. Additional calcifications were noted on mammography in the retroareolar region. Magnetic resonance imaging performed for extent of disease assessment. Magnetic resonance imaging demonstrates a solitary mass in the superior breast that demonstrates rim enhancement (arrow). The majority of the mass is similar in signal intensity as the background parenchyma and does not demonstrate enhancement. Techniques to aid in the suppression of background parenchyma may facilitate lesion detection in these cases.

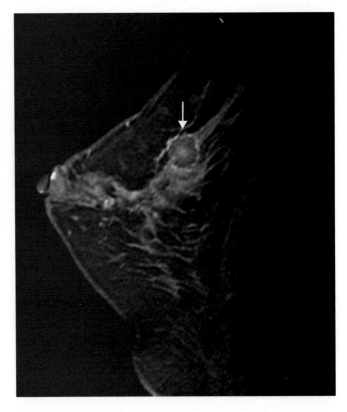

FIGURE 27.9. A 40-year-old woman with lump in upper inner quadrant. Mammogram demonstrates 2.5-cm mass that underwent ultrasound core biopsy yielding carcinoma. Mammogram also demonstrates additional calcifications spanning 3 cm in the upper outer quadrant. Magnetic resonance imaging performed to assess disease extent. An obscured rim-enhancing mass is noted with central enhancement (arrow) corresponded to a 1.7-cm invasive ductal carcinoma not otherwise specified (NOS) type, histologic grade III/III and nuclear grade III/III. Additional surrounding enhancement was noted that corresponded to extensive ductal carcinoma in situ solid/cribiform types with high nuclear grade and extensive necrosis. This was noted in the region of abnormal calcifications. Patient underwent mastectomy after initial attempt at conservation failed.

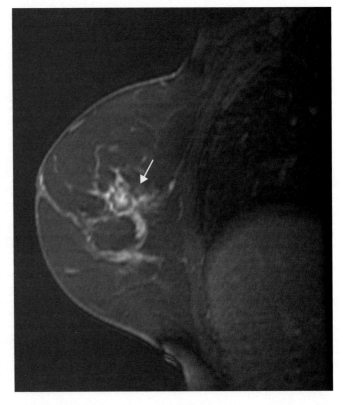

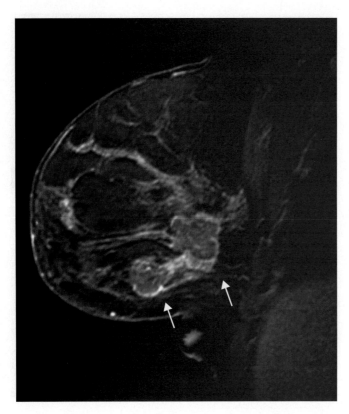

FIGURE 27.10. A 43-year-old woman felt lump in right breast. Mammogram demonstrated a lobulated noncalcified mass that could not be completely imaged. Ultrasound showed a 3-cm mass in the lower outer quadrant that was biopsied yielding poorly differentiated invasive ductal carcinoma with necrosis. Magnetic resonance imaging performed demonstrates large lobulated mass with thin rim enhancement (arrows). A contralateral carcinoma was detected in the left breast on MRI. Staging work up demonstrated multiple hepatic lesions, aspirated and proven to represent stage IV metastatic disease. The patient was treated with systemic therapy.

1.4. Smooth Margin

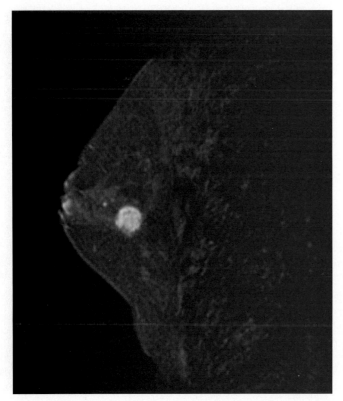

FIGURE 27.11. A 41-year-old woman with history of skin puckering of left breast. Mammogram negative. Ultrasound demonstrated solid suspicious mass that was aspirated yielding carcinoma. Magnetic resonance imaging demonstrates round mass with some smooth as well as irregular margins. Pathology was invasive ductal carcinoma, histologic grade II/III and nuclear grade I-II/III with DCIS cribiform/micropapillary with low nuclear grade and minimal necrosis. Patient treated with breast-conserving therapy. Note predominantly round shape and smooth margins.

FIGURE 27.12. A 46-year-old woman with abnormal right mammogram that demonstrates an irregular mass with pleomorphic calcifications. On MRI this mass demonstrated rim enhancement with some smooth margins though internal enhancement was heterogeneous. Excisional biopsy demonstrated DCIS solid type, high nuclear grade with moderate necrosis presenting as a dominant mass. A few foci of microinvasive DCIS in the form of single cells and microscopic clusters were also identified. Nodes were negative.

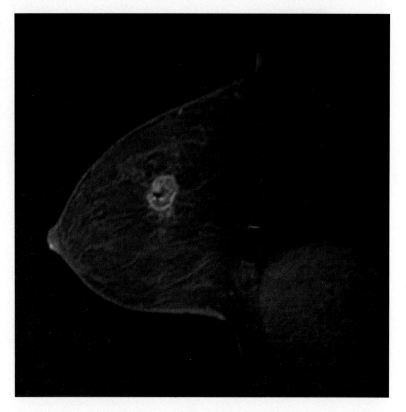

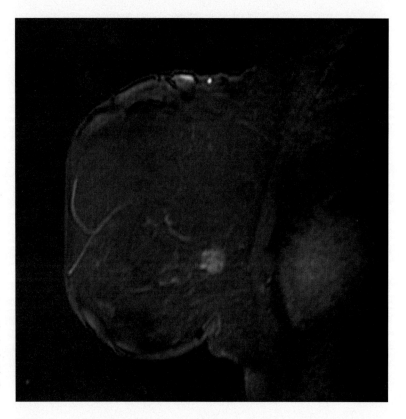

FIGURE 27.13. A 40-year-old woman presents with palpable abnormality. Magnetic resonance imaging demonstrates lobulated partially smooth mass. Heterogeneous internal enhancement is seen. Pathology invasive ductal carcinoma.

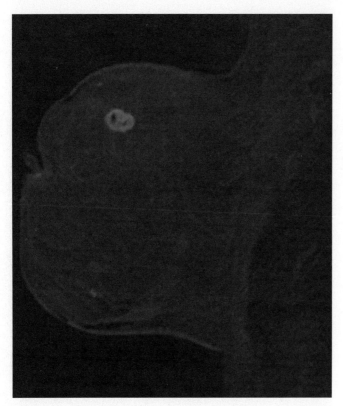

FIGURE 27.14. A 30-year-old woman presents with a palpable abnormality in the left breast. Mammogram negative. Ultrasound demonstrated suspicious solid mass and core biopsy proved carcinoma. Magnetic resonance imaging demonstrated unifocal oval well-circumscribed mass with heterogeneous enhancement. Pathology was invasive ductal carcinoma, histologic grade III/III, nuclear grade II/III, and DCIS, cribiform, intermediate nuclear grade and minimal necrosis. Note that carcinomas can demonstrate smooth margins. Most suspicious feature of the lesion used to determine need for biopsy.

2. Suboptimal Positioning

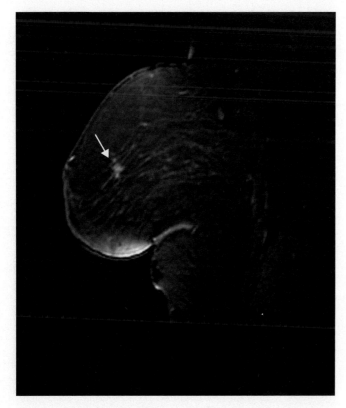

FIGURE 27.15. A 59-year-old woman with left breast invasive ductal carcinoma. Magnetic resonance imaging performed to exclude the presence of contralateral disease. Magnetic resonance imaging demonstrates a central mass (arrow) that was biopsied yielding radial scar. Note coil artifact inferiorly and skin fold in the inframammary region. The breast was not pulled into the coil and the patient positioned herself.

FIGURE 27.16. A 53-year-old woman with unknown primary. Magnetic resonance imaging performed to exclude breast primary. No enhancing masses were identified. Note the inferior artifact and skin fold from allowing the patient to position herself.

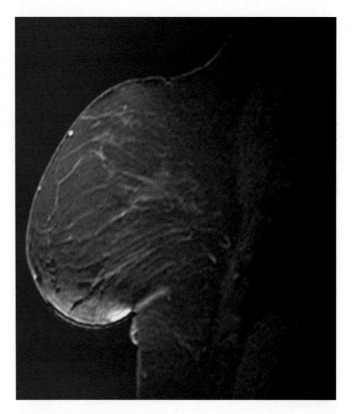

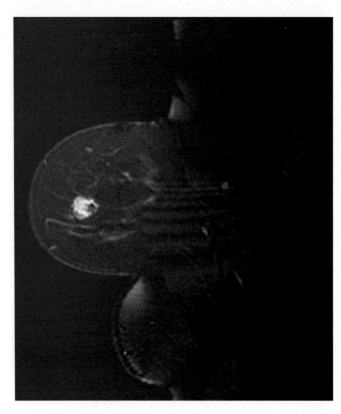

FIGURE 27.17. A 55-year-old woman presents with mass noted on mammogram. Pathology yielded moderately to poorly differentiated invasive ductal carcinoma and DCIS cribiform type. Magnetic resonance imaging performed for extent of disease. Note suboptimal positioning with artifact. Breast needs to be pulled into the breast coil to eliminate redundant tissue and to center breast within breast coil.

3. Suboptimal Windowing

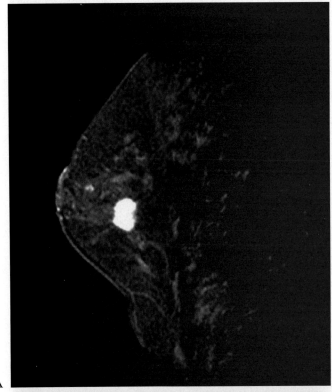

FIGURE 27.18. A 41-year-old woman with palpable breast mass proven to represent invasive ductal carcinoma. (A) Suboptimal windowing demonstrates homogeneous enhancement and the suggestion that the mass has well-defined borders. (B) More optimal imaging demonstrates the mass to be heterogeneous in enhancement with spiculated margins.

A

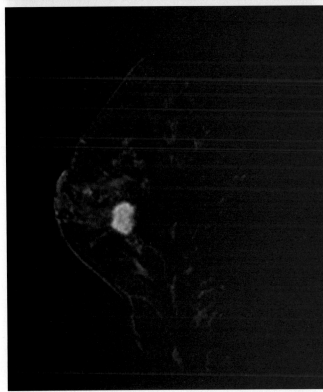

B

FIGURE 27.19. A 55-year-old woman presents with a mass noted on mammogram and ultrasound. (A) Suboptimal windowing demonstrates a well-defined homogeneously enhancing mass. (B) More optimal imaging shows the mass to be irregular with heterogeneous enhancement. Pathology yielded invasive lobular carcinoma.

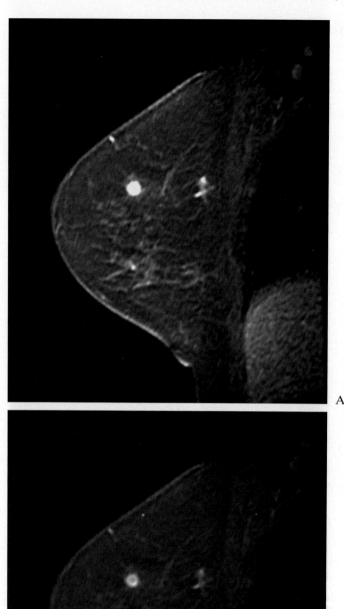

4. Coil Artifact

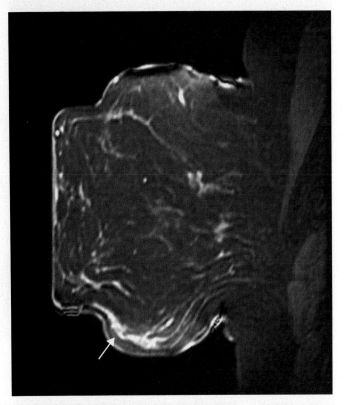

FIGURE 27.20. A 38-year-old woman with prior benign breast biopsy and no family history has outside MRI demonstrating suspicious enhancement. Scan performed for needle localization demonstrates a large breast that contacts the coil producing artifact inferiorly and superiorly. The abnormal linear clumped enhancement along the 6 o'clock axis (arrow) proved to represent atypical ductal hyperplasia.

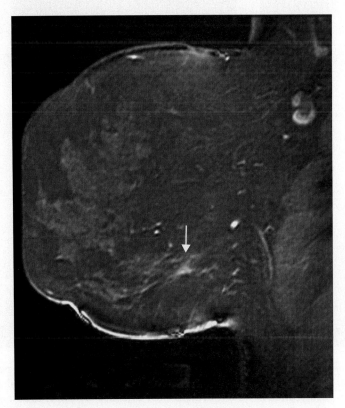

FIGURE 27.21. A 52-year-old woman with a prior history of biopsy yielding atypical ductal hyperplasia presents with palpable axillary adenopathy. Aspiration yielded malignant cells suspicious for breast primary (not shown). Mammogram was negative. Magnetic resonance imaging demonstrates a small irregular mass inferiorly in the breast that proved to represent the patient's primary (arrow). On directed ultrasound it was identified, biopsied, and proved to represent invasive lobular carcinoma. Note inferior coil artifact.

FIGURE 27.22. A 51-year-old woman presents with a palpable mass in the upper outer quadrant (not shown). Magnetic resonance imaging performed prior to surgery. Clumped linear enhancement is identified in the 6 o'clock axis (arrow) proved to represent ductal hyperplasia without evidence of carcinoma. Note adjacent artifact limiting interpretation.

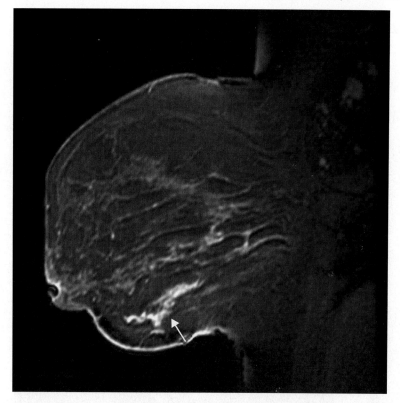

5. Metallic Artifact

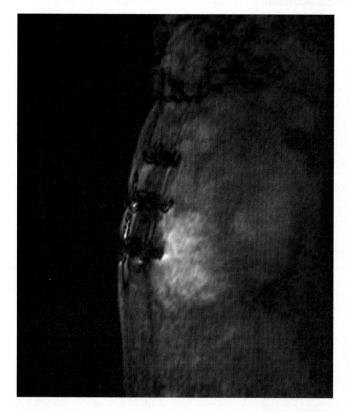

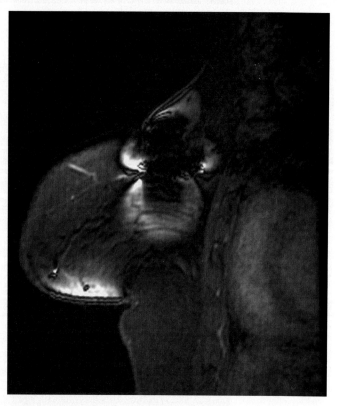

FIGURE 27.23. A 35-year-old woman status post ventricular septal defect at age 11. Mother had premenopausal breast cancer. Screening MRI examination. Artifact from sternotomy wires is noted.

FIGURE 27.24. A 55-year-old woman status post right lumpectomy yielding invasive ductal carcinoma and DCIS. Follow-up MRI demonstrates evidence of artifact from a mediport catheter placed for chemotherapy.

6. Misregistration

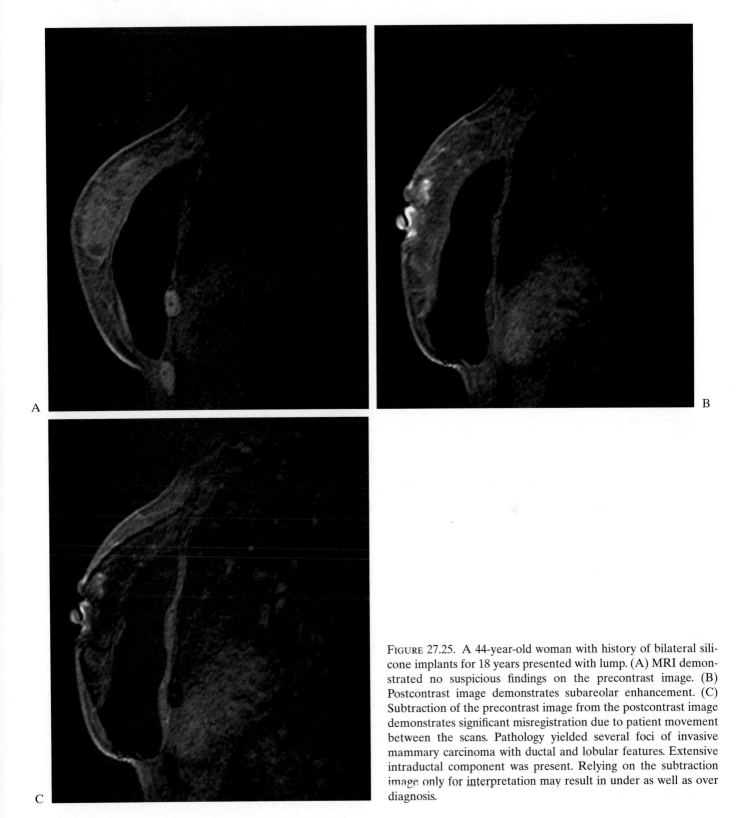

A

B

C

FIGURE 27.25. A 44-year-old woman with history of bilateral silicone implants for 18 years presented with lump. (A) MRI demonstrated no suspicious findings on the precontrast image. (B) Postcontrast image demonstrates subareolar enhancement. (C) Subtraction of the precontrast image from the postcontrast image demonstrates significant misregistration due to patient movement between the scans. Pathology yielded several foci of invasive mammary carcinoma with ductal and lobular features. Extensive intraductal component was present. Relying on the subtraction image only for interpretation may result in under as well as over diagnosis.

Index